birth:
countdown to optimal

information and inspiration for pregnant women

Michel Odent:

❝ Often, women who talk a lot about the birth of their babies are those who had a difficult birth, problems and so on. And women who had a very easy birth tend not to talk about that. I have a very good example: my daughter, who has three children. Although she has a strong intellect—she's a professor of medical genetics—she would never talk about the birth of her babies. Never! Because for her it has always been so simple. The last one: contractions begin at 7 o'clock, baby born at 7.55. So I think it might be good to say somewhere that this book is special. It's full of accounts we can learn from. Usually, I recommend that pregnant women should not read too many books. I tell them they should rest their intellect, listen to the music they love, go swimming, do whatever it is they like to do. That's much more important. They don't need to know too much because they lose their sense of proportion. If they read a medical dictionary they will find all sorts of... well... But this book is an exception. It's a book written by a mother with experience of undisturbed birth, who knows what birth can be like. And that's different. It's unusual.

A former Head of Midwifery:

❝ The stories about caesareans are particularly moving, especially where one woman describes a feeling of being burgled! This is nicely balanced with a positive story of a caesarean, which demonstrates that high risk women can have a positive birthing experience, even in a medicalised environment.

The section describing what happens week-by-week is fantastic and I have not seen such detail in a book or paper written by a non-medical/midwifery person. The detail is perfect and written at a pitch which anyone can appreciate. I think this section is invaluable. Life in utero is described extremely sensitively and much more meaningfully than in most pregnancy books.

Antenatal teachers:

❝ A wonderful and necessary piece of work.

❝ I love this approach to pregnancy, labour and birth, and the more women who are introduced to it, the better. Bring it on!

❝ Reading this almost made me want to have another baby!

birth:
countdown to optimal

information and inspiration for pregnant women

Sylvie Donna

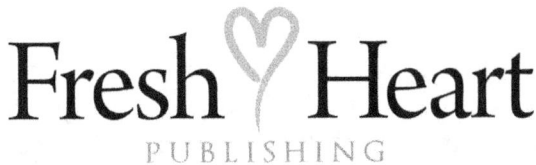

Fresh Heart
PUBLISHING

2nd British edition

First published in Great Britain in 2011 by
FRESH HEART PUBLISHING
a division of Fresh Heart Ltd
PO Box 225, Chester le Street, DH3 9BQ
www.freshheartpublishing.co.uk
1st edition published in 2008

© Sylvie Donna 2011

The moral right of Sylvie Donna to be identified as the author of this work has been asserted in accordance with the Copyright, Designs and Patents Act 1988.

All rights reserved. No part of this publication may be reproduced, stored in a retrieval system, or transmitted, in any form or by any means, electronic, mechanical, photocopying, recording or otherwise, without the prior permission of the publisher. Nor may this publication be circulated in any form of binding or cover other than that in which it is published and without a similar condition being imposed on the subsequent purchaser.

A CIP catalogue record for this publication is available from the British Library

ISBN: 978 1 906619 19 0

Set in different fonts to reflect different 'voices' as follows:
- Franklin Gothic Book—for all the author's commentary
- Bookman Old Style—for all commentary from experts
- Comic Sans MS—for all other contributors' commentary

Printed in the UK by Lightning Source UK Ltd
Cover photo of Nuala OSullivan and Ciara © Jill Furmanovsky
Cover design by Fresh Heart Publishing
Designed and typeset by Fresh Heart Publishing
Photo opposite page by Sylvie Donna: Pithiviers hospital

Disclaimer

While the advice and information contained in this book is believed to be accurate and true at the time of going to press, neither the author nor the publisher can accept any legal responsibility for loss, damage or injury occasioned to any person acting or refraining from action as a result of information contained. The advice is intended as a guideline only and should never be used as a replacement for consultation with midwives, doctors or consultants.

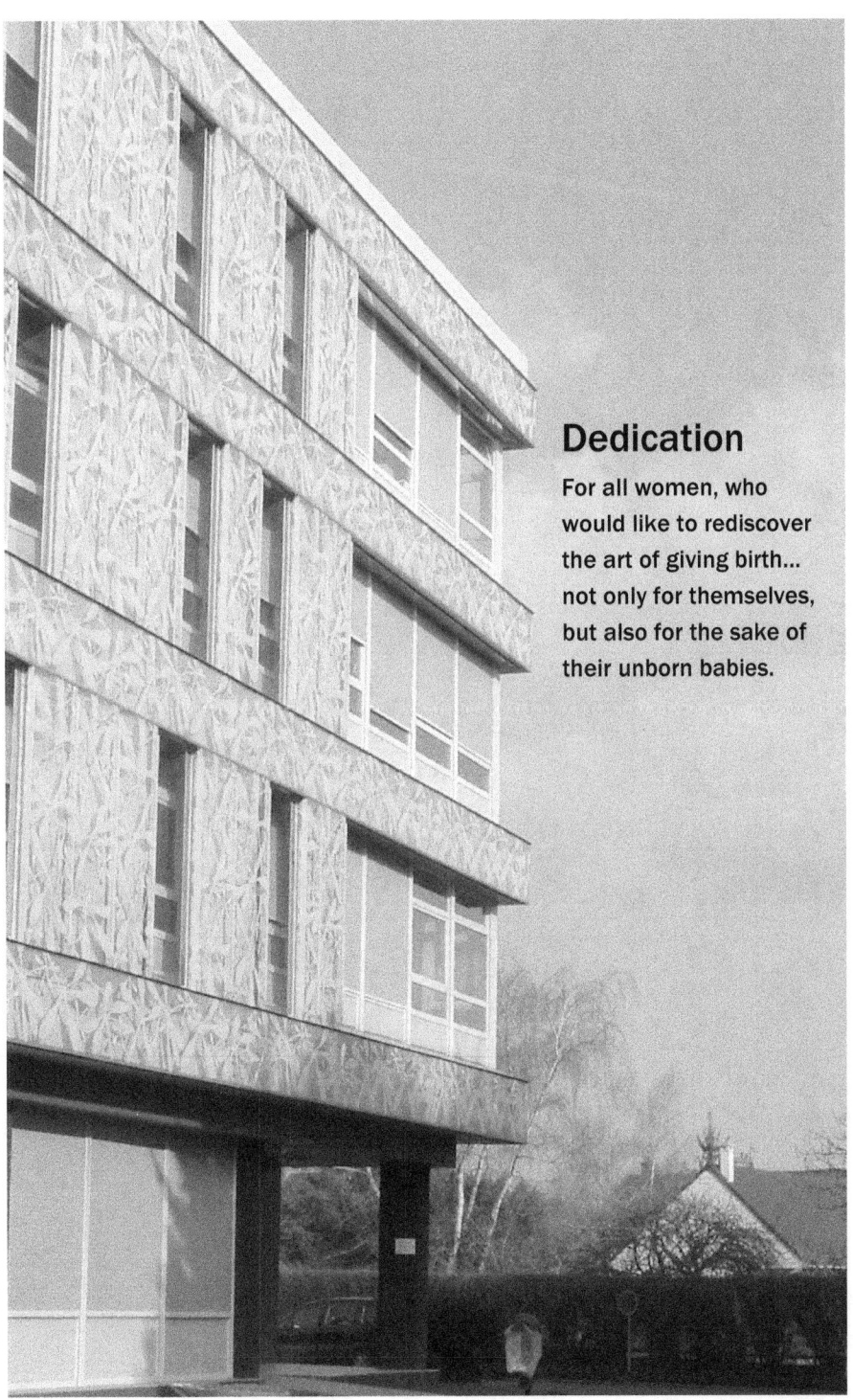

Dedication

For all women, who would like to rediscover the art of giving birth... not only for themselves, but also for the sake of their unborn babies.

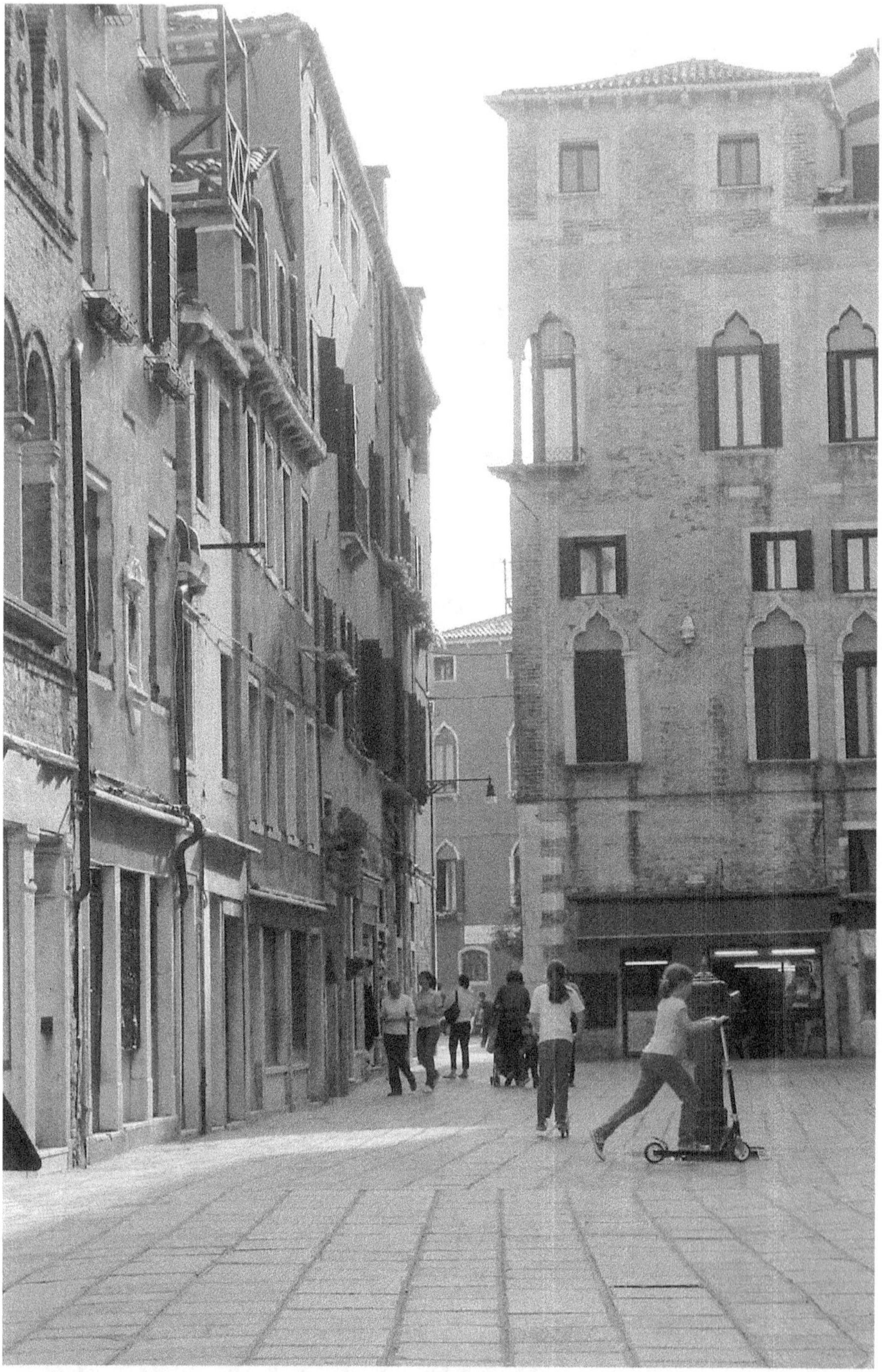

Hey! Where are you going? And why? Do you have enough information?

Contents

Acknowledgements x

A few words from Sheila Kitzinger... xiv

... and a few words from Michel Odent... xv

Introduction: An interesting challenge 1
Your need to know ◆ Your need for perspective ◆ Your right to choose ◆ Your right to be reassured

10... Understand 'optimal' 6
What is an optimal birth? ◆ Why try for an optimal birth? ◆ How can you have an optimal birth? ◆ The reality of 'optimal' (in pregnancy, labour and birth, and immediately after the birth) ◆ In the words of a few other people... (comments about the onset of labour, first stage, second stage, third stage, cutting the cord or not, after the birth) ◆ Life-saving intervention ◆ Infertility ◆ The healthy normality of birth (a surprising secret) ◆ Learning from experience

9... Consider your assumptions 58
The ubiquitous 'high risk' patient (multiple sclerosis, twins, triplets, breech position) ◆ The caesarean conundrum (the facts, the fashion, the feeling) ◆ Are caesareans really necessary? ◆ Assumptions reviewed

8... Do not disturb 97
The delicate cascade of hormones (the hormonal cocktail of pregnancy, the hormonally triggered switch to 'instinctual', the hormones of labour and birth, hormonal production shortly after the birth) ◆ What constitutes a disturbance? (in pregnancy, labour, birth) ◆ Facing the modern reality ◆ Why drug-based 'pain relief' really isn't a good option (epidurals, opioid analgesics and sedatives, gas and air) ◆ What about complementary approaches? (aromatherapy, herbs, TENS, acupuncture, massage) ◆ Where does it all leave us?

7... Help your baby 139
Pregnancy (the first trimester, second trimester and third trimester, including a week-by-week guide to fetal development in pregnancy, Weeks 1-43, being on the safe side, maximising your baby's chances of existence, wondering whether you're pregnant, checking your due date, sharing your news, resting while you're pregnant, getting your baby well-positioned for the birth) ◆ Putting theory into practice ◆ Accidental unassisted birth ◆ The birth

6... Care about care   195

Why worry about antenatal care? ♦ What kind of antenatal care do you really need? ♦ Shouldn't you worry about things going wrong? ♦ What can you do constructively? (Check your own due date, maintain good relations with your caregivers, be clear about your view on tests and abortion, consider your view on ultrasound, decide how you feel about monitoring, consider your view on other tests, think carefully about antenatal classes, prepare a care guide and get it accepted) ♦ Why worry about care when you're in labour? ♦ Why is there a tendency to be interventionist? ♦ What kinds of intervention take place now? ♦ Intervention all women may experience without realising it ♦ Good reason to be careful...

5... Think ahead   259

What can happen when people don't prepare? ♦ Proactive planning (what you could have, what you need, what you don't need) ♦ Care guides (What if your caregiver objects to your care guide? What if it isn't taken seriously? Sample care guides) ♦ When things don't go well ♦ When things go just fine! ♦ When the worse comes to the worst

4... Choose who   301

The importance of having the right caregiver ♦ Variations in quality of care ♦ What should a caregiver be like? ♦ Why is it sometimes difficult to find support? ♦ Women's experience of searching ♦ Caregivers who were appreciated ♦ Taking practical steps to find support ♦ Other birth attendants (doulas, your partner, children, friends) ♦ The most important people of all

3... Choose where   333

A very practical decision... ♦ The historical shift toward the hospital (cost, conditions and cleanliness, pain relief, equipment, statistics, fashion) ♦ Is the hospital the best place to give birth? ♦ What about giving birth at home? ♦ Land or water?

2... Help your body   366

In case you're not yet pregnant... ♦ While you're pregnant... (Relax and breathe well, consider what might be crossing the placenta, think about useful and harmful supplementation, enjoy your changing shape, help your skin, minimise physical discomforts, help your reproductive organs, enjoy your sexuality, respond intelligently to scares, accept your physical situation) ♦ While you're in labour and giving birth... (Eat and drink whenever you want to, make as much noise as you like, adopt helpful positions, use hot water and *lean forward*, continue to move as you wish, don't let anyone disturb you, avoid tearing) ♦ After the birth...

1... Help your mind   410

Sort through the psychological junk (identify feelings and make decisions, deal with any major psychological issues) ♦ Protect your mind ♦ Respond effectively ♦ Find friends ♦ Learn from past mistakes ♦ Solve any practical conundrums ♦ Visualise a good birth ♦ Embrace the unexpected ♦ Stay focused! (What if I suddenly start doubting everything? Why did I opt for no drug-based pain relief or management? How am I going to know when I'm in labour? When should I tell someone else I'm in labour? What should I do while I'm in labour? What positions should I use while I'm in labour? How am I going to cope with any pain? Should I eat and drink something? When shall I get someone to look after other children? When should I call my birth attendants? When should I go in (to the hospital)? How should I relate to anyone who's around? What can I ask of other people? What must other people not do? How am I going to refuse drug-based pain relief? How will the birth work in very practical terms? What position am I going to use to give birth? What do I need to have ready for my labour? What if I keep having contractions but nothing more happens? What if I'm told my baby is posterior? What if something just doesn't feel 'right'? What if my caregivers suggest cephalo-pelvic disproportion is the cause of a long second stage? What if people put pressure on me to accept drugs, procedures or interventions which I don't want? What if I feel strange in the days, weeks or even months leading up to the birth?)

0+1... or 2, or 3   472

Reminders and tips for a smooth start (Avoid early disruption, Get help, Love yourself) ♦ Breastfeeding ♦ Mothering ♦ Surviving as 'you'

Summary of the 10 countdown steps...   487

Special circumstances   488

Key decisions to make   489

Useful contacts   490

Further reading   493

Bibliography   495

Notes & references   497

Glossary   563

Birthframes index   585

Index   588

About the author   612

What inspired this book?   614

What this book can do for you...   615

Acknowledgements

I would like to thank everyone who helped me and contributed to this project on behalf of all the women, men and babies who might be helped by it. I consulted with everybody on how material would be used and even the rather critical or analytical introductory blurbs and commentaries did get approved.

My reason for writing blurbs, incidentally, was to place each birth story in the context of the book and make the overall message of the book consistent and clear. My consultation with contributors was useful in many cases because it allowed me to identify misunderstandings, which might otherwise have been left unresolved. Of course, I also took the opportunity to request many explanations and additions, which is why some accounts, which had initially appeared elsewhere, appear in this book in much longer form. Most of the accounts and comments are original, though. I did, incidentally, decide to adapt the spelling (and occasionally the wording) of some accounts to British English for the sake of easier reading but only vocabulary or spelling changes were made.

As you will see, many of the contributors were very happy to be named. Initially, I thought almost everybody would want to be anonymous. Then, one day, very early on in the process, I received an email from a woman who said: "I don't want or need to be anonymous!" Other contributors said "I'd love to be named" or similar, and explained why they wanted to contribute towards this project. In the words of one contributor: "I would be really pleased for you to use my story in the book. I do think that it's important for other mothers, who may be in the same situation, to feel that they can be in control and make their own decisions about what they want for their birth." It soon became clear that this was a subject on which people wanted to 'stand up and be counted'. Perhaps, also, they wanted it to be clear to readers that their contributions were totally authentic.

In cases where contributors did request anonymity this was sometimes at the request of husbands or children and sometimes because the content of what had been written was sensitive or potentially embarrassing in some way. I must admit, there were cases where I suggested to people that they should be anonymous where they simply refused. Of course, I generally respected people's decisions on this, although I have taken two names out for legal reasons. Please forgive me for making this compromise.

Birth stories were contributed by Bhavna Amlani, Phil Anderton, Helen Arundell, Janet Balaskas, Elaine Batchelor, Debbie Brindley, Sarah Buckley, 'Tina C from the UK', Sarah Cave, Marion Chatfield, Jeannette Clark, Ruth Clark, Kathryn Clarke, Krisanne Collard, Esther Culpin, Mave Denyer, Beth Dubois, Pauline Farrance, Amanda Fergusson, Sarah-Jane Forder, Helene Gee, Elise Hansen, Janet Hanton (along with Caroline Flint and Pam Wild from www.birthcentre.com), Sarah Hobart, Jenny Hodge, Tracy Hoekema, Angela

Acknowledgements

Horn, 'Iona and Laura from California', Deborah Jackson, Jennifer Jacoby, Nina Klose, Tanya Kudryashova, Liliana Lammers, Nicolette Lawson, Alan Low, Cara Low, 'Christina from the UK', Ashley Marshall, Nathalie Meddings, Steve and Olga Mellor, David Newbound, Nuala OSullivan, Sue Pakes, Gaia Pollini, Monica Reid, Justine Renwick, Justine Rowan, Clare O'Ryan, Jenny Sanderson, Joanne Searle, Maria Shanahan, Laura Shanley, Debbie Shaw, Gemma Shepherd, Jo Siebert (and Lawrence Impey), Sarah Stanley, Fiona Lucy Stoppard, Fiona Taylor, Georgina Taylor, Jan Tritten, Caroline Turner, Rachel Urbach, Ulrike von Moltke, Janet Walshaw, Carol Walton, Michael White, Liz Woolley, Rebecca Wright, Heba Zaphiriou-Zarifi and several anonymous contributors. Thank you too to Esther Culpin for her account, a version of which originally appeared in *The Practising Midwife* in January 2003. A special thank you to Michel Odent for allowing me to print his comments on the births of his own children.

Extracts from birth stories, diaries, birth plans, letters or emails, interviews, self-standing comments or information texts were contributed by Helen Arundell, Celina Barton, Elaine Batchelor, Paula Bays, Wendy Blumfield, Debbie Brindley, Bill Bryson (with CARE International), Sarah Buckley, Emma Cameron, Amanda Chalfen, Ruth Clark, Kathryn Clarke, Kathy Cleere, Rachel Cockburn, Janine DeBaise, Beth Dubois, Sarah-Jane Forder, Mary Frankland, Jill Harradine, Jenny Hodge, Kris Holloway, Angela Horn, Eleanor Jackson, Jennifer Jacoby, Libby Kelly, Eliza Klose, Nina Klose, Liliana Lammers, Dr Nicolette Lawson, Julia Lockwood, (and Melanie Milan), Karen Low, Liz Perry, Anne Phillips, Ashley Marshall, Shari Henry Rife, Justine Rowan, Hazel Rymell, Katya S from Moscow, Jenny Sanderson, Kay Sawford, Claire Saxby, Amanda Sealy, Joanne Searle, Gemma Shepherd, Teri Small, Sarah Stanley, Fiona Lucy Stoppard, Clare Swain, Fiona Taylor, Georgina Taylor, Jan Tritten, Jill Unwin, Rachel Urbach, Juliana van Olphen-Fehr, Ulrike von Moltke, Carol Walton, Julie White, Clare Winter, Sonia Winter, Rebecca Wright and by numerous anonymous contributors. A very special thank you to everyone who asked to remain anonymous!

Thank you, too, to everybody who contributed photographs. Particular thanks to Richard Bailey, Elaine Batchelor, Sarah Cave, Jill Furmanovsky, John Huson, Nina Klose, Christa Lloyd, Ashley Marshall, Jenny Matthews (of CARE International), Nuala OSullivan, Nancy Radford, Jenny Sanderson and Colin Smith, as well as to my pregnant models Sarah Morris and 'Linda' (who asked me not to reveal her surname) and to one anonymous, naked, pregnant woman. Thank you, too, to the other anonymous contributors of photos.

I would also like to thank Sarah Buckley, Esther Culpin, Angela Horn, Sheila Kitzinger, Nina Klose, Liliana Lammers, Christa Lloyd, Nancy Radford, Dr Claire Robson, John Rowell and Adrian Rowell for practical support. I am particularly grateful to Dr Sarah Buckley for allowing me to use adapted extracts from her excellent research articles. Thank you too, to Dani Zur of *Mother and Baby Magazine* for letting me use some of the results from the survey conducted in association with Persil in 2002. An enormous thank you to my various anonymous advisers in the realms of midwifery and obstetrics.

A very special thank you to my reviewers and editors (in alphabetical order) Nina Klose, Liliana Lammers, Michel Odent, Clare O'Ryan, Theresa Prentice, Nancy Radford, Jenny Sanderson, Jenna Shaw-Battista, Liz Woolley and Rebecca Wright. (There was also another editor, who asked to remain anonymous... Thank you, mystery mother of four!) Thank you also to Nancy Radford for her invaluable advice and to Clare O'Ryan for acting as a perfect sounding board to my ideas. My thanks are also due to my husband and to our daughters for encouraging me over the years and for allowing me to spend many, many hours at my computer. My mother has also been a wonderful source of support and I really appreciate the interest my mother- in-law and sister have taken in this project too—not to mention my friends.

A heartfelt thank you to Sheila Kitzinger and Michel Odent for their forewords and to Michel for all the other material he contributed or checked for me. A very special thank you too, to my various anonymous contacts at the Royal College of Midwives, the Nursing & Midwifery Council, Doula UK and the National Childbirth Trust, whose informal advice and encouragement at conferences, via email or snail mail has been invaluable; thank you too, to the midwives, obstetricians, professors and senior lecturers of midwifery who have been in touch with me by email or letter to offer support or encouragement and to Betty-Anne Daviss from Canada for her comments on page 615. Thank you, too, to Denis Walsh, Soo Downe and Sarah Buckley for reviewing research evidence and therefore providing me with a great starting point for the notes and references at the back. Any errors in this text remain my own, of course. And special thanks to Robin Russell, anaesthetist at the John Radcliffe Hospital in Oxford, for helping me to understand pain relief issues.

Finally, I would like to mention the obstetrician who attended the birth of my first child in Sri Lanka and to all the staff who supported me. Thank you! I am also grateful to Elaine Batchelor for helping me to work out a backup programme for my second labour for the period when Michel wasn't available, and to the NHS for providing my routine antenatal and postnatal care. Thank you in particular to Jo Farrington for that wonderful, long, reassuring pre-birth chat we had one afternoon, and to my doctor for not striking me off his list! Thank you to the NHS midwife, who helped smooth the path to my third and final labour by not hassling me and at the same time offering me invaluable support. (It's a great shame you weren't able to attend the actual birth.) My thanks to the midwives who did arrive for the last few minutes and went along with my requests. A big thank you to Lawrence Impey in Oxford and Donald Gibb in London, both consultants who appeared out of the blue in birth stories. Along with all the other supportive professionals I came into contact with while researching this book, you really do seem to be working to optimise conditions for mother, father, baby, family and society at large each and every time a new child is born. Perhaps my first obstetrician was right when he said he was convinced that violent births result in a violent society, while gentle births result in gentle, loving societies. Let's hope we find out the outcome of a mass move towards gentle birth over the next few decades. Our world needs a bit more peace and harmony.

Acknowledgements

The publisher would also like to thank the following for the use of previously published material:

- CARE International and Bill Bryson for the extract from the *African Diary* (Doubleday 2002) (page 199 and pp 202-203)
- Clairview Books for allowing the reproduction of extracts from *Birth and Breastfeeding* by Michel Odent (Forest Row, 2007)
- *LLL GB News* for allowing the publication of adapted and extended versions of accounts (Birthframes 23 and 60)
- *Midwifery Today* for the care guide prepared by Janine DeBaise, which first appeared in, Issue 37, Spring 1996
- *New Beginnings* for allowing the publication of a longer version of an account which appeared in the May/June 2003 issue (Birthframe 86)
- *Reader's Digest* for information and ideas which appeared in an article in the July 2003 edition of *Reader's Digest* magazine (page 335)
- Shufu no Tomosya for the photographs of Liliana Lammers, taken by Jill Furmanovsky (www.jillfurnamovsky.com), which were originally published in the Japanese-language magazine *Balloon*—and thank you too to Jill for allowing me to reprint these photographs (pp 192, 193 and 372)
- St. Petersburg: Pioneer / Moscow: Astrel, 2001 for the extract from *Rody bez travm: kak rodit' zdorovogo rebenka (Birth without Trauma: How to Birth a Healthy Baby)* by Marina E. Svechnikova (page 375)
- *The Practising Midwife* for Esther Culpin's account (Birthframe 52) which first appeared in the January 2003 edition (2003 Jan 6(1):10-1)
- *Woman's Weekly* for giving permission to publish an abridged version of their article about the Down's syndrome child described in the book *Sally, Face Like a Flower* (Dent Dale Publishing 2004), which originally appeared in *Woman's Weekly* on 21 September 2004 (Birthframe 38)

The publisher was unable to contact the copyright holders of the following material, after repeated attempts. If you are the copyright holder, please make contact and corrections will be made in future editions of this book.

- The photos of Mave Denyer and her triplets (page 68). (Access to the originals would be really appreciated.)
- The extract from the book *Sally, Face Like a Flower* (Birthframe 38), published by Dent Dale Publishing.

If any material has been used accidentally without appropriate acknowledgement, or if any details are incorrect, please contact the publisher with details so that amendments can be made in future editions. Every possible effort has been made to ensure that all details of contributions are correct.

A few words from Sheila Kitzinger...

It is difficult to write a book about birth drawing on research, analysing the effects and side-effects of interventions and also acknowledging that in the right setting and with loving, sensitive and unobtrusive support birth is a psycho-sexual process which can bring ecstasy. Sylvie has achieved this splendidly. She writes with energy and passion. Her book is rich with women's accounts of pregnancy, birth and after. Readers who do not relish childbirth may find it hard to take it all on board, but the tone, both of the women whom she quotes lavishly, and her own enthusiasm, is so compelling that many could be converted to a radically different view of birth. If they are brave enough to explore what she has to say, with another pregnancy birth may turn out to be a very much better experience. This is a book that can help its readers be adventurous. Breaking the barrier involves not only getting information on which to base choices, or of acquiring the knowledge to make a birth plan, but also getting our inner confidence to grow and blossom!

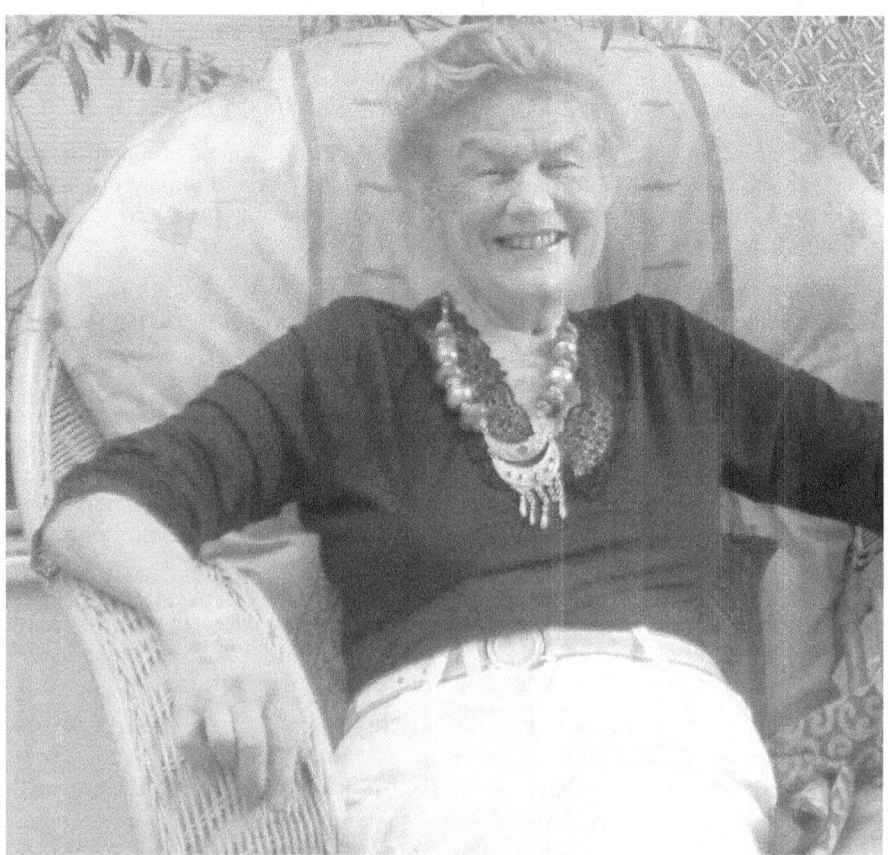

Sheila Kitzinger, author of Birth Crisis *(Routledge 2006) and* New Pregnancy and Childbirth: Choices and Challenges *(Dorling Kindersley 2008), as well as* Birth Your Way *(Fresh Heart 2011) and many other books on childbirth.*

... and a few words from Michel Odent...

There are many reasons why this book is special. One of them is that Sylvie has become a real expert in childbirth. Thanks to her first-hand experience, she is immune to the countless received ideas that abound in magazines, newspapers and books.

I must admit, though, that I was sceptical when I first heard of her idea to write a book. My immediate and tacit reaction was: "Yet another book about childbirth. If I had kept all the manuscripts and books that have been sent to me over the last 20 years, I would need to have an extension built onto my study!"

It was only after several conversations with Sylvie that I started to change my mind. I realised that, thanks to her personal experience, Sylvie was aware of what very few people have understood. Here she tells you what she's learnt... In this book you'll absorb some authentic knowledge transmitted by an authentic expert.

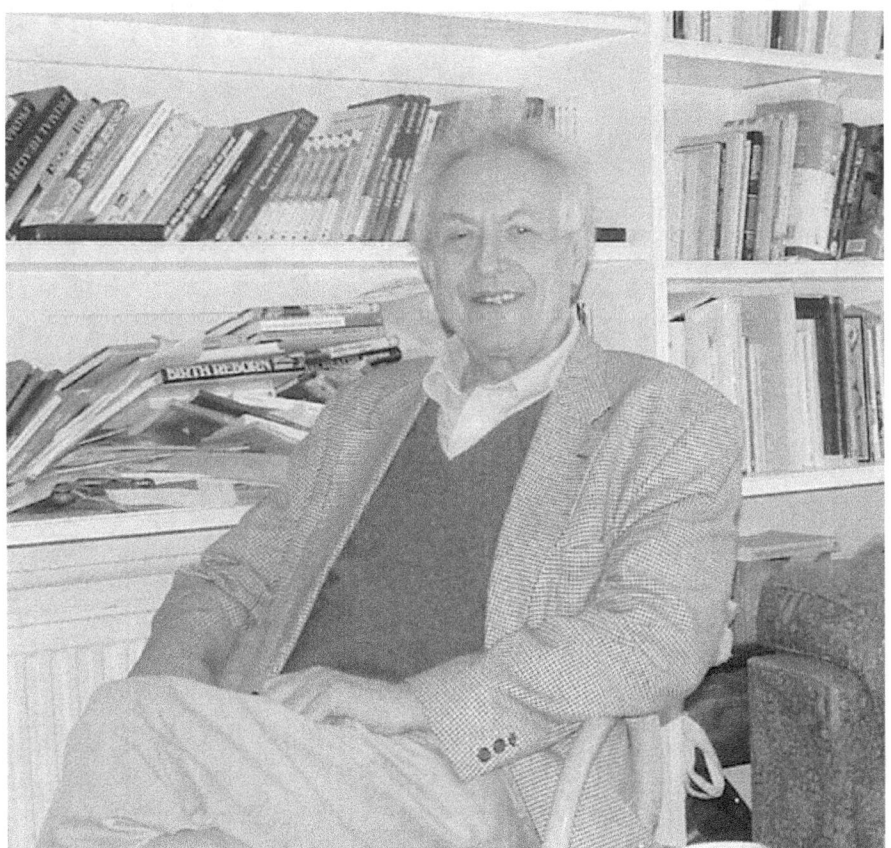

Michel Odent in his study at his home in London.
We'll be calling him 'Michel' in this book—pronounced 'Mee-shell'.

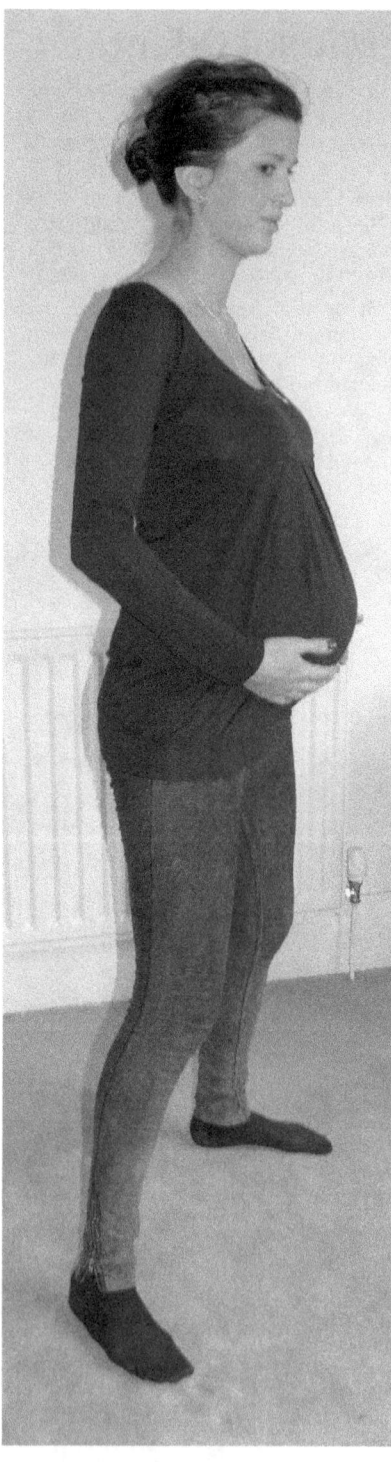
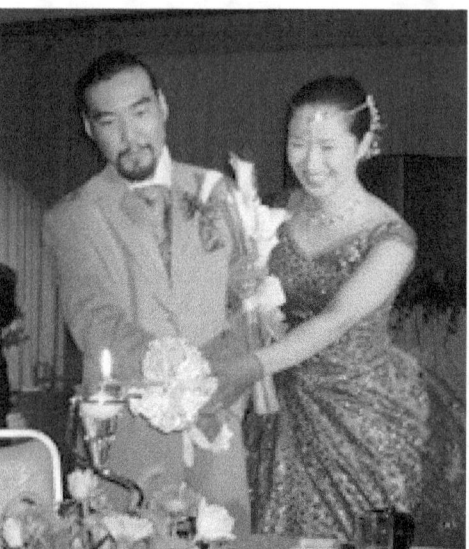
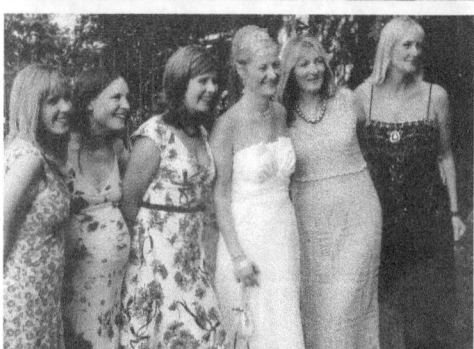
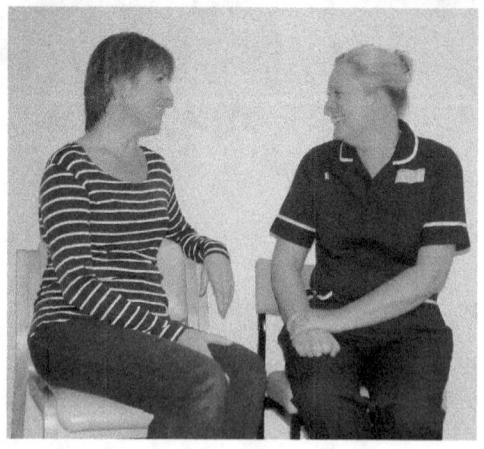

Whoever you are, whatever your situation, you need to know your choices and your rights

Introduction: AN INTERESTING CHALLENGE

Your need to know

If you're pregnant or thinking about getting pregnant soon, you may well benefit from finding out more about pregnancy and birth—even if you've done it all before. This book will help you learn from other people's experiences, find out about key research findings and also understand your rights.

I called this book *Birth: Countdown to Optimal* because I think pregnancy is a bit like a countdown... and it should be, in fact, if we are to prepare ourselves adequately for a safe, happy labour and birth. The 'optimal' bit is about taking decisions during pregnancy and labour which are best for you and your baby.

If you get information which is normally difficult to find *before* you get too far along in your pregnancy, you will have more power and choice. After all, you'll then have more understanding of key issues and will be able to participate in discussions and decision-making. This book will help you, not only by providing easy-to-read explanations and discussions from page to page, but also by providing quick-reference definitions in the Glossary. It will also point you to resources to check out issues or choices—because the assumption underlying all the discussion in this book is that you are interested in making your own birth as safe and as enjoyable as possible. In short, this book is designed to give you information because there really are things you need to know—and inspiration, so that you will act on whatever you find out.

Your need for perspective

When you start finding out about pregnancy and birth, you may have a few surprises in store. Talking to women, midwives and other professionals, you may find you're getting a lot of mixed messages. You'll find that most official organisations—including the Royal College of Midwives (the RCM) and the World Health Organization (WHO), to name just two, seem to be encouraging the kind of births recommended in this book—perhaps because of the negative aspects of other approaches, which research has revealed over the last few decades. Nevertheless, you're likely to discover that many friends and even some caregivers are encouraging you to have what seems to be a less than 'optimal' birth, with as much questionably safe intervention and pain relief as possible. And people who've had very different birth experiences might all be evangelical about their particular views. What on earth is going on?

The answer is partly to do with our recent history and partly to do with fear. Midwives used to be the main caregivers and experts in facilitating healthy birth but their role has been temporarily eclipsed in recent years in Britain. This is because techniques and drugs were used experimentally over the last couple of hundred years, usually with the very best intentions, of course, and because women were increasingly opting for hospital birth and the drug-based pain relief options available, especially epidural anaesthesia. *Pushed* by Jennifer Block (Da Capo Lifelong 2007) details how women increasingly came to be pressurised to have the type of highly managed birth which resulted.

Since research has revealed problems with an unnecessarily interventionist approach,[1] policy makers are realising how important midwives are and there is growing enthusiasm for natural birth practices. These are based on the idea that pregnancy and birth are healthy processes, which will mostly proceed smoothly, or with minimal intervention (often by midwives). Many researchers and mothers are also expressing enthusiasm for natural birth, after discovering that various problems are associated with unnecessary intervention.

However, a woman who chooses a more natural approach (because she correctly sees it as being safer) may well find she has no friends or colleagues who've had a natural birth which worked out, or a birth they saw as 'optimal'. Women's mothers—who probably experienced very experimental obstetric practices—are often particularly apprehensive about childbirth because they see it as a process which requires medical intervention. (Often it does, in fact, after anaesthesia or analgesia have been used because drugs do change the naturally occurring processes.) In other words, our recent history of unnecessary intervention has effectively socialised women into believing that childbirth is a sickness and that it is impossible to accomplish without drugs and lots of other medical intervention too—so many people may be pessimistic.

This outlook makes optimality a near impossibility quite simply because fear interferes with the effective production of the main hormone of birth, as we shall see later. The tiny minority of women who we do need to worry about (and who need intervention) have unintentionally distracted us all from healthy care patterns and an atmosphere of fear and excessive caution has been the result. This has stopped the vast majority of women from labouring and birthing their babies successfully. The culture of litigation has also made many consultants and midwives fear the consequences if they should ever be accused of *not* intervening—which means they tend to intervene over-readily. Reinforcing everyone's fear, films and soap operas continue to portray birth as a dangerous event, involving practices which have now been widely discredited (such as giving birth lying down and pushing on command). This means we're now at a critical point in history where many caregivers are turning away from common practices which have been found to be unhelpful.

Your right to choose

Whatever the views of people around you, you can certainly influence the outcome of your own personal birthing experiences.[2] You need to choose whatever is best for you, understanding a few important things about birth. First, you need to understand that pregnancy and birth are normal, healthy, *natural* processes and that they are in no way similar to diseases or ailments which usually take us to health professionals. Secondly, you need to understand—on a very real level—that you are the person who is going to be giving birth. No matter how wonderful your midwife or consultant, the fact remains that your baby has to pass through, or out of, your very own body. Your caregivers may be relieved if you have prepared yourself for this event and if you responsibly make the choices available to you, which suit you personally and seem *optimal* from your point of view. Finally, you need to understand that you really do have to choose—and that *not choosing* is also a choice, which will probably have consequences. (It's you and your baby who would be affected.)

There are complicated reasons why a) we consult health professionals *even though pregnancy is a healthy process* and b) health professionals allow us to make certain choices ourselves which relate to our own health. (Don't they know best?) Obviously, there are opportunities for screening processes and tests and also there are treatments available if any problems or *potential* problems are discovered. However, *we still have a choice.* Hopefully, having regular antenatal care will also reassure us (because for most of us pregnancy and birth are not everyday experiences) and having a professional birth attendant (a midwife or obstetrician) will help to ensure that nothing goes wrong—or that effective treatment is given if it does.

Making your own decisions at every stage is important because outcomes vary enormously, depending on the choices you make, either actively or through ignoring certain issues. Looking at just one aspect of the birth process, if you choose to give birth without any pharmacological pain relief (drugs, basically) there will probably be a certain amount of pain and you will have a new type of psycho-sexual experience. (Really!) If on the other hand you choose to have a very managed birth (with drug-based pain relief, which necessitates medical management) you will have to accept all the risks and consequences involved. All choices are valid for different women and all are acceptable in modern society, but you may sometimes have to fight for your right to choose!

Having said all that, as you may know, there are some women who choose to give birth without the support of health professionals. (This has become known as freebirthing. It seems to work well for some women, but obviously there are greatly increased risks because there is no fall-back option.) There are also many women who refuse to make choices regarding their professional care. It must be said that because they are unprepared, these women usually 'end up' having all kinds of problems and experiences which they would rather not have had. There are occasional happy exceptions, of course. Usually, though, decisions are made on the spur of the moment and previous vague preferences are forgotten as the realisation dawns that birth is something which can't be brushed aside and as fear actually *causes* the birthing process to go wrong. (As I mentioned before, the hormone which accompanies feelings of fear quite simply stops the main hormone of birth from being produced.) You therefore need to work through your own fears and emotions, by finding out about birth and discovering how wonderful—how optimal!—it can be. That's what this book is all about. To sum up, this book could be very useful to you if...

- ♥ You decide to learn about birth beforehand so you're not afraid when it actually happens
- ♥ You decide you want the support of health professionals both before and during the birth
- ♥ You choose to give birth in the way which research and first-hand accounts suggest is optimal, for both mother and baby

And what is optimal? In a nutshell, it seems to mean having antenatal care, choosing a suitable birthing place and caregiver, then having a physiological birth without any anaesthesia, analgesia or unnecessary intervention, in an undisturbed environment which feels safe, with a professional in attendance. (Please turn the page... it's not as bad as it sounds! Quite the opposite, in fact.)

Your right to be reassured!

In case you're shocked to read this, please be reassured that physiological birth (i.e. natural birth) is a wonderful process. I like to say that it's 'fantastically fizzy' and logical too. (Fizzy logical... physiological... Get it?!) The fizz comes from the feeling both mother and baby naturally experience directly after the birth. The logical bit is about how it all makes sense. As you'll discover from personal experience, if you respect the natural processes of pregnancy, labour and birth, the results can be really amazing—fantastic, in fact! Actually, it seems strange that so few people seem to know how fizzy and logical birth can be these days. The art of giving birth really does seem to have been lost and although science is repeatedly confirming its safety, people seem reluctant to rediscover it. Fear of pain has forced women into a position where they are actually doing things which could harm their babies—even though they will later go to extreme lengths to help their children. Is it simply that women no longer realise that putting up with the pain during labour actually means less pain overall in the end? Don't people see the exhilaration of women who experience this kind of birth—exhilaration which lasts not just for hours, but months, if not years? Is the art of giving birth *really* in danger of becoming completely lost?

That's where I come in. Although I'm not a midwife or doctor, I've discovered some interesting things about giving birth, mainly through having three births myself, which I consider to have been optimal. Talking to other women after each birth, I gradually realised that I was a bit unusual and that most women wanted what I'd experienced but for one reason or another hadn't had the same outcome. So I decided to do some research into why things didn't work out for so many women and then write a book to communicate what I'd learnt about how it all works. My research included a scouring of the academic literature, consultation with various professionals and also many conversations with 'ordinary' women who had often done extraordinary things.

One of the professionals I came into contact with was Michel Odent. I'd been looking for a caregiver to attend the birth of my second baby and I knew, from what I'd read, that he would do nothing to disturb the natural processes. He's a well-respected doctor, who was responsible for some 15,000 births earlier in his career, and he's written 12 books and over 50 academic articles for medical journals—so I was very glad to have his support. (He did in fact attend my second baby's birth and that was an interesting learning experience for me, which prompted more thought and research.) Michel has always been open-minded in his approach, and his conclusion—after many years of research, clinical practice and discussion with midwives—is that birth needs to be left alone as much as possible if it is to be a safe, healthy and happy event for mother, baby and everyone else concerned. His most recent research has even revealed long-term negative effects of intervention in labour and birth.

Nevertheless, Michel has always recognised that intervention is necessary in some cases, for a small minority of women. This perhaps explains why he is apparently such a whiz at caesareans in an in-labour emergency! (His caesarean rate at the maternity hospital near Paris, where he was the manager, was always below 8%.)

Personally, of course I also recognise that intervention is life-saving in many cases and I am enormously relieved that modern medicine has made it possible for certain problems to be identified and solved. However, it seems to me that in too many cases nowadays, caregivers intervene too hastily, perhaps out of fear or over-cautiousness, or because they don't know how best to facilitate the physiological processes, for normal, healthy women and even for women who are considered high risk. Too often the processes of pregnancy, labour and birth are disturbed with profound and damaging effects. So, to me, it's not a question of whether or not intervention is good or bad in general terms, but whether a particular intervention at a particular time, for a particular woman or baby, is appropriate and helpful or not. And I feel that intervention in the form of drug-based pain relief is misguided because the sensations of labour and birth are not only useful, they also lead to very positive feelings postnatally. Too many women, it seems, are experiencing the negative effects of drugs, while missing out on the empowering, joyful aspects of childbirth.

Like me, many other women have also experienced the joy of giving birth without the help of drugs or unnecessary medical interventions and their babies have experienced the benefits. You can read some of their stories in this book, as well as stories about intervention. There are also comments from people from all walks of life who've 'been there, done that', and have something to say. Actually, I didn't originally intend to include birth stories and comments in this book—I only wanted a couple to give you a clear picture of the kind of birth I'm talking about. However, I soon found myself deluged with material, so I decided to be systematic about collecting it. The good thing about this process was that literally everything I read confirmed my belief in the countdown steps I've outlined in this book. At first I was scared that wouldn't happen! So I confess to being a bit relieved. And of course I'm very grateful for all the support I've had. My detailed thanks are in the Acknowledgements. I apologise to the many people whose material I was not able to include.

I hope *Countdown* (*Birth: Countdown to Optimal*) will help you to make your own choices. I hope it will help you understand how you can maximise your chances of having the very best possible birth for both yourself and your baby (or babies, if you're having more than one). I also hope this book will help you find the courage to do the best for your babies, because this is the main reason for avoiding anaesthesia or analgesia in labour and discovering instead the empowering and very possible processes for which our bodies were designed. I even hope this book will help you joyfully think "Baby, be born!"—just as I did, when I gave birth the second time. After all, birth shouldn't be an ordeal or something to be endured. It should and can be a wonderfully empowering, joyful experience, as I said. (It's strange, but true, that birth really can involve profound feelings of pleasure and exhilaration.) Finally, I hope this book will help you to feel that you're not alone on this amazing journey into motherhood.

Thank you for taking the time to consider this idea of 'optimal'. I think you'll be relieved you did. Please do read with an open mind. More is possible than you might believe... that is, until you do it yourself or, rather, *allow* it to happen.

Sylvie Donna

10... UNDERSTAND 'OPTIMAL'

What is an optimal birth?

An optimal birth is a birth which involves the processes which occur spontaneously in the absence of unnecessary intervention in a healthy body. It is a birth which is as good as it possibly can be, for both mother and baby.

An optimal birth in our modern world can actually be very different from *natural* birth as it's been understood over the last few decades. I like to use the phrase 'old natural' to describe that... Occasionally, it resulted in a beautiful birth, but most of the time it resulted in huge amounts of disappointment and feelings of failure. Often, plans for a water birth were ditched and the woman was rushed in for a caesarean. Or she may have ended up with a highly managed birth, with plenty of interventions and drug-based pain relief, for all the wrong reasons. At the end of most failed 'old natural' births the new mother felt disillusioned, disappointed, angry, even guilty—all feelings she could well do without. If you're one of those mums, please read on. There's something better out there.

'Optimal' basically means giving birth as our bodies are designed to do, while at the same time using all our knowledge of what makes birth safe, with ready access to life-saving intervention in case it's needed. In a nutshell, a modern optimal birth means an ultra-natural approach, backed-up by all the best our society has to offer. No drug-based pain relief or intervention is used, unless absolutely necessary, because anything done is likely to disturb the normal, healthy physiological processes and increase the level of risk to both you and your baby. This means no induction, electronic fetal monitoring, TENS, pethidine, diamorphine, spinals or epidurals. It means no complementary therapies (acupuncture, homeopathy, etc)—precisely because they can be so incredibly powerful. Unlike 'old natural', which didn't facilitate the natural processes, but often tended to disturb them instead, optimal birth really is possible for most women, as long as a few basic principles are respected.[1]

Why try for an optimal birth?

Research has shown the kind of birth described above really is safest for both you and your baby.[2] Anecdotal accounts also tell us it results in a much better overall experience, not just at the time of the birth, but also for a long time afterwards.

If you choose optimality, i.e. a normal, healthy birth—which the World Health Organization associates with minimal intervention in terms of maternity care—in other words, if you leave your body to go through its natural, healthy processes, undisturbed, your new baby is likely to be completely alert and able to breastfeed.[3] He or she will then be able to relate to you as nature intended so as to facilitate the bonding process.[4]

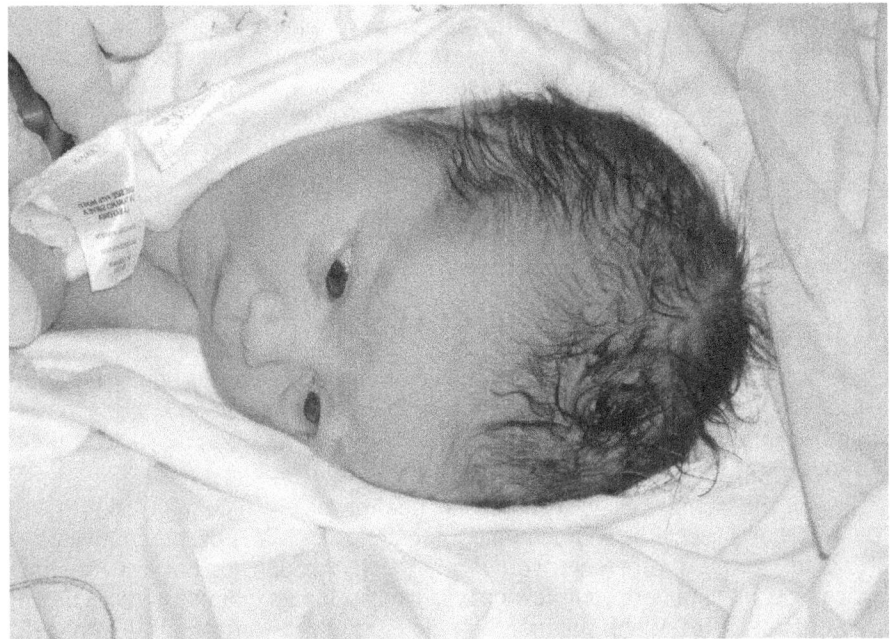

The biggest reason to go without drugs is the prize of a super-alert baby at birth. This optimally-birthed baby was just two hours old when this photo was taken.

What is an optimal birth?

An optimal birth is a birth which involves the processes which occur spontaneously in the absence of unnecessary intervention in a healthy body. It is a birth which is as good as it possibly can be, for both mother and baby.

An optimal birth in our modern world can actually be very different from *natural* birth as it's been understood over the last few decades. I like to use the phrase 'old natural' to describe that... Occasionally, it resulted in a beautiful birth, but most of the time it resulted in huge amounts of disappointment and feelings of failure. Often, plans for a water birth were ditched and the woman was rushed in for a caesarean. Or she may have ended up with a highly managed birth, with plenty of interventions and drug-based pain relief, for all the wrong reasons. At the end of most failed 'old natural' births the new mother felt disillusioned, disappointed, angry, even guilty—all feelings she could well do without. If you're one of those mums, please read on. There's something better out there.

'Optimal' basically means giving birth as our bodies are designed to do, while at the same time using all our knowledge of what makes birth safe, with ready access to life-saving intervention in case it's needed. In a nutshell, a modern optimal birth means an ultra-natural approach, backed-up by all the best our society has to offer. No drug-based pain relief or intervention is used, unless absolutely necessary, because anything done is likely to disturb the normal, healthy physiological processes and increase the level of risk to both you and your baby. This means no induction, electronic fetal monitoring, TENS, pethidine, diamorphine, spinals or epidurals. It means no complementary therapies (acupuncture, homeopathy, etc)—precisely because they can be so incredibly powerful. Unlike 'old natural', which didn't facilitate the natural processes, but often tended to disturb them instead, optimal birth really is possible for most women, as long as a few basic principles are respected.[1]

Why try for an optimal birth?

Research has shown the kind of birth described above really is safest for both you and your baby.[2] Anecdotal accounts also tell us it results in a much better overall experience, not just at the time of the birth, but also for a long time afterwards.

If you choose optimality, i.e. a normal, healthy birth—which the World Health Organization associates with minimal intervention in terms of maternity care—in other words, if you leave your body to go through its natural, healthy processes, undisturbed, your new baby is likely to be completely alert and able to breastfeed.[3] He or she will then be able to relate to you as nature intended so as to facilitate the bonding process.[4]

You yourself will also feel alert and you'll be able to respond to your new baby in whatever way you feel prompted to do so. All the hormones you need in order to do what new mothers have to do will be produced efficiently in a cascade of hormones. You're likely to feel very peaceful—even exhilarated—after an optimal birth and you're likely to easily resume daily activities within minutes of giving birth. Sex will probably be much easier too as your heightened perception during the birth will mean less damage to you know where![5] This also means you'll probably have less pain after the birth, because the risk of tearing and bruising is lower. Your experience of breastfeeding is likely to be much better because many drugs used for pain relief weaken a baby's suck. With a healthy suck, a newborn can easily get the colostrum and milk he or she needs, without hurting you. In short, you'll avoid all the risks and side-effects of unnecessary drugs and interventions.

So 'optimal' means a less painful experience for you overall, both physically and psychologically, fewer health risks and a better deal for your baby.

In case you're wondering... the alternative means being turned into a patient, so that the whole healthy process of giving birth is turned into an illness, which needs to be carefully managed for safety reasons. This is what happens when drugs or interventions are used unnecessarily for anything but safety reasons, because they make the process of birth much more dangerous.

The first trimester (Weeks 1-12)

The first two weeks of pregnancy actually take place before conception in this strange counting system. Week 1 is the week beginning with your last menstrual period so you will only ever think about these weeks retrospectively.

The first three months are often a time of heightened emotions and physical unease due to occasional bouts of nausea and tiredness, and unfamiliar bodily changes. The upheaval is caused by the different hormones circulating and the effect of the growing placenta. Emotions are often coloured by reactions to the pregnancy and they might even stimulate shockingly vivid dreams. There might be an overwhelming need to sleep at any time of the day and the pregnant woman usually also needs to go to the toilet more often because of hormonal changes. It is in this period that the new baby is going through one of its most crucial stages of development—all the major body organs are formed.

> It is in the first trimester that the baby is going through one of its most crucial stages of development

The second trimester (Weeks 13-28)

Most women experience fewer discomforts during this phase of pregnancy. Any nausea usually disappears completely by Week 13 or 14 because the placenta is now fully functioning. Hormones settle down and fewer trips are needed to the toilet. The slowly emerging bump is often perceived positively because it's tangible proof of the pregnancy. Some women will by now have adjusted emotionally to the fact of being pregnant, but many will still be grappling with strange thoughts and feelings.

More blood is now circulating around the woman's body (meaning more work for the lungs, kidneys and heart), thanks to the work of the placenta. This will sometimes mean that women are mistakenly diagnosed as suffering from anaemia, when really the lower percentage of haemoglobin in their blood is simply an indication that the placenta is functioning healthily.[8]

Typically, women feel much more alert and energetic in this trimester but they sometimes worry about the idea of giving birth or about impending motherhood. They may also have all sorts of fears about the welfare of the baby at this stage. All this is perfectly healthy—optimal, in fact!—because it's a sign the woman is tuning in to her baby and his or her needs. From Week 18 or 20 on, most women can feel the baby kicking and moving about now and then.

The third trimester (Weeks 29-40+)

Often women experience no particular changes as they enter the third trimester, except for a dramatically increasing girth. The fact of getting bigger may bother some women, though, especially if poor posture is causing backache. Tiredness, because of the increased weight and uncomfortable nights, may also be a problem and once again the baby will probably be putting pressure on the woman's bladder. The pregnant woman may well feel a need to drink more water than usual, which is logical considering that the amniotic fluid (around the baby in the womb) constantly needs to be replaced. Stretch marks may appear and nipples are likely to look different.

Most women find themselves thinking a lot about the upcoming birth. The constantly-changing cocktail of hormones in the woman's body is gradually preparing both her and her baby for the big day on a physical level too. Quite spontaneously, some of these hormones, as well as other processes (which are as yet little understood) will trigger the beginning of labour, approximately nine months after conception took place. Some women go into labour earlier, and some later. All kinds of things probably influence the timing: genetics, health, diet, lifestyle, psychology, circumstances... as well as an incorrectly calculated due date.

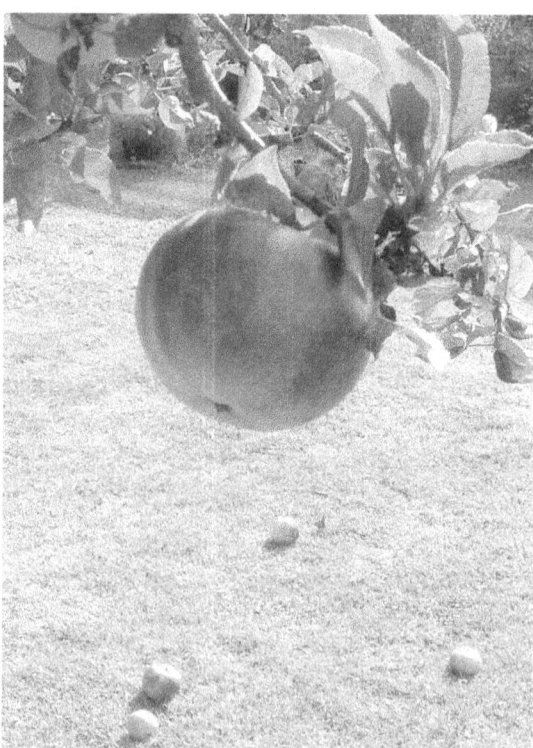

Apples fall from the tree at a certain stage of ripeness. Our bodies know how to release babies in a similar way.

Hormones gradually prepare your body for giving birth

LABOUR AND BIRTH

How does a woman know she's in labour? Sometimes, she might notice a 'show', a discharge of a jelly-like substance, which may be smeared with blood. Seeing this jelly would be a sign that the cervix—the muscle at the base of the womb—is beginning to open so as to eventually release the baby into the outside world. Sometimes, but less frequently, a woman might suddenly experience a gush of 'water' from between her legs. Most often, a woman will become aware that something is changing within her body in a less dramatic fashion when she suddenly has either a bigger or a smaller appetite, when she becomes restless and has a sudden spurt of energy or when she experiences a bout of diarrhoea which will indicate that her body is 'clearing the way' for the new baby—or babies (in the case of twins or triplets).[9]

Eventually, the woman will notice that her uterus (her womb) is gradually—or suddenly—becoming active as it flexes so as to fully open up the cervix and push the baby down through her pelvis, out into the world. These rhythmical 'flexes' of the uterine muscles are frequently—rather unhelpfully, it must be said—called 'contractions' in most books on childbirth, or 'rushes' in some others, which is again sometimes an undescriptive, unhelpful term because in some phases of labour a woman may not always feel that things are 'rushing' anywhere. Having said this, if a woman has not interfered with the physiological processes taking place within her at any point during her pregnancy or labour, she is certainly likely to feel that an enormously powerful, absorbing, irreversible process is taking place, and 'sweeping' her along toward a predetermined biological end. That end is, of course, the birth of the baby... or babies, in the case of a multiple birth.

Are the sensations of labour and birth painful? As you no doubt know, most women experience 'contractions' as extremely painful, but not all do. Some only experience pain for a short part of their labour and some don't experience any pain at all during the birth itself, i.e. the second stage. (I didn't the second time I gave birth, which is the time I was least disturbed.) A few women experience the whole process as interesting, rather than painful.[10]

> I have done some exciting stuff like parachute jumps, wing-walking, trips to war zones, but giving birth was definitely the most intense thing ever. My body felt totally out of control.

If you just observe what is happening within your body you may be surprised to find that it is not exactly pain in the normal sense of the word. You may even experience it as being pleasurable or at least interesting for most of your labour. And because of the hormones and endorphins that are naturally produced in your body while you are experiencing contractions in a complete-ly undisturbed environment, you will be surprised how you will find the resources within yourself to withstand difficult sensations.

Most women have no experience of finding these resources because only a very small number of women nowadays actually labour in an environment which they perceive as being totally safe and unthreatening, with absolutely no disturbances of any kind. The kind of labour I am describing is, after all, a completely physiological labour, the kind of labour we are designed to experience as mammals. Other mammals instinctively seek out complete privacy and even in a modern hospital environment we need to do the same.

Towards the end of labour the cervix will have opened up fully to about 10cm dilation, which is sufficient to allow the passage of the baby's head. Then, thanks to the powerful, rhythmic, muscular contractions which have been taking place and which still continue, the baby descends through the woman's pelvis and down through the soft, fleshy folds of her vagina. (There is sometimes a short break between the cervix becoming fully dilated and the baby descending, which may last anything up to an hour for first-time mothers. During this break the woman experiences no contractions whatsoever. Other women continue on without a moment's break.) When the woman is in an upright position one of the bones which would normally block the baby's downwards passage—the tailbone (or coccyx)—moves out of the way.[11] (It is much more likely that this will happen during an optimal birth because the woman will be entirely conscious, unanaesthetised and responding to her body's cues. These will prompt her to move around, squat down or stand up.) [12]

When the baby's head stretches the perineum the woman experiences a sudden burning sensation, often called the 'ring of fire'. (This may feel extremely 'vivid', rather than painful.) Then, suddenly, first the baby's head, then its body emerges through the woman's vagina—provided, of course, the baby isn't being born breech, in which case the feet or bottom emerge first!

If the woman has not been disturbed in any way during her labour, she is likely to be in a pleasant 'submerged' state of mind and just before the moment of birth it is possible she may experience what Michel Odent calls a 'fetus ejection reflex', i.e. a sudden and compelling rush of energy which makes birth simple, safe, active and intuitive. She will suddenly flick her hips forwards so as to release the baby's head, then body into the world.

No commands are necessary to tell her how to push. There need be no straining, no fear, no control and no management.[13] After the baby slips out of the woman's body (hopefully onto something soft) it will spontaneously take its first breath just a few moments later, sometimes crying as it does so, and sometimes not.

At this point, both mother and baby are usually in a state of heightened alertness and the woman will typically instinctively put the baby to her breast—or the baby will slowly make its way there on its own. Usually, the baby's suck feels very strong and the mother is struck by something about the baby—its tiny size, its hands, its hair, its gaze…

In her own time, the mother can check the baby's gender herself, if she is not being disturbed. Actually, it's very important indeed (from a safety point of view) that she isn't disturbed while all this is happening. Any disturbance can inhibit production of the hormones which will release the placenta, which needs to be born safely as soon as possible—probably within two hours of the birth, but usually much sooner—either moments after the birth, or 30-60 minutes afterwards. The umbilical cord is cut when it stops pulsing or can remain intact until it spontaneously breaks away from the baby's body a few days later. (Sometimes it breaks as the baby is born. This happened to me when my third baby was born.[14]) Then suddenly, provided there is no disturbance, the placenta is born too—usually in one smooth, slippery movement. In an undisturbed physiological birth, this happens very soon after the birth of the baby (even one or two seconds later). Breastfeeding also stimulates the production of the hormone (oxytocin) which makes the birth of the placenta possible.

As we've already noted, if the woman was upright (squatting, semi-squatting, or on her hands and knees) at the moment of birth, it's very likely that her vagina, and indeed all her sexual organs, will be undamaged after all these processes have taken place because the perineum—the muscles which support all the organs in that area—is naturally stretchy and the woman's complete awareness of every sensation will help her to make sure the birth does not cause any injury. This means she'll have no pain after the birth, beyond a little discomfort doing her first wee and poo and the experience of her womb contracting back to its normal size. She will feel essentially normal when sitting or walking around.

Often there is some mess during the whole birthing process. There might be blood or faeces involved because the baby is, after all, emerging through a fairly narrow passageway, near other passageways, and the placenta is attached by a network of blood vessels before the birth. However, Michel reports that after a true fetus ejection reflex there is dramatically less blood loss. I hadn't realised this myself because obviously I didn't look down and think, "Oh, less blood," but Michel has seen this phenomenon countless times as a birth attendant. The reduced blood loss after a true fetus ejection reflex occurs because the placenta detaches so fast and efficiently. It means not only that the woman is extremely strong after the birth, but also that the risk of haemorrhage—a concern to any midwife anywhere—is minimised substantially. So if the woman is not disturbed in any way while she is giving birth and immediately afterwards she is at an enormous advantage. (In Africa and elsewhere, traditional practices mean that the woman is *ritually* disturbed at the moment of birth, before the 'birth' of the placenta.) Even when there is no true fetus ejection reflex and consequently more blood is lost (because the placenta detaches more slowly), a haemorrhage is still very unlikely, especially when the woman breastfeeds immediately or soon after the birth because breastfeeding stimulates production of the right hormones to help the placenta detach smoothly.

Despite any mess which may occur (faeces or blood), since both mother and baby are fully conscious and active during and after a completely physiological birth, a number of pleasant mind-body states are typical. These include wonder, alertness and euphoria—and it seems, from both the babies' facial expressions and research evidence, that the baby experiences these too. Perhaps it's a bit like good sex... it's so absorbing that the mess becomes acceptable. Who cares about puddles of clothes, dampness and wet hands? And who thinks about mess on first locking eyes with a new baby, who smells wonderful, whose skin is deliciously silky soft and whose every feature and action seem like a tiny miracle? Actually, when they're truly undisturbed, natural labours are even more absorbing than sex. This is because hormones produced in these special circumstances transform the woman's state of mind. A woman who is usually self-conscious about being naked will happily strip off her clothes and get into unusual positions. This happens when she has 'gone to another planet', as Michel Odent puts it, when the normally inactive, instinctual side of the brain takes over. Every woman has this ability to transform herself so as to be able to give birth, it's just been forgotten in modern obstetrics, although thankfully research evidence is now helping professionals to rediscover what was once taken for granted in some places.[15]

Another interesting thing about physiological birth is that the baby does not need to be 'caught'. The mother-to-be can simply prepare something soft for her baby to land on and can position herself above it. (Actually, my third daughter went clonk onto the bathroom floor and suffered no ill effects.) The woman can also be alone—in fact some people would say it's better if she is—or supported by just one very unobtrusive and sensitive midwife. (Another could wait outside if two are required by law.[16])

Although it's wise to have a back-up system in place, no help of any kind is needed after most completely physiological births because all the baby's reflexes will help him or her to adjust to life outside the womb. Coughing, sneezing, rooting* and sucking all take place completely spontaneously, when necessary, and the newborn will almost always breathe without assistance in a completely undisturbed, natural birth.[17] If something does need to be done by an outsider—for example, if the umbilical cord is wrapped around the baby's neck—the mother herself, who is fully conscious and active, often spontaneously does it herself. (A few mothers who contributed to this book reported doing this.)

An optimal birth can be very fast (perhaps a couple of hours in total) and at the same time perfectly safe. Or it can take longer—anything up to a whole 24-hour period. A lot depends on the birthing mother and the circumstances in which she gives birth, including, crucially, the number of people who may be with or near her and how they behave. (Michel has observed that the more people there are, the longer the labour.) Perhaps the baby has some influence over the whole process too.

*If any words are new to you, just use the Glossary at the back of the book.

This is Nuala OSullivan and her baby (see Birthframe 27)
Photo © Jill Furmanovsky

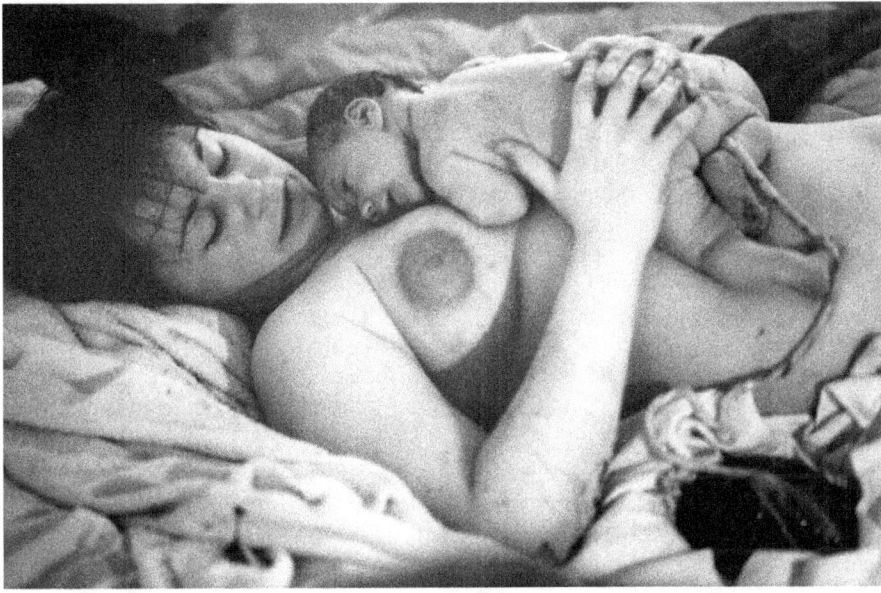

Your baby will spontaneously try to find your breast... you can help him or her to latch on

IMMEDIATELY AFTER THE BIRTH

After-birth scenarios obviously vary enormously. Mother and baby are usually both very alert for about an hour after the birth. In that time, the baby usually starts breastfeeding to get the creamy health-sustaining substance 'colostrum'. This is available to the baby at birth and the milk comes a few days later. Mother and baby—and often the father too—start bonding, as the baby gazes, cuddles up, sucks and drifts off into a contented sleep. (Of course, since many hospitals still tend to take the baby away from the mother, you need to ensure in advance that midwives or other staff know your preference to have your baby with you at this time, as long as he or she is obviously vigorous and well.)[18]

While you're breastfeeding your new baby (which is the most likely scenario after an optimal birth) your birth attendant—let's assume it's a female midwife—will need to check that your baby's OK. First she'll give him or her a brief examination while he or she is lying in your arms. If all seems well, she'll write 'NAD' (no abnormalities detected) on the birth records, as well as an Apgar score. This is a score out of 10 which was originally devised by Dr Virginia Apgar. The table overleaf shows how the points are awarded—your baby can score a possible two points for each of five categories. This score is calculated one minute after the birth and then again at five minutes. (You yourself probably won't be aware of anything being done.)

There is an obvious limitation to this scoring system for naturally birthed babies. After all, many natural babies don't cry when they're born and they don't cough or sneeze either. If there's nothing blocking their nasal passages, they simply smile contentedly as they start breathing and latch on to breastfeed.

Your midwife will also want to check that you yourself are well and in no need of treatment. The placenta will be examined and your blood loss will be estimated. Your blood pressure will be checked too. (If it's low, as mine was after my first birth, you may simply need to lie down for a while until the pressure increases again—perhaps for an hour or two.) Your vagina and perineum will also be checked for damage. As we've seen already, tears are unlikely after a completely undisturbed physiological birth because this kind of birth involves complete awareness. If there is slight tearing (known as 'first degree tearing'), no stitches are needed because healing will take place spontaneously. You would simply need to make sure you avoided spreading your legs for two weeks. Stitching for worse tears is usually carried out under local anaesthetic.

After this examination you may want to rest or continue breastfeeding. (I find it amazing that newborn babies know exactly how to breastfeed when they've been born without drugs. It's so lovely to see their alert faces and curious gaze.) Your baby will probably still be naked at this stage, perhaps draped with a blanket.

You will probably want to have a wash at some point because labour can be quite a sweaty business. Your baby, incidentally, will almost certainly *not* need a wash. You needn't really wash your newborn properly for a week or so, so that you can enjoy his or her beautiful newborn scent. It really is something special, to be enjoyed for as long as possible. Any blood or mucous can simply be wiped away. If there's any creamy vernix, this can be rubbed gently into your newborn's skin. And dirty faces and bottoms can be cleaned with a flannel or cotton wool dipped in tepid water.

SIGN	0	1	2
Heart rate	Absent	Slow (below 100)	Over 100
Respiratory effort	Absent	Weak cry, hypoventilation	Good strong cry
Muscle tone	Limp	Some flexion of extremities	Well flexed
Reflex response	No response	Grimace	Cough or sneeze
Colour	Blue, pale	Body pink, extremities blue	Completely pink

Apgar scores explained

On the subject of dirty bottoms, you may also want to help clear up yourself if you've given birth at home. I'm not generally someone who is keen on housework but postnatal tidying up is something I can now do with joy. I suppose this is because it puts me in touch with the site of such a special event all over again and because I generally prefer to wipe my own bottom, now that I'm an adult! It's important to rest and tune into your baby, but involvement in the processes and dignity may also seem important to you, as they did to me.

What else will you want to do after the birth? Eat, probably. The work of labour along with your new energy requirements for breastfeeding might combine to make you very hungry indeed. A cup of tea is often also very welcome at this time and you may find you have plenty of appetite for cake!

Beyond that, you should find you're up and about within minutes of giving birth. Breastfeeding will suddenly occupy a great deal of your time, though, and will force you to sit down and rest every now and then. It will give you an appetite and it's also likely to make you feel very thirsty—so you'll need to have plenty of water on hand.

Breastfeeding will also trigger afterpains for the first few days. They occur when your womb is gradually shrinking back to its former, pre-pregnancy size and are triggered by one of the hormones you produce when you're breastfeeding. (Afterpains would happen even if you bottle-fed, but the whole process would take a lot longer.) Afterpains are especially strong after a second or subsequent birth. They're just something we have to put up with, again hopefully without drugs because any drugs would pass straight into the baby through your milk. They don't last long—a day or two at most—and only the first couple of feeds are usually really painful. At least they have the positive side-effect of helping your tum get back into shape.

Your life with a new baby—or babies—will have begun.

BIRTHFRAMES

I present 'birthframes'—birth stories—in this book so as to help you visualise real life scenarios. Incidentally, I've created the word 'birthframe' to refer to any true account of a birth experience, part of it, or even only part of the labour or pregnancy—or it may cover more than one birth.

The word 'birthframe' reminds me of 'window frame', through which you can get a glimpse into someone else's world, and 'frame of reference', which helps put other things in perspective.

The first three birthframes are about me because I thought you might like to know exactly where I'm coming from in terms of my own experience. They're just a starting point—soon you'll hear about lots of other people too.

Here are some comments on my own birth journey... **Birthframe 1**

I didn't meet the man who seemed to be my life partner until I was 36.
By the time we decided to stop using contraception, I was 37. This meant that I was 38, 40 and 43 when I had my three daughters. We were living in Sri Lanka during my first pregnancy, and both of us were working full-time.

Way back then, I had no particular pre-conceived ideas about birth. However, the fact that I was in Sri Lanka prompted me to consider many issues and I soon found myself taking a stand on things I'd never previously considered. This was because there was a tendency in Sri Lanka (and in many other developing countries, I later found out) to copy the outdated 'Western' model of medicated birth, which is now being seriously debated by many people in the field of birth and which evidence from countless research studies is proving to be misguided.

My first inkling that this might be the case was when the first consultant I registered with disagreed with something in the birth plan I'd drawn up—following the advice in one of my pregnancy books. Episiotomy, he said, was a routine procedure, so I would have no choice but to accept it. Only a few weeks before I hadn't even known the meaning of the word 'episiotomy'. Now, not only did I know that it meant cutting a woman's perineum (see the Glossary!) with a pair of scissors, just before a birth, I also knew that research had shown it to cause more problems than it was supposed to solve. Instead of *preventing* a nasty tear to a woman's intimate parts, it turned out it *caused* worse problems when the cut turned into a tear. The girl I had been, who'd learnt dressmaking at school and at home, felt this made sense... And the logical woman I had become felt that a cut which was *certain* seemed a worse option than a tear which was only a *possibility*. As a private patient, I felt that I should be able to demand the treatment of my choice, so I started looking for another consultant.[19]

Not finding a replacement consultant, I nevertheless continued with my antenatal appointments and hit various other problems. EFM—another new term—would also be a requirement, apparently, and again it was completely non-negotiable. This monitoring, carried out by means of straps across my belly, while I laboured lying back on a bed, seemed to be bad news. It was almost certain to mean I wouldn't be able to move around as I wished. It would put me in a position which even a basic understanding of physiology and gravity seemed nonsensical, and—reading up on the research—I found that its only reliable effect was to increase the caesarean rate.[20] According to respectable research studies, it caused no improvement in 'outcomes', i.e. it didn't reduce the death rates of either mothers or newborn babies and it brought about no improvement in health for either of them.[21] Frustrated, I continued my search for another caregiver. Since I was in a small place and unwilling to go to a government hospital I had few options open to me.

I reconsidered my position again and again, but acquiescing to 'the protocols' seemed my only option. (It was unrealistic to fly back to the UK... I could not afford the time off work and in any case it would be far too expensive.) It seemed unlikely I'd be able to persuade a midwife or consultant from the UK to fly out for an extended holiday. And I didn't feel happy about the idea of having a 'freebirth', which in some circles was all the rage. No... What I wanted was to let my body function as I felt it would spontaneously do, with the backup of medical help *in case it was needed.* All that was necessary to make this possible was a wise caregiver, who was up-to-date with the scientific research and sensitive towards women.

A few months later, still not finding another caregiver who would accept my birth plan, I continued to reconsider my position... It seemed to me that all the procedures I was arguing against having would turn me into a patient if I accepted them. I didn't want to be a patient. It seemed to me that birth must be a healthy process, so why should it need to be medicalised to such an extent? Why couldn't I only have intervention if it was really necessary? My research had convinced me that the mortality rates in poor areas of the world were due not to lack of intervention, but to all kinds of other things:

- traditions of early marriage (from age 12) and lack of contraception
- unsafe abortions and/or overlarge families, with inadequate incomes
- lack of clean water, poor sanitation and inadequate housing
- health problems or threats (anaemia, malnutrition, which often meant an undeveloped pelvis; malaria, HIV, AIDS, Strep B, sexually transmitted diseases, such as gonorrhoea)
- traditions of female circumcision, which involve cutting away more or less of a girl's genitalia and sewing up the wound, to leave only a tiny hole—which, unsurprisingly, creates physical difficulties when it comes to birth
- lack of access to good screening procedures in pregnancy (to detect problems) and lack of care facilities to deal with problems that arise
- misunderstandings about how to facilitate the processes of birth, which often result in births being disturbed by inappropriate intervention
- lack of skilled medical care for both routine births and problematic ones
- lack of health care facilities and well-maintained or modern equipment
- lack of *access* to health care facilities because of poor road networks or transport systems, not to mention problems with power cuts on arrival
- shortages of drugs and medicines as well as fresh blood for transfusions
- lack of money to pay for care in countries where no free care is available
- superstitious 'traditional' practices during labour, birth and afterwards (such as 'smoking' newborn babies so as to drive away 'evil spirits')
- lack of breastfeeding, because of the use of opiates in labour (such as pethidine or diamorphine) and/or superstitions about colosturm (the first milk), and marketing campaigns to promote formula in recent decades... contaminated water used for the formula often causes diarrhoea and babies can die as a result

I had a certain understanding of these issues even before I started to do my research because I'd already lived in Morocco for two years and had travelled extensively in Asia, while living in Singapore and Japan. Although I'd had little contact with babies or children over this time, I knew what the hospitals were like in poorer countries and had come across many rituals and unhealthy traditional practices, which seemed to be entrenched in the collective psyche. I'd also experienced what it was like to be without water for three days (in Morocco) or electricity (in other places), what it was like to be in houses with terrible sanitation (in poor homes in the Philippines and India) and what it was like to get stuck in an inadequate transport system (in Thailand, when I injured my back on a trek and had had trouble getting back to a relatively civilised bed). In my travels, I'd also met many people who'd had 'unusual' health problems: a man who, for nine months, had been nursing a tiny cut on his big toe, which had become infected and which was refusing to heal in the tropical heat; a friend who'd given birth without water in the medina (the 'old town') of Casablanca; a colleague who'd 'gone native' in Malaysia after falling in love with and marrying a local... Her lifestyle, when I visited her a few times afterwards, was far from modern and I began to realise what it might be like to live without modern cleaning materials, laundry facilities and easily accessible medical facilities. Even the weather often affected access to facilities at times, I found—when my plans were affected by typhoons, monsoon rains, flooding and even earthquake damage.

Accepting pain relief in labour would turn me into a very needy patient, I discovered. Rather than being the means to a painfree birth—the popular fallacy—I discovered that accepting an epidural represented a method for undermining my body's ability to give birth and even my own autonomy...

- Since an epidural tends to slow down labour if given too early, I learnt it's often given *after* the woman has endured several hours of labour.
- Since it tends to slow down the pushing stage (or, indeed, make it impossible), I found out that most caregivers prefer to let it 'wear off' before the actual birth. Of course, this means a sudden whammy of pain!
- In 10% of cases epidurals don't work at first and it apparently takes up to an hour to sort out the anaesthesia levels so that it *is* effective.
- If the woman moves while it's being administered—bearing in mind that she's in intense pain at this time—the consequences can be severe. In a few cases women are left paralysed after the birth. In other cases, where the anaesthetic gets into the wrong place, a 'reversal' is required postnatally, which is described by women as being horrendously painful.
- In many cases, even if the epidural has apparently been successful during labour, afterwards women experience a severe headache continuously for up to six weeks. (I didn't like the idea of this, since this would be my first few weeks with my new baby.) Other women complain of backache every time they have a period for the rest of their lives—and they are convinced the epidural is to blame.

- Most importantly, I gradually came to realise that accepting an epidural would also mean an implicit acceptance of all kinds of other interventions... My blood pressure would need constant monitoring because one of the inevitable side effects of an epidural is a lowering of blood pressure. (Dangerously low blood pressure would mean that blood—and therefore oxygen—was not circulating around my own and my baby's body fast enough.) I would need to be on a drip in case, as would be likely, I'd need to have contractions artificially accelerated, because epidurals usually slow down labour. A urinary catheter would probably be needed to drain off my urine because I would probably be unable to recognise any need to urinate. Electronic fetal monitoring (EFM) would be necessary because the effects of the anaesthetic and the drip might be unpredictable as far as the baby is concerned, and put him or her at more risk. Forceps, ventouse or a caesarean would be more likely—and I would have to accept them if this were the case. After the birth, breastfeeding might go less well... In short, in accepting an epidural I would have to accept the status of a passive patient and would be signing up to a full 'managed' birth because it would mean my natural bodily processes would be disturbed and would not function properly.

My aversion to the idea of all this was clear in my own head. Nevertheless, I discovered—to my surprise—that epidurals and other forms of analgesia or anaesthesia were being hailed as a symbol of women's liberation by many women. They saw drugs as representing a path to painfree birth. Clearly, I thought, these false women's libbers hadn't done much research into birth. Other forms of pain relief also came with all kinds of significant drawbacks.

Drug-free active birth, on the other hand, seemed to promise something entirely different. Women I met who'd had an entirely unmanaged birth seemed strong and exhilarated when they spoke about their experiences. There was no militancy and no evangelism because their decisions to 'go natural' had clearly not been made with any religious or masochistic motive in mind. They'd opted for 'drug-free' for the sake of their babies' well-being. (This seemed a good reason.) And the sense of womanly empowerment that seemed to go with these women's experiences was quite unlike the *dis*empowerment, resignation or trauma I observed amongst women who'd opted for drugs. (Most of these women seemed dismissive when they talked about their birthing experiences.) I felt drawn to the serenity and joy of the women who'd birthed their babies drug-free. I was intrigued by their ability to manage any pain, which they said built up gradually, or was even pleasurable instead of painful—even orgasmic for some! I wanted to find out more...

The upshot was that I persevered and found someone who would support me. Then, and when I gave birth to my other daughters later, I experienced the wonder and beauty of drug-free, intervention-free births... and I decided to write a book about something I felt sure represents optimality. Fortunately, I'd also discovered the research generally agrees with me on this.

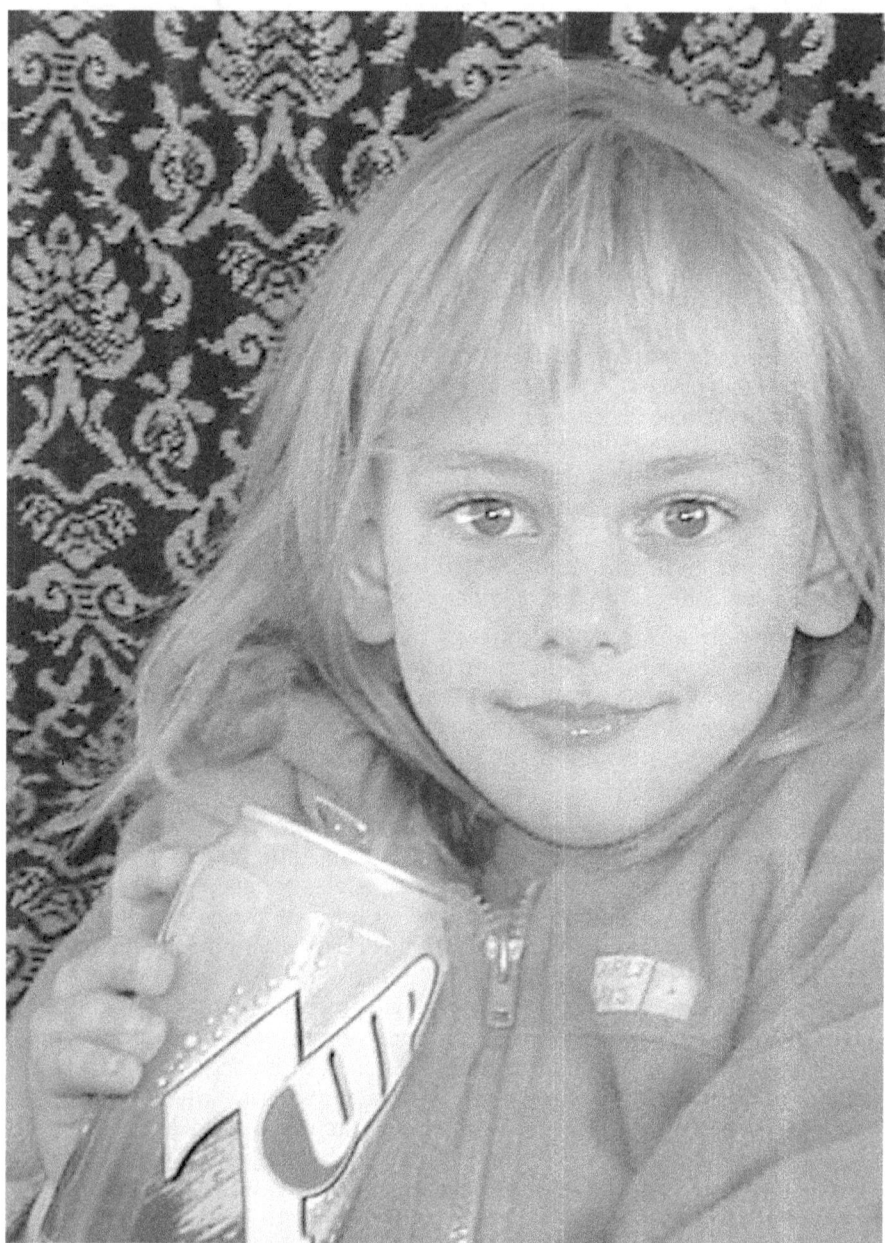

Here's a photo of my first-born daughter, Anjula, when she was 5. I've included photos of babies and older children in this book with the idea of reassuring you that optimally birthed babies are not weirdos—but they do often seem surprisingly full of joy! I also included photos because I think that when we think of having children we are thinking of precisely that—i.e. children, not babies.

I'd like to tell you more about one of my births in detail... **Birthframe 2**

I look back on my second child's birth with a great feeling of peace, happiness and even wonder. Nina-Jay was born on 15 December at 11.30 in the evening, just two hours after I experienced the first contraction; the placenta came out painlessly with another contraction, a few moments later. Her Apgar score was 10 and she weighed in at a very healthy weight. There was no problem with blood loss and no need for any stitching—I only had a little superficial tearing, which healed in a couple of days. I started breastfeeding my new baby moments after she was born and we continued —with breaks!—until she was nearly 2 years old, without any problems.

In the three weeks before the evening of her birth I had experienced numerous painless or low-pain contractions. The contractions which started at 9.30pm on her 'birth day', while I was doing the washing up, came on very suddenly. They were much stronger than any I had felt in the days and weeks before. In fact, they were completely absorbing. I was immediately on my hands and knees on the kitchen floor.

Fortunately, Michel Odent, my caregiver for this birth, was already in the house when these contractions started so there was no problem with this being a short labour. Just before I'd started doing the washing up, he and I had sat at the kitchen table after an enormous dinner, talking about my life and all my problems and I realise that something in me had relaxed during that conversation. I'd been worried about the future but Michel had somehow reassured me. The day before this, I had called him, thinking I was in labour, and had had to apologise when he arrived since my contractions had stopped. He decided to stay at our place that night and in the morning said he would like to come to dinner again later that day and again stay overnight. (We were living a long way from his home in London.) I must say, I wasn't keen when he said this because I had visions of cooking for him and apologising for the next two weeks—but it turned out that he was right to return so soon. When he arrived at around 4.00pm, I was fast asleep, having had a huge and wonderful lunchtime curry. My partner was at home that day because of a quirk in his timetable, so I hadn't needed to look after 2-year-old Anjula—I could rest.

With these sudden, overwhelmingly powerful contractions, I soon felt the need to stagger upstairs and start some sonorous groaning. Michel, hearing the noise, emerged from the room we'd assigned him—next door to the bathroom, where I was—and asked if he could please check the baby's heartbeat and position. His brief examination reassured him that conditions were ideal for me to labour undisturbed. Firstly, palpation of my bump had told him I had a full bag of waters. This meant there was little danger of the umbilical cord prolapsing or becoming compressed.[22]

Secondly, he established that the position of my baby was fine—LOA—see the Glossary for an explanation. (Later Michel told me his 'treatment'—i.e. to leave me to labour undisturbed—would not have been different if she had also been in a posterior position, like her big sister. He said he has found that women find better positions for helping the baby turn if left alone, undisturbed.) Thirdly, Michel confirmed with a fetal stethoscope (a Pinard) that the fetal heartbeat was strong. He was also reassured to see that on my return to the bathroom I was spontaneously labouring in favourable positions—leaning forward, either standing, on my hands and knees, or on my knees in front of the toilet when I was throwing up! He knew this would mean avoiding compressing the vena cava, which would happen lying down, and which is important for the baby's oxygen supply. While I laboured alone, in peace, Michel waited and listened from the room next door. He even waited outside while I gave birth.[23]

Phil, my partner, helped me throughout my brief two-hour labour. As each contraction ripped into me I fully understood why some women choose drug-based pain relief or a caesarean—but I knew I must not even mention any of these thoughts out loud. A few contractions into my labour I said to Phil, "Two children are enough! We really don't need to have a third one, you know." Wisely ignoring my comment, he ran up and down the stairs fetching things for me—candles for candlelight, something to tie my hair back... (We'd agreed he'd do this in advance.) Meanwhile, Michel continued to keep watch from the next room, without making himself seen. He knew from long experience that the best support would be to leave me completely undisturbed, with a feeling of being unobserved.[24] The sounds I made would be enough to tell him if all was going well. Of course, he administered no drugs and insisted on no routines. Nature had her own routines in mind...

Then, within two hours of feeling that first contraction, I gave birth. Moments before, Anjula had woken up so Phil had had to go and console her. After sitting on the toilet for a few minutes, straining to do a non-existent poo, I suddenly stood up, lifted up my arms, flexed my knees slightly and gave birth! Between my feet, bundled up in a large ball, was a plastic sheet which I'd been 'relocating' around the house in a preoccupied manner for the few days before I went into labour. So much strength was coursing through my body when I was ready to give birth that I didn't need anyone's help or support. I thought about various things I'd read... I thought of Inuit (Eskimos)—supporting their wives from behind and pushing down on the bump so as to help the baby, and I focused in on my own baby within me. Then I thought, "Baby, be born!"—calm, joyful words which passed through my head quite spontaneously. Then suddenly, I gave two wonderful strong, clear, purposeful painfree pushes. The ring of fire I then felt made me consciously realise my new baby's head must have crowned.

I momentarily felt worried I would tear. Then—thinking, "Oh, I don't care if I rip in two"—I flicked my hips forward. Reaching down to feel what was going on I was shocked to feel a head. "Michel!" I shouted, anxious that I should be giving birth without his help. Knowing it would be dangerous to disturb me at this point, he ignored me and carried on simply silently watching through the crack in the door. There was a moment's pause, then again I flicked my hips forward. In a sudden gush my baby was born and, confused, I felt another gush seconds later.

I looked down, transfixed for what must have been only a few seconds, admiring my new baby's features. Suddenly she let out a cry and saying, "Don't cry," I took her up in my arms and instinctively put her to my breast.

There was none of the hesitation I'd expected to feel. Having read about so many problem situations, I had wondered whether breastfeeding would be so easy the second time around. My new baby sucked as if for the thousandth time, not the first. As I looked down it dawned on me that the second gush had been the placenta... It was all so fast! Beautifully alert, my baby was gazing quizzically into my eyes as she breastfed. Michel came in at this point and was reassured to see the placenta lying by my side, born and whole, a sign that all was properly finished and safe. My husband was sad to have missed the birth and 2-year-old Anjula, who'd just woken up, looked amazed at her mother holding a new baby in her arms.

It was wonderful not having someone else 'catch' the baby for me. It was also wonderful being able to discover her sex myself and pick her up for the first time without anyone observing or 'checking' on me. The most wonderful aspect of this birth, though, was the feeling of strength I had. I felt so strong, both physically and mentally. I didn't need anyone to support me as I suddenly stood up, swung round, raised my arms in the air, elbows bent, feet planted firmly on the floor some distance apart, knees flexed. I certainly didn't need anyone to tell me I was fully dilated. Somewhere deep inside, I knew it was time to push. The feeling of pushing—two long, clear, happy pushes—was very positive and also completely painless, as I said before. The ring of fire which I immediately became aware of at the end of these pushes was also not painful or 'weak-feeling'. There was never any need to 'pant' or control my breathing—I just felt poised, focused, very alert and decisive. And I was strong physically in the sense that I had no problems with low blood pressure and no feelings of weakness after the birth. This had been a truly authentic fetus ejection reflex.

After this birth, and my third a couple of years later, I realised again the enormous advantages postnatally of giving birth like this. I understood on a very deep level how *optimal* this type of birth is, physically and psychologically and how little pain there was overall. Most importantly, I saw the advantages for my babies, who were alert, breastfed easily, and *thrived*.

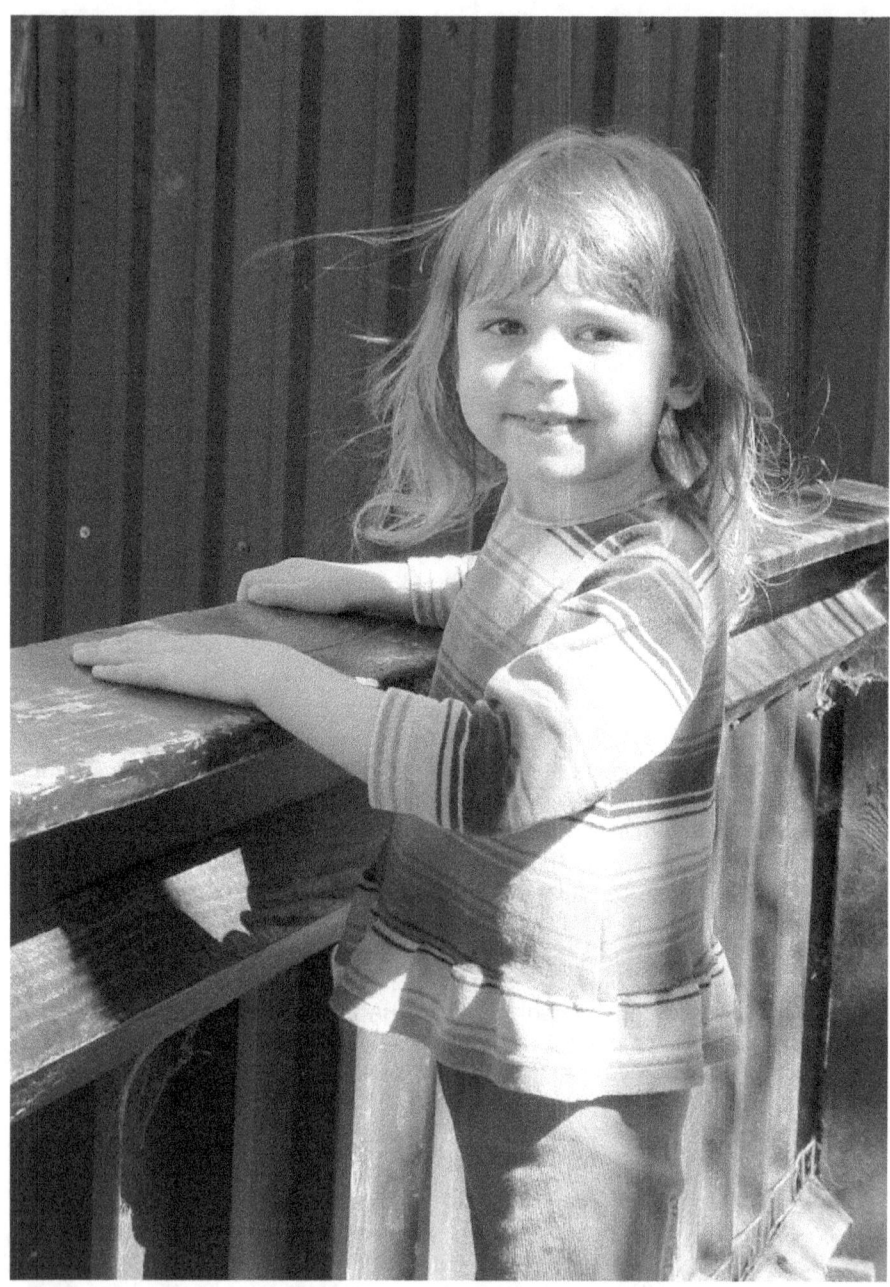

Nina-Jay, aged 3, born by fetus ejection reflex. (Jumeira, my third baby, will have to remain a mystery for the time being. I'll tell you about her labour and birth in a while.)

In case you're suspicious because it all sounds too easy....   **Birthframe 3**

I'd also had a lot of trouble finding a caregiver who would support me when I became pregnant with my second daughter. By this time we'd moved back to the UK and I initially assumed there would be no problem. However, although the first time I'd given birth vaginally, with no complications, my first midwife refused to consider me low risk because of my age: I was 40.[25]

I asked around and visited various midwifery practices. Eventually, I registered with a different GP because I'd heard the midwives at the attached community midwifery practice were very supportive of healthy, unmedicated birth. Nevertheless, after a while it became clear that the support I was receiving was rather half-hearted, even though the pregnancy was progressing smoothly with good test results at every antenatal appointment. A great deal of worry was going on about everything possible which it was thought 'might go wrong'. After various pregnancy scares (which inspired a section later on in this book), I decided to explore my other options. I was worried the fear might escalate when I was in labour.

Eventually, when I was 30 weeks pregnant, I enlisted the support of Michel Odent, a person I'd previously only read about in books. (Somehow I got hold of his phone number and plucked up the courage to ring him.) Even then, since he was only available from two days *after* my due date I still had to find backup care I was happy with. This I found in the form of an independent midwifery practice. My husband and I had to take out a bank loan to afford all this and even then could only afford partial private care! Nevertheless, I felt sure that having the right people to support me during labour was the most important factor in helping me to cope with the pain...

In my third pregnancy, I had even more trouble. Not only was I thought positively geriatric by this time, I was also in another very interventionist culture: Oman. It was a real battle to avoid interventions, which seemed unnecessary, so I was not at all optimistic about the upcoming birth.

When—after much deliberation—my husband and I decided to return to the UK for the birth, I still had a little trouble finding a midwife who would enthusiastically support me. I did find someone who worked within the NHS this time. She very helpfully carried out all my antenatal care in my own home and prepared the way for her colleagues to support me while I was in labour, because it seemed likely she would not be on duty then. Although I'd never met the two midwives who turned up to attend the birth, they did support me and provided excellent care. I had to assert myself in various respects, as usual, but it did all go relatively smoothly and everyone was happy afterwards. Thanks to my preparation, I was able to cope once again.

Since then, I've met many midwives who are enthusiastic about what I'm defining as optimal birth because research data is causing a real change in attitudes...[26]

In the words of a few other people...

Here are comments from a range of contributors, including Michel Odent, to give you even more insight into the physiological processes, as they are typically experienced in an optimal labour and birth.

Onset of labour

This is where it all starts... or is it? I asked Michel:

What would you say to a woman who says she's in labour?

Unless it's absolutely obvious, I always doubt the diagnosis of labour. I usually say, "You don't look like a woman in labour." That's one way of avoiding a very long labour.

How can you tell whether or not a woman is in labour?

You can't really. Often, a midwife will do a vaginal exam and pronounce the woman in labour if she is already 1 or 2cm dilated. But being a little dilated does not mean that the woman is in labour. Actually, you don't need to diagnose labour unless it's absolutely obvious. There was a midwife in Pithiviers who used to say, "I never admit that a woman is in labour as long as she's not at complete dilation." She was joking, of course, but there was some truth in what she was saying. Basically, what she meant was that it's very difficult to tell when a woman is really in labour.

So what's your definition of labour?

In retrospect, when the baby's born you can say the woman was in labour. It's a bit of a joke, of course, but what I'm saying is you can only be sure in retrospect. Contractions every five minutes do not mean labour. Perhaps they will stop and start again another night. That's why the stories of women who've been in labour for five days aren't really stories of long labours. These women were having a pre-labour in the days leading up to the birth. Saying a woman is in labour puts pressure on her to give birth soon. So it's better not to diagnose labour at all until it's totally obvious—when contractions are very strong and coming very close together.

> The night before Arion was born I had an innate sense that it would be the following day. I woke a few minutes to 6pm and had to get up to go to the loo. Shortly afterwards, I had a show and things started to happen. I felt a tightening in my stomach that felt like a contraction. I had been unaware of anything up till this point. Very soon, I was having contractions every five minutes, lasting approximately 30 seconds. [Arion was in fact born a few hours later.]

> I woke up needing to pee, and made it to the loo with clear liquid coming down my legs. The odd thing was that I had no control over this liquid, it just sort of fell out when I stood up. [The baby was born the same day.]

> Well, time went on. Due to finish work soon. On Sunday, 25 June 2000 I was a little off, and I slept like a baby. Must have needed it, as Darren could not believe I had slept so well due to the noise going off outside—neighbours. Thought nothing of it.

On the Monday, I took my son to school, as normal, and waddled off to work for my last week. I was up and down like a yoyo, going back and forth to the bathroom. Well, something was happening and I was just not ready. Rang the midwife, but by the time I had finished talking I was huffing and puffing...

[Twins were born just after 3.00pm the same day.]

" At 32 weeks I had an antenatal check-up and was told the babies were roughly 6lb each in weight, so you can imagine my surprise and shock. The next few weeks I got bigger and bigger and everyone was hoping for an early delivery... even the doctors at the hospital couldn't understand after 36 weeks how I was still carrying them. Then 40 weeks approached and my due date. I attended another antenatal clinic, where I saw the consultant. He told me there was still plenty of room for them to grow so he would not induce me! 40 weeks + 3 days, my contractions started and I went to hospital, where they told me it was the first time they had ever seen a twin pregnancy overdue. By 6.00am the first baby was ready to arrive: I pushed for about 15 minutes and Megan Victoria was born at 6.19am, weighing 7lb 1oz, then six minutes later after pushing came Thomas William, weighing 7lb 12oz, both perfectly healthy.

Clare Swain

My contractions stopped. Apparently, this is very common.

" I had a whole night of very strong, regular contractions 24 hours before Asya was born. I was sure this was the real thing, but at 6am they petered out. Apparently this kind of 'false labour' is very common, because the body produces the most oxytocin at night. It didn't feel false! The good news is that false labour does help to open the cervix, so your labour will probably be that much shorter when it does get going for real.

" Perhaps what I experienced was false labour, or perhaps it was interrupted labour. All I know is that my strong, regular contractions suddenly stopped after I'd been talking to my mother on the phone for five minutes. She sounded horrified that I was in labour when I answered the phone. She then immediately switched to a totally boring, irrelevant topic for the rest of the conversation... er, monologue. No amount of relaxation exercises could restart the contractions when I came off the phone. However, the next day, when my contractions started again, they were even more purposeful and my 'real' labour lasted less than two hours.

Michel says:

" Relax! Don't worry about going into labour. It is sometimes very worrying for a woman to be told a date for induction. Waiting for labour is the best way to become inhibited. Just relax and enjoy the last phase of your pregnancy.

First stage

This is the bit where your cervix gradually opens up so the baby can come out.

" I did not want to leave the top floor of our house, I did not want the curtains open, and I did not want the lights on. Almost as soon as labour had begun I had started to withdraw into what I see as a sort of animal protective state.

" At the beginning my temperature perception was going up and down, so during a contraction all my clothes came off, then I was freezing in between, and they all had to go on.

" In the middle of the night my waters broke. I was asleep. It was about 1 o'clock in the morning and I woke up and I was just lying in bed and it was all wet. I called the nurse and she said, "No, you've probably just wet yourself," which made me feel really bad—it was really horrible. But I was certain it was my waters that had broken and so I insisted and she came and checked then called the doctor who was on call that night. He examined me and I was already 7cm dilated. But I hadn't felt any pain or anything—just pressure. I'd been feeling that for some time when I was standing up.

" Before my labour I ate voraciously. Part of my first stage I then spent throwing up into the toilet! This felt fine, actually. Afterwards, I rationalised that I must have digested most of the food I'd had beforehand anyway.

" You asked how I felt about shouting but to be honest it was more like a cow 'mooing'. It felt good to me and I reached a point where I stopped even caring what anyone else may have thought of it.

" Found standing up and leaning over the bed on a beanbag, rocking and having someone massage my lower back excellent for pain relief.

" Baby turned from posterior position to anterior a short time after I adopted an all-fours, bottom-up position.

" When they checked me over, I was 9cm dilated. The twins wanted out. There was nothing I could do but go with the flow.

" I had now been on my feet for about nine hours with nothing to eat since the night before (my breakfast having hit the stairs some time before), and I really wanted to lie down. I did not care if labour stopped for half an hour; I just wanted a rest.

" I went from Stage 1 to Stage 2 in about five minutes. From being able to hold a normal phone conversation one minute, I was suddenly only capable of screaming blue murder the next. My husband has never shown a cooler nerve as he drove me to hospital. By this time I was screaming so loudly I was sure the whole of London could hear me. Incapable of sitting in the car I was raging around the back seat like a werewolf. I was in the grip of elemental forces that were telling me to go and find a lair, a den, a quiet place to do this really important job. An overwhelmingly strong instinct was telling me to get my trousers off so that this being could come out. I would have done it in the lift. I would have done it in front of a million people. As it was, they found me a room and a couch and I was told the very encouraging news that I was already fully dilated.

" My midwife used a Sonicaid (a waterproof one bought especially for my water birth), but I can hardly recall it. I think she only listened once to the heartbeat at the same time as she examined me internally.

Second stage

The bit where the baby comes out.

I was in the grip of elemental forces!

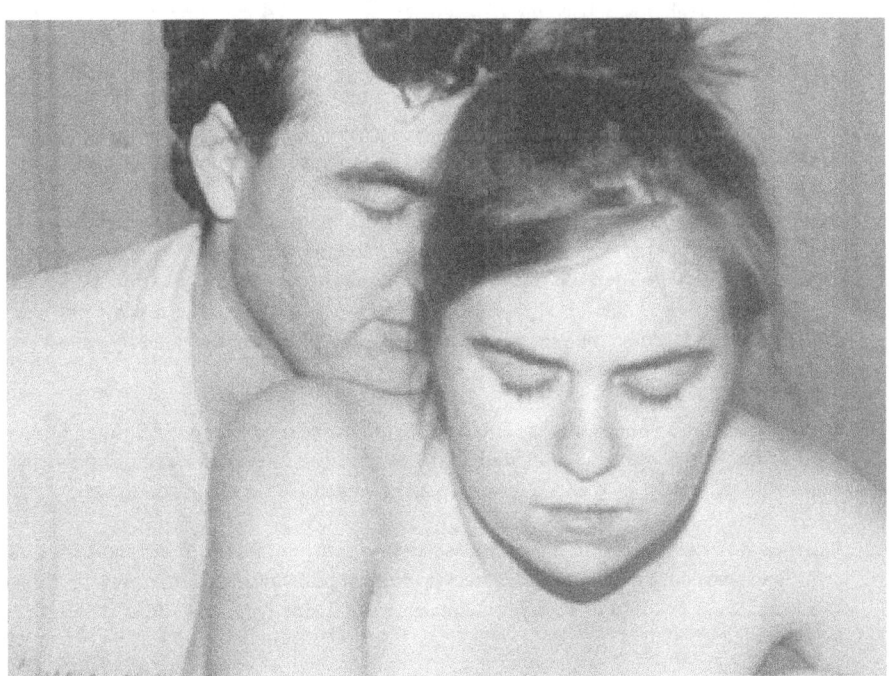

I refused all photos of women in labour and actually giving birth except this one and one other from Ashley Marshall (see Birthframe 4). Don't let anyone use a camera until after the placenta has been born—it may well cause a disturbance.

> In second stage my body seemed to know when I should push, to pant or hold back, and I didn't need the midwife's help to control the delivery.

> At the next contraction I said that I could feel the head crowning; I don't think anyone believed me. My next comment was "Ah that's better, the head's out." I then remember someone saying that they needed to get me off the toilet; once again I had my own ideas. I also had another contraction and the body was born. With this contraction I lifted myself off the toilet seat and caught our baby. I brought her up between my legs and sat back down to cuddle her for the first time. It was 10.30am, and she straightaway went to my breast.

> I had gone from no baby to baby in about three minutes. This was a truly shocking experience, and I remember screaming as this thing fell out of my body.

> As I lifted the baby up, just after he'd been born he didn't cry, just opened his eyes and looked around curiously. I felt like superwoman—amazed, empowered and overjoyed that birth could be such a wonderful experience!

> My daughter Isabel was born on 9 December 1999, at 8.43pm. She was born in my bedroom just by the door. I had told the midwives I would make it to the end of the bed but when push came to shove I didn't want to get any further into the room.

> I asked for an enema during my first labour because I felt blocked up. I was given a pessary and just a little poo came out a short time later. At the time, I didn't feel I'd been disturbed by this procedure but looking back I wonder whether I was in fact because I had a very long and difficult second stage. In my second labour, I again felt constipated, but my request for an enema was ignored. A few minutes later, I suddenly decided I'd stand up and do my 'poo' straight onto the floor! As I pulled myself up I also knew I was going to have a baby—not do a poo at all—so I think I wasn't really the least bit confused. The baby came out easily—she was obviously ready. It didn't even hurt!

> From what I'd read about births, I had expected pushing to feel good. It didn't feel good to me. But it was really weird and interesting. The best part was definitely the moment after the pushing ended, when here she was at last, a whole new person!

> Rebecca was delivered in a supported squatting position, Ros in a leaning forward crouching position, Juliet and Natasha in a kneeling position. Third stages were all in the kneeling-up position except for Rebecca, when I was lying down (and it was the least comfortable).

> Keeping upright keeps the tailbone out of the way making the pelvic area wider so that the baby has a little more room to get out.

> This time I wasn't lying down when I gave birth. I was squatting. Michel asked David to hold me under the armpits while I squatted—which was, in fact, difficult for him to do. I think Michel wanted me to get into that position because he knew she was going to be a big baby. But I didn't have to do any pushing at all. There was never any need to push… it was all just coming slowly but surely—and then fast.

A midwife's account:

> As the last few barriers to Jenny's relaxing disappear (the last of the children are taken out), contractions become more painful, impinging on her concentration. Contracting strongly, every four minutes for 30-40 seconds. Jenny feels she needs to move away from things happening around her. Darkened bathroom, candles. I remove all offensive smells (cooking in the kitchen). She's out of the bath kneeling now, leaning over. Tim's applying pressure to Jenny's back. Things have hotted up. **15 minutes later:** Pressure increases, intensity increases. Jenny thinks it's a boy—only a man would muck her about like this! Tim looks on, not making any comment. **30 minutes later:** Shoulders and baby and all. Together Tim and Jenny investigate what their new baby looks like. "A girl," says Tim. "I'm glad you're a girl". Tears! Placenta born into the plastic bowl. All present and correct. Jenny has a bath with herb infusion. Baby checked and all there—not a *little* girl at 9lb 5oz (4.22 kg)!

> I felt no pain at all during the second stage, just an incredible surging strength.

> With two clear pushes the baby came down the birth canal. I did this in about two seconds, between two contractions. I'd say it was like doing a very easy, but big poo—not diarrhoea exactly, but very easy and even more satisfying than producing two long, plump turds. What I produced, after I'd then felt the 'ring of fire' and had flicked my hips forward twice, with the next two contractions, was a beautiful, baby, who now lay at my feet on a crumpled up sheet, looking up at me with rapt attention. When she suddenly burst into tears, I picked her up and put her to my breast. She seemed relieved and suckled with gusto.

> As I pushed the baby out, my whole body was rising up in the water. That took me by surprise, but it did not make the birth difficult. The midwife said, "Julia, get ready to catch the baby," and I said, "but what should I do with it?"

> I found the whole experience of a natural birth very exciting and satisfying. It hurt like hell, but it was bearable (just). I would be happy to go through the whole thing again next week if I could. It was a real peak experience for me.

I found the experience of a natural birth very exciting and satisfying. It hurt like hell but it was bearable (just).

Third stage

The placenta comes out...

❝ I was surprised when the placenta shot out from between my legs as I reached down to pick up my new baby. So fast and easy!

❝ My physiological third stage was surprisingly painful, but very fast. Then suddenly, it was all over.

A midwife's notes:

10.24 Baby delivers, brought straight out of water by Georgina and G. Baby cries instantly.
10.35 Baby lying in Georgina's arms.
10.40 Baby still attached to placenta but cord ceased pulsating now. Georgina has period-like pains and feels the placenta beginning to come. Water temperature increased after the birth (temperature now 37.3 degrees centigrade). Baby feels warm. Baby is lovely pink now.
10.50 Baby is feeding from Georgina now.
10.55 Placenta membranes delivered spontaneously in the water. Baby still feels OK but has been covered up with a towel now. Cord clamped now and cut by his daddy.
11.00 Georgina out of the water. Bleeding minimal, estimated all in all at approx. 100 ml. Perineum observed, no tears at all. Georgina just feels sore and bruised but it all looks healthy and well.
11.05 Placenta looks complete. Membranes x 2 present and 3 vessels in cord.

❝ The placenta had a strange smell and didn't look as I imagined it would.

❝ I got out of the birthing pool for the third stage and had a small tear, which didn't require stitching.

❝ There was no need for stitches afterwards.

❝ It might be of interest to note that although I had what seemed like a lot of blood loss when the placenta was expulsed (without the use of syntometrine), this large loss of blood is considered a good thing in many so-called undeveloped countries and this seemingly large quantity of blood was followed by very little lochia. On Day 1 I seemed to be soaking sanitary towels fairly consistently but from Day 2 onwards I have had very little discharge.

❝ Postpartum, I just needed 'mini' sanitary napkins.

❝ Postnatal problems? I simply didn't have any. I think problems can sometimes be triggered by drugs given in labour, catching infections, unnecessary interventions, etc

Cutting the cord, or not

This is when the umbilical cord is cut (or not), making the baby independent.

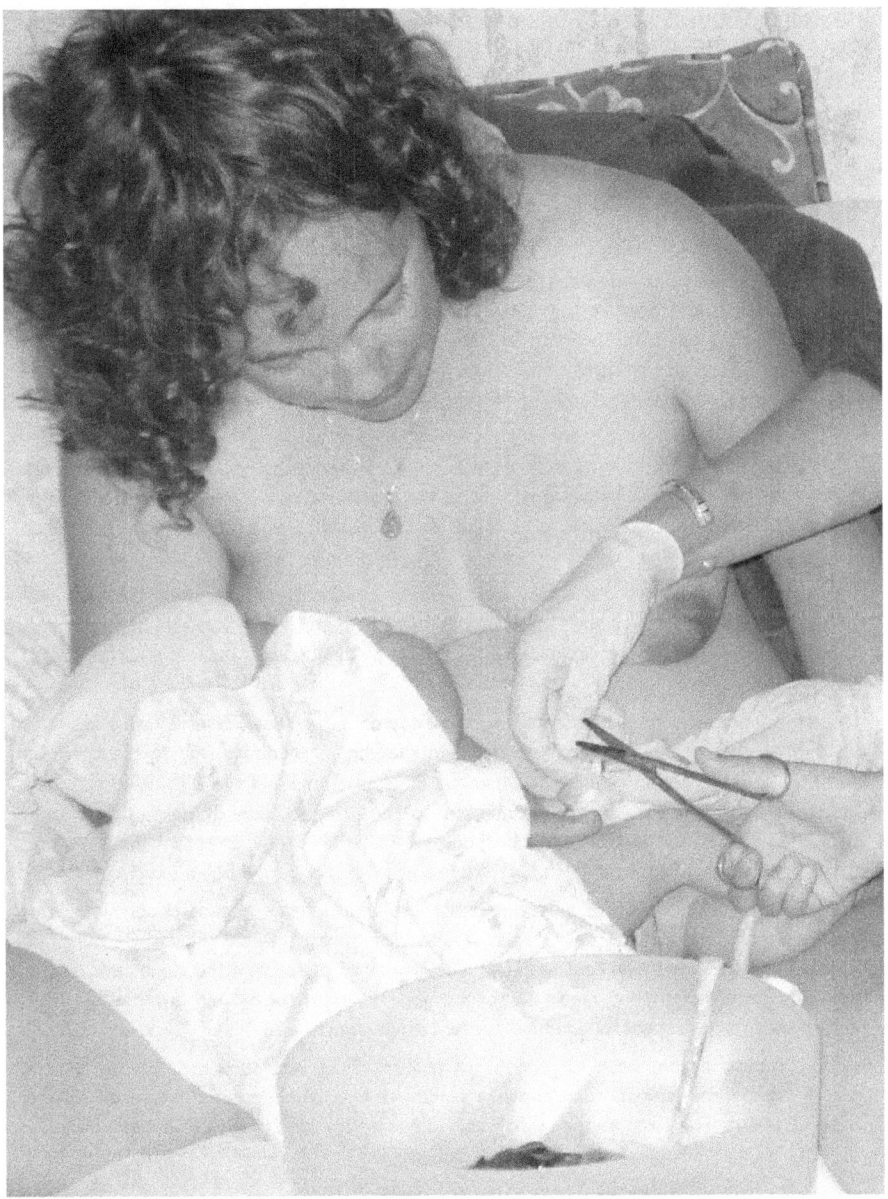

It's entirely up to you when the cord is cut—or whether it's left to fall off naturally. Here, the midwife is helping the baby's big brother to cut the cord.

Birthframe 4

Some people question the widely-held assumption that it is either necessary or helpful to cut the cord.[27] (Is it part of the natural process or not? What about in situations where knives and scissors are not available?) These people see both psychological and spiritual reasons to leave the baby attached to the placenta for however long it takes to drop off naturally. 'Lotus birth'—the term which has been given to this practice of leaving the umbilical cord undisturbed—is explained and exemplified through the following birth, which took place in the USA in 2001.

Harper's birth at home was sweeter than I could have dreamt it. I laboured easily and powerfully with loving support from my husband, doula, and midwife. When Harper's bag of waters popped, birth energy rushed through me and soon his little head began to emerge. There was a slight case of dystocia and a tight umbilical cord but we were safe in the skilful hands of our midwife. Then, all of a sudden, there he was—pink, alert, and beautiful.

As I sat in awe of this perfect, wise being I rubbed the creamy coating of vernix into his delicate skin and knew we had made the right decision to give him a lotus birth. It was the most blissful beginning to follow the culmination of pregnancy and the sense of loss that often ensues.

Lotus birth is the process of leaving the baby's placenta attached via the umbilical cord until it falls off of its own accord. Its purpose is both physiological and spiritual. Physiologically, the baby receives 43% of the blood left in maternal/placental circulation.[28]

Ever wonder why cord blood banking has become so popular? It is known that cord blood—or blood left in the cord and placenta that hasn't made its way to the baby—is useful in helping to fight childhood leukemia later in that child's life.[29] Why not stop denying a baby this vital blood and allow it to pass to the baby after birth instead? Also, the placenta is the baby's life preserver before breathing is established. As long as the cord remains intact and while it still pulsates the baby is being oxygenated.

Long after the cord stops pulsating and the physical transference is complete, the spiritual transference has only begun. This quiet time is when the baby's aura, or spiritual presence, is being realised. The placenta originated from the same cells as the baby and because of this bond they are a genetic identical of one another. A lotus birth allows for a respectful goodbye to the baby's womb mate.

How does a parent care for an intact placenta? It was surprisingly easy. After Harper's birth my husband and midwife placed it in a colander and rinsed all of the blood clots out. Then we rubbed it with sea salt and sprinkled it with lavender flowers.

A lotus birth allows for a respectful goodbye

Harper's placenta wore a cloth nappy just like he did and we changed it daily. We swaddled the 'placenta package' right along with him so we were free to pick him up, nurse and cuddle without the fear of tugging at his navel.

On the third day after his birth, Harper let go of his placenta. He was content and whole and ready to be free. We said goodbye to the organ that had nourished and protected our son for his first nine months but we will see it again when we plant it at Harper's first Blessing Way ceremony. In case you don't know, a Blessing Way ceremony is a Native American ritual used to mark significant life passages in one's life, frequently held to commemorate a birth, a marriage, a death or a woman's journey into motherhood. It is a more spiritual ceremony than the traditional American baby shower, where the focus is on showering the mother with gifts for the baby. A Blessing Way ceremony honours the mother and helps her draw upon her own inner resources that she will need to later give birth. My husband and I decided to offer our children a Blessing Way ceremony to celebrate their first year of life as well as my first year postpartum. We also planted their placentas at this time. (They were kept in the freezer up till then.)

Harper is our second child to be born at home, but our first lotus birth. We now know that we would never have another baby without giving them a lotus birth. It was three very mindful days that enabled us to remain in that warped sense of time that follows birth. We were surrounded only by love and close family while Harper made his earthly transition. There was plenty of time for lively celebration later that week but I will always be grateful for those precious days when Harper was lotus-born.

Ashley Marshall

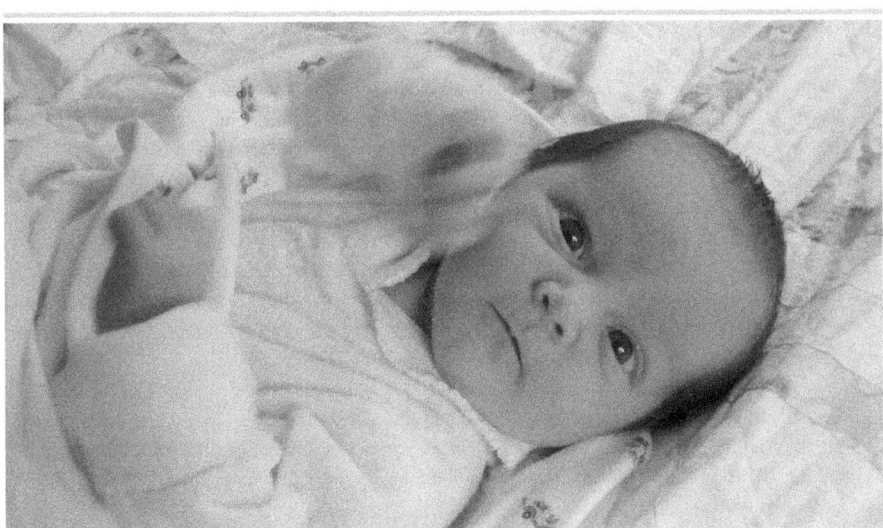

A super-alert newborn baby whose birth you will read about soon. She was born with absolutely no drugs or unnecessary interventions—and was also a VBAC baby.

After the birth

That strange time, which may seem difficult to imagine if you're pregnant now, when you have your new baby...

" I can't tell you what an amazing feeling it is to hold him, touch him, look at him making funny, suspicious faces and wrinkling his brow. I can see Mum was right when she said romantic love is nothing compared to this feeling of utter astonishment and prostrated adoration of this minute creature. My husband and I both feel it. My husband went home to get a few things and run some errands the next day. "I got home to the empty house and it all seemed so pointless. All I wanted was to be back with the two of you." He is utterly taken by the baby. We haven't needed any name for our son in these timeless days at the hospital, with no one but the three of us, a tiny universe.

" Somehow the house feels entirely different now. We have a home now where we're sheltering somebody infinitely precious. Before it was just a post-college pad for two of us to hang out in and amuse ourselves. Now it all has a point.

" I was a bit confused after the birth for a while. I almost felt like I'd failed because it wasn't totally enjoyable. I kept having to remind myself of what I'd achieved, which wasn't hard—I just had to look at my baby and I knew I'd done something wonderful! Being just me and my husband at the birth made it very special and intimate, we didn't need anyone else. After the birth it was all very peaceful and beautiful.

" Babies are such a wonderful way to start people!

" Mum left on Sunday. That afternoon we took him for the first walk of his life, in Regents' Park. All the other parents with children looked calm and collected. We got hot around the collar trying to put the pram together with him in it.

" My husband and I rowed horribly in the first weeks after our baby was born, partly because she was so incredibly interested in everything all the time and so disinterested in sleep! We constantly criticised each other's attempts to care for her and I felt tremendously alone and unloved. Fortunately, things eventually settled down and our second baby was incredibly easy and obliging, although also clearly as bright as a button.

" I really threw myself into the childrearing and I remember at least one person said to me "What about you? You have to give some time to yourself" and I remember saying "This is me. This is important." Not to say, there were times when I didn't get exhausted.

Life-saving intervention

Of course, it is occasionally necessary to intervene in pregnancies or births... While, for the vast majority of women pregnancy and birth really are very healthy, physiological processes, which take place smoothly, for a small minority they present unusual physical challenges. This needn't mean that the processes become highly managed; it may simply mean some judicious use of interventions at key stages of the pregnancy and/or the birth, or more careful monitoring, so that intervention can be made, if necessary. If the intervention is wise, it may indeed optimise outcomes and even reinstate an air of normality to the processes. The objective, of course, with any intervention is to help both the woman and fetus or newborn have the safest and best possible experience. From this point of view, many of the principles described in this book remain true for pregnancies or births which require intervention.

Birthframe 5

Here, we have a clear case of obstetric knowledge being used to ensure an optimal result. Although the woman giving birth used a TENS machine for pain relief, she did manage to avoid all other drugs and interventions while she was in labour. Clearly, both she and her caregivers realised the advantages— from the babies' point of view—of minimising interference in the natural, physiological processes.

I found out I was expecting twins when I was only 10 weeks pregnant and was immediately put under the excellent care of Lawrence Impey and his team at the Feto-Maternal Medicine Unit at the John Radcliffe Hospital in Oxford, England.

Due to the twins being identical—sharing a placenta and monochorionic—I was informed straightaway of the complications that could occur, particularly of the risk of twin-to-twin transfusion syndrome. I was told I would be monitored closely and have regular scans.

Throughout my pregnancy I was healthy and reasonably comfortable until at 32 weeks I developed obstetric cholestasis. I was given medication to control this [ursodeoxycholic acid] and my pregnancy continued as normal.

[Obstetric cholestasis is a rare condition of late pregnancy which can develop when the liver doesn't function as well as it needs to. The main symptom is intense itching, especially on the hands or feet, and the condition is confirmed or ruled out through a blood test. Cholestasis needs to be taken seriously because it can result in stillbirth.]

At 36 weeks I went into labour and I gave birth to healthy twin boys, weighing 4lb 6oz and 4lb 8oz, with no caesarean, no epidural and only the use of a TENS machine for pain relief.

I was very lucky to receive such outstanding care at the hospital. I believe that it was the positive attitude of the medical staff toward vaginal twin births and natural pain relief that enabled me to have such a wonderful natural birth experience.

Jo Siebert

Birthframe 6

Here's an account where medical support became necessary even when the mother and all those around her were hoping for a completely physiological birth. Perhaps it's never possible to know the real reasons for undesired events in our lives. I find it interesting that there is a clue in the following account for what follows even in the first line—in the phrase 'all being well'. The feelings of the mother's *mother* are intriguing...

My daughter had planned, all being well, to give birth at home.

The very strange thing was that months in advance I couldn't see it happening. I never said a word to anyone, but on a few occasions when it was quiet, I sat down and wondered... Why? What could happen? Was my daughter to change her mind? Would something go very wrong? Impossible to tell, I just could not see her home birth a reality. But don't think I was full of fear or negative thoughts, it was more like a fact, a reality that I could not comprehend.

Three weeks before her due date she went into labour. Michel Odent came at 10pm and we all went to rest. At 2.00am Marisa woke me up. She was fine. She wanted to be by herself, but thought Michel had better know she was still having contractions. Michel, after listening to the baby, asked if he could do an internal. Marisa had no problems with that. I wondered why, but I didn't ask questions. No words, but Michel looked different, a bit tense. Marisa decided to go back to her room, where her boyfriend was asleep. At 5.00am I saw Michel was nervous. I questioned him and his reply was: "Footling breech. I can't wait any longer." I had no time to think, he was pushing us into a taxi. Marisa said she was having contractions every 20 minutes. She looked lovely. What to do? Michel could not take it any more.

You probably know, Sylvie, that for footling breech the policy is elective caesarean. For a breech birth Michel will only accept a home birth if it is quick, between four and five hours. They can be very quick. Some of these babies are born on the way to hospital. The worst thing to do is touch them when you see the lower part of the body appearing—any stimulation can get them 'stuck', so there are many deaths or brain damaged babies. I suppose you know all this. But quick undisturbed, undiagnosed breech births can go very well.

So I talked to Marisa and she said, "That's fine. Let's go". Baby Ryo was born two hours later by caesarean. To me it was a shock. First time in my family.

Marisa, with her 18 years, took it quite well. She is fine, the baby is adorable, and she had plenty of milk from Day 1. They all sleep together. Even in hospital after a C-section, they were happy for mum and baby to be together all the time.

We will never know what could have happened if we had stayed at home. One of the risks is cord prolapse. With their feet they kick so much that if the membranes rupture, cord prolapse can follow, although not necessarily, of course.

Sometimes, it is a problem to know all this.

Liliana Lammers

For more on breech birth, see Birthframes 17, 18, 19 and 52.)

Infertility

Of course, some people find themselves in an even more difficult situation. It's important to consider this, I think, if only to be able to relate compassionately toward other women who have a completely different experience. Whatever our ethical or moral standpoint, we need to remember that a great deal of pain is usually involved in other people's life choices...

I'm not sure where to start really... **Birthframe 7**

The next contributor, an old playmate of mine, made a special effort to write something which might be helpful to women in a similar situation. If you are one of the majority of women who can conceive easily I hope that reading this might help you to have more empathy for women who cannot have children.

I'm not sure where to start really. I have spent the last few years trying hard NOT to think or talk about my endometriosis and subsequent infertility. I'm not quite sure whether I am really the right person to ask/talk to about this, but I will have a go. If you're thinking, "It may help to talk/think about it," I don't agree. I've had counselling, treatment and more counselling and I still find that it's best not to talk or think about it for me.

I was diagnosed when I was about 26. I started my periods when I was 12 and, although I can't say I actually enjoyed them, I just got on with them, like all women do. By the time I was 16 I was experiencing so much pain and taking so many painkillers that Mum took me to the doctors and, to her horror (she's Roman Catholic), he put me on the Pill. Mum was very anti this and she often said that the pain was one of the 'joys of being a woman', etc, and that I had to learn to live with it. Neither of us realised that what I was experiencing was actually NOT normal, so I just tried to get on with it as best I could.

By the time I was in my early 20s, having stopped taking the Pill due to high blood pressure, I was in so much pain for about two weeks out of every four (and sometimes more) that I was again taking heaps of painkillers. I went to my doctor again—a different one as I had moved house by this time. He referred me to the Elizabeth Garrett Anderson Hospital in London; they ran loads of tests and for the first time I realised that the pain I had been experiencing was not 'normal' and there was something wrong. I then started a long haul of new types of painkillers, diary-keeping, etc, and eventually had a laparoscopy and was diagnosed.

By this time I had met and married my first husband who, looking back on it, was really not very supportive. We decided to start trying for a baby and after a year did not conceive. I had a strong feeling that my endo was causing this. More tests followed and I was then told, somewhat brutally, that I would not be able to conceive.

The rest is history. I won't go into what happened then, but my marriage started to break down. I had loads of hormonal treatment over about three years...

One drug made me grow a moustache! I eventually resigned myself (now single again) to the fact that I would not have children and was stuck with endo. I have tried various diets and loads of different drugs.

I joined a self-help group, which helped a bit. I have accepted it now and made a conscious decision that I am doing nothing more now and will have a hysterectomy, which I have been told will be necessary, when I am a bit older.

When I let myself, I feel quite angry that it took so long to be diagnosed and that I took so many painkillers over so many years. But that's life, I suppose. I wouldn't want anyone else to go through it if it could be avoided because I found it so painful. I still have endo and sometimes feel quite unwell but it rarely stops me doing what I want to do in life and I have so many wonderful things in my life (like a new and very supportive husband) that I don't complain, I just keep it to myself. I don't intend to have any more treatment, except for my hysterectomy... and that's a conscious decision. I met a number of women who let it take over their lives and I will NOT let that happen to me.

" My husband and I had been trying for a baby for just over two years, when we started IVF treatment. I had two embroyos implanted. I fell pregnant immediately. At my six-week scan they told me it was twins. I always knew it could be a possibility, so I wasn't shocked, but it took a long time to properly sink in. It still hasn't really... and they are now 4 months old!

Birthframe 8

Of course, when couples don't conceive quickly and easily, IVF is not the only way forward. (In any case some people object to it because it involves creating embryos, then selecting only 'strong' embryos and discarding the rest.) Here, one woman explains why she and her partner chose the adoption route instead of IVF and how it turned out for them.

My first daughter was born in 1979, an unplanned surprise. My relationship with her father ended when I was five months pregnant. The rest of the pregnancy was full of ups and downs and stands out as one of the most intense periods of my life. Claire entered the world at 7.00pm on October 11th . I shall never forget that first look into her eyes.

I met the person I am with now and we became a family of three. After a while we started to think how nice it would be to have another child. But after about a year we realised it was not going to be as straightforward as we had hoped.

Our first daughter was about 9 years old when we thought about adopting and we had been trying to have a baby since she was 3 years old. I had watched programmes on TV about infertility, read self-help books and we had some preliminary investigations into why I might not be able to conceive.

Then one Sunday, I discovered an article on adoption in the paper. I asked my husband what he thought about adoption and passed the article onto him. We were both interested in finding out more. I didn't like the idea of IVF as it could mean lots of hospital visits, painful examinations and possibly a lot of trauma and disappointment. Neither of us minded if we were making a child between us—blood wasn't thicker than water to us. To us, a child was an individual who would grow up to lead their own life whether they came from us or somebody else, There was no way of knowing what your own child would be like anyway. They may look like you or inherit physical things such as health issues but their personality would be their own. Our influence would be to provide opportunities, experiences and happy memories. We wanted to be parents again above all else. My husband had not been the birth father of my daughter but he didn't think he would feel any different if he had been—he was being her parent anyway. He could live with the fact that he would never see me being pregnant or giving birth and I could certainly live with the fact that I would never be pregnant again.

The process was long and our daughter at 10 was not particularly interested in having a sister or brother—she couldn't see why she wasn't enough for us. This was the hard part; if I had been pregnant she would have had to come to terms with it in another way. As it was, she had to be questioned by social workers about her thoughts and feelings and she didn't like it. We desperately wanted her to agree with us so that we could go ahead and have a bigger family. However, it was years before our second daughter was placed with us. Our first daughter was 13 and had been persuaded round to the idea of adoption, although perhaps only to please us at first.

We had to go through a three-month trial period to see if the adoption would work. Thank God it did. Our second daughter was 20 months when she moved in but nearly $3\frac{1}{2}$ by the time she was finally adopted. This was because the birth mother was contesting, which meant we had to go through a court hearing, which took time. She had been unable to respond to the help and support offered to her by the Social Services until finally her daughter had been placed for adoption. She contested at this stage as she wanted to be given another chance to keep her daughter, but the child's life comes first. Social Services make every effort to keep birth families together, but there comes a point when the child's life is at too much risk and they need to move forward before it is too late. Social Services then start searching through their information to find the most suitable family for a child. In this case we were seen to be the most suitable match. We agreed on letter box contact with the birth mother, which means that once a year a letter is exchanged between us and the birth mother via the Social Services. We are saving these so that in the future our second daughter will have some information about her roots and if she does want to contact her birth family she will have something to get her started. She will always be able to ask us questions about being adopted rather than going through a great shock as some children had to in the past.

Our influence will be to provide opportunities for the child

We agreed to go ahead with the adoption before meeting our second daughter for the first time in her foster home. The adoption process began as the foster mom said, "Come and meet your new mummy and daddy." Our second daughter moved in with us, but for a long time we were visited regularly by the Social Services and our new daughter was also visiting her birth mother at a family centre once a month. It was approximately two years later before everything was decided at a court hearing and we became the adoptive parents of our second daughter. Everything worked out well in the end and we really enjoyed having two daughters. The only problem was that it was a bit like having two only children as they were so far apart in age. Their needs and interests were totally separate. We started to think how nice it would be to have another child so that our second daughter had someone to play with. So we started the process again.

It all moved a lot faster for the second adoption and now we have three daughters. As older parents, we decided to request a 4-year-old child. Our second daughter needed to be at least two years older than a new child according to the Social Services. We thought it would be best to avoid the baby stage as this would mean starting right from the beginning again, giving up work for a while and so on, so we were very surprised when we had been matched up with a 14-month-old baby. It was approximately a year and a half after we had been approved so we had carried on with our lives hardly expecting anything at all to happen at this stage let alone being matched up with such a young child. It was almost like being pregnant unexpectedly when you are older. We had to decide quickly over a school half-term, so we discussed it and thought about it non-stop. Our second daughter was very keen to go ahead. Our eldest daughter, who was living away from home at this stage was also very interested. The extended family were encouraging us to consider a third child as they had seen how well the previous adoption had worked out. So we went ahead and were introduced to our third daughter. Within a few weeks she was living with us. The process went quickly and smoothly, partly due to a great foster mum who handled the transition from her home to ours very sensitively. There was a brief court hearing then all three daughters and the extended family got together, bought presents and celebrated 'Adoption Day'.

If you're thinking about adopting, it's important to remember that it can be a long and intensive process. This is necessary in order to find the right family for the child but it also helps potential adopters to analyse themselves and their relationships in a way they may not if they have a child naturally. By the end of this preliminary process I felt I had a good idea about what it would mean to take on someone else's child and be their parent for always. I also realised that every child is an individual whether they come from me or not. Nobody really knows what a child will be like, but as a parent I felt I could be there to support, help, enjoy and share my life with a child as he or she would grow up. Parenthood is one of the most important and special relationships in life and, speaking as a parent of both natural and adopted children, I think it is definitely possible to love all children in a household equally as one family.

Another possibility is surrogacy... **Birthframe 9**

Another modern possibility is surrogacy. Actually, this is not so modern in a way, given the interesting solutions to marital and fertility problems that can be found in the Bible. The following woman decided to be a surrogate mother so as to 'give something back'. Here, she explains a bit more what it was all like.

I've been in two minds about whether to write this—I'm far from being the only person involved, you know? But I've just read an article written by a woman who was on the cusp of changing her mind and taking the baby back from the couple whose baby she'd had, so that makes me want to write about the other side—I didn't change my mind and, while I have regrets in life, that's not one of them.

My reasons for doing it were fairly complicated. I had one child, and was grateful that she was bright and healthy, even though I lost full-time custody of her when my marriage broke up. My ex-husband's unwillingness to contemplate surrogacy was also now a factor in its favour. I was in a relationship I considered to be short-term, although he later revised his plans to travel the world, and stayed home with me, which I'm very glad about. If I remember right, I was being unreasonably independent—"I'm doing this, it's really nothing to do with you. If you want to dump me, go ahead," sort of thing—which makes it to his great credit that he was actually hugely supportive. I had a superstition that you pay for luck either by doing good, or by balancing bad luck. I was broody, I was emotionally insecure... I wouldn't say it was a fully thought-through, rational decision on the part of a woman who had her life sorted out, but I've always been glad I did it.

I'd already done egg donation because that had been pointed out to me as an easier and more likely option than surrogacy, if I was really serious about helping someone else have a baby. If I had my life to live over and had to choose one or the other, I'd definitely choose surrogacy over egg donation, although it's possible that my reactions are very unusual. After all, I don't drink alcohol or smoke, I avoid painkillers and I'm something of a control freak. I also have a tendency to react badly to chemicals of many kinds. I am the type of person who would rather sit next to one of the great unwashed than next to a woman who's just gone overboard with Chanel.

My strongest memory of egg donation was of waking up alone on a trolley, not remembering who I was, or where I was. I sat up and noticed that, while I had a top on and there was a towel over my body and legs, I wasn't actually wearing anything from the waist down. My next discovery was that there were reddish stains on my inner thighs and that my lower abdomen was achy. Egg donation was not one of the many possibilities that occurred to me!

A nurse came in and told me that my friend was here to take me home. "Good!" I thought, "I have a friend. That's something." The friend in question was kind-looking and seemed a complete stranger. I got into his car and nodded every time he asked me something.

About 20 minutes into the journey I remembered who I was and where I worked, although his name was still not available to me. I remember asking to be dropped off at work, rather than at home, because it was still early afternoon. And I remember being quite put out when he said he'd take me home, and if I wanted I could get a bus back to work. Work I could face, but a bus seemed out of the question.

With egg donation they do a two-part process because it's only really worthwhile if they can harvest several eggs at once. First, they 'zero' your own hormones, by inducing a mini-menopause. When I did it, this required use of an inhaler two times a day for two weeks. Then you inject different hormones to make your ovaries work overtime. As I remember, there were three injections and, because of the timing, they had to be either self-administered, or administered by someone who lived with you. Because I was in my 'I will survive' phase, I chose self-administered. As a needle-phobe, that was a big challenge. Each injection was an 'Everest' moment for someone who's spent a lifetime being hopeless at blood transfusion sessions. Two of the injections were at reasonably civilised hours, but the third had to be 12 hours before the 'harvest'. I remember after my first injection, telling my daughter (who was with me most weekends) that if I sang while I was doing it, and did it fairly slowly, it hardly hurt at all. She suggested doing it even slower, so it didn't hurt at all—which worked. Not bad for an 8-year-old.

On the plus side, I found out that I was actually capable of giving myself the intramuscular injections. On the minus side, the clinic I visited had a policy of not telling women if any of their carefully harvested eggs ever turned into a baby, so I still feel like I'm waiting to find out what happened. Not ideal for a closure junkie.

The surrogacy was for a couple who were already fostering a little boy, so Social Services were involved from the outset. For a very brief period I had a skewed vision of what life must be like for Madonna—the entourage, you know? This is my social worker. This is the other couple's social worker. This is the little boy's social worker, and this is the social worker of the fetus. Shall we begin? I have nothing but praise for all of the social workers involved, who were very honest and forthright about all of the risks we faced and about the options open to us. I was fairly sure from the outset that I wasn't going to change my mind. What I hadn't realised was that I would be giving the baby into the care of Social Services, who, technically, could decide that another couple altogether should adopt the baby. I could take the baby back at any point during (if I remember right) her first six months of life, but I couldn't make any other solid decision.

At the same time, the couple who wanted the baby were applying to adopt the little boy that they were fostering, who'd been with them for most of his life. The parents originally planned to have him back after six to eight weeks—and until he was $2\frac{1}{2}$ the plan was still to just keep him for a few months more—oops, not ready yet, a few months more again. After a few years of this, they did decide the best thing was to give him up altogether, and he was freed for adoption.

They decided the best thing was adoption…

It was pointed out to me by one social worker that, since there are dozens of couples who'd like to adopt a healthy toddler, and not that many who want to foster, it might be that 'their' little boy would still end up being offered for adoption to someone else. Since both cases were heard together, when the child I gave birth to was just under a year old, for some time they were looking after two children who could both be taken from them. This is not for the faint-hearted!

I took only a month off work. I stopped work on my official due date because that was the last day possible, believing from experience of my first birth, that my real due date was still almost two weeks away. It made my boss nervous, but it worked out as I expected.

The birth was the easiest I've ever had—I'd had one baby before and have had two since, two early miscarriages, one at five months, and in retrospect, I think I was handled as a special case with the surrogacy... 'Handle with care. Likely to explode without warning'. I do honestly believe that every expectant mother should be treated as a VIP—but it only felt that way on that one occasion. I shook doorways until I was pretty much fully dilated. Once I was taken downstairs, I had a midwife who was with me until the baby was born. Since we hadn't met before, she conducted the whole thing from the far side of the room, while my husband did the hands-on things. She positively encouraged me to adopt whatever position I was comfortable in, which hasn't always been my experience.

However... the baby had an infection, which meant she was kept in the hospital until it was cleared up. I have vivid memories of this beautiful, relatively huge 9lb baby in Intensive Care, surrounded by tiny dolls of premature babies. Like Gulliver in Lilliput. I stayed with her for 10 days, not wanting to leave without seeing her on her way. I breastfed her, which probably caused problems when she had to change diet very abruptly. At the time, though, it felt like the best thing to do for her. I wanted to be wholeheartedly with her, and then wholeheartedly gone.

It helped that Social Services encouraged me to write letters, both before and after giving birth, and to think about what legacy I would like her to have—books, pictures and so on. The other couple were really positive about me being a third parent with, I suppose, a cultural contribution to make as well as the biological contribution, and that made the whole thing feel better. It was more like telescoping parenthood into a relatively short space of time (the pregnancy plus 10 days), rather than losing it altogether.

Afterwards, I went to stay with my partner's mum (now my mum-in-law), who was great. I spent a few days just crying my eyes out non-stop, hiccupping, "It's just hormones" whenever someone asked how I was.

Since then, I've had letters and photos once a year via Social Services letter box contact, and we send letters back by the same route. That's like an extra Christmas in September—and a really useful chance to stop and take stock of the previous year.

> I spent a few days just crying my eyes out non-stop

I wouldn't do it again, mainly because of the demands it makes on everyone else. My daughter at the time was 8—I think she grew up a whole chunk as a result of me having a baby for someone else. Just fending off questions like, "Are you looking forward to having a little brother or sister?" from perfectly well-meaning strangers, is a hard one to deal with, and on the whole, she coped very well. I remember the difficult thing being finding brief answers to questions that were only meant as token well-wishing... and finding that I'd get it wrong sometimes.

I think most people will recognise me from the circumstantial evidence in this account... but can you withhold my name? People feel quite strongly about surrogacy, and while I'm quite happy to talk about it, I do consciously pick who I talk to about it. I'm not expecting to be stalked, exactly, I'd just feel very silly if I had to spend weeks fending off people who think I did something insanely stupid, or something I should do again, only for *them* this time.

The healthy normality of birth

Thankfully, most of us do not have problems conceiving. We also manage to carry our babies through pregnancy and give birth without drama.

Most of us have no problems... **Birthframe 10**

To remind us of the optimal, healthy processes as they usually take place, here's an account by a first-time mother from London, Jenny Sanderson. This account provides some clues as to how the physiological processes can be facilitated effectively. (There'll be more on this later.) Incidentally, Jenny started out planning a hospital birth and she only started considering a home birth when she learned about typical hospital procedures. She says that while some people felt she was making a brave choice, she herself felt it was her best option, after all the research she'd done. Labouring undisturbed with Michel in attendance, Jenny experienced a typical optimal birth.

My first labour:
On the morning of my EDD [expected date of delivery] I didn't feel too good, not very well—but not bad enough to cancel friends who were coming to lunch—an arrangement deliberately made for this date, on the assumption that the first baby would be 'late'. I ate a normal breakfast.

Our friends arrived about 11.00am. Soon after, I began to feel that I didn't want to sit still and went round the garden and up and down the house. We called Michel; I spoke to him but he wasn't anxious, especially when he heard about the breakfast. By lunchtime, I didn't want to be sociable or to eat anything and went upstairs.

Tim phoned Michel again and everyone had lunch, leaving by early afternoon just as Michel arrived. He saw that I was not in 'hard labour', felt the baby's heartbeat and pronounced everything to be normal.

During the afternoon and early evening I spent some of my time walking round the bedroom but mostly in the bath or on the toilet. Later on I found leaning against the towel rail useful but I didn't want to use Tim for support and the one time I tried lying down on some cushions felt stranded and found the contractions harder to manage. I spent a good deal of time on the toilet, though I'm sure my bowels were long since empty.

During this time Michel listened to the baby's heartbeat several times with his Doppler machine and confirmed that the mucous plug had been ejected into the bath. He spent most of the time upstairs in the spare room with a book and occasionally talking to Tim.

Shortly after 8.00pm Michel could hear that my breathing had turned to grunting and suggested that I move out of the bathroom into the bedroom. Tim supported me for two or three contractions before Rebecca was born at 8.25pm, by candlelight. Michel laid her on a towel and used his mucous extractor.

[This was simply the funnel of a hand-held stethoscope. The procedure is explained in detail on p107 of *Birth Reborn* (Souvenir Press 1984).] Then Rebecca and I lay down on some cushions. She didn't want to breastfeed but didn't cry much either. Michel lay on our bed for half an hour or so; Tim made drinks. At about 9.00pm I delivered the placenta into a hastily found casserole dish; we did not eat it! Michel weighed Rebecca (8lb) and did the necessary paperwork before leaving us to a leisurely meal.

The next morning he returned and we phoned the hospital, my doctor and the midwives. Both Michel and a midwife visited for most of the following 10 days.

The one time I tried lying down I felt stranded

By the way, in case you're wondering, Michel was mainly using a medical approach here called 'watchful waiting' while Jenny was in labour. In other words, he was monitoring her not by using any electronic equipment, but by observing how she was moving, what sounds she was making and how she was behaving generally. Having observed other women in labour, Michel was able to identify that Jenny's labour was following a normal, healthy pattern.

His initial examination of her bump had reassured him that the fetal heart was beating as it should be (i.e. that there was no fetal distress) and that there was an appropriate amount of amniotic fluid—not too much and not too little. He will also have noted, at that point, the position the fetus was lying in.

Michel's interventions during the birth and afterwards are not routine but he obviously felt they were necessary in this particular case. His actions were minimal but wise under the circumstances.

He could hear my breathing had turned to grunting

My second labour:
About three days after my second baby was due I went out in the afternoon with Rebecca (my first daughter), experiencing occasional indigestion-like twinges. By the time Tim came home I thought I was probably in labour but didn't mention it until about 6.30 or 7.00pm. We put Bec to bed and I phoned Michel at around 8.30pm; this time he said he'd come straight away. Tim and I then had dinner, though I ate only moderately. After Michel arrived we had a cup of tea. Tim and I went for a short walk and when I returned I went at once to the bath, where I stayed for most of the rest of the labour.

From about 10.15pm contractions were getting very strong. At approx. 10.40pm I thought I needed to go to the loo, but after straining for a bit, I reached down and felt the head. Rosamund was born all in one go with the next contraction, at 10.45pm; Michel caught her as she came out and laid her on a towel.

I lay in the bathroom with the baby for half an hour or so and then squatted to deliver the placenta with no assistance. Michel checked me, weighed Ros (7½lb) and did his paperwork before leaving us together.

This labour was certainly the shortest; I was out visiting friends at about 5.00pm when I felt the first early contractions and Ros was born just over five hours later. There obviously was a second stage but it was very short and I didn't need to do any strenuous pushing as I did for the other three. But it was quite a shock for the baby to be born so quickly.

My third and fourth labours:
For me there were overwhelming advantages in having home births and I went on to have two more (which, unfortunately, Michel was unable to attend) with an excellent midwife. [Of course, these were two more optimal births.]

Jenny Sanderson

Having had Michel in attendance for her first two labours, Jenny felt confident to have two more births afterwards with another (female) midwife. Both she and Michel were creating the perfect conditions for optimal births by not disturbing the normal processes and at the same time, by facilitating them with their reassuring presence and silent monitoring. (We'll come back to this idea of having an undisturbed birth in Step 3.) Just like sex, birth is a process which can be easily affected by environmental factors, which include speech from anyone in the same room, or nearby. It's an intensely private process, which is why it's so important that it does remain undisturbed and protected from the outside world. And if you're reeling from shock because these births all took place in someone's home, please suspend your disbelief and read on...

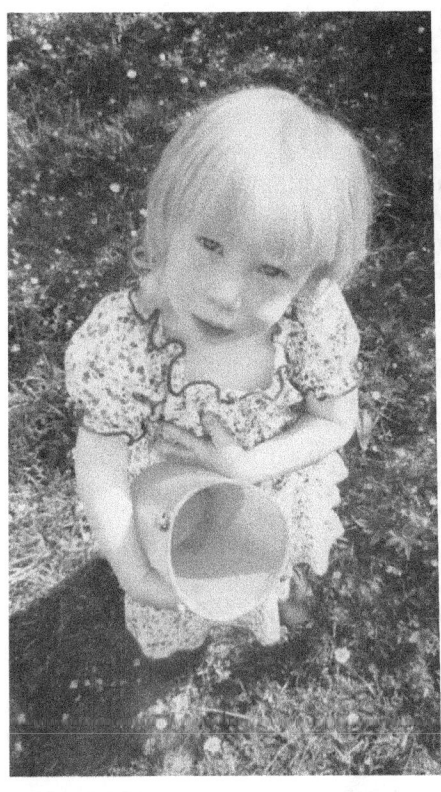
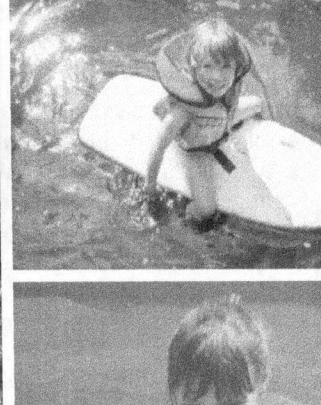
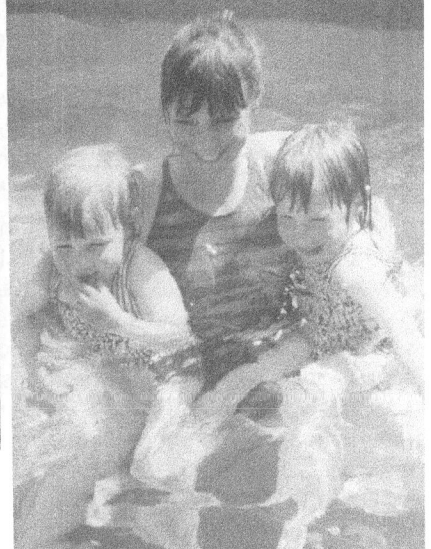

*A few photos of the Sandersons:
a family of optimally-birthed children*

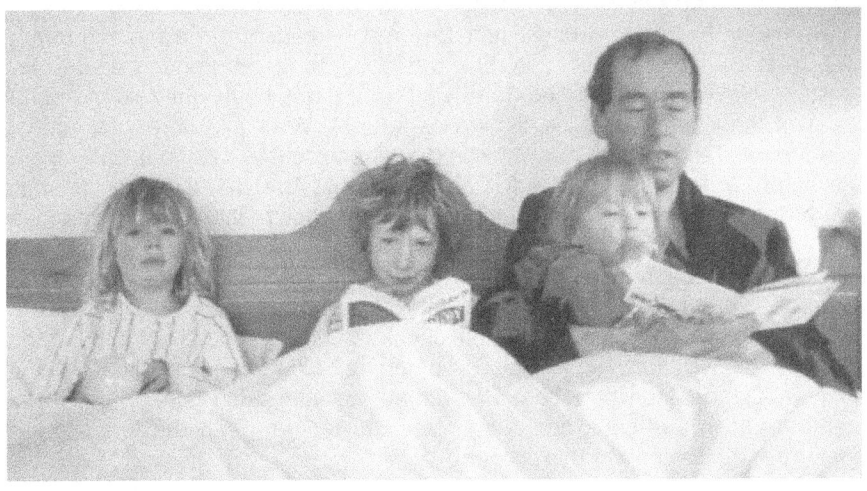

A surprising secret

Do you find yourself doubting that Jenny's experience really is the norm for a person who is generally healthy ?

If, like most people, you read magazines, watch TV and read newspapers, you might be forgiven for thinking that optimal births almost never happen. Media coverage is inevitably unbalanced, though, because editors are looking for unusual things to report. I was reminded of this when I contacted a Features Editor of a well-known women's magazine, when I was researching this book. At the time I was looking for a vaginal breech birth story. She initially seemed enthusiastic to pass material on to me, but completely changed her tone when I said I was also interested in any births which had involved life-saving intervention. "Ah no," she said. "You wouldn't be able to have any of that. That's precisely the kind of story *we're* interested in." It was clear that the magazine's aim was not to portray reality, to present a balanced picture of what childbirth is for most women, or to help women consider what it might be. It was to catch people's interest through the sensational.

Perhaps as a result of our constant media exposure, perhaps because of our fear of failure and desire to control everything in our lives, the present-day climate in hospitals is one of worry, habitual intervention and insensitivity to a labouring woman's needs. So it's not surprising that many women don't experience optimal births. Of those who do, most feel no need to talk, precisely because they haven't been traumatised in any way. When I chanced upon somebody who'd had optimal births, it was usually rather difficult to get an account. The women concerned were quite open about their experiences, but they didn't make a 'big deal' of them. Sometimes my 'potential contributors' did realise there was something special about their experience, but they clearly felt no driving need to talk about it. As a result I had to do quite a bit of hassling to get hold of many of the optimal birth stories in this book.

Here's an example... I met Fiona Taylor, a herbalist from a farming family, on a train on my way to London. She was going to a conference that day. We chatted and when I mentioned that I was writing this book, she told me about her own three optimal births. It didn't take long. After all, there was nothing much to tell. I then asked her why she thought her births had gone so well and she said, "Well I wasn't expecting any problems. After all, I've seen animals give birth loads of times. They don't usually have any problems, so why should we?" When I then asked her if she would write down what she'd said to me, she said: "Oh, there's really nothing much to write down. Don't worry, you'll remember what I told you." "Aaargh!" I thought. "But I want authentic contributions which have been double-checked and approved by the authors in writing!" This well-dressed, articulate woman just didn't see her births as being a big enough deal to write about. She did at least say she was happy for me to mention her in this book and I later tracked her down via the Internet and persuaded her to confirm this account.

Eventually, I also obtained some other accounts to show that it is not only primitive women who know how to give birth. Modern women are very good at it too!

Birthframe 11

Here are some comments from Nina Klose, a Harvard graduate, who works in the financial industry.

> I consider myself a modern woman. To the casual observer, I might appear to be an office drone. I've been working in a big investment bank for eight years now. A happy cog in a vast organisation. I hold various academic and professional degrees that ostensibly aid me in performing my duties. When it came to giving birth, though, none of them helped in the least. Degrees of all sorts are irrelevant for giving birth. In fact, what you do for a living doesn't have much bearing on how you give birth. Sure we've trained ourselves to sit in offices for hours on end, talk on the phone instead of face-to-face, etc, but we're all human animals. When the time comes to give birth, we know what to do. It's instinct.
>
> That makes it sound like birth was easy for me. In a way, it was. I didn't need to do anything specific to be able to give birth. I just did it. But it was essential to be in a calm, familiar place and to be attended by someone I knew well. On some level, certainly, I was anxious about whether I'd be able to pull it off. But deep down, I think I had great faith in my body. The body is wise. It could grow a fetus without my even thinking about it. What more complicated task could there be? I have to admit to having grave doubts when it came time to push. But pushing was so powerful a reflex, there was nothing I could do to stop it once it got going. Giving birth was the most powerful, elemental—and stupendous—event I have ever participated in.

Learning from experience

Do you still have doubts about your own personal ability to give birth? Is it because it went wrong last time?[30]

Many women go on to have an optimal birth after a bad first experience. Women of the !Kung San tribe in Botswana have an interesting viewpoint. Their ideal is to manage to give birth alone by their third child. Before that they are only 'practising'.

There are plenty of women in the developed world who do the same—they improve their birth stories each time they give birth, simply by learning from their experience. So, even if it didn't work out last time, it's perfectly possible for things to be wonderful this time round.

On the next page, a few women comment on this phenomenon of 'learning how to give birth'....

> After having forceps and a postpartum haemorrhage the first time round, my second birth was totally straightforward with no time for the TENS, birthing pool or gas and air, which I had planned. I stood up for delivery, supported by my partner and pushed the baby out myself, the midwife 'catching' her well. I had no injection [of syntometrine] to speed up the placenta and control the blood loss as it was just not necessary and this third stage was completed in about 20 minutes.

> For my first child I'd planned a water birth but ended up with a four-and-a-half hour labour that was very traumatic. I was rushed into hospital and into a very clinical environment, with bright lights and at least six people standing around me. Jamie was a forceps baby and I ended up having to be stitched. It was almost enough to put me off having any more children. So when I got pregnant again I knew I wanted things to be quite different and I was prepared more. After Arion's birth I felt so empowered that it had gone right the second time.

> This time round I was in control the whole time and I knew what was going on, I was more prepared mentally and physically.

So you don't need to expect any high drama for your own personal case. Why would Mother Nature intend birth to be high drama? It just wouldn't make sense for the great majority of births—obstetric difficulties simply aren't practical or efficient from the point of view of procreation.

It's understandable if you're still terrified of what childbirth might mean for you personally. This is a very common feeling and I certainly had it too. The idea of a whole baby emerging through such a small and private place is shocking or at least worrying to most women. But a woman's vagina really can increase in size in just the same way as a man's penis enlarges in response to psychological and hormonal stimuli. And it shrinks back afterwards—just like a man's penis! Our female bodies are designed for childbirth and letting them function without drugs, intervention or disturbance makes us feel strong, fulfilled and motherly. Unlikely as it may seem, the seemingly impossible vaginal feat of expanding to allow for the birth of a baby is not only possible, it is often both exhilarating and fulfilling, just like any other sexual act.

Even if you're the kind of person who is a little (or a lot) self-conscious about natural processes, don't worry—you can still have an optimal birth. If you find it difficult to relax when you make love, if you get constipated or feel self-conscious about even *asking* to use the bathroom at a friend's house, rest assured your hormones will come to your rescue when you have a baby. As long as you make sure you're not disturbed during labour, your hormones will do all the work—they'll trigger the necessary physical changes, put you in a helpful frame of mind and bring your intuitive knowledge to the surface. Really! We'll talk about the practical ramifications of this in other chapters.

Birthframe 12

In case you're still in doubt about your own abilities, I'll leave you with another birth story. This is the story of a woman full of ideals, who became disillusioned after a bad first initial experience of birth when all kinds of intervention had seemed inappropriate. Would she be able to rediscover her innate, instinctual ability to give birth if left to her own devices?

I was very frightened about my ability to give birth properly, and questioned all my ideas about home and water birth. I called the Active Birth Centre in London and explained my experiences at the hospital when I had my first baby, Fiohann. I asked if there was anyone I could talk it through with. They gave me a few names, and then suggested Michel Odent. I couldn't believe that I actually had my revered Michel Odent's phone number.

Before I could think about it, I forced myself to phone him. I explained to him what had happened, and although, understandably, he wasn't prepared to comment on the hospital treatment, he did explain that not many midwives had experience of water births, and could panic, thinking the baby would drown. I told him it was a dream of mine that he would deliver our baby, and after hearing when the conception date was, he found that it did fit in with his schedule of international conferences, and that yes he would. I had to pinch myself!

He came around to meet us and I cannot describe what a gentle, intuitive and passionate man he is. He filled me with a quiet confidence and reassurance, and was so different to our doctor, who had originally told me that if I wanted a home birth I would have to find another doctor. Another difference was that he had absolutely no problem with calculating the due date from the conception date: it was a simple nine months later. The community midwife could not cope with anything more than the date of my last period, which I did not know exactly, since I never paid any attention to my cycle. Her date was two weeks before Michel's estimate. The pregnancy went well in that I was fit and healthy, but my partner and I started to have problems and when I was six months pregnant he left home for a month. I felt desperately insecure and cried through most of my pregnancy. Another pregnancy filled with grief, but so different to the first. We went on holiday and decided to try again.

I hired the birthing pool two days before the earliest due date and waited. The midwife got increasingly agitated and by 21 July was telling me that I would be causing the fetus brain damage because my placenta was past its sell-by date. Michel calmed her by telling her it was due on the 26th, which she could not comprehend. Sure enough, on the 25th, which happily was a Saturday, I went into labour. I called Michel and he promised to be over in a couple of hours.

We filled the pool, put the low music on and had candles ready, and I tried to relax, but found it difficult because of my doubts in myself. Michel arrived and asked me how I was, felt my tummy, and said he would go to sleep in the next room, because I had a few hours to go yet.

My partner went to sleep in our bed, and I spent most of the night sitting on the loo having contractions; it felt the most comfortable place to be, looking at the stars through the bathroom roof window, and going back to bed trying to doze before the next one.

Early next morning, things started hotting up and I decided to get into the birthing pool to ease the pains. It did ease them immediately, and as soon as he heard the change in my noises, Michel got up and came in. He can tell where a woman is in her labour by the noises she makes, and just that small change had indicated to him a change in me. I told him I didn't know what to do, asked him what I should be doing, so different from my first birth, and he told me just to listen to my body, just as I had done in the first. I yelled that I didn't know what it was saying, and was very fearful. How different to the first time, with my confidence now in tatters. He calmly created an environment where I would have to listen to myself, by leaving me alone and getting my partner to go and have some breakfast. Our Brazilian au pair was beside herself that I could be moaning and wailing alone with no doctor, and took it into her own hands to go and tell Michel in no uncertain terms to go in to me and induce me! In Brazil, apparently, over 40% of women have caesarean sections because it keeps their passages honeymoon fresh! He handled her sweetly and reassured her.

Things really got going at about 8.30am. I was gnawing on the side of the birthing pool, thinking about the benefits of knives and drugs, half hoping that she wouldn't come out at all, would go back and stay safe inside me.

But that doesn't happen, and finally I got that huge push urge, when all you can do is that colossal push and your whole body is intent on turning itself inside out.

It did know after all what to do, I just had to get my doubts out of the way. Her head came out in the water, just like Fiohann—my son. Michel reached down and checked the umbilical cord was not in the way, and then said that because she was so big, we needed gravity to help us. With her head still between my legs, he lifted my legs, and my partner lifted my torso out of the pool, and I hung from his arms, with Michel ready to catch her.

I held her close... soon she was nuzzling at my breast

Two more big pushes and out she slid, our beautiful girl. I flopped to the floor and Michel gave her to me immediately. I held her close and within a few minutes she was nuzzling at my breast ready to suckle, still attached to the umbilical cord.

Michel was delighted at the perfection of it, but said that before she settled into it he would tie off her cord with string rather than the metal clamps because it was more comfortable for the baby. I lay on our bed with our wonderful baby and as she suckled I realised that it would have been no different for Fiohann. If only.

Michel left me to deliver Eowyn's placenta naturally, which came easily shortly afterwards. What I hadn't expected was the sharper pains as my uterus contracted back again, but apparently this is a normal feature of a second childbirth.

10... UNDERSTAND 'OPTIMAL'

The following day I felt so happy. I'd just had a baby!

Michel wrote to our doctor to inform him of the birth and our baby's 'top' scores, knowing that we would be left undisturbed until Monday. Once again, I had no tears and was perfectly fit. The day following Eowyn's birth we had a celebration barbecue, and I walked around Tesco shopping for it, feeling so proud and happy, as if everyone must be able to tell that I had just had a baby! Michel came with his son, and was thrilled to see us so clearly well and happy. It was perfect.

Our doctor and his doctor wife arrived Monday morning, demanding to know how long she sucked on each breast and making appointments for paediatricians to see her. I had no idea how long on each breast and I declined the paediatrician offer, which they seemed a bit put out about.

Finally they left, leaving the midwives and health visitors to do their checks, etc. and eventually we were left in peace again.

Eowyn is now a very fit and healthy 4-year-old.

Maria Shanahan

[For more on 'learning from experience' also see Birthframes 41, 46 and 47.]

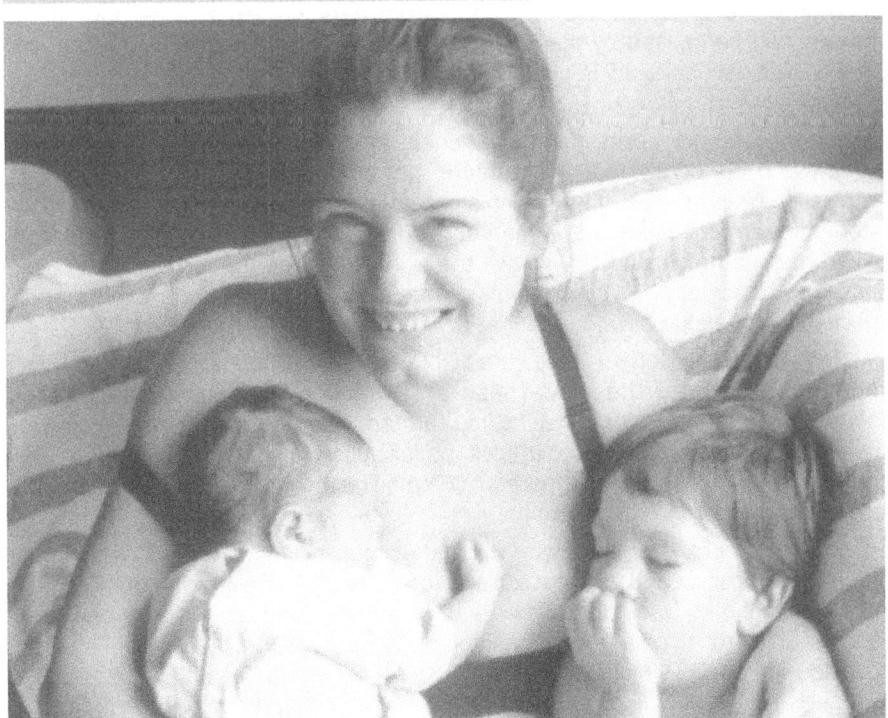

Maria with Eowyn and Fiohann

9... CONSIDER YOUR ASSUMPTIONS

By this stage, you may be thinking, "Yes, that's all very well, but what if..." Optimal birth is possible in many more situations than you might expect. That's why I'm asking you to consider your assumptions.

Sometimes, because we're doubtful we limit what we're able to do. Often antenatal care doesn't help us in this respect because assessments may leave us labelled 'high risk'. The problem is that the label we're given is likely to affect the type of care we're offered or put under pressure to agree to.

The ubiquitous 'high risk' patient

In practice many women are considered 'high risk' at some stage of their pregnancy. The end result is that most women spend a lot of time worrying about 'things which can go wrong'. As Michel has pointed out, this is far from ideal because a pregnant woman should ideally feel relaxed and confident in her own body so that she goes into labour with the right attitude. (Of course, her emotions may well have an effect on her growing baby throughout the months of her pregnancy too.) I know from personal experience how much anxiety can be caused by these labels because my age automatically put me in the 'high risk' category in all my own pregnancies.[1]

Focusing on ways of facilitating best outcomes actually seems to be more important than risk assessment. In Michel's opinion, the same principles apply to low and high risk labouring women: the amount of disturbance a woman experiences and the extent to which she feels safe are most important. In other words, leaving the labouring woman undisturbed might be more important than close monitoring because it will give the woman and her unborn baby the best possible conditions for successfully orchestrating the cocktail of hormones necessary for a safe birth.[2]

I'm asking a lot of you here, aren't I? Let's read about a few women who put these ideas to the test. These are women who dared to believe in something more. My aim in asking you to read their accounts is to help you to begin to reassess the concept of 'risk' as it applies to childbirth in general and to your personal situation in particular. What might really be possible for you and your own baby?... or babies!

In the rest of this chapter, you will find accounts and comments about twin, triplet and breech births and we'll also consider the caesarean solution. You know, sometimes twins or triplets are undiagnosed until after they're born and some babies turn into a breech position at the last minute, so maybe it's worth considering all possibilities. Should all these categories of risk be automatic caesareans? Or should mothers be 'allowed' to try for an optimal birth? Please read with a very open mind... You may well be surprised!

MULTIPLE SCLEROSIS (MS)

As we can see from Michel's account of his own son's birth, sometimes medical conditions bring their own advantages...

Birthframe 13

Women with multiple sclerosis (MS) usually give birth easily, although they are more often than not classified as high risk, which is a handicap. I might offer many anecdotes.

One of the most demonstrative and typical examples I can relate is the birth of my own son, Pascal, in London in 1985. His mother, Judy, was 38 and a half, she had never given birth previously and had been diagnosed as having MS at the age of 26. During her antenatal visits at the local hospital she was classified as high risk. However she wanted to give birth at home.

A week before the official due date, she suddenly woke up after an afternoon nap, at 5.30pm.

She immediately had strong contractions suggestive of real labour. At that time I was not registered as a doctor in the UK. In order to be legal we called a pair of independent midwives. They thought they had plenty of time for the first delivery of a career woman. They eventually arrived at 8.30pm, at the same time as baby Pascal, who was born on the floor, by the toilet.

Of course, there are other factors that can explain such an easy and fast birth. Judy's mother and sister had uncomplicated births. During labour Judy had complete privacy. She was on her hands and knees, screaming on her bed, while I was the only other person in the house, constantly busy in another room. I did one internal exam and I listened to the heartbeats once.[3] Although the labour had been intense and noisy, even violent, Judy claimed afterwards that it had never been painful. We might add that Judy probably had one of the best possible childbirth preparations: she had had two opportunities to attend straightforward births in the home-like birthing room of our hospital in France.

Because Judy was involved in MS associations and self-help groups, I met and interviewed many mothers with MS and I attended the home delivery of several of them. This is how I drew the conclusion that, in general, women with MS give birth easily. There are several plausible interpretations. One of them is that such a disease is associated with deviations of the system of prostaglandins (a variety of cell regulators involved in birth physiology) that might facilitate the birth process.

The labour had been intense and noisy, even violent, but Judy claimed afterwards it'd never been painful

After the birth Judy published a book called *Multiple Sclerosis and Having a Baby* (Judy Graham. Healing Arts Press. 1999). When researching her book, she could not find any study about how difficult or how easy it is for women with MS to give birth. Until now we must rely on anecdotes.

Michel Odent

TWINS

Here Steve Mellor, an American, explains how he and his wife unexpectedly came to give birth to twins at home.

Birthframe 14

Toward the end of April I was out shopping for some new shoes when my mobile phone buzzed. It was Olga (my Russian fiancée) calling with a big surprise. It seems our last visit together had been more productive than either of us thought. Yes, she was pregnant and we were going to have our first baby. So within one year I went from being single to finding my life partner and expecting my first child.

Because of the visa processing time I was not around for the first few months of the pregnancy as Olga was still in Moscow. It was hard for both of us as we did not get to celebrate like most couples, but what we did do was start the process of preparing for our child coming into the world. This is where it got a little interesting.

It was by no means anything like the Cold War of our two nations but, because of our different life experiences, our ideas about how to have a baby differed. Myself, having been born and raised in America, knew exactly how to have a baby: you get pregnant, wait nine months and then go to the hospital where the doctor can give drugs to get through the pain and then he delivers it.

Olga had a completely different plan. Having been raised in Russia and not always having faith in the medical system, she didn't want to have a hospital birth. She wanted to have a home birth, as did many of her friends, with no medication, as she understood that any drug she took, the baby would receive 10 times as strong.[4]

Now I had neighbours years earlier who had had a home birth and at the time I had thought, "How interesting", but I had never thought to myself, "Yes, that is what I want." So Olga wanted to have a home birth and I knew nothing about it. One of my good friends, who was a chiropractor and who had studied a lot about natural ways to heal the body, gave me a book on natural childbirth. So I read the book cover to cover and learnt all I could. The book had me questioning a lot of the traditional things I had heard about giving birth or had seen in films or on TV, when they were showing a woman having a baby. At the same time Olga was attending a series of classes in Moscow, where the main idea was to do everything as naturally as possible, without any interference.

I'd think something was crazy, but then do some research...

Olga's classes were great as she was not only learning how to deliver, but also talking about birth on a physical, emotional and spiritual level—something I think is missing in the typical American system. So as she would tell me about the classes I would think to myself that some of the stuff she was learning was crazy. But then I would do some more research and find out for myself that it wasn't really. I remember our first conversation about having a home birth. I was scared of the possibility of things going wrong.

And then I would find statistics stating that most C-sections were done on Fridays—wouldn't want to ruin the doctor's weekend!—and that women were actually scheduling their C-sections before they even gave a regular birth a try. It started to appear to me that the medical system seemed just as crazy.

There were many other questions that I found myself asking. Olga didn't want to have any scans and that again concerned me. Then I started to ask around to find out the purpose of doing them. No one could really give me a good reason. I heard things like: "To know the baby's sex", "To help predict the due date" or "To find out if the baby is healthy".[5]

But then I would also find out that even though they could find some things out, in most cases there was nothing that could be done. I further learnt that there have been cases of couples who, learning about some defect, chose to abort the pregnancy, only to find out afterwards that the baby was perfectly healthy. And I loved the way Olga always told people that if she were meant to know the sex of the baby or know how it was going, God would have installed a window on her belly. Also, I read in one book that 94% of women could deliver naturally without any problem. So I decided to trust the process and be responsible for creating an environment where everything would live up to the vision I had created.

Finally Olga's visa was approved and we got married in a small ceremony in Oregon. We didn't have time to arrange a big ceremony as we were given 90 days to get married from the day she arrived, and we had no idea when the 90 days would start.

One night, when we were out shopping there just happened to be a farmers' market going on. Right outside the shop we were in was a woman advertising a home birth collective, run by a group of midwives. We got a lot of information that night and ended up contacting them later in the week to interview our potential midwives. Ellen and Kenna came over the next week and we talked through what we wanted to create in having our baby and what they could do for us. It really helped me more than anything to see that they had lots of experience and training and could handle the most common problems, should any occur. So Ellen would be our primary midwife and Kenna would be her back-up. They would come by the house every other week to do checkups. Also, at that time Ellen was training Julie in midwifery, which would later prove to be a blessing.

For the next three and a half months we went through the basics of daily living. I worked, and Olga worked hard at being pregnant. And I mean this in the most positive way. Every day she took the time to walk a mile to the gym and swim for an hour in the pool. She took the time to eat really healthy food that would provide our child with a great source of natural nutrition. Olga took this time because she didn't want to take man-made, antenatal vitamins, which to her were not as good a source of nutrition as real healthy food could provide. She wanted our child to have only food that was from nature and full of life.

We took Bradley natural birth classes and this became one of my biggest learning experiences. We were in a class with five other couples who wanted to have their babies born naturally, but they were having hospital births. It was amazing for Olga and me to experience this class, where we spent half of each meeting learning how to defend ourselves from a hospital and their possible interventions when not needed or wanted. I remember in one class Olga was actually in tears hearing about all the problems with hospitals and we were not even going to one. It was an eye-opener to hear how they would tempt women to have some drugs regardless of what their wishes were. I was never more thankful for Olga's strength and determination to have our child at home in a loving environment.

We spent half the classes learning to defend ourselves

Then came the big day. We were actually about two weeks from the projected due date, sitting in a cinema, watching *Star Wars I*. The big battle at the end was just starting when Olga got this very funny look on her face. I'm sure I would look like that too if my waters had just broken and my trousers were all wet. Well, needless to say, Olga never saw the end of the film and wouldn't do so for a couple more years. We headed home, just a couple of blocks away, and called the midwives...

Olga gave birth the next day to her first baby in a birthing pool, supported by her midwives and husband. Back to Steve for the rest of the story...

It was 3.40am in the morning, 29 hours from when Olga's waters first broke and Olga gave one more push and out came our beautiful baby girl right into my hands. We slowly brought her out of the water of the birthing pool and onto Olga's chest so mother and baby could start the bonding process.

It was great to have this time. No one carried her away, cleaned her up, probed or weighed her. We all just held each other and experienced the miracle we had just been given. I remember at one point about 13 minutes into working on the placenta Olga jumped and asked Ellen if she had long fingernails. She said, "No," and we went on. Then about a minute later Ellen was checking the progress of the placenta when she uttered those now famous words to us: "This is too hard for a placenta. Oh my god, you're having another baby!" And just as those words were leaving Ellen's lips Olga gave a push and out came another baby girl. Everyone in that room was completely amazed, and moved in quickly to deal with the extra child. For nine months no one knew there were two babies. I have to say the excitement in the room was pretty wonderful. Truly, we had a small miracle on our hands.

Everyone in that room was completely amazed

After some time, Olga delivered the placenta and we eventually brought the girls out of the birthing pool. Having Julie as an apprentice was again just perfect, as we needed three people to take the girls and the placenta out of the pool, while Ellen attended to Olga. We also had to remember which child came out first.

We had happened to wrap up the first girl in a yellow blanket and the second one in a blue one, so we created the rhyme 'blue two' which to this day still holds true. Olga had originally wanted to keep the placenta attached for 24 hours. This was to allow all the blood that is pushed into the placenta during the birth process to return to the child and also because of an old Russian spiritual tradition that recognises the placenta's importance in the development of the child. Well, with having just one placenta and two babies connected to it, this was not a good option. But we managed to go a couple of hours before I cut the cords. We then wrapped them up in blankets and brought Olga and the girls into the bedroom and put them in our bed for a well-deserved rest. Also, during this time the midwives took the time to get all the statistics like weight, height, and do all the other checks they do on newborn babies.

We spent the morning talking about the shock and beauty of what had just occurred, about the signs that had been there but that no one had picked up on, and for good reason. Ellen had, of course, never delivered twins at home and told us had she known that we were having them she would have sent us to a hospital. Knowing Olga like I do, I know she would have refused to go, as she wanted the birth experience she had and really was fearful of what would have happened to her in the hospital.

We don't think hospitals are bad places, they are just not for us as we understand they have two goals: do the best they can to help women deliver babies, and make sure they avoid lawsuits. We had our girls 29 hours after the waters broke and if we had been in a hospital we would have had only 18 hours to deliver before they would have started to intervene and force the girls out.[6] In reality, we had twins born perfectly, head first, with no complications. We didn't spend the nine months worrying about all that could go wrong, we focused on how it would go just right, and it did.

We focused on how it would go just right, and it did

A lot of people ask us how we could not have known we were having twins, and all I can say is it was a series of events that helped us to create the birth experience we wanted. Throughout the birth Olga only gained 15 pounds and was actually six pounds lighter after the birth than the day she found out she was pregnant. So she had about 21 pounds total for the pregnancy and the girls weighed 4½ and 5 pounds. This was because she ate right, exercised and just took excellent care of herself—something most working women are not given the time to do these days. Also, Olga had really strong stomach muscles from many years of riding horses, which made the midwives' job of examining [palpating] her bump very difficult. The midwives didn't ever think to look for multiple heartbeats and, since we had chosen not to have a scan, the girls were able to support our goal by hiding from us all, so that they could be born at home in a beautiful, loving, peaceful and drug-free environment.

They were able to support our goal by hiding from us all!

64 birth: countdown to optimal

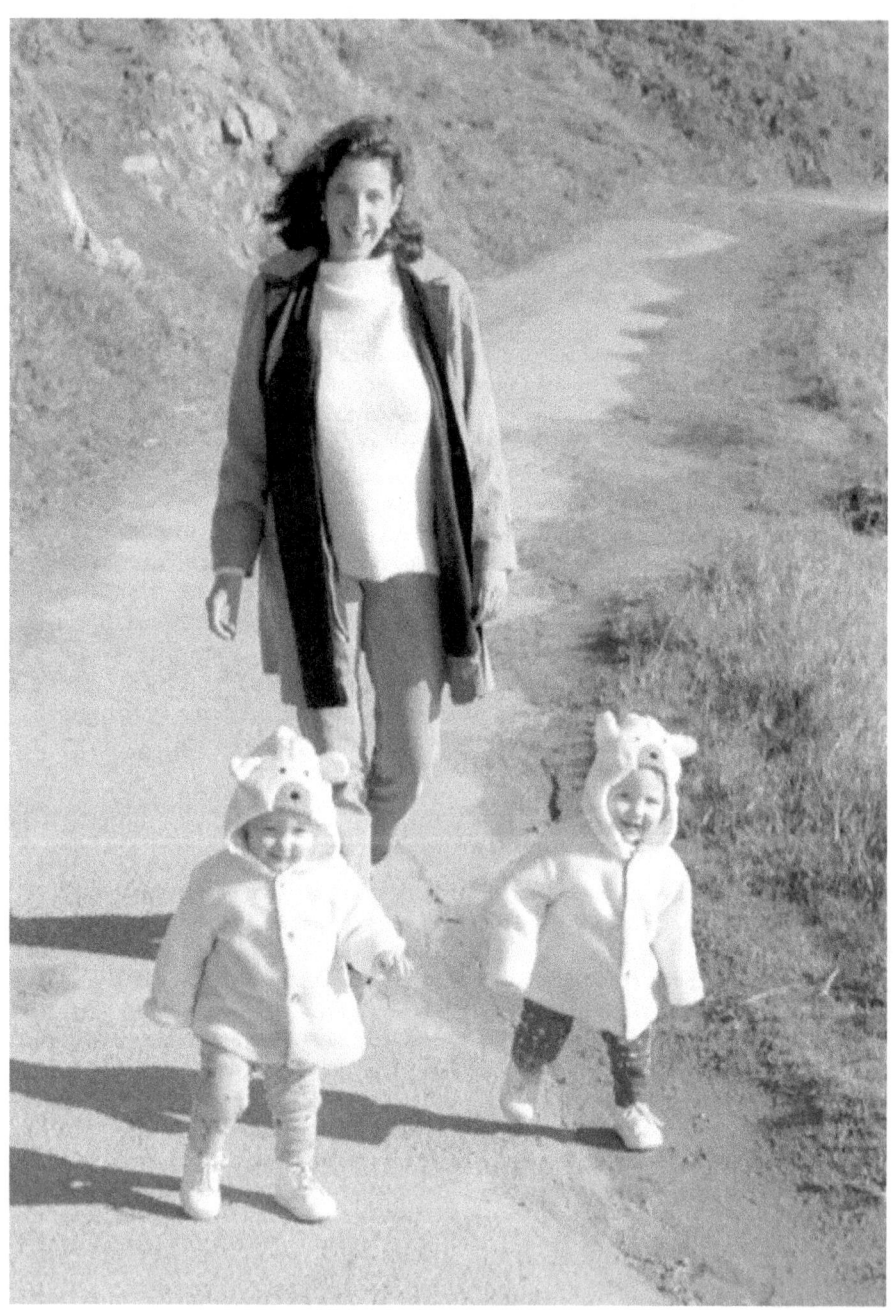

Olga with her two little girls

Olga's comments...

I had a beautiful and wonderful birth experience. I was very grateful for all the workshops I attended in Russia and for the Bradley classes in the USA. I was very conscious and confident about what I was doing. I think what helped me most on this journey was the deep belief that everything would be fine. I was taking care of my body—exercising and feeding it well—and it did a great job of getting through pregnancy and giving birth with all the wisdom of nature that it has inside it. In the classes in Moscow we discussed the process of birth through the experience of a child, which makes you understand that natural childbirth is the best way to bring a child into the world.

> I think what helped me most on this journey was
> the deep belief that everything would be fine

I am very grateful to Steven because he gave me a lot of love and support, which helped me to gain strength and confidence. During the birth we worked together like a great team. I am sure that creating a loving relationship in the family is very important for having a healthy, easy pregnancy and birth. It is not a rule but I believe that a happy woman with a positive attitude has a better chance to have an easy birth. Creating good relations depends on the people themselves.

In my opinion, these are the most important things, if you want to have a great, natural birth:

- ♥ Have a deep knowledge of the benefits of natural childbirth for both the child and the mother and make a conscious choice to do it 100% naturally. It is very important to select people (especially midwives or doctors) who will support and encourage you in your choices. It will never work when the woman says: "I will go to the hospital and try to do it." There is a big chance that there will be a nurse who, after several hours of labour and pain, will say: "And now this is your last chance to get an epidural. Would you like it?" It's terribly hard to answer "No" when you're in pain.
- ♥ Have a deep belief in yourself that you can do it, trusting your own body with all its wisdom. Have a very positive attitude and a lot of gratitude for all the processes that are taking place within you.
- ♥ Take good care of your body. Have a very healthy, natural diet and do a lot of exercise (like swimming, walking, stretching).
- ♥ Consciously accept who you are and work to develop positive thoughts and a peaceful state of mind, and nurture a deep feeling of love for your child, yourself and the world. Work through the problems in your relationships with others (especially in your family) and within yourself.

Steve and Olga Mellor

For other references to twins see 'twins' the Index.

TRIPLETS

If you're pregnant with triplets—congratulations!—you need to decide whether or not having a caesarean could be sufficiently advantageous (to yourself and your babies) to balance out the risks which might (or might not) be involved in a vaginal birth. And you also need to take into account, of course, the fact that a caesarean also carries with it risks (for both the woman and her babies) and that breastfeeding and general childcare might be more difficult after a caesarean.[9] Finally, you need to remember that if left to your own devices your babies might gestate within you for longer than a pre-scheduled caesarean might anticipate, which would be to your babies' advantage.

There are apparently two reasons why many consultants recommend a caesarean for women expecting triplets. Firstly, there are stories of problematic second or third deliveries and even accounts of emergency caesareans following a successful vaginal delivery of a first or second triplet. These cases invariably involved a great deal of disturbance and obstetric intervention so it is impossible to ascertain what might have happened if the labouring woman had really been left undisturbed, with a feeling of being unobserved. However, this risk obviously does exist, whatever the circumstances. Secondly, it seems to be very difficult to monitor multiples effectively—if, indeed, it's ever possible to effectively monitor babies who are in the process of being born. One doctor mother of triplets I spoke to told me she'd decided to have her triplets by caesarean after seeing on television a prospective mother of twins in labour: the first twin was born successfully and the second was stillborn. In this case, the mother was certainly not given any privacy—since her labour and births were being televised—and there were also undoubtedly interventions of the kind that many hospitals take for granted as 'harmless'.

So the decision as to whether or not to go the caesarean route seems to depend on a woman's attitude toward monitoring and, consequently, disturbance (since monitoring involves disturbance) and also on her concerns about, or confidence in, the normal, healthy processes.

I would like to dream that gentler, less invasive but safe births might be possible for future triplets. Why is it considered necessary to give a woman expecting triplets a running commentary on potential problems? (How much focus is there on what's going right?) Is it really necessary or helpful for so many people to be present at the births of triplets? Could mobile phones not be used, or could staff not wait discretely outside the room where the mother is labouring? Alternatively, for extremely high-risk cases how about installing glass which can only be seen through one way? Is it not time we recognised every woman's need for silence, privacy and sensitivity? What about the babies' need for gentle treatment too? Can we not find better ways of providing intensive care so that the experience of birthing premature triplets is less stressful for the parents... and also the babies?

Birthframe 15

Here's an account of a vaginal triplet birth which took place in the UK in 1961.

I found out I was expecting triplets a few weeks before I went into labour. I was a bit shocked and I didn't quite believe it. I was having visits from the district nurse and she put on my card "Lots of limbs, go for an X-ray". That's how they discovered it. It wasn't as a result of infertility treatment and there was no family history of multiple births.

I already had two children. My son was then $3\frac{1}{2}$ and my daughter was 20 months. I'd chosen to have them at home, as most people did 50 years ago. They'd both been very good experiences. As for the triplets' birth, obviously I would have liked to have had them at home too but when they discovered it would be triplets, they said it had to be hospital. There was no talk about having a caesarean, though. Nowadays, people seem to do caesareans at the drop of a hat. They are necessary at times, of course, but there was no need for one in my case.

It all started a week before Christmas, when I began having pangs, you know, contractions. They were born a bit early, as multiple births almost always are, but I can't remember how many weeks—about three, I think. Anyway, I went into hospital for about 24 hours or so and they said, "Nothing's happening. Go home and come back again after your Christmas dinner." So I did.

I went back into hospital that night, when the waters broke. It was a case of "Call the ambulance immediately!" I'm not sure of the exact time but it was probably about 3 or 4 o'clock in the morning that I went in. And they were actually born just after 2 o'clock in the afternoon, about 12 hours later, the day after Christmas, within about 45 minutes of each other.

They were all born vaginally. I'm very happy that they were as normal as possible. No caesarean. No messing about. For both the babies' sake and for mine, too. There were no instruments or tearing or anything like that. No, I was lucky—when you hear of what some people have. Afterwards I felt as if I could push a bus over—I felt as if I could leap out of bed and do anything. But I didn't. There were no buses going by at the time. Yes, it was very exciting.

> Afterwards, I felt as if I could push a bus over!

Now the triplets are almost 50. Jon's a bachelor with his own house and a Physics degree. His job involves the testing of many materials used in the building and construction industries. He plays badminton and meets his brothers and mates in a pub at least once a week. Tim now has three children—two boys and a girl—while Greg has three sons. They started their own gardening business a few years ago, with much help and support from their wives, and are now extremely busy. I often wonder if any of their customers think they are seeing double, which of course they are!

Mave Denyer

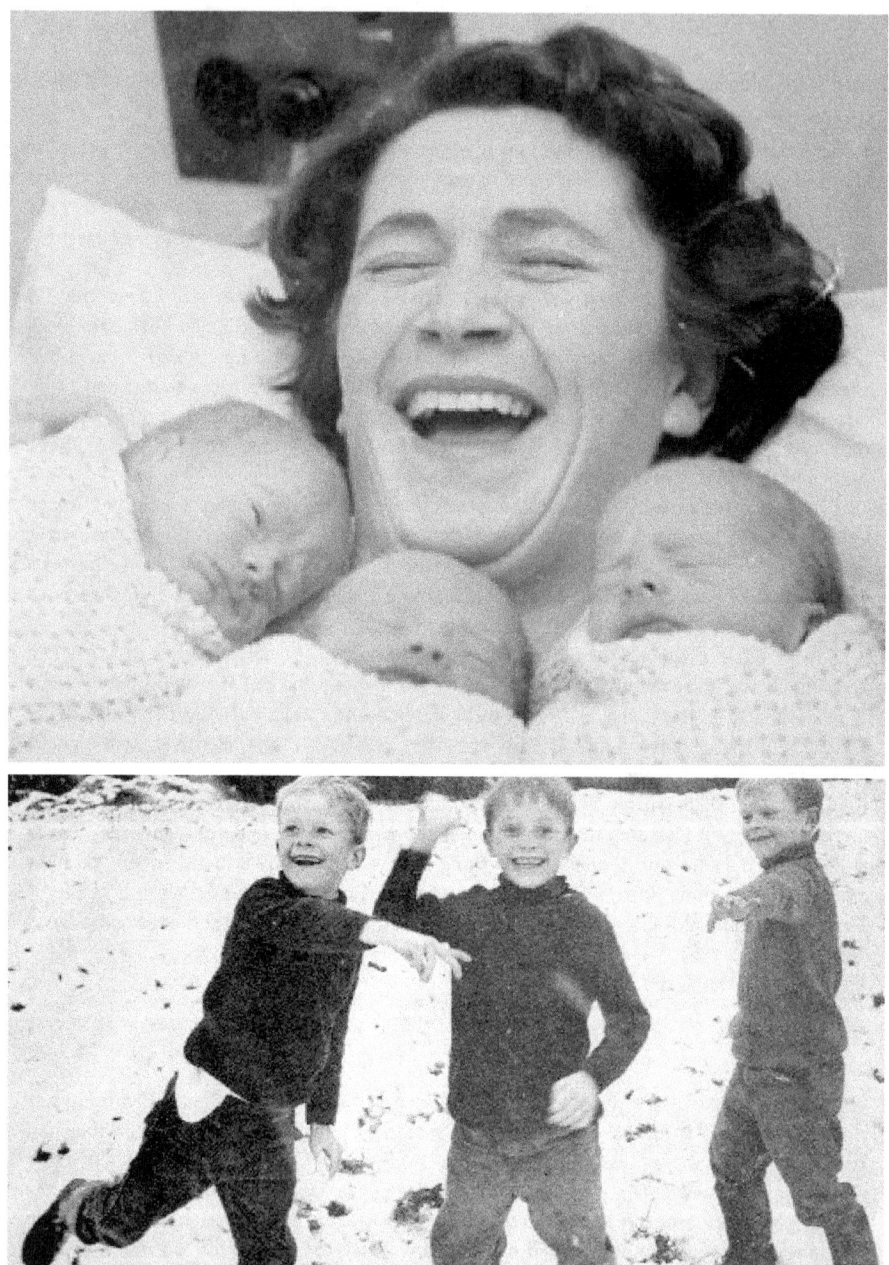

Top: *Mave with her newborns* Bottom: *The triplets having fun in the snow*

Birthframe 16

The next account is of a vaginal birth which took place in a London hospital.

No IVF, no family history, we simply were that freak statistic—a spontaneous triplet pregnancy

In August 1999 in a small scanning room in a London hospital we were told some life-changing news. At 35 years old I was pregnant with my third child. Actually, third and fourth children as I had discovered at a previous scan that it was twins.

Since then, we had been away on holiday for three weeks, and had got used to the idea that things were not quite going as we had expected. We returned that day, just off the plane and very jet-lagged, for a further scan. My husband jokingly said, "Just don't tell us there's another one!"—at which we were stopped in our tracks by those unforgettable words, "Um... well, actually there is." I was pregnant with triplets. No IVF, no family history, we simply were that freak statistic—a spontaneous triplet pregnancy.

At 9.00pm on 30 November, the evening of my daughter's fifth birthday, my waters broke. I couldn't really believe it. I was only 28 weeks pregnant. Though tired during the pregnancy, things had gone well. I had been resting in bed for two hours each day, and had been feeling healthy and full of confidence. I had been told at the hospital: "As long as you get to 32 weeks, we're not too worried." I had been so sure that this pregnancy would go way beyond that date. I rationalised that I had already had two full-term pregnancies without any problems or complications. Clearly, my triplets would be born later rather than earlier. So confident was I that I used to pass over the 'premature baby' section in the books on multiple birth, sure that I wouldn't be needing that information.

We had taken on Caroline Flint to be our independent midwife as soon as I became pregnant with what we assumed to be our single third child. Caroline had been our midwife for our second child, and I had given birth to him at home. When planning to have a third child, I had thought that we would probably have another home birth. However, with the news that I was expecting triplets everything had to change.

Caroline tried, on our behalf, to find a consultant who was willing to consider a vaginal delivery of triplets. She did not have any success. Whilst we were not against the idea of having a caesarean if it were necessary for the babies' safety, we wanted my case considered on an individual basis. I had given birth two times before without any need for medical intervention and wanted someone to look at my particular case, consider all the options, and make a safe and sensible judgement about the mode of delivery. The view seemed to be that triplets should always be born by planned caesarean and the fact that two of our babies were 'monochorionic' was given as a further reason for not having a vaginal delivery. (Incidentally, we have since discovered that all three babies are identical.)

['Monochorionic' means that two (or more) babies are developing in one chorion (bag), each in its own amniotic sac, inside the single chorion.]

One consultant, Donald Gibb, was prepared to consider a vaginal delivery, but his contract with my community hospital was to expire before my due date, and so he was unable to take my case on. We accepted that the babies would be born by caesarean.

When my waters broke, I immediately phoned Caroline, who said that she would come to the house and check me over. 15 minutes later I started to have contractions and so we arranged to meet at the hospital. The contractions were very quickly becoming regular and urgent-seeming. I felt panic-stricken, every minute seeming an eternity as we waited for my mother-in-law to arrive to look after our older two children.

We arrived at the check-in desk of the labour ward...

"I'm having contractions. I'm having triplets—I'm only 28 weeks."

"Take a seat. We don't have any rooms at the moment."

"But I think it's an emergency—I'm meant to be having a caesarean."

"We have other emergencies to deal with. Take a seat in Reception."

The situation seemed surreal. I was certain that I was in established labour and that things were happening at speed, and yet we couldn't seem to persuade the hospital staff to take us seriously. We went down to the reception area, which was out of sight of all staff. I felt quite despairing, pacing up and down, convinced that I would give birth to our babies right there.

Then, to our utter, utter relief, Caroline arrived, took one look at me and dived off down the corridor. She came rushing back, looking relieved. "Donald Gibb is here."

By a quirk of fate Donald Gibb was there on his second-to-last night at the hospital. Immediately, everything started to happen. We were rushed into a room as some poor woman was wheeled out into the corridor, and I have a hazy memory of Mr Gibb tearing the sheets off the bed. There were no intensive care cots available at the hospital and the plan was to transfer me by ambulance to another hospital, where there would be places for the babies once they were born. However, on examination I was already 9cm dilated (this only one hour after my waters had broken). It was then inevitable that the babies were to be delivered there and then.

I felt disbelief that this was happening to me. I was full of fear at what might happen to the babies, and indeed to me, and yet couldn't quite take the situation seriously. I found myself giggling inappropriately at Mr Gibb's wellington boots. The room filled up with people and equipment, and I felt as though I was appearing in some bad hospital TV drama. At the same time, I was terrified. Instinctively, I turned my back on the room and knelt on all fours on the bed. This was the same position in which I had delivered my other two children, and I couldn't imagine any other way. I remember Mr Gibb saying, "Do you want to deliver the first one like that?" and replying that I wanted to deliver them all like that. He said that he would see how things went.

> Instinctively, I turned my back on the room and knelt on all fours. This was the same position I'd used for the others.

The paediatric registrar kept appearing by my head to report on progress in the search for intensive care cots for the babies. It was mostly bad news. They couldn't find three intensive care cots available in one hospital, the babies might have to go to different hospitals, one might have to go to another town, etc... I became very agitated about this and remember Mr Gibb telling me not to worry, that it was their job, not ours, to sort this out, that our job was to get the babies out safely.

From that moment on, I felt a sense of calm. I felt that I had done everything I could. I was in expert hands and what now happened to the babies was out of my hands. I felt totally focused on giving birth. Although the room was full of people and I had a tube in my hand in case I needed a caesarean, I was able to block almost everything out. I had a scan during the labour, but it was so unobtrusive that I hardly noticed it. I knelt on the bed with my back to everyone and was aware only of Bruce (my husband) in front of me, Mr Gibb's voice, and Pam Wild (the other midwife) rubbing my back and reassuring me. I felt such faith in the people looking after me, and in my own ability to give birth that in spite of everything I felt calm and relaxed. I leant on Bruce, used gas and air, and concentrated on counting my breaths, keeping them long and even. Exactly the same as I had done in giving birth to my other two children. I remember saying to Pam and Caroline, "I'm pretending to have a home birth here."

At 10.30pm Kate was born. She was so tiny that it was not like the second stage of labour with my other children. It was more a question of trying to hardly push at all, to make her delivery really gentle. I didn't see or touch her, as she was taken straight to the resusitaire to be surrounded by a paediatric team and ventilated. I just had a chance for a quick look at her as she was wheeled past me on her way to SCBU [the Special Care Baby Unit], a scrap of humanity amidst a mass of tubes. I wasn't really able to focus on her birth as my mind and body both knew there were two more ahead. Then everything stopped. There were no contractions, and I lay against Bruce and felt as though I was almost asleep while we all waited. I had no sense of time at all, though in fact it was 40 minutes before Sophie was born. After 30 minutes Mr Gibb ruptured the membranes because she had some bradycardia [an abnormally slow or unsteady heart rhythm], and she was born shortly afterwards. 10 minutes after that, Louisa was born. All were born head down, and I was able to deliver all three kneeling on the bed with my back to the room. As with Kate, Sophie and Louisa were taken away immediately by their paediatric teams to be ventilated and we caught a brief look at them as they were wheeled away to SCBU. They weighed 2lb 9oz, 2lb 10oz and 2lb 11oz.

I asked for syntometrine [similar to ergometrine—see the Glossary], and shortly after the placenta had been delivered Bruce and I found ourselves alone in the room wondering whether it had all been a dream. We had no babies with us, all the medical staff had gone. It was only two and half hours since my waters had broken.

A little later Caroline and Pam took us down to SCBU to see the babies, where they

I was able to deliver all three kneeling on the bed

were being held until transfer to another London hospital. We had been lucky as three intensive care cots had been found in one unit. I was in a wheelchair and felt as though I couldn't breathe properly. I couldn't really take it all in. The birth had left me feeling on a high, as though I could do anything. I felt fantastic, exhausted and confused. I couldn't relate emotionally to the three tiny bright red bodies in their incubators, covered with tubes, and hooked up to all kinds of machines. These didn't seem to be my babies. I was given a Polaroid picture of each one, and taken back to the ward. I didn't want to think about what had happened, and asked for a sleeping tablet. That night, Kate and Sophie were transferred and Louisa was transferred the next morning.

The babies spent the next two weeks in the neonatal intensive care unit. It was a very difficult and frightening time. The almost hourly ups and downs of each baby's progress meant an experience which could be likened to being on three roller coasters at once. And during this time we could do nothing but watch and wait. We couldn't hold them for many days and could do very little to help them. I was sustained during this time by the memory of their birth. The way in which I had given birth to them gave me a physical connection with them which I was not able to have during the first weeks of their lives. I also found it helpful that I was able to start expressing breastmilk for them. This was frozen until they were ready to begin breastfeeding.

After two weeks the babies were transferred back to the hospital where they were born. They spent a further five weeks in hospital before being discharged home at 36 weeks' gestation. I continued to express milk for them throughout their time in hospital, and for some weeks once they came home. For 10 weeks they were exclusively fed with breastmilk, initially by tube and later from a bottle.

Kate, Sophie and Louisa are now happy, healthy $3\frac{1}{2}$-year-olds.

Janet Hanton

For other references to triplets see 'triplets' in the Index.

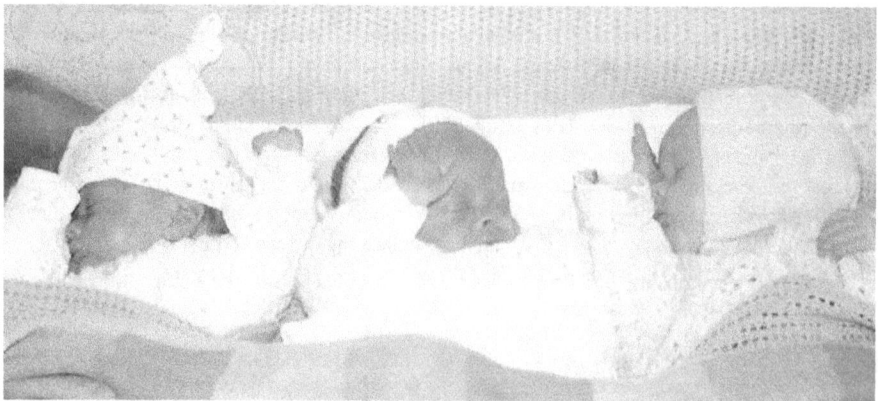

Kate, Sophie and Louisa (left to right) at 7 weeks old, just after they had come home

BREECH POSITION

Approximately three in every 100 babies are in the breech position as they are about to be born. Of course, the number is much higher a few weeks leading up to this time, but many babies do eventually turn round to the more common 'head-down' position by the time their mum goes into labour. If you find your baby is in an unusual position before you are 32 weeks pregnant, don't panic! This is perfectly normal. It's only as the baby gets bigger that he or she has to limit movements and assume a position in readiness for the upcoming birth. If you are informed after 32 weeks that your baby is breech, you will need to consider carefully whether or not you want to try and help him or her turn round to the more conventional 'head-down' position—see ECV in the Glossary.

Birthframe 17

Some people don't worry when a baby is breech, they simply continue as originally planned.[10] In the following interview, Elise Hansen—a midwife, working in Oregon—explains how and why she had an optimal birth.

Elise, I understand you gave birth to your baby vaginally, even though she was breech. Why did you decide to do this? Why not simply have a C-section?

I gave birth to my daughter in 1977. At the time I was not a midwife. The only thing I knew about breech birth was that it could be difficult, but I didn't know anything more specific than that. I was living in France at the time and it never even OCCURRED to me to have a C-section. I had had two easy and fast vaginal births before that. (When I returned to the States, I then found out that she would have been an automatic C-section here.) I had searched out a local doctor who specialised in 'Leboyer births' and who attended at a very small clinic.[7] Once we knew that my daughter was breech, I asked this doctor about the difficulty associated with a breech birth, but he responded that there really wasn't any difficulty at all, just that it was 'a little more complicated'. His matter-of-fact, no-fear response just reinforced my trust in my ability to birth easily.

When did you find out your baby was breech? What kind of breech position was your baby in?

I think she was breech from the very beginning. I don't remember her ever being vertex. She was a footling, but I'm not sure we knew that part before the birth. If the doctor knew, he didn't mention it.

Did you try to turn her at all?

No, the issue never came up. If there was no difficulty associated with a breech birth, why bother changing it?

If the doctor knew, he didn't mention it

Did you have any trouble finding someone to attend the birth?

No, as I mentioned before, I had chosen the caregiver because he was a 'Leboyer' doctor; the breech position seemed incidental to him (and, consequently, to me).

And how did the birth go?

GREAT! My partner woke me up in the middle of the night wondering if I was OK because I guess I was moving around in the bed. I woke up but didn't notice anything unusual. Got up to wee and my waters broke. Went and took a shower, then we woke up my 4-year-old daughter and got into the car. We had to stop by the post office to use the phone (we had no phone in our house) to call a friend to meet us at the clinic to take care of the 4-year-old. By the time my partner got back into the car, I could no longer sit down, so I grabbed onto the cross bars on the inside of the roof of our car (an old 2CV with a peel-back roof) and just hung from them for the 10-minute ride.

By the time we arrived at the clinic, I could feel my daughter's foot at the entrance of my vagina. However, I had to walk up two flights of stairs to get to the birthing unit. During the whole walk up with a foot dangling out under my dress, I had images in my head of my baby bouncing down the stairs behind me! It was kind of funny, really, but that was the only time I was a little nervous, wondering if I would be able to catch her. As soon as I hopped up onto the exam table, the resident midwife lifted my dress and shouted in a very surprised voice (in French, of course), "But, Madame, you didn't tell me this baby was breech!" I replied, "But, Madame, you didn't ask!" By then, she just had time to grab a towel and hang onto my daughter as she came out in one quick contraction. About 45 minutes had passed since my partner had shaken me awake.

Would you do the same again?

You bet! (Though, knowing what I do now about breech birth in general, I would probably have a little more fear.) But I would have a midwife AND a home birth! And probably STILL do it outside this country.

> Continue to have faith and trust that your baby knows how to give birth. Also, find a caregiver who will honour your choices, who has experience, not fear

Do you have any advice for women whose baby is presenting breech?

Just that they continue to have faith and trust that their bodies know how to give birth. There is nothing abnormal about a breech birth. Those babies just choose to come into this world walking. Find a caregiver who believes in healthy birth and who honours every woman's (and baby's) choices and who has experience, but not fear.

> Find a caregiver who believes in healthy birth

I have had two breech babies... **Birthframe 18**

Here's another beautiful, courageous story from a woman who decided that the way risks are usually assessed might not always take all the facts into account. It's interesting how she mentions thoughts and states of mind at various points in her account. Perhaps these are more powerful than we usually assume, whatever the potential physical constraints.

I have had two breech babies. The first, a boy, was born in 1999 by caesarean, the second, a girl, was born naturally in 2001.

I was a breech baby and so was my brother, so it shouldn't have been a surprise when it became clear that my second child had no intention of turning round, but I kept thinking she would. I tried external cephalic version (ECV) and moxabustion, as well as lots of undignified bum-in-the-air positions.[8] But as nothing was working, my midwife and I began to plan for a breech birth.

With my first baby, I had encountered a lot of opposition to having my son vaginally at the hospital where I was registered. As he only turned breech a few days before my due date, I had little opportunity to find any alternatives, let alone research whether what I was being told about risks was accurate. After he was born by caesarean I felt very upset emotionally, as well as physically. Obviously, I was happy to have him, but I felt 'all wrong'. I had gone into labour and then had an emergency section and my body felt strange, literally as though it was still pent up, still had something left to do. I can't explain it in words. I felt like I had let my body down and let my baby down.

Second time around I had an independent midwife, Judith, with lots of experience of breech birth and had also switched hospitals and booked with a consultant who was prepared to support my efforts for a vaginal birth. Both Judith and the consultant felt that the studies on breech birth had not given enough weight to the impact different skills and experience of midwives/doctors had in determining outcomes. However we were all clear that whilst we were trying for a breech birth, at any sign of problems we would go straight for a caesarean. Given this, and the small risk of a problem with my previous section, we felt we had to opt for a hospital birth.

A couple of days before my due date, my waters broke as I was cooking the evening meal. There were no contractions so we went ahead with our dinner with my partner's brother, who then took our son to his grandparents. I phoned Judith, who called round to test if it was definitely amniotic fluid. I was happy for her to leave while we awaited developments. At about 10.00pm I started having contractions. They were anything from 10 to two minutes apart and quite strong. In between, I tried to read to keep calm. We wrote down times. Past midnight I was sick a few times and my partner managed to doze off for a bit. As it approached 6.00am I decided I wanted to leave for the hospital. Although it's only about 12 miles away, I wanted to beat the terrible rush-hour traffic jams.

Judith met us at the door of the hospital. Walking brought contractions thick and fast; I had one in the three yards between car and door, one in the elevator and a couple in the corridor. We went into a large room with a long row of windows, giving a good view over the city—we were four floors up. I said to Judith that after a whole night of contractions the last thing I needed was to be told I was only 2cm dilated. She said, "Shall we not look then?" So we didn't.

For a long time, I crouched on the floor and held on to a metal chair leg with each contraction, staring intently at the pattern on the hard tiles. After a while, Judith said she wanted me to get things moving by walking about more. With her on one side and my partner on the other we processed up and down the long room, lifting our feet up as high as we could. As before, walking brought a rush of strong contractions.

At around midday Judith examined me and pronounced me 6-7cm dilated—good job she hadn't checked earlier. We kept walking but I refused to leave the room to take to the corridors. We had been left completely alone by the hospital staff and I couldn't bear the idea of seeing anyone else. Every now and then I was sick. As the afternoon wore on, Judith started getting me holding the end of the bed, squatting and imagining the baby moving down. At this stage, I don't think I actually believed that this baby would really be born and be born through my efforts.

Another examination showed that I was almost fully dilated. Judith quietly told me that the next part would be very hard work, but that if I wanted an epidural I could still do that. Having done so much already, I felt determined not to do this and risk the interventions that could follow. I told her I was scared of what was to come. She said being scared would make it harder, so I decided not to be. It seems incredible that you can decide not to be scared, but that is what I seemed to do.

I was very hot and sweaty and Judith suggested changing clothes. Once I got my big T-shirt off, I refused to put another one on. It felt like it would be a distraction.

Judith told me to start pushing with contractions. I couldn't get the hang of it at all. I felt no urge to push, I felt like I was pretending. I tried to think about a beautiful baby coming down. After a while I started to understand that I needed to push really hard and for a long time each time. I think the penny finally dropped that it was really up to me to do this and that I would have to work harder than I believed possible.

Judith said she could tell what sex the baby was (a quirk of having a breech). Then, after a big push, I finally felt the baby moving through me. I was leaning over the back of the chair when another push brought the baby's bottom out. I shouted to Judith as I was scared the baby would drop out onto the floor. The consultant was now in the room. She, my midwife and partner all lifted me onto the bed. This felt awful as it felt like the baby was being pushed back inside. Judith said to me: "The more of this you can do yourself the better."

> It felt like the baby was being pushed back inside.
> She said: "The more you can do yourself the better."

The next contraction I gave a big push and the legs came out; the next brought the arms and shoulders spinning out.

Then there was what felt like a very long silent moment. I could see the sunset through the big windows. I could see the midwife and consultant looking at me. I wondered if they were worried, if there was a time limit on this bit. I didn't wait for a contraction but decided to push with all my might, to get the baby's head out as quickly as I could. Then she was in my arms. A bit blue but soon pink, not crying, very calm, big eyes open in the dimly lit room as night began to fall.

I felt a bit sore for about half an hour and then felt fine. Physically and emotionally I felt great then and for about three days afterwards. Really great, super-happy, full of energy. I awoke each morning with what felt like a hangover. Judith said it was coming down from the endorphins. Partly, I felt great too because I was amazingly proud of myself. I had no pain relief, no interventions and no stitches and a breech baby! Particularly after having a section for breech position the first time around, it seemed almost incredible.

Liz Woolley

Birthframe 19

A growing number of women are choosing to give birth without the assistance of medical personnel. These women—who are usually highly educated women (in particular in the USA and Russia)—are proving that modern woman still has the inborn ability to birth her babies, without instruction or support from caregivers. Laura Shanley, who has birthed all of her four children 'unassisted' (at least by the medical profession)—and who contributed the following story—suggests that *every* woman (modern or primitive) has the inborn ability to give birth, provided any ingrained fear, guilt or shame can be overcome. She helped overcome her own negative feelings through what she calls 'belief suggestions'; in other words, she repeatedly 'thought' statements which reflected what she wanted to believe—either on an ongoing basis or at key moments. Her husband completely supports this approach; he also believes that natural, undisturbed, home-based birthing is best because he says traumatic childbirth diminishes the mother-child relationship, starts a person off on a rocky start and is ultimately to blame for many of society's ills.

Of course, the practice of intentionally giving birth without medical assistance is highly controversial, even though its safety record is good. Laura has worked to publicise the advantages of 'going it alone' through her website www.unassistedchildbirth.com, her book *Unassisted Childbirth* and her film *A Clear Road to Birth*. Whatever our personal position on this issue, it is truly remarkable to consider how straightforward a birth can be—in this case an unexpected footling breech—when a female body and her baby are left to labour entirely without disturbance, and when both mother and baby experience birth without fear.

A year and a half after giving birth to my first son John, I realised I was pregnant with Willie. Once again, I had a very healthy pregnancy. I never experienced morning sickness or had any of the other so-called 'symptoms' of pregnancy (which I believe are often fear-induced). I decided I would give birth on my hands and knees because that had worked so well with John, but in a dream I was shown otherwise. In the dream, I was watching a woman giving birth standing up. She was straddling a little plastic baby bathtub and catching the baby herself. As I watched her, I heard another woman very gently say to me, "Tell her to remember not to do too much." I understood what the woman was saying and the peaceful feeling of the dream stayed with me for the remainder of my pregnancy.

I want to say, at this point, that I don't follow every dream I have, but this dream was different. It seemed to be coming from the deepest part of my being. And so, I decided to follow it faithfully—I would catch my baby myself as I stood over my little bathtub, and I would move out of the way and essentially do nothing to interfere with the process.

On the morning of August 17, I began to feel contractions. David and I made love and I remember feeling an orgasm followed immediately by a contraction. The rhythmic contracting of my uterus during the orgasm felt almost identical to that of the contraction. They seemed to have the same pattern, although I must admit the orgasm felt better! A few minutes later, I was walking across the room when my waters broke. I took out my little bathtub and stood over it as I had been shown in the dream. At that point I couldn't feel the contractions, but I knew I was having them because when I put my hand inside my vagina I could feel my pelvic muscles rhythmically contracting around it. A few minutes later a foot appeared between my legs. I wasn't expecting a breech birth, although a friend of mine told me during my pregnancy that he had dreamt he saw the baby inside me standing right-side-up.

David and I said 'belief suggestions' that everything would be all right, and then we patiently waited for Willie to be born. Little by little his foot got lower and soon his other foot popped out. When I felt the time was right, I gave one push, and gently pulled him out by the feet. David and John had been in the other room but walked in just as Willie emerged. David yelled excitedly, "You did it!" and Willie immediately began to breastfeed. Incidentally, 12 years later I read that Michel Odent says that for a breech delivery a woman should always be in a 'standing squat' or 'upright' position and an attendant should do absolutely nothing to interfere if at all possible. This was the message of the dream.

Soon after the birth I dreamt that Willie was speaking to me. He told me that part of the reason his birth had been so fast and easy—he was born two hours after the first contraction—was that he hadn't been afraid either. Babies are always picking up on our beliefs, both before and after birth, so a fearless mother means a fearless baby.

Today, Willie is a happy and fearless 22-year-old!

Laura Shanley

Babies are always picking up on our beliefs

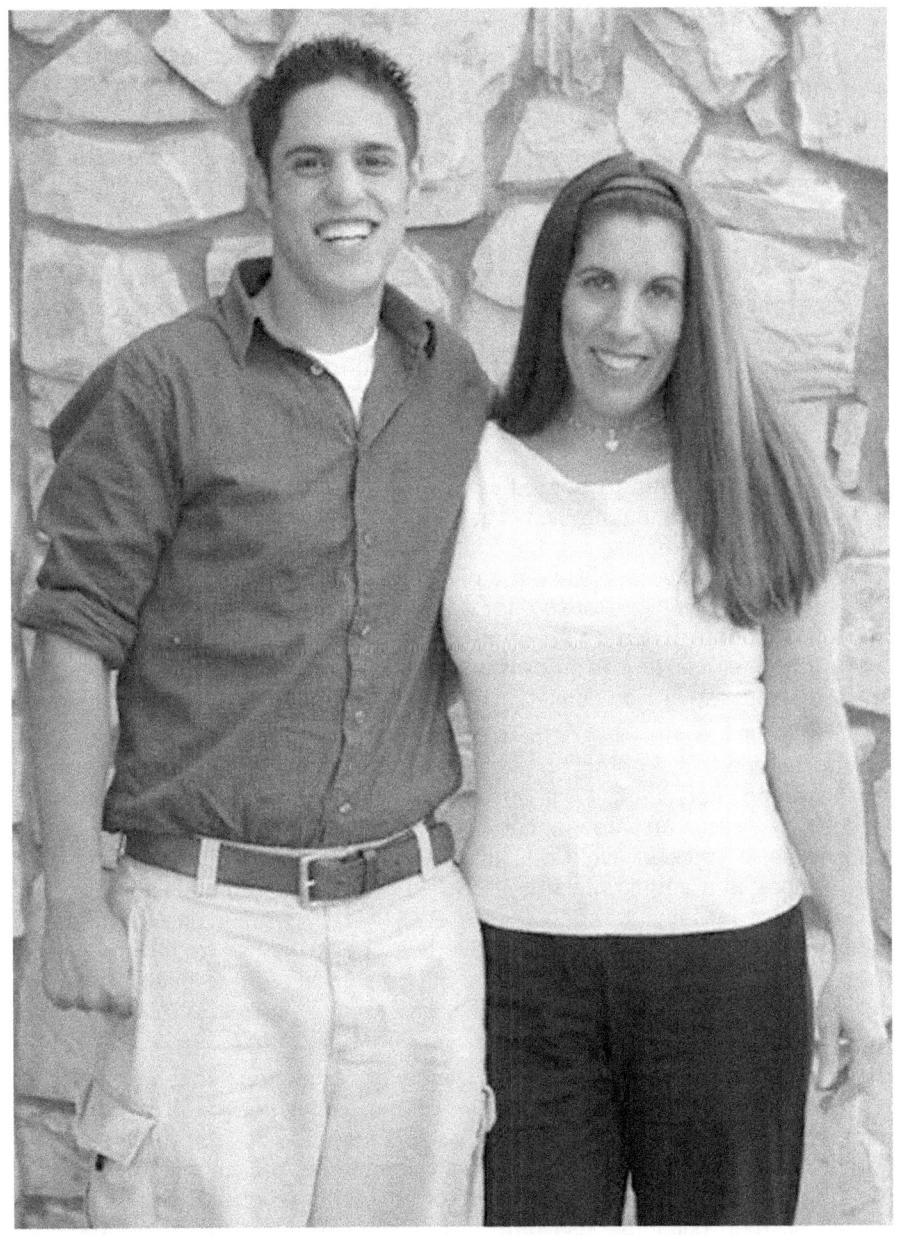

Willie and Laura—summer 2002

The caesarean conundrum

Some people might protest: "But isn't a caesarean the ideal way to give birth?" Actually, in the light of current research it's quite absurd to suggest that the modern caesarean represents an ideal. The modern C-section is simply an extremely effective rescue operation, which is now mostly safe, for cases where things would otherwise be likely to go wrong, for whatever reason.

A caesarean represents a great departure from the normal, healthy processes and is less pleasant, less safe and less healthy for both mother and baby, unless of course the operation really is lifesaving.[11] It's likely that being born by caesarean has long-term effects on the psychological development of the baby firstly because of the enormously different hormonal environment present when a woman has this kind of major abdominal surgery, secondly because of the experience itself and thirdly because of the disruption to the normal bonding processes after the operation.[12] The absence of oxytocin (dubbed by a researcher, Niles Newton, 'the hormone of love') is the key concern here and may interfere with the baby's development of the ability to love.[13] Michel has discussed this at length in his book *The Scientification of Love* (Free Association Books 1999). Of course, efforts can be made to counteract this potential problem but the point is that a caesarean birth is not ideal for the baby, unless of course it saves his or her life, or that of his or her mother. It is also not ideal for a mother in terms of minimising damage to her sexual anatomy firstly because damage to the pelvic floor (which includes the muscles around a woman's vagina) usually occurs during pregnancy and secondly because of the enormously important psychological aspect of arousal, response and orgasm.[14]

In the light of the current fashion for C-sections it might be difficult for you to believe this. In order to show you just how enormous an intervention a caesarean represents, I'll give you a detailed description of the surgical procedure. In an attempt to convince you you'll be better off without a caesarean, if you can avoid one, I'll also give you some facts and figures, birthframes and comments from contributors. These represent a range of viewpoints. Initially, I received material mostly from women who had caesareans which shouldn't really have been performed or from women who later had the experience of an optimal birth. Later, in order to balance out the accounts and comments I already had, I made an effort to get hold of some other views, as you will see.

In approaching this topic in this way, I sincerely hope that women who really do end up needing a caesarean will not be frightened. In cases where either mother or baby is in serious danger it is obviously best for this life-saving intervention to take place because it is currently the only means we have of dealing with certain obstetric problems and emergencies. The risk of the operation then becomes less than the risk of the alternative, i.e. potential death of either the mother or baby.

So the small minority of women who really do need to have this operation are best advised to focus on the life-saving properties of the modern C-section than on any negative aspects and to be thankful that they can be helped in a difficult situation. If, as is likely, you're one of the vast majority of women who are capable of having a physiological birth, being cut open is far from ideal.

THE FACTS

In 1998 research data was summarised in the *British Medical Journal*. According to this summary, women who have a caesarean (rather than a vaginal birth) open themselves up to all kinds of dangers.[15] In the short term, they have a far greater risk of haemorrhage, infection, ileus, pulmonary embolism and Mendelson's syndrome. (Check the Glossary to find out what these are!) Long term health problems faced by caesarean mothers apparently include the formation of adhesions, intestinal obstruction, and bladder injury. Uterine rupture is also a possibility in a subsequent pregnancy, especially if labour is induced or augmented.[16] Research also shows that women who've had caesareans are more likely to have fertility problems, an ectopic pregnancy or a placenta praevia later on.[17] It's also more likely that there will be a need for a hysterectomy, which would also have an obvious impact on fertility. There is even evidence that the health of caesarean mothers' future children may be affected by having an older caesarean-born sibling. Psychological problems, such as postnatal depression, are also more likely for caesarean mothers, especially if the operation was carried out under general anaesthetic, and these psychological problems are likely to affect the mother's ability to bond effectively with her baby, or babies.[18]

Research has also shown a significantly higher death rate for caesarean mothers, but it's impossible to determine how high the risk is.[19] This is partly because it would never be possible to carry out a randomised control trial (the 'gold standard' of medical research) and partly because the level of risk would depend on the reason for the caesarean and the woman's general level of health. Some writers and researchers claim that a woman having a caesarean is two times as likely to die as a woman giving birth vaginally, and some even say she is 16 times more likely to die. The imprecision of these estimates is obvious if you consider any other risk in life—such as the risk of crossing the road, which is affected by numerous personal and situational factors. The estimates are also absurd in a sense because without the operation any one woman might have died anyway, or her baby might have. For a complete review of recent research relating to the effects of caesareans, see *Pushed* (Da Capo 2007). The caesarean is real rescue surgery in high risk cases but for low-risk women who are capable of having a safe vaginal birth the evidence shows it's far from ideal. This is not really surprising, when we think that it constitutes major surgery and a lengthy disruption to the normal mother and baby bonding processes.[20]

The operation itself

Elsewhere in this book you'll find out about vaginal births so here is the equivalent level of detail for a caesarean birth. For the following account, I am indebted to *The Caesarean* (Free Assoc Books 2004), *Obstetrics by Ten Teachers* (Hodder Arnold 2000), *Myles Textbook for Midwives* (Churchill Livingstone 2009) and *Abdominal surgical incisions for caesarean section* (Mathai and Hofmeyr 2004).[21] Some details are vague because of the variation in protocols in different hospitals.

Before the operation...

- The pregnant woman (or her partner) is required to sign a consent form.
- In the case of an elective caesarean, the evening before the operation some glycerine suppositories may be given. These will help the woman do a poo, which will empty the rectum.
- The woman's abdominal and pubic hair is removed.
- An antacid may be given so as to prevent the contents of the woman's stomach from becoming acidic.
- Drugs to prevent thrombosis are sometimes given as well as antibiotics, in case infection develops. An intravenous drip (IV) is set up for the further administration of drugs.
- A catheter is installed so urine can be continually drained from the bladder.
- A blood pressure cuff is placed around the woman's arm.
- Jewellery, nail polish and make-up are removed, so that small changes in colouring can be observed. Contact lenses are also removed. Teeth are checked so that no loose ones are inadvertently swallowed during the operation!
- The woman is asked to change into a clean operation gown.
- The woman is asked to lie down on her left side and a wedge is placed under her right buttock.
- She is then asked to curl up into the fetal position if an epidural is to be inserted or topped up, or a general anaesthetic is injected via the IV.

During the operation...

- The surgeon wears a double layer of plastic gloves and a clear plastic shield around his or her face. This is to protect him or her from exposure to the pregnant woman's bodily fluids.
- The woman is turned onto her back so that her abdomen can be easily accessed. At the same time, the operating table is tilted slightly so that the woman's head is lower than her feet. This is to help establish a level of anaesthesia which will be high enough to make the woman's abdomen numb, but not so high that it will affect her ability to breathe.

- A nurse then paints the skin on the woman's abdomen with an antiseptic solution. Someone on the surgical team will then cover the abdomen with drapes and sterile plastic—leaving exposed only the area which is to be cut. The drapes are put over a bar above the woman's chest so that she cannot see the operation itself... er, except in the reflection of the light above in some cases!
- In one clear motion, the obstetrician then makes a horizontal, crescent-shaped incision, just above the usual site of the pubic hair. In the standard technique, the incision is made deep into the skin, so as to cut through all the superficial layers. In a more recently proposed technique (developed by Michael Stark in the 1990s), which Michel considers to be optimal, the scalpel only sinks one inch into the layer of fat and the so-called lateral tissue underneath is torn apart using two fingers. (Techniques involving tearing, rather than cutting, are generally recommended, where possible.)[22]
- Continuing to use fingers and a thumb, or using a scalpel and tiny forceps (which are like tweezers), or even electrocautery (if the 'Pelosi' technique is used), the obstetrician then tears or cuts deeper into the subcutaneous tissue. He or she then reaches a thick layer of fibrous tissue, called the fascia. After that the mucous membrane called the peritoneum, which is the last layer of the abdominal wall, is opened. This is done either by cutting or tearing in order to gain access to the abdominal cavity—which, of course, contains the uterus.
- After the bladder is pushed away, another peritoneum (which loosely lies over the 'low segment' of the uterus) is cut. The so-called 'low segment' of the uterus is then also cut open using short, careful strokes of a knife.
- The small original cut is then extended to a length of at least 15cm with the use of fingers or blunt-ended scissors.
- If the membranes around the baby are still intact—they may have burst open by this time—they are punctured and opened.
- The obstetrician then places one hand inside the uterus, under the baby's head and exerts pressure on the upper end of the uterus with the other hand so as to push the baby through the incision. (An assistant usually helps with this.)
- The baby's throat may be immediately suctioned with a small ear syringe and then the shoulders and the rest of the baby are eased out.
- Held up in the air, the baby usually begins to cry. When this happens the new baby is frequently held over the mother (if she is conscious) so that she can see the baby's genitals! The assumption is that her first priority will be to know whether she has a boy or a girl.
- The cord is clamped and the baby handed over to a nurse holding a warmed towel. Mothers and babies usually also have some skin-to-skin contact at this stage because modern caesareans rarely require general anaesthesia.

- There have been reports of some women complaining of pain during the next few stages of the operation, or of having difficulty breathing, although both are probably rare occurrences nowadays. Some women also vomit while their organs are being handled and the damage repaired. If any of these occur in the next stages of the operation, the woman will be immediately sedated.
- The placenta is then pulled out and passed to an attendant, who gives it a thorough check. He or she may well be soaked in blood and amniotic fluid by this stage.
- Next, the uterus is sutured (sewn together), either while still inside the abdomen (as advised by *Obstetrics for Ten Teachers*) or after being taken out to rest on the outside of the abdomen.
- The loose peritoneum covering the uterus is sutured closed, or left open for spontaneous healing if the obstetrician considers this to be preferable. Then the fascia (the thick fibrous layer) is brought together with heavy thread stitches because it is this layer which holds all the abdominal organs inside and keeps them from coming through the incision. The subcutaneous tissue (which is mostly fat) is sometimes also closed using loose stitches. The skin, the final layer, is sewn up with silk or synthetic thread, or joined with metal staples.
- A dry bandage is placed over the woman's incision and taped to her skin.
- Finally, the drapes are removed.

After the surgery...

- Both the woman and her baby are transferred to the postnatal ward together as soon as possible.
- Wherever she is, the woman's blood pressure and pulse may be recorded every now and then and her temperature noted every two hours or so. Whether or not this is done, and the frequency with which it is done will depend on the woman's apparent condition. If she is talking and alert, no checks may be considered necessary.
- The woman's wound is inspected every 30 minutes to check for blood loss and her lochia is also inspected. If the woman has had a general anaesthetic, she is left in the recovery position until she is fully conscious because she is still at risk of airway obstruction or regurgitation and silent aspiration of her stomach contents.
- Analgesia is prescribed and given. This may take the form of an epidural opioid, rectal analgesia or intramuscular analgesia (i.e. an injection). If the epidural route is chosen, the woman's breathing also needs to be carefully recorded.
- The baby is put to the mother's breast as soon as possible in such a way that the mother is disturbed as little as possible.[23]

The woman is reassured if she feels drowsy, which is common

- Even if the woman feels very hungry, she is only allowed to have fluids at first because there is a risk of something called paralytic ileus. (See the Glossary, if necessary!) The woman still needs to have an intravenous infusion for a while after the operation.
- The woman is helped out of bed and encouraged to walk around as soon as possible so as to reduce the risk of deep vein thrombosis. She is also encouraged to perform breathing exercises. A physiotherapist usually teaches these and may also give chest physiotherapy. Low-dose heparin (an anticoagulant drug) and TED anti-embolism stockings are often prescribed to prevent thrombosis.
- Blood pressure, temperature and pulse continue to be checked periodically. The intravenous infusion continues and the urinary catheter remains in the bladder until the woman can get up and go to the bathroom. The wound and lochia are observed hourly.
- When the urinary catheter has been removed, urinary output is monitored carefully because some women have difficulty passing urine at first or emptying the bladder completely.
- A woman is reassured if—as frequently happens after a general anaesthetic—she feels tired and drowsy for hours or even days after the operation. If, as often happens, the woman complains of feelings of detachment and unreality or feels she cannot relate well to her new baby, she is encouraged to talk freely and is again reassured.
- Painkillers are given as often as the woman asks for them. This usually means giving intramuscular opiates for up to 48 hours (i.e. injections) and oral analgesics (tablets) after that. Some women don't feel they need any painkillers at all.
- The woman is encouraged to rest as much as possible and visitors may be discouraged. Because she is likely to tire quickly, the woman will probably need help looking after her new baby.
- Finally, the woman is not allowed to drive a vehicle or carry other children for six weeks after the operation.

The woman is encouraged to rest as much as possible.
She will probably need help looking after her baby.

As you've seen, a caesarean is a complicated surgical procedure, with all kinds of risks, indignities, discomforts and inconveniences. So why on earth has it become fashionable in some quarters to have a caesarean section instead of a vaginal birth?

THE FASHION

Caesarean rates have been steadily increasing around the world. In the UK, in England and Wales in 1960, only 2.8% of births were achieved by caesarean section, but the figure had risen to 24.3% by the end of 2007. In 2001 in the US, the rate was 22.9% and in the same year in Australia it was 21.9%. (In the USA the rate had risen to 31.8% by 2007.) In Brazil the overall rate for the country is well above 50% and in private hospitals in big cities such as Sao Paulo and Rio de Janeiro the rate is a staggering 80%.

> The modern fashion for caesareans is easy to understand

This modern fashion for caesareans is actually quite easy to understand.[24] Choosing a caesarean section appears to mean choosing to have complete control over a natural process. As one midwife explains...

> " The C-section has sadly become part of our culture and an acceptable, if not desirable, way to give birth. Women find the control element of caesareans, particularly elective [maternal request] caesareans, appealing (in my opinion). In our society, generally, women are used to having control of their own bodies and their lives and to give up their body to labour and birth is very frightening to some women. Having 'a date' for their delivery day is another example of control—being able to plan it into their life/husband's holiday leave, etc, as opposed to waiting until the baby is ready.

It's interesting, though, that women who have both elective and emergency caesareans report feeling a *lack* of control when they comment on their own experience, as we shall soon see. In some sense then, the idea that a caesarean gives women control is just a fallacy... Although women might have superficial control in terms of timetables, when it comes to emotions they tend to feel out of their depth. And of course, although the birth itself may be scheduled, post-operative recovery for both mother and baby is highly unpredictable—far less so than with a vaginal birth.[25]

Apart from wanting to control the processes, why else do women actually choose to have a caesarean? One reason is that it appears to mean choosing to blot out pain and discomfort because anaesthesia and painkillers have to be used. It is a fallacy, unfortunately, that no pain will be experienced, mainly because postnatal pain is usually a feature of a caesarean. If physical pain is not experienced (thanks to strong painkillers), often there is emotional pain, so one way or another caesarean mothers seem to get the short straw. Another common reason to have a caesarean is to avoid damaging the sexual organs. Unfortunately, this is also misguided because damage to a woman's pelvic floor usually occurs mainly during pregnancy.[26] The best way of avoiding damage to the vagina and perineum generally (the muscles which support everything 'down there') is actually to have a completely drug-free,

THE FEELING

What does it actually feel like to have a caesarean?[27] Here's an account of an in-labour emergency caesarean. (Incidentally, you can read this same woman's VBAC account for one of her subsequent births in Birthframe 82.)

Birthframe 20

First they put me on the strange, narrow, tipped operating table and increased the anaesthetic in my epidural. I was so terrified my teeth were chattering. Two kind young anaesthetists stayed with my husband and me at the head end of the drape so we wouldn't see me being wrenched open. The operating theatre had one of those strange, fly-eye, seven-faceted, non-glare lamps overhead, lots of monitors checking my heart rate, blood pressure, blood oxygen, etc. They put an oxygen mask on me, to give the baby extra air, they said. When my lower body felt like nothing but lumps of dough, they got to work putting in a catheter and then slicing open the abdominal wall.

"What's happening now?" I asked, because it felt like I was being tugged in all directions. I wondered if the baby were coming out. "Oh, they're pulling apart some of the layers of your muscle wall," the anaesthetist said brightly. "It heals better than when they cut it." I wished I hadn't asked.

Not much later we heard a small cough and a phlegmy squall. "There he is! He's breathing!" I said, and burst into tears. We didn't get to see him right away, because the paediatricians had to check him for any problems related to the meconium and the long labour. We heard him screaming for his life for several minutes. Then they brought him to us wrapped in a blanket. My husband held him and showed him to me. All I could see was a bit of tiny face in a big white blanket. I didn't know what to do.

(If this ever happens to me again, I will make sure that the drape is lowered so that I can see the baby lifted out, and have him brought to me right away to be comforted.)

"Can I feed him?" I asked, since I knew that was what you were supposed to do. They said maybe not yet, since I was still swathed in operating sheets to my chest.

"Shall I give him his Vitamin K?" asked the midwife. I said no, I didn't want that to be the first thing he ever tasted.

"How much does he weigh?" I asked. Nobody had weighed him yet.

"Would you like me to weigh him for you?" the midwife offered.

I said OK, since I couldn't think of what else to do. So she took him away and I could hear him shrieking in terror as he was made to shiver for the sake of his parents' idle curiosity. I berated myself for being so thoughtless as to allow him to be taken away again so soon. Finally, he was returned to us, still terrified. My husband was led away with the baby to the delivery room. The anaesthetist stayed with me while the doctors finished putting me back together. They lifted me from side to side to wash away the blood and iodine disinfectant that had sloshed onto the table, then they lifted me back onto my wheeled bed, and rolled me back along the corridor to the delivery suite.

Having a caesarean was like getting burgled

Having a caesarean was like getting burgled. Strange burglars, who ransack the house and leave behind world's most priceless gift, my baby son. But a burglary nonetheless. I was robbed of an experience that I had been anticipating my whole life.

Sometimes life forces us to face our worst fears. Perhaps it was necessary for me to go through the caesarean first so that I would be able to appreciate the gift of a healthy birth at home. I can't take it for granted. Now over three years later I can say it was a valuable experience. After all, now I've been in an operating theatre and have experienced major surgery. Gee whiz. Kind of interesting.

I've experienced all those hospital interventions and I know what it's like. If it's happened to you, I can relate. It is possible to do it another way the second time! From the day after my son's birth, I comforted myself by thinking about what I was going to do differently if I got a chance to try again. The day after I discovered I was pregnant a second time, I started looking for an independent midwife. I really did my homework.

I still regret the terror and pain that my son must have felt being yanked out into bright light by strangers. He is happy and healthy and no one could say, "Here is a child who had a difficult birth." But these things are not visible to the naked eye. Wouldn't it have been so much better for him if I had been able to welcome him to the world in a gentler way? Is that why he cried inconsolably for 36 hours after his birth? They say some babies 'just are' more unsettled than others. How can I help wondering if the caesarean was the cause? Maybe I was the cause of his distress, because I was so upset. Maybe if I hadn't wanted a natural birth so much, I wouldn't have caused him such distress. But I can't be different from who I am. My husband and I were both overjoyed about the baby, nothing could change that. It was a more abstract feeling than after the second, natural birth. After the second one, I felt a physical joy. My whole being was happy. The first time, we were filled with love and wonder for our beautiful son. But my body felt sad.

Nina Klose

Birthframe 21

After the caesarean I was in a state of shock. Weeping uncontrollably for weeks and months. I became agoraphobic (normally I have to be outside), and couldn't travel in a car because it was far too scary. I was more vulnerable than a cream cake at a Bulimic Congress and the gory nightmares I was having were beyond the fright that most people are required to endure. Worst of all, I thought this was permanent. The good side is that everyone who has this Dark Night of the Soul learns from their experiences and gets stronger, and that's just what happened to me.

Birthframe 22

Post my caesarean with my first baby, I was in pain for a very long time. Even three months after the birth my scar was still nagging and painful by the end of the day or if I went out for a long walk. I remember the horror I felt when the prescription drugs ran out. After five weeks, a string came out of my scar. The soluble stitches had in fact not dissolved, and my body had had to reject them by sending the length of suture up through the scar and to the surface. I hadn't been warned of this possibility. I was so squeamish and horrified by the whole thing that somehow I managed to ignore this, and didn't even visit the doctor. I think it could have been one of the reasons for the continuing pain. My scar didn't really heal properly and became keloid.

And then it was my daughter's turn. When I became pregnant with her I suddenly realised the downside of an elective caesarean—it makes it much more likely that you'll need one the next time, only this time round you have a heavy child who you're not allowed to pick up. I really debated whether to go VBAC but was told that I would be allowed only an hour in the second stage labour, and effectively as a first timer my chances of an emergency section were considerable. So I booked a maternity nurse and went for it again.

Second time round was incredibly different. After 10 days I felt better than I had after three months with my first—I was going up and down stairs, I was off the prescription drugs. My scar healed fine. It made me realise how rough the first time had been, now I had something to compare it with.

Retrospectively I think I'd have done better to go for natural childbirth the first time round: that six weeks after the second child is born when you can't pick up your jealous first child, or put them into the bath, or change them, is really hard.   I didn't even think of it when I was making the original decision. However, it's not the end of the world. My pelvic floor and perineum are intact and my son doesn't seem too traumatised.

Birthframe 23

In case you happen to be one of the women who needs a caesarean for medical reasons, here's a positive birth story. (This account is reprinted with kind permission from La Leche League in the UK, since it first appeared in the magazine *LLL GB News*.) It's the story of a woman who was initially in favour of a vaginal birth, who changed her mind after a difficult first labour, which resulted in an emergency caesarean. She describes how she managed to optimise outcomes for an elective caesarean (for her second child), by taking an intelligent, caring and proactive approach. As you will see, this account demonstrates how even major abdominal surgery can be optimised, when it is needed for medical or psychological reasons.

I feel happy for those mothers who have experienced normal births but concerned that mothers who have experienced other births might feel that their experiences may be seen as somehow less honourable, less heroic. I've had two caesarean deliveries: each time I felt that this birth was an incredibly heroic act. I think all births must be. The first was performed as an emergency after an incredibly traumatic labour. When my beautiful baby, Tom, emerged he weighed in at almost 12 pounds! After having such a traumatic time, I chose to have my second baby by caesarean. I asked other mothers to share with me their experiences of planned caesareans through a La Leche League newsletter.

I wanted advice in general and also particularly wanted to know how well breastfeeding had gone for other caesarean mothers, without the hormonal kickstart of going through labour. I was touched and impressed to receive many letters in reply. We are all so busy bringing up young families, with very little time that we can spend writing letters, and yet here were all these La Leche League mothers taking the time and trouble to write long and detailed letters to a complete stranger! It was such a treat to read these handwritten, deeply personal stories and lovely to find that almost all these mothers reported a positive start to breastfeeding.

The day for my elective caesarean arrived and my husband and I arrived at the hospital, as planned, at 7.30am—thanks to one tip I got from a letter to sleep at home the night before. Our hospital's policy is normally to admit a mother the night before for tests and to meet with an anaesthetist, then they simply keep the woman in hospital overnight. The hospital was happy to comply with my request so Tom, our 3-year-old, had his granny with him to take him to playgroup and give him lunch afterwards.

I'm writing this account 17 months later and find I can scarcely remember the hours before Louis' birth. I think I was very excited and also very anxious. When birth begins with labour, one gets swept along in the unfolding experience. Without labour, there is lots of room to reflect on what a truly extraordinary and somehow unbelievable miracle is about to happen—wonderful, but scary. A lovely midwife welcomed me at the door when I arrived back at the hospital, showed me where to put my things and took me down to the operating theatre. She joked and chatted with me as the anaesthetist did his work and informed me of what was happening all the way through. She knew I wanted to be well-informed as I'd shown her my birth plan on my visit the night before. [See page 274.]

Once prepared, I lay on the operating table, numb from the waist down... well not quite numb, actually, but unable to feel pain. It's a strange sensation, hard to describe. My husband was beside me, dressed up in his little operating theatre hat and clothes. It was a moment of intense feeling. I was aware that someone was about to cut into my body—OK, I couldn't feel it, but somewhere inside us all must be an instinctive sense that we should not let ourselves be cut. I was aware that of course I was about to meet my baby... Would it be a girl or a boy? Would it look like Tom? Would it be healthy?

I could feel the baby moving about inside me—it had been awake and vigorous all through the preparations. I felt rather pleased that it wasn't being roused from slumber! I also was aware that it would be quite a few weeks before I would begin to feel really recovered from the operation—it's hard to welcome the prospect of weeks of discomfort and limited mobility. And I was aware that here I was, about to begin an entirely new phase of my life as mother of two. I also realised that I was lying in exactly the same spot where I had been when Tom was born, exactly three years and two weeks before. Except that this time I was conscious, it wasn't an emergency and the circumstances surrounding the birth were different.

Suddenly, here he was! Our beautiful baby boy, perfect and chubby, and screaming. The midwife wrapped him up immediately and put him on my chest for me to hold while I was being stitched up. Some mothers are able to breastfeed at this point but I was quite happy not to, feeling a bit strange and particularly immobile. After a little while, we went through to the recovery room where, as I'd requested, I was able to watch as Louis was washed, checked and weighed (9lb).

Then came the breastfeeding... It's not the easiest thing to breastfeed a baby when lying flat on your back with drips and tubes in the backs of your hands and no movement in your lower body, especially when it's a newborn baby who has never breastfed before. It was agony! I kept taking him off to see if I could improve the positioning but nothing particularly helped. (Breastfeeding continued to often be quite painful for a couple of weeks or so. I have a private theory that some mothers like myself are particularly sensitive to the pressure that the baby's suck exerts on the breast and we interpret it as pain until we get very used to it.) Louis didn't want to feed for the next 15 hours, although I kept offering him the breast. I was getting anxious. Would the staff insist he should have a bottle of formula? Would my milk take five days to 'come in' the way it had with my first baby? A midwife approached with a bottle of water and I squawked a protest. But she said she only wanted to drip a few drops on my nipple to encourage Louis to latch on. I'd never heard of this before (or since!) but, miraculously, it worked. The milk 'came in' early on Day 3 (and, of course, Louis had the valuable colostrum when he breastfed in the first two days). Maybe there was no delay because I did not start off exhausted after a long labour. Louis grew steadily and has been such a delightful baby. I'm proud of us both.

Birthframe 24

Of course, it's necessary to consider the possibility of an *unplanned* caesarean... With so many positive second-birth accounts and so much publicity about the feasibility of a vaginal birth after a caesarean (a VBAC), it's sometimes assumed that it must *always* be possible. However, as the next account shows, sometimes a planned VBAC turns out to be another caesarean. This can be very disappointing, as the following account illustrates. Here we meet up again with one of the anonymous contributors we've met before, earlier in this book.

For my second pregnancy and birth, I had wonderful, skilled, loving care from a home birth midwife. Labour started naturally, I dilated quickly, and the urge to push came after just a few hours.

But then I pushed... and pushed... and pushed... and pushed... The three different midwives reached in to try to turn the baby's head to facilitate delivery, to no avail.

After six hours of pushing, as the sun rose, my midwife said my scar just didn't look right, and I walked down the stairs with my midwife and husband, got in the car, and we drove to the hospital in rush hour traffic! (At the time I lived in a western suburb of the nearby city.) I was having immense and powerful pushing contractions, kneeling backward in the car with my midwife helping me.

I was admitted to the hospital, and we all agreed that after the now 7+ hours of pushing, that perhaps an epidural was in order so I could rest a bit. Everyone was very calm and professional. My midwife stayed with me the whole time. I and the baby were both doing fine according to the monitors. They catheterised me to empty my bladder, as I had been unable to urinate much during labour. That was a relief, actually.

In three or so hours, at 3.00pm, a doctor came in to check me. The baby had not moved down at all, to everyone's great surprise. I had continued to have pushing contractions. I was able to keep that up because I had been so well fed and watered during labour! I was informed that a caesarean would be necessary. I knew they were right and even my midwife, who was an expert on VBAC births, agreed. I cried. She cried. My husband held me. The nurses were confused, but polite. The anaesthetist was kind and professional, as was everyone else.

My midwife sat with me and described to me what was happening step by step. The doctor opened me, looked up and said, "Who did this?" I for some reason thought it was funny he asked, but his voice was dead serious as he repeated, "I mean it, WHO did this? Who did the previous C-section?" I told him, and he kind of snorted angrily. As my daughter's head was exposed and pulled out he said, "WOW, look at the size of that head!" I think he said it just to make me feel better. Her head just looked like a baby head to me! She was beautifully chubby and healthy, (three ounces heavier than my son at 8lb 14oz) and her Apgar score was perfect.

I held her after they fiddled with her for a few moments. Of course, I would have preferred to hold her immediately, but it was wonderful to see her. Then my husband held her as they stitched me up.

My recovery was much less painful and traumatic than after the first C-section. There was one nurse who came in and lectured me as I emerged groggy from my anaesthesia. She told me I was lucky I came in when I did and said how dare I try a home birth after a 'failed' first birth. She also said the uterus was so thin when they did the operation I was lucky it hadn't ruptured. I laughed. Did she know I had been in the hospital for over eight hours before the operation was performed? I didn't actually say anything, I was too groggy. She huffed out.

> I didn't actually say anything. I was too groggy.

I had massive scar tissue from the previous operation

The doctor came in and told me that I had massive scar tissue from the previous operation, which he had managed to 'clean up'. My bladder had been abnormally adhered to my uterus after the first C-section, which is why I could not urinate during labour. I was catheterised for five days so that the bladder could heal properly. The doctor was amazed that I hadn't had any symptoms from that problem. Neither doctor nor midwife could give any specific reason why I could not deliver vaginally. It was apparently possible that the scar tissue had caused an impediment. My bone structure seemed normal. I dilated normally. My contractions were very strong and coordinated, for hours and hours and hours! She was a baby on the large side of things, but certainly not abnormally large.

I put up with a few annoying staff comments such as "She'll never sleep in a cot if you keep holding her." But as a better-informed second-time mother no procedures were performed or drugs given to my daughter that I did not want. I wish I hadn't had to have any drugs, but I'll take what good things I can.

I cannot describe that feeling of loss—really a physical ache in my vagina, as strange as that sounds. The great expectation of holding the baby there, but then not, again. I don't know what to make of it emotionally. I sometimes don't even want to think of it, the disappointment is still strangely fresh. At least this time, I wasn't pressured into anything, I didn't make decisions out of fear. I had the antenatal care and labour I wanted until the very end. My care was respectful and loving, and I was NOT a particularly 'good' patient! Thank heavens.

I am trying to accept that even when I do everything right, there are some

---

At least in this case, both mother and baby were well. Sometimes this may not be the case. Amazingly enough, in these days of high technology and information still approximately 1 in every 100 babies is born dead... and there is still a fairly high maternal mortality rate, which varies from country to country.

According to the World Heath Organization, a woman's chance of dying at some point in her life as a result of pregnancy or childbirth can range from 1 in 6 (in Rwanda or Sierra Leone) to 1 in 8,700 (in Canada or Spain). Interestingly (or worryingly) neither the UK nor the USA statistics are particularly good: 1 in 4,600 and 3,500 respectively. Would the rates improve if more people knew how to prepare for and facilitate optimal births?

> Interestingly—or worryingly—neither the UK nor the USA statistics are particularly good. Would the rates improve if more people knew how to facilitate healthy, vaginal births?

Are caesareans really necessary?

Dystocia (also called 'failure to progress') and fetal distress are reasons given for a great number of caesareans.[28] While caregivers are right to monitor the progress of a woman's labour and her baby's safety, it is essential that they do so without actually causing a labour to become extended or a baby distressed. Most of the practices and interventions which are common on labour wards all over the world actually disrupt women's labours and cause fetal distress.[29] Lack of privacy, interruptions, alienation through the use of machines and impersonal practices, deprivation of food and drink, continuous or constant monitoring... all these are practices which disturb and therefore lengthen a woman's labour. An atmosphere of fear and tension, fetal scalp monitors and inappropriate physical positions—such as when the mother lies on her back— are ways of causing fetal distress.[30] It seems incredible that the needs of a labouring woman, not to mention the fetus, should be disregarded in the name of safety. It is not surprising that dystocia and fetal distress are the result.

One of the emailed conversations I had with Michel while writing this book relates to this problem. I had been wondering how often caesareans might need to be performed, in an ideal world...

Michel, if every woman were to begin labour spontaneously and were to labour undisturbed and unobserved, without pain relief or interventions, what do you imagine the rates of mortality and morbidity, and caesarean might be?

Imagine that the prerequisite to be an obstetrician or a midwife would be to be a mother who has a personal experience of vaginal unmedicated birth. I guess that the caesarean rate would drop below 10% with the same perinatal mortality rates and lower rates of transfer to paediatrics.

Is nature really that inefficient, though? Surely even a 1% caesarean rate would indicate extreme inefficiency in nature...

... or would be a reminder of the laws of natural selection. The huge development of the part of the brain called the neocortex (the brain of the intellect) is a handicap where childbirth is concerned. As long as the neocortex remains active, it tends to inhibit the activity of the primitive brain structures that are supposed to work hard during labour (releasing all the necessary hormones). That is the main reason why a difficult birth is an aspect of human nature. There are other reasons why human beings are condemned to have difficult births. One is that the fetal head is so large that it has to spiral down in a complex way inside the maternal pelvis. If we add the deep-rooted cultural misunderstanding of birth physiology, one can explain why the rates of caesarean sections are far above 1%.

Can you explain what you mean by 'the deep-rooted cultural misunderstanding of birth physiology'?

I mean a widespread, deep-rooted failure to understand the basic needs of women in labour. Recently, I attended a birth that could be used to illustrate my assumption that the current rates of caesareans would drop dramatically if the basic needs of women in labour were better understood.

Here's Michel's account of the birth... **Birthframe 25**

The woman who gave birth belongs to a family that is familiar with caesarean birth. Her brother, her sister and herself were born by caesarean. When she gave birth for the first time, it was decided after a long trial of labour in hospital that the baby was too big for her and that she needed a caesarean: the baby was 9lb (4kg). While she was expecting her second baby, she asked me if I would come to her home when the labour started, because she wanted to try to give birth vaginally. My answer was: "Yes, if I'm not in Costa Rica".

The labour started during the night preceding my flight to Costa Rica. I could stay in her home until she was in advanced labour, so that when she arrived at the hospital with Liliana (her doula), she was not far from a point of no return. She eventually gave birth with the help of ventouse to another 9lb baby.

When she was expecting her third baby, she asked me again if I might come to her home when she was in labour. My answer was: "Yes, if I'm not in Italy".

The labour started two days before my flight to Italy. There were ideal conditions of privacy. I was following the progress of labour from another room, through the sound. Liliana who, as a doula, behaves like a cat, was around, evaluating the progress of labour with her own criteria—postures, sound, breathing patterns, etc. I did only one vaginal exam.

At 12 noon, the father left in order to make some arrangements so that the children could stay in the house of friends. Soon after, there was a series of powerful contractions—a real 'fetus ejection reflex'. At 12.45 the ecstatic mother gave birth to an 11lb (5kg) girl... no drugs, no tears, no episiotomy.

For more accounts about Liliana, see Birthframes 6, 60, 61, 73, 77 and 91.

Assumptions reviewed

As we've seen, a caesarean does not seem to be the best way of giving birth unless it really is medically indicated. In fact, it is very far from being the ideal way of giving birth.[31] Having a normal, healthy birth will not affect your sex life as long as you follow the guidelines in this book so as to avoid drugs, episiotomy, tears and forceps. An optimal vaginal birth will be safer and more pleasant for both you and your baby—or babies!—both during the birth and afterwards. [32]

On the other hand, when caesareans are performed in order to safeguard the well-being of either the labouring woman or the baby, they are to be welcomed. It is, after all, thanks to the caesarean (as well as improved nutrition and sanitation and advances in the fields of antibiotics and anaesthesia, in particular) that childbirth is no longer the potentially life-threatening rite of passage for women that it once was.[33]

With this operation as a safety guard, we can now confidently leave the physiological processes to take place and have an unmedicated vaginal birth, knowing that if we or our baby are in danger, there is fast and effective surgery to rescue us. This represents a new vision of obstetrics, as Michel explains:

> My idea is to introduce a sort of futuristic strategy of childbirth which is partly what I have already practised. It is based on having a good understanding of physiology and of the basic needs of human beings in labour—for privacy, a sense of security, etc. If the midwife behaves in a motherly way and disturbs the woman as little as possible, either it works or a caesarean is necessary. This strategy makes it possible to avoid the two main alternatives as much as possible: drugs (which all have side-effects) and difficult interventions by the vaginal route (difficult forceps and so on). If we avoid these alternatives, there are really only two possibilities: a completely undisturbed physiological labour or a caesarean section.

But what if you still find it hard to think about giving birth vaginally? I suggest you read the rest of this book and note the feelings that women express after different kinds of births. Perhaps you should also focus particularly on the last chapter of this book... Help your mind!

If you feel you're rightly categorised as being high risk, do your own research, consult your heart and discuss your options with both experts and friends—not to mention your partner. While you're doing this, remember that risk assessment is always subjective, even when carried out by professionals. Even the opinions of the most senior midwives and consultants are influenced by personal experience, training, familiarity with research and personal levels of fear.[34] After you have come to some kind of conclusion as to the best approach, find a caregiver who will support you. There will be more on this in a later chapter... but for now we need to consider a few other key steps in order to prepare for an optimal birth. Surprisingly, perhaps, the next step is the most important one in terms of understanding and putting everything into practice.

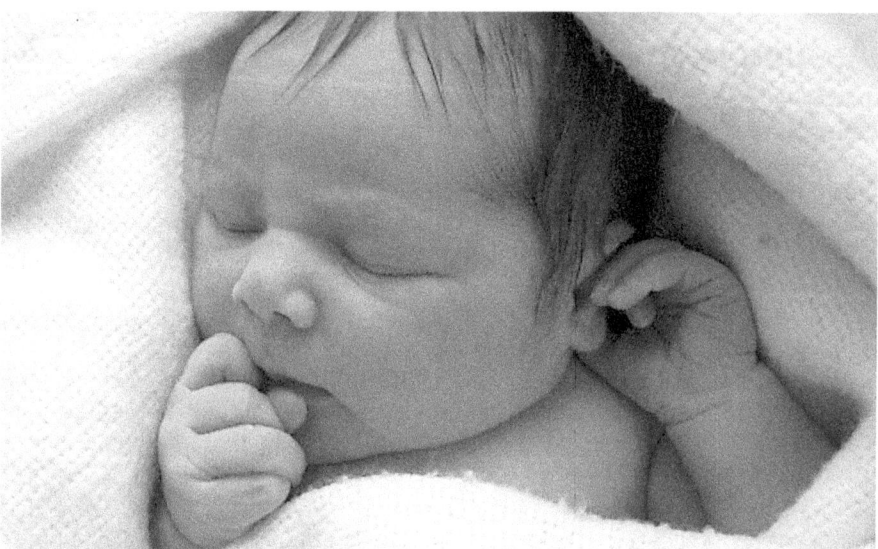

One of the optimally-birthed babies you will read about soon—another VBAC baby

8... DO NOT DISTURB

This is really a very simple step. It means not disturbing the processes at any stage in any way unless there is an extremely good reason for doing so. Of course, there are two problems. First of all, it's necessary to establish what constitutes a disturbance. Secondly, there is rarely full agreement as to when a disturbance is really necessary.

I get the impression many people think that nothing much constitutes a disturbance when it comes to birth... All kinds of people are invited along to watch, cameras and even camcorders are used, and medical personnel come in and out, frequently with no respect for the woman's privacy.[1] People freely talk to the labouring woman, unaware that this might have a profoundly negative effect. Midwives and consultants interrupt the labouring woman whenever they perform vaginal examinations or listen to the fetal heartbeat and they sometimes suggest hooking her up to an electronic fetal monitor, which usually limits her movements. Caregivers issue commands or make suggestions, they offer drugs and other options for pain relief and if they actually administer any they completely change the woman's internal chemistry.[2] They touch the woman and usually catch the baby, they offer comments and information without being asked (e.g. on the baby's gender) and they often interrupt early mother-baby interactions. All these things are done without any real concern that disturbance is a possibility.[3]

Reasons for these and other procedures are numerous and influenced by institutional or personal cultures. Although at times, there are excellent safety reasons for stepping in, sometimes caregivers, relatives or friends of the woman disturb things out of impatience. Sometimes their speech or actions are prompted by worry or fear, sometimes caregivers are following protocols and sometimes people do things out of habit. At times it may even be a desire to control a seemingly wild experience which prompts someone to cause a disturbance. And, of course, very often the processes of labour and birth are disturbed by attempts to alleviate pain. The idea that a woman is entirely capable of giving birth without anyone else's help is shocking to many people... even though it's true.[4]

The delicate cascade of hormones

The processes of birth are so delicate that many things can disturb a labouring woman and make her labour slower and more dangerous.[5] Just as one small jolt changes the pattern in a kaleidoscope or one mistake at work might have enormous repercussions, affecting numerous people, even one inappropriate action, comment, intervention or therapy can have a dramatic effect.

Disturbances can make labour slower and more dangerous

Disturbances can be very subtle because labour and birth are sexual experiences, and emotions are intricately intertwined with hormones—as the adrenaline produced in response to fear proves. As you may know, even a mistimed comment or wrong movement during sex can take a person 'out' of the mood. If a person outside the experience should also come along... well that might *really* change outcomes. States of mind are very important and things proceed most smoothly if people involved drift off into a different, totally absorbed state of mind. To do this, a feeling of privacy and security is necessary... in other words, the labouring woman needs to be undisturbed!

So often women have told me they wanted a natural birth, but it didn't work out. After listening to them it has been quite easy to pinpoint the disturbance which occurred in their labour and in almost all the cases I've come across it was a disturbance which wasn't at all necessary from a safety point of view. I have been amazed by the predictability of this element in 'failed' natural births. What has saddened me is people's apparent unawareness of disturbance. Again and again, the assumption that nothing can possibly 'disturb' birthing processes emerges. In one article I read in a popular women's magazine, a woman expressed disappointment and sadness at not having the natural birth she'd wished for *after being induced.* What did she expect? Induction is an enormous intervention, whether by ARM, sweeping of the membranes, prostaglandin pessaries or administering syntocinon. In the same way, I've been repeatedly amazed that women who've had epidurals have then expected the physiological processes to proceed smoothly. After any major intervention, such as induction or the use of drug-based pain relief, medical management is essential for the sake of safety. In his book *Birth Reborn* (Souvenir Press 1994) Michel commented that the more medicine gets involved with childbirth, the more complex and difficult everything becomes. It's no wonder that the phenomenon of the 'cascade of interventions' has become so well-known. Often what started out seeming 'helpful' ends up being a trigger for another problem and another intervention. By definition, disturbing things means changing them in some way, and this is particularly the case with birth.

The outcome of disturbance is a disturbed birth, which is less safe, less beautiful and less peaceful. The labour is usually much longer, the birth more traumatic for both mother and baby and postnatal experiences are usually entirely different. There are short- or longer-term side-effects to all the drugs and interventions which are now commonly used during pregnancy, labour and birth.[6] Everything—even herbal 'remedies' and acupuncture—may have side-effects. The pain relieved by drug-based 'pain relief' is replaced by numerous other problems either during or after the birth and these problems involve physical and/or emotional pain for either or both mother and baby. This is why I think the phrase 'pain relief' is a misnomer. The experience of so many mothers seems to suggest that both mother and baby have a less fulfilling experience of birth when drug-based 'pain relief' is used. The mother simply replaces one type of pain with another, which usually lasts much longer.

There's another problem with a great deal of approaches to pain relief of either a conventional or a complementary kind: it is usually necessary to bring an extra person into the labour room. This is not good because it's bound to disturb the labouring woman. As I've already pointed out, Michel has observed that the more people are around during a labour, the longer the labour.

Does this all surprise you? It's true that sometimes things do proceed toward a happy conclusion despite any number of disturbances... but usually they don't. We can only be sure we will produce all the right hormones at the right moment if we leave the processes of pregnancy, labour and birth undisturbed. The physiological processes are so complex that changing just one aspect of what's going on affects everything else.

When processes remain truly undisturbed, the outcome is usually beautiful for both mother and child... and perhaps for a wider circle of people too.

Healthy, physiological childbirth can help to initiate us into motherhood— or renewed motherhood if it's not our first baby. This initiation embraces psychological, physical and practical aspects of the mother-child experience because both our own and our baby's hormones and instincts are allowed to flow as nature intended.

It's understandable if you find it difficult to accept this at this stage. In order to really understand the complexity and be able to respect the delicacy of the normal, healthy processes, you need to know more about them. It's true that many pregnant teenagers have fast, easy labours precisely because they have no expectations, but others are paralysed by fear because they're afraid of what they don't know. Let's find out more about the precise hormonal processes of pregnancy and birth. Basically, as you'll see from the summary on the next few pages, each hormone seems to trigger specific events or behaviour. Instead of a 'cascade of interventions', there's a helpful cascade of hormones.[7]

For the following details, I'm indebted to Sarah J Buckley, who originally researched this area. Sarah is a trained GP/family physician, an internationally-acclaimed writer on gentle choices in pregnancy, birth, and parenting, and mother to Emma, Zoe, Jacob and Maia, all born gently at home, 1990 to 2000. Sarah's writing critiques current practices in pregnancy, birth, and parenting from a scientific as well as a personal viewpoint. She encourages us to be fully informed in our decision-making, to listen to our hearts and our intuition, and to claim our rightful role as the real experts in our bodies and our children. She has experienced almost everything that she writes about. Sarah has been writing about pregnancy, birth and parenting for more than 10 years. Her book *Gentle Birth, Gentle Mothering: A Doctor's Guide to Natural Childbirth and Gentle Early Parenting* (Celestial Arts 2009) contains her distilled wisdom, as well as a complete overview of research in these important areas. (Other texts by Sarah are reproduced here with her kind permission, provided before the above title was planned. See her book for the full texts.)

THE HORMONAL COCKTAIL OF PREGNANCY

The first hormone noticed in pregnancy tests is, of course, human chorionic gonadotropin (hCG). Progesterone, which is initially produced by the ovaries (stimulated to do so by hCG) and later by the placenta, will already have prepared the womb for pregnancy by stimulating the uterine lining to thicken (so that the fertilised egg can implant itself).

Progesterone also has the important functions of stopping the uterine muscles from contracting (thus allowing the fetus to grow undisturbed) and of stopping lactation from beginning until after the birth. It also protects the placenta by fighting off unwanted cells and strengthens the mucous plug, thereby preventing infection.

Fetal growth and maternal breast development, is supported by another hormone called human placental lactogen (HPL) and this hormone also has the important job of ensuring that the mother doesn't absorb too much glucose. Oestrogen, a group of hormones, is also vital and is thought to trigger the maturation of fetal lungs, kidneys, liver and adrenal glands, the production of prolactin, which prepares the woman for breastfeeding, and to regulate bone density in the fetus, amongst other things.

Other hormones—calcitonin, thyroxine, insulin, relaxin, cortisol and erythropoietin also play key roles. Oxytocin has a key role in pregnancy too, although is 'drowned out' by progesterone until the woman goes into labour. However, as well as stimulating the mammary glands to produce milk, it enhances nutrient absorption and helps the woman conserve her energy by making her sleepy![8]

THE HORMONALLY TRIGGERED SWITCH TO 'INSTINCTUAL'

According to research, since the hormones of birth are produced mainly in the 'middle' brain (sometimes called the 'mammalian' brain or limbic system), an important switchover needs to take place sometime in the early stages of labour. Instead of being controlled by the neocortex (which makes us rational beings), as is normally the case, the woman must suddenly surrender control to this more primitive part of the brain. Hormones which she spontaneously produces will allow her to effect this important switchover.

Interestingly, these hormones (which allow a woman to experience labour as positive and even enjoyable) also trigger appropriate mothering behaviour after the baby is born, so they have two important purposes. What's more, beta-endorphins, which are produced during pregnancy, begin to be produced at much higher levels, along with CRH (another hormone produced in stressful situations) at this stage. Rising levels of beta-endorphins now and during labour, which peak at birth and subside one to three days after the birth, help the mother to cope with pain and perhaps even experience it as positive. And they also help her to get into an appropriate instinctual state of mind.

THE HORMONES OF LABOUR AND BIRTH

Despite all we that we know about birth, it is still not known precisely what triggers the onset of labour, but both oestrogen and progesterone are thought to play a part, perhaps because of their changing ratios.[9] Of course, oestrogen is the main hormone which prepares the uterus for the contractions of labour[10] and both hormones also serve the important function of activating the woman's normal opiate-producing mechanisms which operate in the brain and the spinal cord.[11]

Produced in the hypothalamus and released into the bloodstream in a pulsatile manner, oxytocin is associated with positive emotions and sensations. Often called 'the hormone of love',[12] it is produced during orgasm, birth itself, breastfeeding and also in social situations such as eating with other people.[13] (Interestingly, perhaps, the baby produces this hormone as well as the birthing woman and even the placenta, so the fetus is swimming in oxytocin-flavored amniotic fluid![14] Because of this strange fetal hormonal production at the onset of labour some researchers have suggested that the baby may be responsible for triggering the onset of labour.)[15] Wherever it comes from (i.e. baby, mother or placenta), while oxytocin is thought to be the main initiator of rhythmic contractions, some researchers have hypothesised that prostaglandins assume this same role later on in labour.[16] Interestingly, oxtytocin has been shown to relieve pain in pregnant rats and mice.[17]

Oxytocin is responsible not only for the contractions which open up the labouring woman's cervix, but also for those which push the baby down and out of her body[18] and for the contractions which make her uterus contract back to its pre-pregnancy size after the birth. Intriguingly, though, something interesting occurs just before the moment of birth in the case of a woman who has been completely undisturbed while in labour. Catecholamines—the fight-or-flight hormones adrenaline and noradrenaline, along with dopamine—are produced alongside oxytocin.[19] (These hormones are usually antagonistic, but they aren't when they are produced spontaneously and smoothly in labour.) Instead of stimulating the body to fight or flee (as they usually do), just seconds before the birth these hormones activate what some researchers (particularly Michel Odent) have called the 'fetus ejection reflex'. From the labouring woman's point of view, there is a rush of energy which makes her want to stand up and perhaps also grab hold of something. (Any birth attendants, including a much-loved midwife, might be abused or shouted at around this time! Frequently, the woman expresses intense fear, anger or resentment.) The woman then flicks her hips forward and gives birth! The intense, highly efficient contractions stimulated by the high levels of oxytocin combine with these catecholamines to produce the perfect cocktail for birth. As for the baby, the sudden surge of catecholamines (especially noradrenaline) has a beneficial effect because it protects him or her from the effects of oxygen deprivation, helps metabolistic processes and temperature regulation and improves respiration—which will come in handy outside the womb, in the big wide world.[20]

HORMONAL PRODUCTION SHORTLY AFTER THE BIRTH

After the birth, uterine contractions are made possible because the newborn baby helps the mother to continue producing oxytocin. His or her stroking, licking or sucking actions, alongside skin-to-skin and eye contact, trigger a loving response in the mother, which results in continued hormonal production.[21] Most importantly, perhaps, all this pleasant 'bonding' which facilitates efficient uterine contraction has a safety function because it prevents a woman from suffering from a postpartum haemorrhage (PPH). (On this point, though, it's important to remember the role of catecholamines. While they were useful at the point of birth, their usefulness disappears straight afterwards. If levels do not drop—which is likely to occur if the new mother feels cold—oxytocin production will be inhibited, which will obviously increase the risk of PPH. When they do drop, although this is positive in terms of safety, the mother typically feels shaky or cold. Research has found that oxytocin levels in the mother peak when the placenta is born and then subside over the next hour.[22] Levels of oxytocin in the newborn baby peak around 30 minutes after the birth, but are still high for at least four days after the birth.[23] This generally means that both mother and newborn baby enjoy the pleasant effects of oxytocin in the first hour after the birth and afterwards. High catecholamine levels at the moment of birth also cause extreme alertness in the baby.[24] Levels typically remain high for around 12 hours,[25] then subside so a much-needed rest is possible. Noradrenalin, another hormone which is produced spontaneously at this time, is thought to promote mothering behaviour because mice who were bred to be deficient in this didn't care for their young unless they had an artificial injection of the hormone. (It's interesting to note that smell probably also plays a key role in early mothering behaviour.[26] One research study discovered that monkeys who were given caesareans rejected their babies unless the newborns were swabbed with secretions from the mother monkey's vagina.)[27] Prolactin, the main hormone stimulating breastfeeding, also causes mothering behaviour,[28] as well as an increase in appetite (in the mother), suppression of fertility and changes in sleep cycles (which suddenly include more REM sleep), amongst other things. Of course, these changes support the new mother's abrupt shift in lifestyle, which is bound to include a need for a focus on the newborn baby (even in sleep), to the detriment of the mother's own needs.

Finally, the beta-endorphins which began rising at the onset of labour[29] continue to play an important role in the mother-infant breastfeeding relationship.[30] With their ability to induce feelings of pleasure and dependency, they usefully help cement the mother-baby bond. Since they peak around 20 minutes after a woman starts breastfeeding at any one time, they continue to enhance the mother-infant relationship long after the birth took place.[31]

Given the extreme complexity of all the processes described here—which, we must remember, only take place like this in a completely undisturbed labour and birth—it's easy to see how easily things might be disturbed.

What constitutes a disturbance?

A disturbance is any event or action which changes the course of events during conception, pregnancy, labour, birth or the postnatal period.

PREGNANCY

During pregnancy in particular there's enormous scope for 'disturbance' because we're constantly ingesting food, drink and chemicals and we're usually offered lots of tests too. In very practical terms, how can we leave the physiological processes undisturbed?

The answer is to only allow your caregivers to give you tests which you perceive to be non-invasive, unless you are convinced they are vital for either your own or your baby's health. What kind of test is invasive? Many caregivers have a very broad definition, but I personally decided to refuse ultrasound scans, amniocentesis, chorionic villus sampling, electronic fetal monitoring, Doppler Sonicaid (the device which is often used to check the baby's heartbeat during pregnancy and labour) and fetal scalp blood sampling—because these all disturb the baby in some way or other. (You may wish to choose to accept infrequent monitoring with a Sonicaid during your actual labour if you feel this will disturb you less than the use of a Pinard stethoscope. I chose the Pinard but only had it used once or twice during each of my labours.) I also agreed to only very few internal vaginal examinations because of the risk of infection. Examples of non-invasive tests include any test which involves the use of a urine or blood sample—from you, not your baby—or external, unobtrusive observation of you or your baby's behaviour without the use of ultrasound.[32]

> The obstetrician said, "Unless we have a reason to examine you, I don't really want to because it might cause you to start opening." So I hadn't been examined for a while.

> When I was in labour I had a strange feeling. I was in another state of mind, yet at the same time rational thoughts occasionally passed through my head. I didn't speak any of them, they were just something I was aware of. Fortunately, no one spoke to me either. And while I was in this deep state, my body just did what it had to do. It was very powerful. Thank goodness nobody disturbed me.

In a way, in order to make sure our pregnancy isn't disturbed, we need to give up the idea that we can control everything—or that our caregivers can. If we're basically healthy, the best we can do is nothing at all. After all, doing something is likely to disturb the delicate balance of what's going on. And even if we can ascertain the effects of one antenatal test, we can't be sure what kind of cumulative effect tests might have on the physiology and psychology of the baby growing within us or on our own body and mind. We need to have confidence in our body's ability to grow a baby. It really can do it without help!

Ensure that no powerful herbs, hormones, chemicals or medicines enter your body in any way. This means being careful about herb teas which are marketed as harmless, caffeine-free alternatives to coffee and tea; it means reducing your use of herbs in cooking—especially fresh ones, which are stronger than dried ones; it means avoiding foods which are naturally high in oestrogens (e.g. liquorice) because these might make you go into labour prematurely; it means staying clear of complementary treatments, including those which are marketed as 'harmless' to pregnant women; it means steering clear of most beauty treatments; it means stopping using all over-the-counter or prescribed drugs—even innocent-sounding aspirin.

Avoid any activities or treatments which may disturb your mind or body in some way. This means avoiding any dangerous sports while you're pregnant; it means no acupuncture or shiatsu; it means no horror films or psycho-spiritual practices which could upset you or your baby. Use your own intuition to judge what is acceptable and helpful and what constitutes a disturbance to what is going on within you. I personally decided not to have my legs waxed while pregnant!

Above all, make sure nobody brings your pregnancy to an abrupt end by breaking your waters, sweeping the membranes or inducing you with syntocinon, which is artificial oxytocin.

Birthframe 26

The practicalities of asserting my wishes were difficult...

During all my pregnancies I was repeatedly asked to justify why I was refusing invasive tests and often people tried to force them on me. The idea of leaving the baby to develop at his or her own pace, undisturbed and undistressed, was apparently not considered important. The priority was to disturb the healthy processes so as to 'check' that everything was OK. At every antenatal appointment I had to remind the midwife (whoever it happened to be that time) that I didn't want her to use a Sonicaid. Sometimes a midwife would make a fuss about having to find the fetal stethoscope which didn't use ultrasound. They all seemed reluctant to honour my request for no ultrasound unless absolutely necessary.

I was instructed to go for an ultrasound once because my midwife at that time was concerned about inadequate fetal growth. I refused, mentioning that it was in the previous week that both my overcoat and my maternity trousers had become too tight. I felt sure I must be growing out at the sides, rather than straight out at the front. This suggestion was, of course, mocked and I was made to feel irresponsible and uncooperative. Several weeks later my baby was born at a very healthy weight. A friend who was also asked to have a scan for the same reason agreed to go along; she was simply reassured the baby was growing fine, after all.

LABOUR

A medical examination can trigger a physical reaction—either prompting your cervix to dilate or to stay firmly closed. Watching a hilarious or frightening film can trigger labour. Even a comment from an insensitive caregiver can constitute a disturbance while you're working through contractions because a labouring woman is especially sensitive at this time. It is better to be left alone while you are labouring and giving birth than to spend time amongst people who are likely to disturb you.

Here, in an adapted extract from *Birth and Breastfeeding* (Clairview Books 2007), Michel explains why our minds need to remain undisturbed and how it is that our bodies tap into their instinctual knowledge about giving birth:

The activity of the primitive brain prevails during the process of birth. We share this primitive or archaic brain with all the mammals. It is old also in the sense that it reaches maturity very early on in our lives, at the age when we are still dependent on our mothers. It cannot be dissociated from the hormonal system and the immune system, with which it forms a complex network. This network itself represents the adaptive systems involved in what we commonly call 'health'. The archaic brain, which governs the emotions and instincts, can also be looked on as a gland releasing the hormones necessary for the process of birth, inducing efficient uterine contractions, and protecting against pain as well.

The process of birth is all the easier when the other brain, the new brain, takes a backseat. This new brain—the neocortex, whose huge development is the main feature of human beings—does not reach maturity before adulthood. Its activity during the process of birth only hinders the activity of the old brain. All inhibitions come from the neocortex during a delivery (and in any other event of the sexual life, as well). That is why, in a very spontaneous birth according to the method of the mammals, there is a stage when the woman seems to be cut off from our world, as if on her way to another planet. This changing level of consciousness is obviously related to a lesser degree of control by the new brain. Then the labouring woman is freed from any sort of inhibition. She dares to scream out; to open her sphincters; to forget about what she has learnt, what is cultural, even what is decent. That is why the best way to make a birth longer, more difficult, more painful (and more dangerous) is to stimulate the neocortex where all the inhibitions originate. The labouring woman needs to be protected from any sort of neocortical stimulation.

The neocortex can be stimulated by light, or by having to listen to people talking logically and rationally, or by being surrounded by people who behave like observers. A feeling of privacy, on the other hand, accompanies a reduction in neocortical control. The need for privacy, along with the need to feel secure, is a basic mammalian need in the period surrounding birth.

Let's be clear about this. Here, Michel is talking about a complete lack of disturbance. It is very different from a situation in which there is a lack of care or inappropriate care... where a woman's labour is disrupted, neglected or mismanaged.

Lack of disturbance is very different from lack of care

I remember once speaking to a very bitter German woman who'd given birth in Japan. Not speaking any Japanese, she'd nevertheless communicated her wish to have a natural labour. After three days in labour, she gave birth to a brain-damaged baby. I listened carefully to what she said and it was only after much reflection that I realised that there were various things that were odd about her account. Certain comments she'd made indicated clearly that her birth had not been at all 'natural'. For example, she'd mentioned in passing that she'd had to drag her drip, on its stand, to the pay phone, and had said what a nuisance this had been. This must have meant either that she was being denied all food and drink and had therefore been put on a glucose drip, or—a more likely scenario—that she was being administered pitocin in order to accelerate or induce her labour. It's very sad that she insisted on continuing in this situation for a full three days, before finally giving birth. She'd clearly had interventions, so the healthy processes had been disturbed. Her labour was then neglected at her own insistence.

Perhaps this is not such an uncommon scenario, not because of the communication difficulties which were obviously a factor in this birth story, but because lack of understanding on the part of women or caregivers as to what really constitutes disturbance. Very often, midwives will talk about or suggest procedures which disturb the labouring woman, without realising that they are doing anything disruptive. The labouring woman will then insist on continuing in a disturbed situation because of a misguided view about natural birth. This is sad because really we have a choice between leaving nature alone completely or disturbing it and having a very 'managed' labour. Unless we are extremely lucky, there is usually no middle road.[33]

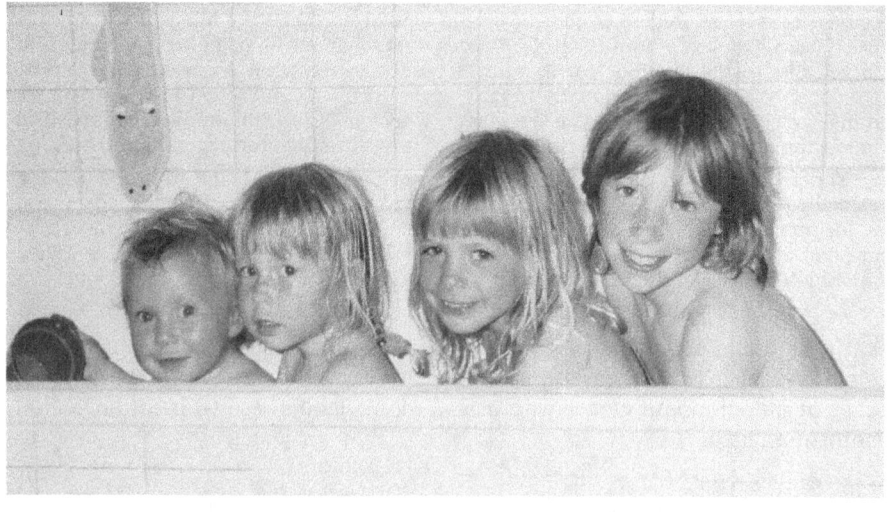

Anyone who's ever let children play in the bath knows the difference between disturbance and negligence...

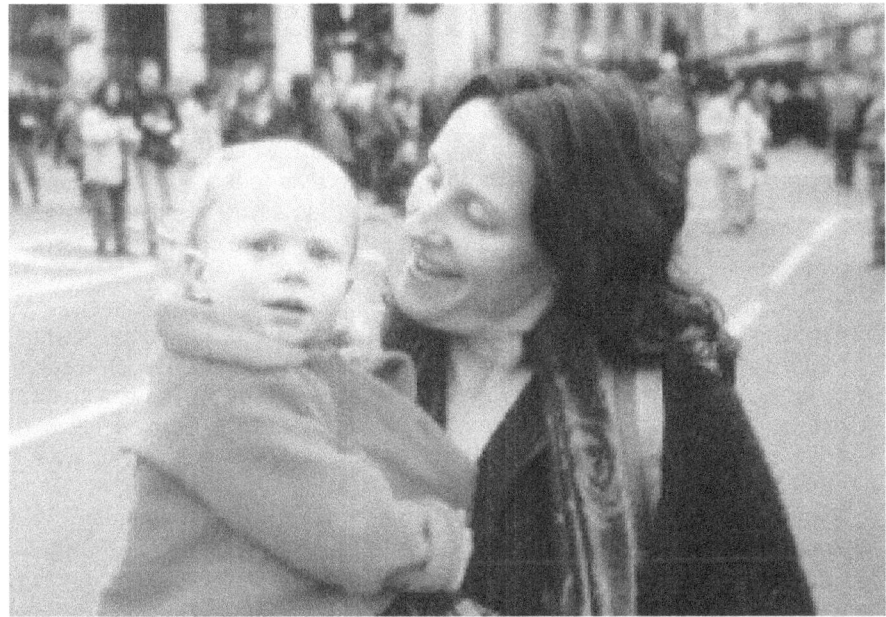

A woman and baby several months after an undisturbed birth. (See Birthframe 95.)

All very well for women who are perfectly healthy, you might say, but what about those who have problems? I asked Michel about this...

I have read that you have said the higher risk the woman the more important it is that she remains undisturbed during labour. The conventional approach seems to be the opposite—i.e. women who are high risk are told they will be monitored very closely. Do you think it is important that all women are left to labour undisturbed, or would you make exceptions in certain cases?

This is the basis of the art of midwifery: to know what is happening without disturbing. I wrote chapters about that, particularly in my book *Birth and Breastfeeding* (Clairview Books 2007).

So I assume you're saying that this can be achieved if (1) the midwife observes without giving the labouring woman the feeling of being observed, if (2) he or she uses a Sonicaid to monitor the fetal heartbeat—or watchful waiting if conditions seem to be good, if (3) the midwife makes sure there is no disturbance between first and second stage and again between second and third stage... and if (4) the midwife stays out of the way at these times too, i.e. throughout the length of the process—for example, by remaining in an adjoining room while the mother-to-be labours and gives birth alone. Have I forgotten anything? Do you think it's always best if the woman gives birth alone, without the help or support of a midwife or other attendant?

The key word is privacy. It does not mean loneliness. Privacy is compatible with the presence of somebody who does not behave like an observer or a guide.

BIRTH

As you may be realising, this is the most crucial time of all, from the point of view of safety, apart from anything else. Tell your caregivers that...

- ♥ Nobody should talk to you while you are in labour, while you're giving birth or before the placenta has been born, unless they feel it's an emergency. Responses to any question you ask or requests you make should be minimal—e.g. 'OK'. Any communication between people involved in your care should take place out of earshot.[34]
- ♥ You want to be left alone unless you specifically request something (e.g. candlelight, a bowl, a hot bath, or some specific music). Some of your requests need to be ignored even then because women often reach a crisis of confidence a few moments before the actual birth. (A request for an enema or for pain relief can be ignored, for example, if you have specified in advance that you do not want these things.) Silence, a few reassuring words or a smile—'You're doing fine'—is all you birth attendants need to give you in the way of 'help'. Your courage is likely to return after a few moments.
- ♥ You want your birth attendants to ensure that you feel completely unobserved. Mainly, this will mean keeping out of your way so that you can gradually sink into another state of mind and 'go to another planet' where your instincts will tell you what to do. There should also be no cameras or camcorders around until well after the birth.
- ♥ For safety reasons, nobody should come towards you or enter the room where you are when your baby has been born until after the placenta has been born. If a midwife has 'caught' the baby, he or she should quietly wait out of sight while you relate to your new baby. No comment should be made or question asked. (You can find out whether it's a boy or girl in your own time.) Your caregiver should only step in to help you if you or your baby are clearly experiencing difficulty. The initial Apgar scoring can easily be calculated by distant observation. This non-disturbance is vital at this stage because disturbance would dramatically increase the risk of postpartum haemorrhage, which used to be a major cause of maternal death.[35]

Does this all seem like an awful lot of non-disturbance? The physiological processes are even more subtle than we may imagine and disturbing them can mean simply not leaving them 'alone' enough to proceed in complete quiet and privacy. As we've seen in many birthframes already, many women do still manage to give birth without drugs and intervention even when they're disturbed to some extent, but many don't. (Their stories are the ones which have become very typical, unfortunately.) When women's births are disturbed to some extent, is their experience as straightforward, safe and satisfying as it could be? Having experienced the difference between disturbance (in the form of talking and observation) and complete non-disturbance, I would say it's definitely better to aim for complete non-disturbance.

You see, in order to give ourselves and our babies the very best chance for a safe birth, we need to change many aspects of birthing environments which have become commonplace. Bright hospital lights, forms to fill in, midwives who 'chat', delivery rooms which women need to be transferred to at a key moment. All these and more need to be changed if we are to cater to our real needs in labour.

Sarah Buckley explains this in more detail...

The term 'undisturbed birth' came to have great meaning for me when I gave birth to my fourth baby, Maia, at home, with only my family—including my medically qualified husband—present. This beautiful experience awakened me anew to the ecstasy of birth, and I realised that the process of birth can be very simple, if we avoid disturbing it. Comparing this birth to my three previous midwife-assisted home births, and to home and hospital births that I had attended, I saw also how ingrained is our habit of disturbance, and that our need to 'do something' so often becomes self-fulfilling in the birth room.

I realised that birth is also very complex, and that the process is exquisitely sensitive to outside influences. The parallels between making love and giving birth became very clear to me, not only in terms of passion and love, but also because we need essentially the same conditions for both experiences—to feel private, safe and unobserved. Yet the conditions that we provide for birthing women are almost diametrically opposed to these. No wonder giving birth is so difficult for most women today.

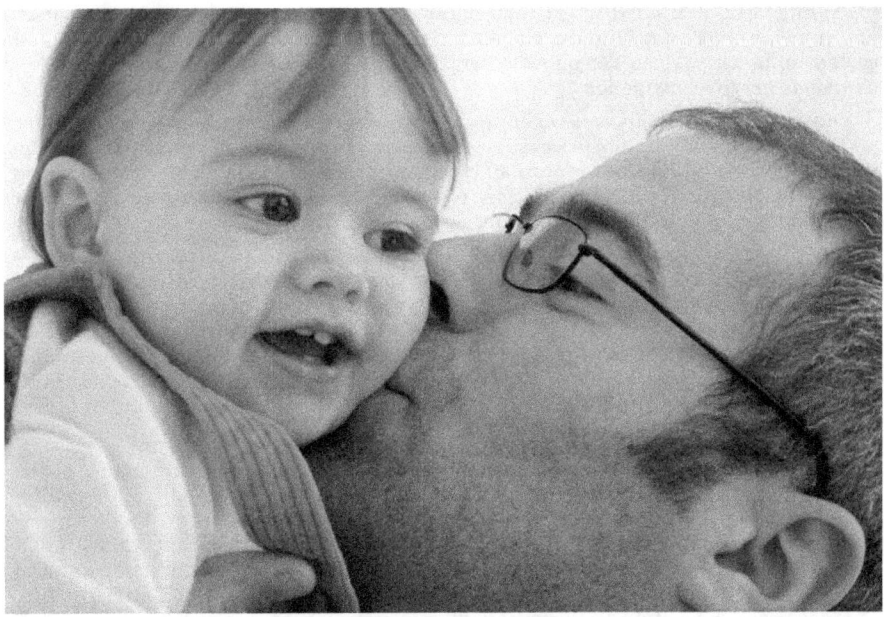

Of course, we need to remember that disturbance may also affect our partner. Early problems after the birth can sometimes affect longer term relationships.

Photo © Colin Smith

The processes are even more subtle than we may imagine

I came to realise first-hand that anything that disturbs a labouring woman's sense of safety and privacy will disrupt the birth process. This definition covers most of modern obstetrics, which has created an entire industry around the observation and monitoring of pregnant and birthing women. Some of the techniques used are painful or uncomfortable, most involve some transgression of bodily and/or social boundaries and almost all are performed by people who are essentially strangers to the woman herself.

All of these factors are disruptive to pregnant and birthing women. Underlying these procedures, is a deep distrust of women's bodies, and of the natural processes of gestation and birth, and this attitude in itself has a strong nocebo (fear-inducing), or noxious effect.

On top of this, is another obstetric layer devoted to correcting the 'dysfunctional labour' that such disruption is likely to produce. The resulting distortion of the process of birth—what we might call 'disturbed birth'—has come to be what women expect when they have a baby and perhaps, in a strange circularity, it works. Under this model, women are almost certain to 'need' the interventions that the medical model promotes and to come away grateful to be 'saved', no matter how difficult or traumatic their experience.

These disturbances are counterproductive for midwives also. When a midwife's time and focus is taken up with monitoring and recording, she is less able to be 'with women' as the guardian of natural birth. When her intuitive skills and simple ways of knowing have been buried in service to the system, more and more invasive procedures will be needed to get information that, in other times, a midwife's heart and hands would have illuminated. And when a woman misses out on the joy and ecstasy of birth, so does her midwife, which will influence her expectations of birth, as well as her job satisfaction.

Our bodies have their own wisdom, and our innate system of birth, refined over 100,000 generations, is not so easily overpowered. This system—what I am calling undisturbed birth—has the evolutionary stamp of approval, not only because it is safe and efficient for the vast majority of mothers and babies, but also because it incorporates our hormonal blueprint for ecstasy in birth.

When birth is undisturbed, our birthing hormones can take us into ecstasy—outside (ec) our usual state (stasis)—so that we enter motherhood awakened and transformed. This is not just a good feeling; the post-birth hormones that suffuse the brains of a new mother and her baby also catalyse profound neurological or 'brain' changes. These changes give the new mother personal empowerment, physical strength and an intuitive sense of her baby's needs and prepare both partners for the pleasurable mutual dependency that will ensure a mother's care and protection, and her baby's survival.[36]

Undisturbed birth, then, represents the smoothest hormonal orchestration of the birth process and therefore the easiest transition possible—physiologically, hormonally, psychologically and emotionally—from pregnancy and birth to new motherhood and lactation for each woman. When a mother's hormonal orchestration is undisturbed, her baby's safety is also enhanced, not only during labour and delivery but also in the critical transition from intra- to extra-uterine life. Furthermore, the optimal expression of a woman's 'motherhood hormones' will ensure that her growing child is well nurtured, adding another layer of evolutionary 'fitness' to the process of undisturbed birth.

Undisturbed birth does not mean unsupported birth, though. Some anthropologists believe that human females have sought assistance in birth since we began to walk on two legs. The change in our pelvic shape that accompanied our upright stance added uniquely complex twists and turns to our babies' journeys during birth, making assistance more necessary than for other mammals.[37] It does mean having supporters who we have specifically chosen as our familiar and loving companions; who are confident in our abilities, and who will intervene as little and as gently as possible.

Undisturbed birth does not mean painless birth either. Giving birth is a huge event, physically and psychologically, and makes demands on the body which are hormonally equivalent to endurance athletics.[38] But when a woman feels confident in her body, well supported, and able to express herself without inhibition, any painful feelings can become just one part of the process and something that she can respond to instinctively from her own resources using, for example, breath, sound and movement.

Finally, we must recognise that having an undisturbed birth will not guarantee an easy birth. There are many layers, both individual and cultural, that can impede us at birth. But when we approach birth with the intention of minimal disturbance, we are optimising the functioning of our birth hormones. This, coupled with our unparalleled levels of hygiene and nutrition, gives us a better chance of an easy and safe birth than any of our foremothers, from whom we have also inherited, through natural selection, the female anatomy and physiology that births most easily and

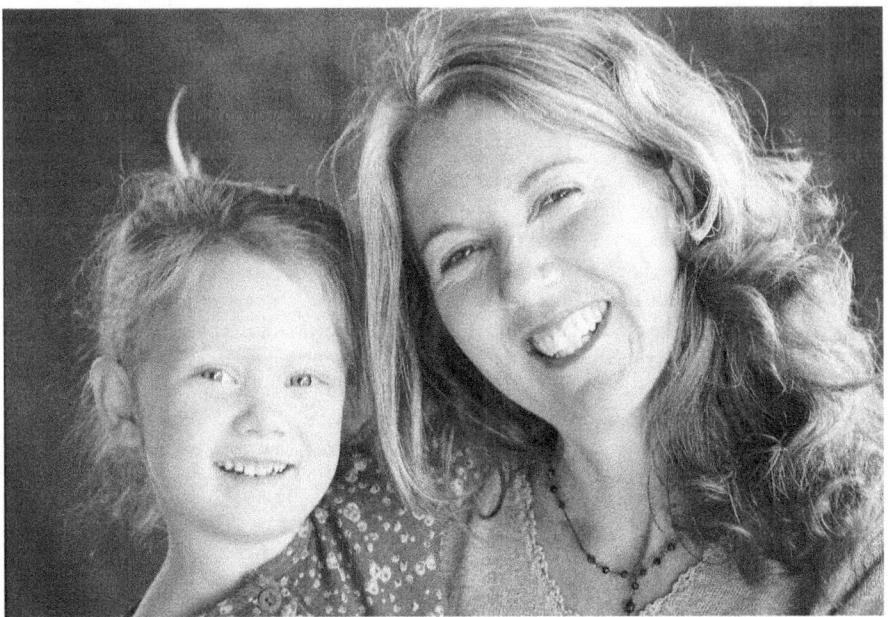

A more recent photo of Sarah with Maia, aged 3.

With minimal disturbance we are optimising birth

Birthframe 27

Next we meet Nuala OSullivan again, the woman whose beautiful birthing photos appear on pp 15 and 332. Here she describes her second daughter's birth and it is clear from her account how much non-disturbance, along with a feeling of security, was so crucial for her during this difficult posterior labour. Moving through the difficult moments in her safe but undisturbed environment, Nuala even managed to continue through to a face-to-pubis birth. (I know from my own first birth experience, just how difficult that can be.) And although Michel had been supremely focused on not disturbing Nuala while she was labouring and giving birth, he was clearly very much there when she needed him—to get her apparently lifeless baby breathing...

I booked Michel Odent for my second daughter's birth, having complete confidence in him and his approach to birth. I had first met Michel when I was being a birthing partner for a friend and watched her beautiful daughter emerging like a lithe Excalibur from the depths of the birthing pool. Michel had then helped me to deliver Ciara, respecting my labouring foibles. He not only accepted that I would soak anyone who came near me but also reassured the local beat police that in fact a child was being born and no one was being murdered despite the scary screams! His gentle consistency and faith in the labouring mother inspired confidence and allowed me to deliver as I had not believed I could.

I had complete confidence in Michel and his approach

Ciara had been 17 days late so when my due date of New Year's Eve came and went, and all the women in my yoga class delivered before me, I wasn't unusually perturbed. On Thursday, 14 January I made the journey to nursery with my toddler dancing forwards and back to keep pace with my slow gait. I was expecting that the 17 hours of Ciara's birth would be divided by three for this baby. Contractions were steady but only 10 minutes apart so I still felt safe and anyway knew people in the shops and houses all the way to the nursery. Her key worker and other parents were all excited for me and still maintained their enthusiasm when a day later we had only progressed to five minutes apart as we made the journey even more slowly. On Friday afternoon we went for a walk with the children and I sat on a see-saw with another parent to try to encourage contractions along. By the evening labour had become established.

Once Ciara was asleep I called Michel and he came

I bathed Ciara walking around our tiny bathroom as she sang to me. Once she was asleep I called Michel, who came to see me, reminding me to call at any time.

My dear friend, Fee, arrived and sat with me. With night and our relaxed energy there seemed to be a lull and, although they never stopped, the contractions didn't seem as powerful as they had been. All night we sat up awake but contractions weren't developing. We looked at the birthing space with the empty birthing pool dominating my bedroom. Located over a cement archway the bedroom was deemed the best room for taking the weight of a filled pool. I had scented oils, the same ones I'd used for Ciara and candles at the ready—remembering how light sensitive I'd been the last time and how I'd craved the cocoon of my room. The freezer had frozen lemon ice cubes for sipping later and there was plenty of cooled water in the fridge.

I was getting worried by the slow development of contractions but by 6am on Saturday contractions had re-established themselves more earnestly. Sally arrived early on Saturday followed by Danuta, my homeopath, and Jill Furmanovsky who had taken such precious pictures of Ciara's birth. Michel dropped in on his way for a swim, untroubled by what felt like established labour to me. I felt partially put out that my 'serious' labour didn't warrant any further attention and partially reassured that he was off for a swim, so delivery wasn't imminent.

Between contractions I dressed Ciara and she went off for the day with friends.

The day passed in a blur. I liked the sounds of the women around me as they talked, prepared meals and got on with other things somewhere on the periphery of my consciousness. I did not engage well with the group by this stage, didn't want people near me. All my social senses dulled, my need for attention became muted. Jill came and gave me a massage at the base of my spine as I had been rocking and could not get comfortable. It was welcome and comforting, and her gentle energy was calming. Mostly, I felt the need to be alone—to have them all somewhere near me, but as background rather than with me.

Michel seemed to materialise as stages progressed and then to fade into the background again. Fee came and sat quietly in the room, when she wasn't making drinks for everyone. Sally cared for Ciara and timed contractions from the kitchen, attuned to my sounds. Danuta checked on me and monitored changes in mood and energy but only sporadically as Michel was keen for me to be left in peace. He instructed that no one should make eye contact with me or disturb me unnecessarily. His protection of the birthing room was useful to me as I took myself out to deal with the contractions. I became acutely sensitive not only to light but even to whispering sounds from the other room.

Nothing was expected of anyone, so each found their own role.

I felt sick. The waves of nausea were welcome as they meant that my body was starting to work and would bring my baby to me. Contractions escalated and I was aware of how tired I had become after two sleepless nights so I began using self-hypnosis. As the contraction began I took myself out and when it released I came back in again. I begged to go into the pool and was heartened when I saw them filling it. It paced me through the next few contractions and gave me something new to focus on.

The police officer resolved never to have a baby!

The light faded and Ciara arrived home. Sally bathed her and I kept going in and out to change her story tape over—I was driven by an odd duty to be there for Ciara, even while labouring.

Because of Ciara, I think, there was no screaming this time and the contractions waned when I shifted attention from them to her. Ciara's birth had been loudly vociferous. As a trained soprano I had released each contraction with treble notes, as round and powerful as the labour itself. My neighbours knew I was labouring and were unconcerned but a passing beat pair called in to ensure that no murderous assault was in progress. Michel had protected me from prying eyes and the presence of extraneous visitors. Although the police wanted to see me, to set their fears to rest, Michel reassured them that all was as it should be and that I was having a baby. They returned the next day to ascertain that a baby really had been born with the police officer declaring that the sound had been 'bloodcurdling' and the woman police officer resolved never to have a baby after what she had heard! Yet Ciara's birth had been beautiful to me.

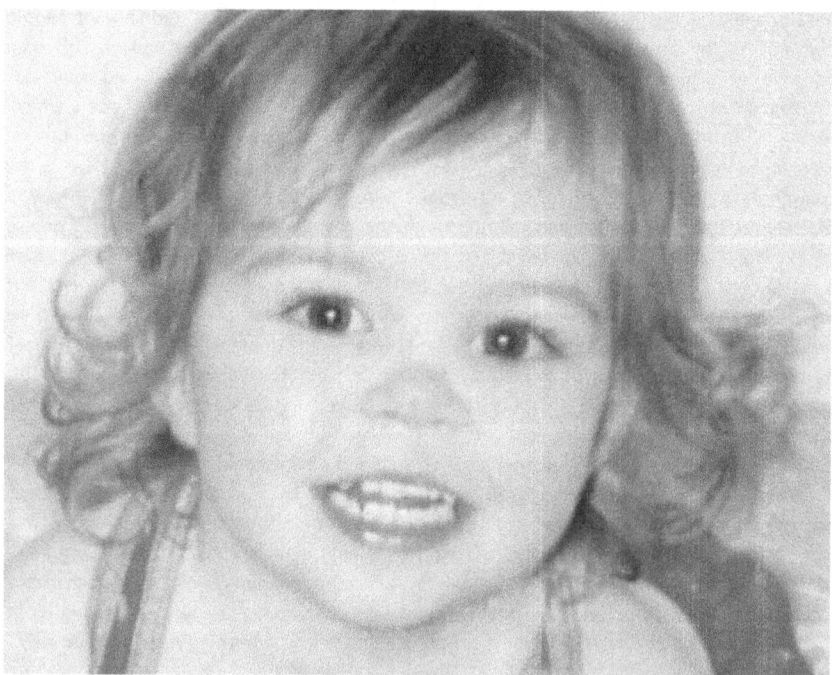

Nuala's 'baby', Isolde, aged 14 months, enjoying a dip in the swimming pool

Sally lay down with Ciara, and I could hear her telling Ciara about the night she was born and answering Ciara's questions until they both drifted off to sleep.

The landscape of pain established. If I had been told two hours or four hours more it would have helped me to put a shape and sense to it but there was no way of predicting. I was 5cm and in the pool. Contractions took me out and when they abated I floated. I kept telling myself I could do 'just that much' again. I drank and sipped ice cubes but couldn't communicate with anyone. I was glad they were there somewhere nearby, but not near me. I tried counting, moving, dancing, going in and out of the water until I was too tired to move from the warm water.

Michel came and monitored me and told me the baby was fine and coping well. That was all I needed to hear. I could keep going if the baby was coping, so this time I stood still to allow monitoring and didn't drench anyone. I could feel my leg wriggling ready to move away. I found the enforced sedentary pose intrusive but I brought all my reasoning to bear on keeping still for long enough for him to take a good reading. Then he moved away again, quietly leaving me to my own space, the journey of my baby and me, unfettered.

Contractions kept challenging me. Just as I got used to one level a new one opened up, demanding my full concentration. Sounds became excruciatingly magnified as all my senses heightened. I shouted to them in the kitchen to be quiet even though my own sounds were louder and they had only been whispering. Still, all complied with the unreasonable request.

> The pool no longer comforted me. I wanted to get out.
> I felt hot, cold and unable to find the centre any more.

My waters exploded like a water bomb in the pool. Sudden, shocking. Danuta was topping up the pool and took the opportunity to ask me how I felt... I told her: "Everything irritates me". "Nox Vomica," she muttered, and went off to find a remedy. I heard the book pages flipping from the kitchen as she studied. It was all too noisy. The pages were like flapping sails to my ears.

Within an hour of taking the remedy I went from 5cm to 10cm dilation and delivered. The last hour I found exhausting. The baby was aligned along my spine and not my front as Ciara had been. The pool no longer comforted me and I wanted to get out. I felt hot, cold and unable to find the centre of the contraction any more. My drive toward the birth and meeting my new baby wavered and I felt emotional and hesitant for the first time in over nine months. My 43-week pregnancy was drawing to a close. From nowhere I started to panic. I believed that I would not be able to bring my baby into the world. Then I felt the baby wasn't capable of going on this arduous journey.

Even as I crossed the bridge of transition I knew that if I could only get through it I would be able to deliver successfully.

Pushing started then and confidence returned. Here was a part I understood. I had a role and something to do with each contraction. I felt myself organising my body's responses and planning how I would greet the new contraction. I got out of the pool thinking that I needed to open my bowels and that once I had I could have my baby. Once in the bathroom I realised that the sensation was confused because my baby was on the base of my spine and was in fact crowning.

> Pushing started then and confidence returned. Here was a part I understood. I had a role.

I called out to them: "She's crowning!" As I staggered back to the bedroom, I noted to myself that even I had started to adopt Ciara's 'little sister' notions. The different voices passing on what I'd said didn't irritate me this time

Michel materialised, allowing me to find my position and my own connection with the contraction. I leant my hands against the wall and pushed. A head emerged with the cord round its neck and an arm up beside it, making the top centile head even wider. Michel deftly slipped the cord over the head. Another contraction and the rest of the baby slithered out, caught by Michel as I collapsed in a heap.

> I collapsed in a heap. Tired out but terrified.

Tired out but terrified. Because there was no sound. No crying.
A little grey daughter with no muscle tone and no sound.
3.6kg, 59cm and inert.
Michel was cradling my baby and sucking out her nose and throat. I splashed water from the pool to baptise her, desperate to do something for her.

> Michel was cradling her and sucking out her nose...

Then I heard the indignant sound of Isolda's own voice. Michel rewarded me by handing me my wailing daughter. Perfect.

Sally took her while the placenta was delivered. Despite having size 4 feet (related to the pelvis size?) and an 8lb (3.6kg) baby I didn't need any stitches![39] Everyone came around me to admire and meet Isolda Lily, each loving face welcome to me now. I bathed with her and then Ciara woke to meet her 'little sister'.

Ciara is 17 and taking 'A' levels now, and hoping to study to become a midwife in September. Isolda is 14 and 5' 6", preparing for GCSEs and aiming to be either CEO of ICI or a catwalk model—whichever happens first! In the meantime, she is curiously delighted with how she has turned out... which is refreshing for a teenager.

Nuala OSullivan

Facing the modern reality

Modern antenatal clinics and hospitals don't usually provide an ideal environment for lack of disturbance. Many medical professionals intervene for the reasons suggested before and more... Perhaps they feel they need to 'manage' the process of pregnancy, labour and birth, perhaps they are afraid of the processes, perhaps they simply lack faith in them, or perhaps they feel they need to be seen to be 'doing something'. Maybe caregivers offer drugs or treatments because they mistakenly believe they will prevent, relieve or eradicate pain. Some even claim their main motivation in operating as they do is a fear of litigation: by tracking everything (irrespective of whether it causes disturbance) they at least have extensive records of the trouble they took, which they feel is helpful in a court case, even if the truth is that it made the birth less safe.[40] And to make matters worse, relatives tend to come in with their camcorders...

> My first baby was a planned hospital birth. I expected to just turn up in labour, have the baby and come home. I did not really take on board the 'cascade of intervention' which can and does happen in hospitals to upset the natural balance of a labour that is going well.

> At some point in transition or second stage, the second midwife arrived—this is normal procedure, just in case both mother and baby need attention after the birth. Next, the contractions became more spaced out, and more painful.

> My husband used the camcorder immediately after the birth. I stopped him filming the birth, even though we'd planned to, because it felt like an intrusion.

> I was put under a lot of pressure to deliver the placenta after Kiz's birth. They had their arbitrary time limit of an hour and were planning on pulling on the cord if I hadn't managed to push it out when I did. I'm sure the fact that they had me sitting on a bed pan on a chair (extremely uncomfortable) meant that it took longer than it would otherwise. I had to lean on my hands to keep all my weight off the bed pan, which meant I couldn't hold Kizzy to breastfeed her. She suckled for the first time— held in position by the midwife—just before I pushed the placenta out.

Birthframe 28

As we've already noted, women often fail to have the birth they want because they don't understand where things could go wrong... where the processes could be disturbed. The birthframe on the next page is an unhappy example of this. 'A woman's intuition' is something that's often mentioned, but usually dismissed. In this case, the woman in question had a strong feeling that her upcoming birth needed to be natural. Unfortunately, though, she did not realise that in order for this to be possible she would have to say 'No' at one or many points in her pregnancy and labour. Not refusing one seemingly small intervention—allowing her waters to be broken—led to a cascade of interventions because her babies clearly were not ready to be born. In a way this woman did have the 'natural' birth she wanted, but it was one which made a mockery of what nature really has to offer. The writer of this birth story has submitted it and approved it (including this blurb and my commentary on the next page) because she wants her story to help other women. Incidentally, when I spoke to her over the phone she said she was glad she avoided a caesarean, even though she did not have quite the vaginal birth she had hoped for. [Names have been changed here, but all other details are exactly as in the original account.]

I gave birth to twin boys, Jamie and Sean, on April 24, 1997.

Ever since I found out I was pregnant with them I always told my husband I was going to have them the most natural way possible, no matter what.

I went for an antenatal check-up at 38 weeks and they told me I was 4cm dilated. They told me I had probably been in labour for a week since my mum and sister took me on a 10-mile walk the weekend before, which gave me backache.

They sent me up to the labour ward to monitor the babies. Around 5.00pm, they decided to break my waters. I was adamant they were not going to intervene but for the babies' sake they had to. For some reason, I was not having any contractions. They found Jamie was the wrong way round, not breech but as the doctors put it 'face-to-pubis' and stuck! He was not budging. All I could think of was not having a section. Under no circumstances was anyone going to make me have these babies unnaturally, after all it may be the only chance I have in life.

I was given an episiotomy but still Jamie was not budging. A while later they took me to the operating theatre. I told them I was not having a section so they decided to give me a spinal injection and as I was hooked up to a contraction monitor because I couldn't feel the contractions, I was told to push when I had them. Jamie came out with forceps at 4.39am and then Sean followed at 5.15am, after forceps and suction. I guess that was as natural as they could have made it for me.

> I didn't start to bond with them until they were about 12 months old. The doctors told me it was probably because of the birth—my body rejected the boys.

I did not start to bond with them until they were about 12 months old. I had a difficult time after it all. The doctors told me it was probably because of the birth. Because of what my body went through, it just rejected the boys. I guess it makes sense really.

Let's consider the interventions which occurred:
- There was no need for the vaginal examination at the 38-week check-up. These 'internals' have become common in some obstetric practices but they often create more problems then they solve. After all, what useful information do they really provide?
- There was no need to break this woman's waters. The waters help to cushion the presenting baby's head as it is pressed against the cervix and as soon as an amniotomy has been performed, since there is a risk of infection, the woman is under pressure to give birth.
- The electronic fetal monitoring, made necessary by the amniotomy, was unhelpful for two reasons. Firstly, the very fact of monitoring in this way must have created anxiety in the labouring woman, whose state of mind must be safeguarded at all times. It's hardly surprising her contractions stopped. Secondly, it would have compromised the babies' oxygen supply because women who are being monitored are almost always asked to remain immobile in a supine or leaning-back position. The fetal distress which the equipment is aiming to detect is actually created by these positions! What's more, a supine or lying-back position would have done nothing to help the babies get in a good position for birth. Leaning forward positions and moving around would have been much more helpful from this point of view.[41]
- The episiotomy clearly did nothing to help the birth of the first baby, so constituted another unnecessary intervention and would have caused the woman additional, unnecessary distress, not to mention pain or discomfort at best, for weeks or months after the birth.
- The spinal would no doubt have relieved the woman's pain but the anaesthesia would have made it difficult, if not impossible, for the woman to perceive what was happening within her as her babies were descending. Given that she was so keen to have a normal, healthy birth and spinals and epidurals, etc are well-known to increase the caesarean rate, precisely because of the lack of sensation that results, this woman might well have refused the spinal if she had not felt so disempowered during her labour and if she had realised the possible consequences.[42]

This woman's labour and postnatal experiences might have been very, very different...

So this woman's labour and postnatal experiences might have been very, very different if nature had been left to take its course. Left to her own devices, this woman probably would have gone into established labour spontaneously hours or even days after her 38-week antenatal appointment.

Birthframe 29

In case you're blasé about the possibility of a labour being disturbed, let me remind you about two forms of disturbance which have become commonplace: cameras and partners. We need to distance ourselves from these two very human kinds of disturbance and remember that we basically have the same needs as other mammals.

Here's an account from Michel...

A week ago on Sunday, I was at a conference in California. I was a keynote speaker. My topic was provocative. It was why and how we should dehumanise childbirth. There were two organisers, two midwives, Iona and Laura. Iona was pregnant and due quite soon—this month—and expecting her first baby. Laura, who herself had three children, was at the same time Iona's partner as a practising midwife, and also her midwife for this birth.

Iona introduced me on Saturday at about 11.30am and while I was speaking some people noticed that she was often touching her back. Then at about 3.00pm she had a rupture of membranes at the conference. So she went back home, which was about 20 minutes from there, with Laura. Luckily there was a third midwife involved in the organisation of the conference.

In the end, real labour started in the middle of the night and Iona gave birth on Sunday morning exactly a week ago. And I just heard before leaving (because I left on Sunday afternoon) that she had had a baby boy. But I called her yesterday to find out more. She told me an interesting story.

She told me there was a time when many women—when the baby was not far away—used to say, "Do something! I can't do it. I can't do it!" But Laura told her, "You can do it. You're a mammal!" [Hearty laughter.] Because of my lecture they had changed their approach. Originally, she had planned to give birth in front of some television cameras but then she heard me talking about privacy and cameras. I'd also said that it was important to be careful about the presence of the baby's father. So in the end she had much more privacy than she'd expected to have. It was her first baby and it was wonderful. And Laura had said twice, "You can do it! You're a mammal!"

"You can do it!" You're a mammal!"

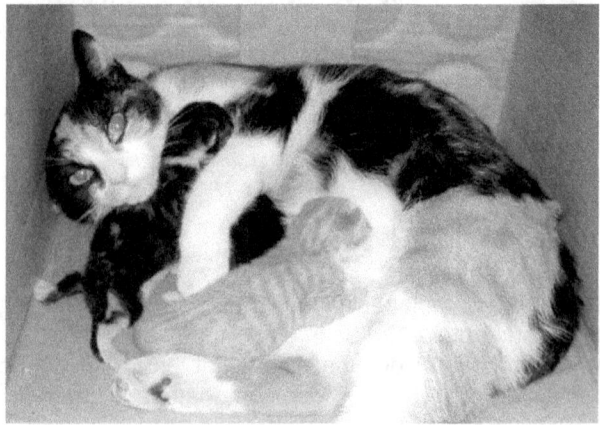

An example of a mammal... cats know how to give birth!

Why 'pain relief' really isn't a good option

Do you ever have doubts about your ability to do without pain relief? Do you ever wonder if you too could just function as a mammal and manage it all?[43] And is drug-based pain relief really such a big disturbance? Yes!

It's not difficult to imagine how using drugs can disturb the normal, healthy processes. Here's an overview of what's used...

- First there are sedatives and analgesics. A sedative (such as temazepam) is sometimes used to encourage a woman to sleep or rest. Analgesics (such as Tylenol and co-dydramol) act as mild to moderate painkillers. Inhalation analgesia (such as Entonox, i.e. 'gas and air') is used in the UK.
- Next we have narcotics—Demerol, Nisentil, Dolophine, diamorphine (which is actually 100% heroin), pentazocine (Fortral) and meptazinol (Meptid). These are even stronger drugs, which function as painkillers. Apparently, though, women widely complain that they don't mask the pain—they say they just make it more bearable. In cases where drugs theoretically have no pain 'ceiling' (i.e. they are all-powerful)—such as heroin—women lose alertness and awareness entirely. These narcotic drugs also weaken the newborn baby's suck, making breastfeeding difficult or impossible.
- You probably know what tranquilisers are. They include Valium, Vistaril and Penergan and are sometimes used in conjunction with narcotics (e.g. pethidine with Phenergen). They're given to women who are considered to be particularly tense.
- Barbiturates are rarely used nowadays because of the depressant effect they can have on the baby. Seconal and Nembutol are sometimes used if it's felt that the mother needs to be sedated.
- Amnestics are drugs which remove the memory of pain. The main example, hyoscine hydrobromide (known as scopolamine hydrobromide in the US), was widely used in the 1950s and is still occasionally used today.
- Local anaesthetics block sensation entirely in certain organs. However, they're not considered totally effective, so they're rarely used. The pudendal and perineal block are examples.
- Regional anaesthetics include epidurals, spinals, saddle blocks and paracervicals. When they're successful, they numb sensation completely in a specific area. However, they are not always successful, they carry risks and are not considered useful or desirable at all stages of labour.
- Finally, there's general anaesthesia, which results in complete unconsciousness. It's used for emergency caesareans because it allows the medical team to work slightly more quickly than they can when only regional anaesthesia is used. It's not used at other times because of the increased risks associated with general anaesthesia over local varieties and also because it's considered desirable for mothers to be alert at the time of their babies' births—for the sake of bonding, of course, apart from anything else.

These drugs have only been around for a few decades so it's important to remember the limitations of what we know. Drugs only began to be used widely for childbirth during the second half of the nineteenth century after Queen Victoria famously allowed chloroform to be used for the birth of her eighth child in 1853. In the twentieth century obstetricians continued to experiment with drugs against a backdrop of debates about religious, philosophical, social and political questions, as well as medical ones. The fact that drugs made women more compliant and less assertive in an age when women were still fighting for basic rights needs to be taken into account. (Ironically, women themselves often mistakenly saw them as a form of liberation.) Also, we need to bear in mind that drugs were primarily selected for their pain-relieving properties: the baby's welfare and the mother's wider experience were not seen as being a primary concern and breastfeeding has only recently been recognised for its health-giving benefits, so the effect on this was also not considered. The most popular pain-relief nowadays—the epidural—has only been widely available since the 1990s (after being developed in the 80s). No form of drug-based pain relief, including the epidural, has been thoroughly tested for its long-term effects on the baby. But side-effects for this and other forms of pain relief are already well-known and widely recognised, as we'll see in the next few pages.

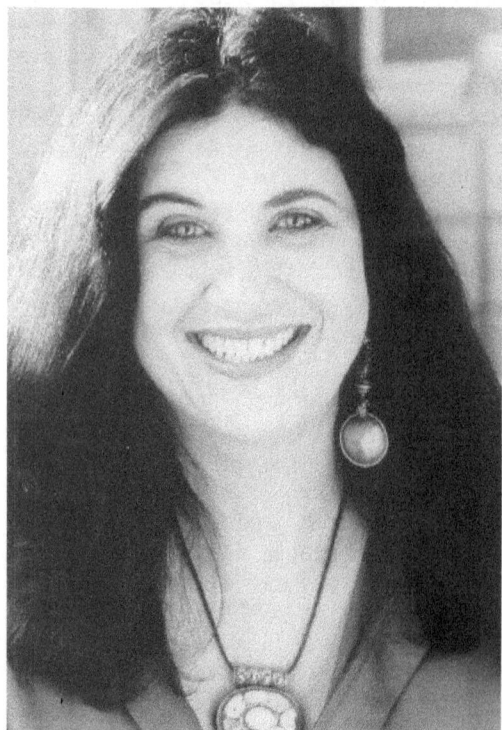

Side-effects for all drug-based forms of pain relief are already well-known and widely acknowledged

Janet Balaskas (left), who you can read about in Birthframe 83, gave birth in the late 1970s and 80s, which was the peak of the hi-tech era. At that time obstetricians actively managed birth: labour was induced at a convenient time, the baby was continuously electronically monitored and the mother wired up to an epidural. This horrified Janet because she felt sure we couldn't be the only mammals incapable of giving birth by ourselves. As you'll read in Birthframe 83, she found a better way of giving birth, which involved no drugs.

EPIDURALS

Epidurals are particularly worth finding out about because—as I pointed out in Birthframe 1—many women mistakenly seem to believe they promise no pain.[44] The reality can be quite the opposite. First, taking a purely straightforward epidural as our reference point, having an epidural involves accepting complete management of labour, which involves a loss of control and dignity... Here's some more detail on what an epidural really means:

- Continuous monitoring is necessary because the drugs in the epidural induce fetal heart decelerations which can be worrying enough to necessitate the use of fetal scalp blood sampling. Electronic monitoring for any reason is associated with an increase in caesarean rates, possibly because caregivers misinterpret or overreact to readings on the monitors.[45]
- The woman's blood pressure also needs to be constantly monitored because the epidural will cause it to fall to possibly dangerous levels. This fall in blood pressure can result in serious fetal distress because less oxygen is circulating in the woman's body.
- Intravenous fluids need to be administered to counteract the fall in blood pressure. These fluids can cause excessive swelling of the woman's feet, legs and breasts. Over-engorged breasts can make it difficult for the newborn to latch on.
- A catheter needs to be used to drain off the woman's urine, because the epidural numbs the woman's bladder too. The catheter must remain in place until the epidural has worn off. (Catheterisation also carries the risk of infection and may result in incontinence for as long as three months after the epidural has been used. A year after the epidural, incontinence is reported to be more common than for mothers who did not use one.)[46]
- The drip which is in place may also be used to administer syntocinon (synthetic oxytocin). This is likely because women's contractions often become weaker after the use of an epidural—probably because the woman feels disturbed, observed and 'managed'. Syntocinon produces unnaturally strong and long contractions which can also cause fetal distress by depriving the baby of oxygen.[47]

On a very basic level, all this 'management' means it's impossible for a woman to 'go to another planet' and experience what Michel calls the fetus ejection reflex, which makes both the labour and birth faster, smoother and safer.[48] And, as we saw above, the newborn baby may have a very different first experience of life—since his or her heart function, breathing, metabolism and ability to adjust to heat or cold may all be affected.[49] According to research, drugs administered by epidural go straight through to the unborn baby at equal and sometimes greater concentration levels than those experienced by the mother.[50] Some drugs go to the baby's brain[51] and almost all drugs take longer to eliminate from the baby's immature system than from the mother's system, after the cord has been cut. In short, babies are inevitably affected.

In case you doubt this, note that one researcher found the drug bupivicaine and its breakdown products in the circulation of babies for three days after their births.[52] Drugs used in epidurals also cause more acidaemia (high levels of acid in the blood) in babies than a general anaesthetic—which is apparently a sign that epidurals compromise fetal blood and oxygen supply.[53]

> I did not want an epidural as I wanted to be able to 'push', for want of a better word. I had been led to understand that the epidural immobilised you, even the mobile epidural to a lesser extent, and I knew that I would want to move about. In any case, the midwife had told me I didn't have to have an epidural unless I wanted one.

> I asked for an epidural after 1½ hours but was told upon examination that I was unable to have one as I was 9½cm dilated and there was no time.

> The contractions then came stronger and closer together, but, due to the effects of the epidural, all I could feel was pressure on my bowel when they were at their very strongest. I had to be told when to push by the other people in the room.

> I was then given a wash by two auxiliary nurses, redressed in my own clothes and put into a wheelchair, due to numb legs.

> A couple of hours later, the anaesthesia began to wear off. I felt as if someone were burying an axe in my back. I heard someone screaming. I didn't even realise it was me until later. I begged and pleaded to be turned over, to be held up on my hands and knees. I screamed again and again. I felt like a beetle, stuck on my back, frantically waving my appendages in a futile effort to right myself, to run from danger. I had a fever, and was given paracetamol anal suppositories.

> After the epidural I could only have ice chips, and I didn't have any because I was too busy screaming and trying to push. I was desperately thirsty, but now was not allowed to have any water because I was being 'prepped'. A few minutes later I was taken into surgery.

> I had an epidural the first time, but didn't the second because there wasn't enough time to get it organised. I was really glad, afterwards, that I hadn't had it. I seemed to recover so much faster after the birth, not having had pain relief while I was in labour.

> Eventually, after three attempts, the epidural was working OK and I felt no pain whatsoever. I had to be told when to push by the two midwives who were there to deliver my babies. (Imagine relaxing your whole body but scrunching up your face.) My blood pressure was monitored continuously and my legs were put into stirrups. I pushed when I was told, which was extremely difficult as I didn't know if I was pushing or not.

You may also like to know that...
- Epidurals interfere with the woman's normal ability to produce endorphins, which are the body's natural painkillers. This is because of the pharmacological products they contain.[54]
- Some women report that their epidural only partially takes effect, e.g. only on one side, or leaves an area of pain. This means they merely experience the pain of labour and birth in a different way. One study revealed that 15% of women who had an epidural got no pain relief at all and another study reported a wide variation in the amount of pain relief obtained. It is suggested that this variation is not because of lack of expertise on the part of anaesthetists but because of the different metabolic rates of the various women.[55]
- Epidurals are usually administered after women have experienced contractions for a length of time and even then they only take effect for an hour or so.[56] Most professionals also prefer epidurals to wear off before the actual birth. This all means that relief is only temporary or partial. If epidurals are given too early, i.e. before contractions become well established, they can have the effect of slowing down contractions.[57] (One research team also reported a higher caesarean rate amongst women who had epidurals earlier on in their labour.) Of course, pain which suddenly returns after epidural relief is bound to be more shocking and difficult to cope with than pain which has gradually built up, along with normal endorphin levels.
- An epidural which takes effect for longer often results in a forceps delivery[58] with an episiotomy because the numbing of sensation that takes place in the abdominal area also means the woman is unaware of any pushing sensations. This means she may not be able to push her baby out or that she will, at the very least, require instructions on when to push her baby out (known as 'commanded pushing'). The drugs in the epidural affect the baby's ability to rotate during the second stage of labour and also prevent the woman from spontaneously adopting the best physical position for pushing.
- In one study[59] babies lying in the posterior position early on in labour were less likely to turn into a more favorable position for the birth when the mother had an epidural. (Without an epidural, only 4% of babies were still in the posterior position when they were ready to be born; with an epidural the percentage was 19%.)[60] Of course, women almost always have a caesarean when their posterior babies do not turn before the birth because the unusual position usually makes the labour and birth more painful. Even when the baby is in a good position for the birth, the birth takes longer with an epidural in place (according to another study).[61]
- Some women have problems urinating after the birth, if they've had an epidural.

- If the mother develops an infection because of the catheter, the drip, the constant vaginal examinations or the possible use of forceps, the baby will also be affected and would need to transfer to Intensive Care immediately after the birth. This would mean additional intervention and stress for both mother and baby, not to mention the father. Whether or not an infection develops, according to one study[62] as many as 1 in 4 women who have epidurals develop a fever after four hours and almost half do after eight hours. This is because of the body's inability to regulate its temperature when half the body is numb.
- After having an epidural some women report having migraine-type headaches which last for days or even weeks after the birth. This kind of headache occurs when the needle goes in too far and there's a leakage into the cerebrospinal fluid.
- A small number of women are paralysed permanently.[63]
- According to another research team, the incidence of third degree tears is three times greater after an epidural. These deep tears can later result in fecal incontinence and chronic pain during sex. Fecal incontinence means having no control over doing poos or passing wind, so they are a cause of great embarrassment and discomfort. The other problem associated with these deep tears is that poo goes into the woman's vagina, which can cause infection as well as unpleasantness.[64]
- In the case of sheep which have been used for experiments, 7 out of 8 ewes which are given epidurals fail to show normal mothering behaviour toward their lambs for at least 30 minutes.[65] Research has even confirmed that the same problem may exist in human mothers.[66] In one study mothers who'd had epidurals described their babies as more difficult to care for one month after the birth.[67] This has led some researchers to conclude that human mothers who have an epidural may have to fall back on their conditioned maternal behaviour, since it may not come instinctively. There were no good studies of the effects of epidurals on breastfeeding until 2005,[68] when studies started finding that epidural babies have a weaker sucking reflex and capacity.[69]

" I had the epidural, my blood pressure dropped and they moved me around until they found a position the 'baby liked'. I dozed in a stupor. I suddenly had a sharp pain on one side, and then a persistent ache. I could not change position: I was too numb. I was utterly dependent. I called the nurse. Now it was somebody different. I hoped she was kind. I was helpless, and I had to rely on her. I tried to be nice, and as unobtrusive as possible. A good patient.

" I was admitted at 4.45pm and by 7.00pm I was getting very painful contractions, an epidural was mentioned and after a few more contractions I decided to have it. What wondrous relief except that you are literally numb from the waist down which makes any form of movement amusing. Things then slowed down as expected, so up went the fluid drip and the hormone drip to get things going again.

Birthframe 30
Even pain which seems 'unbearable' can usually be tolerated if we simply 'hang on in there'. After all, sometimes epidurals cause more problems than they solve...

My twins were born on 7 July 2000. I was two weeks early.

On 5 July I had an appointment with my consultant at the hospital. He stretched my cervix, which was extremely uncomfortable, but he said this would help me to 'get going'. That evening I was fine, as I was the following day. By Friday morning (7 July) I was definitely having contractions.

All through this pregnancy we were recommended to have an epidural, as we were told anything could go wrong with a twin birth. So, as soon as we got into the hospital my husband and I kept telling the midwives, doctors and anyone that I had opted for an epidural and that we should have it before my contractions got too close together. Did they listen? No.

After about three or four hours they got an anaesthetist to give me an epidural, but I was too far gone and I couldn't keep still. They managed to give it to me and my blood pressure plummeted. Suddenly, there were loads of people in the room. Luckily, somehow I carried on giving birth to my first child. He came out head first and was fine, and likewise my daughter, who came out 22 minutes later—she was fine as well. Their weights were 5lb 12oz and 6lb 5oz respectively.

The main point I want to make is that the kids were fine but after 24 hours I could barely move. What had happened was that the epidural had not gone in where it should have and they had to do a 'reversal', basically by taking some blood from my hand and injecting it in my back. It was the most painful experience I have been through in my whole life. I couldn't hold my babies properly for days and I went through so much emotional trauma I wish I had been strong enough to say 'No' to the epidural suggestion, but... well, who knows what may have happened?

Bhavna Amlani

OPIOID ANALGESICS & SEDATIVES

Women have reported feeling drunk and out of control after having doses of opioid analgesics, such as Fentanyl (which is 100 times more potent than morphine) or diamorphine (i.e. heroin). Even these drugs do not fully mask the pain of labour or birth. They can also cause problems for the woman, such as nausea, vomiting, sedation, itching, hypotension or respiratory depression and can prolong labour.[70] They can have dramatic effects on the baby at birth too. Since they go straight through to the baby and are usually still present in the baby's system at birth, they can cause early breathing problems, or convulsions in some cases, they can weaken the baby's 'suck' (so have a dramatic effect on breastfeeding),[71] and they can affect the fetal heart rate and change neonatal behaviour. Research has also established a link between the presence of opiates in the baby's body at birth and later drug addiction in adulthood.[72]

Here's a bit more information about opioid analgesics from a mother, the New Zealand researcher and GP, Sarah Buckley, who now lives in Australia...

Pethidine (Demerol, meperidine) is the usual opiate administered in Australian labour wards; in 1998 here in Queensland Australia, around a third of labouring women used this drug. In the US, other narcotics such as Nalbuphine (Nubain), butorphanol (Stadol), alphaprodine (Nisentil), hydromorphone (Dilaudid) and fentanyl citrate (Sublimaze) have been traditional mainstays of labour analgesia, but have now been largely replaced by epidural analgesia, which may also contain opiates. [In the UK pethidine and, increasingly, diamorphine are often used.] All opiates used in labour can cause side effects such as maternal nausea, vomiting, sedation, itching, low blood pressure, difficulty breathing; for the baby they include fetal heart rate abnormalities, breathing problems, difficulty with early breastfeeding and altered neonatal neurobehaviour.[73]

As with oxytocin [pitocin], use of these drugs will reduce a woman's own opioid hormone production,[74] which may be helpful if excessive levels are inhibiting labour. However the use of pethidine has been shown to slow labour, in a dose-response way;[75] in one randomised trial, morphine (but not naloxone) administered in labour directly reduced oxytocin release.[76] And again, we must ask: What may be the effects for mother and baby of labouring and birthing without peak levels of these hormones of pleasure and transcendence?

The use of pethidine has been shown to slow labour

Some researchers have nominated our endogenous opiates as the reward system for reproductive acts– that is, the endorphin fix keeps us making babies, having babies and breastfeeding.[77] Anecdotally, I notice that women who reap pleasure from these activities—e.g. home birthers and La Leche League mothers—tend to have larger families. On a global scale, also, countries that have embraced the obstetric model of care, which prizes drugs and interventions above birthing pleasure and empowerment, have experienced steeply declining birth rates in recent years.

More serious are the implications of Swedish research into the use of opiates at birth, published in 1990,[78] and recently replicated with a prospective US population.[79] In the first study, researchers looked at the birth records of 200 opiate addicts born between 1945 and 1966, and compared them to their non-addicted siblings. Offspring whose mothers used analgesia in labour (opiates, barbiturates and nitrous oxide gas [i.e. gas and air]) were more likely to become addicted to drugs (opiates, amphetamines) as adults, especially when multiple doses were administered. For example, when a mother had received three doses of opiates in her labour, her child was 4.7 times more likely to become addicted to opiate drugs in adulthood.

Animal studies suggest a mechanism for this. It seems that drugs administered chronically in late pregnancy can affect brain structure and function (e.g. they can cause chemical and hormonal imbalance), which may not be obvious until young adulthood.[80] Whether such effects apply to human babies who are exposed for shorter periods around the time of birth is not known but, as one researcher warns: "During this antenatal period of neuronal [brain cell] multiplication, migration and inter-connection, the brain is most vulnerable to irreversible damage."[81]

Note: You can confirm these references and do your own searches for other relevant abstracts of studies at www.pubmed.com, at www.cochrane.org—or even using www.google.co.uk or www.wikipedia.org.

GAS AND AIR (ENTONOX)

As you probably know, gas and air is very often used in labour wards in the UK. You will read about it in this book in some of the birthframes and if you happen to be in another country you may well find it's available there too. It's portrayed in many old films as being a 'routine' part of birth, e.g. in Ingmar Bergman's film *Secrets of Women* and it is certainly used routinely in Britain. Out of 3,000 women who returned questionnaires in a *Mother and Baby* magazine survey in 2002, as many as 79% of women in the UK reported having used it. Women often say, "Oh, I just had gas and air" when talking about their labours—as if it wasn't anything much. This seems strange, given the way a friend described her experience of using it. She said it was wonderful, like being in a helicopter, circling above her body as each contraction washed over her. Other women find its effect weak and almost unnoticeable. Irrespective of how women report its effects, the fact is that gas and air is a powerful form of pain relief. One manufacturer of Entonox states that it is a very effective analgesic agent, which is rapidly eliminated from the body *once inhalation stops* (the italics are mine). This 50/50 mixture of oxygen and nitrous oxide targets the opiate receptors of the brain, so it must work in a similar way to morphine and synthetic morphines such as diamorphine, even though these are is usually given in higher doses all at once, rather than in short bursts over a period of time.

Why gas and air is perceived as being harmless, with no side effects, is a mystery, given that it is usually used repeatedly for half an hour or so for every one of very frequent contractions. The fact that the main ingredient of gas and air has been associated with increased incidence of drug addiction in adolescents who've experienced it as a fetus during their birth is either little known or inexplicably disregarded—even though, admittedly, this research has only focused on the use of nitrous oxide in isolation.[82] No research has yet investigated the long-term effects of combined oxygen and nitrous oxide, but it seems likely that oxygen is the more 'innocent' ingredient.[83]

Even if the mixture widely used in the UK and elsewhere really is 'harmless' in itself, which seems unlikely, I believe there are other good reasons to avoid it. Personally, I'd even ensure it's not in the house if I were having a home birth—for the same reason as I keep chocolate biscuits well out of my way! Here's a summary of reasons why...

- It is mostly used at a critical time of labour, i.e. in the half hour or so before the baby is born. Although it only remains in the bloodstream for a very short time, if it's used for every contraction over half an hour or so its effect will not be so fleeting... and it's bound to have an effect on the baby.
- Using the mouthpiece or 'mask' to self-administer gas and air, the labouring woman will inevitably be distracted from the sensations she's experiencing.

Why gas and air is perceived as being harmless is a mystery...

She will be unable to tune into what's happening in her body

That's the whole point, after all, isn't it? In a distracted state—which is often more panicky than calm—she will be unable to tune into what is happening in her body. This means she is less likely to be able to coordinate her pushing effectively, which will result in a less smooth journey for the baby and a higher likelihood of injury for the mother. That means a much higher likelihood of tearing and stitches.

- It is very unlikely a labouing woman who is using gas and air will be able to tune into her instinctual knowledge of how to give birth. This means she will not experience an authentic fetus ejection reflex—the natural reflex which enables us to birth our babies quickly, efficiently and, above all, safely.
- Any side effects the mother-to-be experiences while using gas and air will detract from and probably replace the state of mind and sensations she would otherwise have been experiencing. The mother's state of mind and perception of her bodily state is extremely important at this stage because it is just minutes or seconds before she will meet her new baby for the first time.
- If there is a 'break in transmission' in administering the gas and air (either because of the woman's uncoordinated efforts or because of some other factor—e.g. the gas and air running out or being taken away), the labouring woman is likely to be thrown into a panic. This is not the state of mind she should be in just before the birth of her baby. She should be tuning into her bodily sensations in a positive, accepting way—realising that they are a signal that her baby is just about to be born.

Here are a few comments from contributors:

> I began using gas and air through a mouthpiece. It made me feel intoxicated and at first nauseous. I asked myself if I would rather be sick or feel the full impact of the contractions. I decided being sick was preferable so I continued with the gas and air. I found the sickness went quickly and I could focus the pain as a point and make it move further away and distance myself from it.

> When I was fully dilated at 3.50pm the midwife took away the gas and air and told me I wouldn't be able to push adequately with it. I found the instant shock of the pain (when the midwife took the gas and air away) to be devastating. I was in so much pain that I could not speak let alone push. My contractions were without respite and the midwife was constantly telling me to relax. It wasn't until 4.40pm that I could actually push effectively.

A comment from a midwife:

> The Entonox cylinder was empty when they brought it. This happens a lot with hospital gear as staff don't check their own equipment—they rely on the person who used it before to do so. It happened with my first baby too.

I decided to ask Michel for his view...

Why is Entonox used so often in British hospitals but not elsewhere? In a way it seems surprising, especially since nitrous oxide on its own is poisonous.

There were probably some accidents with nitrous oxide, so it is possible that many people in countries other than the UK were not receptive when a safe formula was offered. Before the age of evidence-based medicine, the practice of midwifery and obstetrics was highly influenced by the opinions of a small number of authoritative professors or authors of books. This explains the differences between countries.

Is it a safe drug, do you think?

We have no data on that. Studies into the use of nitrous oxide suggest that this on its own is definitely not helpful from the baby's point of view.[84] We do know that all synthetic morphines—all opiates, in fact—suppress the sucking reflex and since the target of nitrous oxide is the opioid brain receptors, there may be some similar effect in the case of Entonox. Nitrous oxide is not an opiate itself, but it does seem to interfere with the natural production of endorphins, which are natural opiates, probably because it targets the brain's opiate receptors. So in a sense 'gas and air' has something to do with opiates—it's not a separate topic. It may be harmful in the same way as other opiates which are not produced directly by the woman's body.[85]

However, do you think it might be a useful last resort for women who are having difficult labours—e.g. if their baby is in a posterior position?

My feeling is that it is a substitute for privacy. In other words as long as the word privacy is not understood, gas and air will be useful. Once a woman asked us if we have gas and air. Liliana replied with a joke: "I am the gas and Michel is the air!"

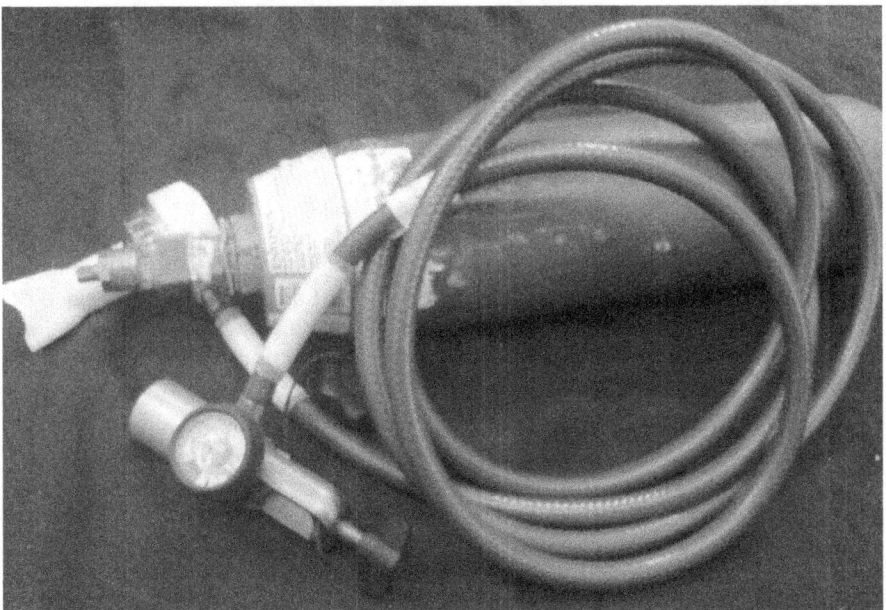

A cylinder of gas and air, also called 'Entonox'

What about complementary approaches?

Aromatherapy, herbs, homeopathy, TENS machines, shiatsu and acupuncture are often associated with 'natural' birth. They're generally assumed to be helpful but harmless. But do they disturb a normal, healthy birth?

The assumption seems to be that complementary therapies are necessary for someone who wants to give birth without the use of drug-related pain relief. A book about natural childbirth is usually a book which gives guidance on the use of complementary therapies. So why—if we want an optimal birth—should complementary therapies be avoided?

The answer is simple: basically, something can't be useful, without also being powerful. Treatments of whatever kind given during the gestation and birth of a baby actually change what is happening. This is why it's extremely risky using them during pregnancy, labour and childbirth. Herbs, acupuncture, TENS machines, shiatsu, aromatherapy and all the other so-called 'natural' treatments may well disturb the physiological processes which would otherwise take place.

There's a problem here, though. What's 'complementary' and what's simply part of everyday life? After all, we're constantly ingesting food and drink and smelling smells... what if these are part of a herbalist's apothecary or an aromatherapist's box? This is a difficult question but, as a rule of thumb, take note of anything which is offered for medicinal or therapeutic use in any way—peppermint tea, a lavender pillow, a shiatsu pressure point—and avoid it. This means no herbal or 'fruit' teas during pregnancy or labour, however seemingly innocuous. It also means no ordinary coffee or tea—or at least very little—and no seemingly harmless luxury treatments. This is simply because they're all too potentially powerful and disruptive.

Having said all this, let me now say that I recommend a handful of exceptions—in particular, two which have survived the test of time and two others which are the result of recent research. One is the use of raspberry leaf tea (a uterine tonic) in the third trimester and possibly also during labour. Another is the use of arnica—a homeopathic tablet (Arnica 30) taken daily to prevent bruising in the last month of pregnancy. The other two are the use of supplementary folic acid in the first trimester of pregnancy to prevent spinal tube defects, and the use of Omega 3 fish oil supplements in the third trimester to help your little one's brain develop.

Everything else is best avoided. When we leave our body alone, in most cases it will redress any imbalances automatically, provided we do not have any major health problems and provided we do everything we can to facilitate the normal, healthy processes. (More on how later!) For now, let's look more closely at a few complementary therapies...

AROMATHERAPY

Have you ever used some bath salts or bubble bath and felt very sleepy afterwards? Some of the aromas used in commercially produced products may have this effect because they are derived from herbs or flora which are used medicinally for the same purpose. Also, there is the problem that organising aromatherapy for a birth usually means inviting another person into the room. What's more, inevitably, it's likely to either distract you or make you feel you 'need' something other than your own resources. You're better off without it.[86]

HERBS

Did you know that some innocent-seeming herb teas (such as peppermint) are produced from herbs from the same family as ones used to induce miscarriage (such as pennyroyal)? If you're not already aware of the power and usefulness of herbs in daily life, you might like to try a few out... after you've had your baby.

TENS

This is generally marketed as a non-invasive method of pain relief—and this, no doubt, explains its popularity, as well as the fact that it's both cheap and readily available. However, it is still very possible that TENS disturbs the healthy physiological processes of labour. And I think women are still better off without TENS machines.[87] Before we consider the reasons why, here's another extract from one of my conversations with Michel...

What do you think of TENS?

TENS is a very minor intervention, perhaps not more than a placebo. In 1975, I described in *La Nouvelle Presse Médicale* the technique of what I call 'lumbar reflexotherapy', which is at the root of TENS.[88] I already gave the physiological interpretations that are given today to explain how TENS works (if it works). With my technique you just need sterile water, while to use TENS you need to buy a device (so it's more commercial). The effects of lumbar reflexotherapy are spectacular, compared with the effects of TENS.

So do you recommend TENS to pregnant women? Surely, recommending a machine such as TENS implies a lack of faith in women's instinctual ability to give birth unaided and couldn't its use distract women and stop them from 'going to another planet', as you call it?

I never took the initiative to recommend TENS, for the reasons that you mention. But when a woman has bought the device and intensely wants to use it, I don't dissuade her. This is true for other non-pharmacological [complementary] treatments too. I am reluctant if the treatment implies the introduction of a therapist, i.e. another person in the birthing place.

I am reluctant if the treatment brings in a therapist...

Here are my own thoughts on TENS:

- As I've already suggested, depending on something 'outside' is likely to undermine a woman's confidence in her own ability to cope. I think a woman's belief that she can give birth is almost as important as her intrinsic ability to do so.
- A woman using a TENS machine is likely to be focusing on technical and practical details, rather than on what is going on within her—so it's less likely she'll 'go to another planet'.
- Inevitably, the machine will restrict her movements to some extent and this will make it less likely that she'll tune into her intuitive knowledge of which positions are best for her baby.
- Research has revealed that women perceive that the use of TENS machines increases, not decreases, the incidence of intense pain later on in labour.[89] No doubt this is because using a machine which is helpful for contractions early on in labour makes later contractions (for which there is suddenly no relief) seem stronger. If using a TENS machine really does make later pain in labour seem more intense, it's likely to be a first step towards other forms of pain relief. (Perhaps this is why it's widely claimed by both women and midwives that TENS is not powerful enough for use through the whole of labour.) Doing without TENS will mean there's a gradual, more manageable build-up of intensity throughout labour.
- There may be other as yet undetected effects on a person and on the birthing process. Just because no research project has as yet uncovered risks does not mean there aren't any.

ACUPUNCTURE

Michel comments on the use of acupuncture in his book *Birth Reborn* (Souvenir Press 1994). In his experience, traditional Chinese acupuncture is seldom used for labour and birth in China, although it is believed to be useful for turning breech babies during pregnancy. He believes the Chinese' avoidance of using acupuncture during labour and birth is probably due to an acknowledgement on the part of acupuncturists of the extreme complexity of the physiological processes, which they realise are best left untouched. I must say, I have actually been told the opposite by an acupuncturist in the UK, i.e. that acupuncture is used by 90% of labouring women in China. Which is true? If acupuncture is being used more nowadays, is there a connection between this and the extremely high level of medical intervention which takes place in births in China?

While I was researching this book I found a couple of birth stories which mentioned the use of acupuncture. The women who sent these had a very positive attitude towards this complementary therapy... despite the fact that they also ended up having a very difficult labour and birth. In one case, the author of the birth account was a potential contributor. When she heard my

Acupuncture is too powerful not to be considered an intervention

interpretation of her birth story, she decided she wanted to withdraw her story. She was worried the detail of the account would identify her acupuncturist, and she didn't want this to happen because she said acupuncture had helped her family in so many other ways. As far as she was concerned, she would never have got through such an awful labour if it hadn't been for the acupuncture treatments. In my view, it was the acupuncture which had disrupted her labour and made it so long and difficult.

Perhaps it's not always dangerous using acupuncture in certain cases, as Birthframe 58 demonstrates, but leaving the healthy processes to take place undisturbed does seem to be the best approach most of the time. Acupuncture, like other types of complementary medicine, is simply too powerful not to be considered a serious intervention.[90]

> I went to a friend's therapeutic masseur, who suggested I rub the acupuncture points on my ankles to induce birth and it did! That night, at 4.00am my waters broke and the contractions started. I'd planned to have a home birth with a government midwife through my health insurance provider and knowing they were probably off duty, I waited until 9.00am to phone them. But they refused to come out as I'd had a show of fresh blood when the waters broke. They said the fetus could be in danger because of internal bleeding around the placenta and I must come to the hospital.

MASSAGE

On the one hand, massage can be an extension of the spontaneous touching which could occur between a labouring woman and her husband, or it could be touching which has been specifically requested by the woman (either from her husband or from a midwife or other birth attendant). On the other hand, if 'massage' becomes 'shiatsu'—i.e. dramatic results are achieved by putting pressure on various pressure points—it can be another form of disturbance. If carried out over many hours massage can certainly be very useful and might in fact rescue a labouring woman who is otherwise having difficult coping, either generally or because of posterior lie.[91]

Birthframe 31

Finally, we have an account, which culminates in the birth story which exemplifies the 'Do not disturb' principle. These are the birth stories of Deborah Jackson, the well-known journalist and writer of books on childcare. (She is the author of *Three in a Bed* (Bloomsbury 2003), *Letting Go as Children Grow* (Bloomsbury 2003), *Mother and Child* (Duncan Baird 2001) and *Baby Wisdom* (Hodder & Stoughton 2002). Her account shows the importance of creating a birthing environment where the healthy processes can proceed undisturbed and unobserved. Perhaps her first labour became established so effectively precisely because people initially took so little interest in her.

A friend of mine always says, "Happy birthday, Mum," to me on my children's birthdays. "It may be the day they were born, but you are the one who remembers it best," she says. My children think this is funny. A birthday isn't something you remember, it's the chance to be at the centre of the known universe.

One of the rituals attached to my children's birthdays is that I recount their birth stories. When they were little, they used to cuddle up close, wide-eyed and excited, thrilled to imagine themselves emerging, cute and lovable, into my arms. Now that Frances is 15, Alice is 12 and Joe 8, they tease me instead. "I know, I know," they laugh, "you've told me that before." Nevertheless, the edited highlights are what they get, and the edited highlights are what will come back to them when they have their own children one day.

Frances: Frances's story became the introduction to my first book. She travelled through the night to be with me, as did her father, who was working away from home in Manchester at the time. What made this birth special was that I was surrounded and supported entirely by women.

I'd had a day of regular but bearable contractions. As I was three weeks early, no one was taking much notice of me. But at 10.00pm, my friend Frederique, who had two darling children of her own, turned up at the door with an overnight bag in her hand. "I think you could be going into labour," she said, "I've come to stay with you."

Lucky she did, because by 11.00pm I could stand it no longer and begged to go to the hospital. It was going to be a long night. I thought I was about to give birth and phoned Paul in Manchester to ask him to catch the next train. "Am I in labour?" I asked the midwife as I stood on the phone, doubled over in pain. "If you know the answer to that, you're a better man than I am," she replied.

I'd written out a birth plan and this, in the end, helped to shape the birth I wanted. Without it, I think I would have been unable to articulate anything but my knee-jerk reactions. I did a lot of stomping around, grunting and dancing and at some time in the night my mother arrived. Fred was going on holiday the next day and had to get some sleep. Mum had driven two hours to be with me and become my emotional support.

There were some interventions: they broke the waters and I had a 'half-dose' of pethidine, before falling into a deep sleep, slumped over a bean bag. When I asked them to remind me what an epidural does, my mother soothed me, saying "It's no more than a body can bear." When I stood up, my baby was born, tearing past me as if she was in a rush to be getting somewhere. The midwife walked into the room and caught her, like a rugby ball, in her hands. Within seconds, she was in my arms.

I looked up to see five women in the room: my mother, a female doctor, two midwives and a trainee. In this large teaching hospital, they had all gathered to see the 'physiological third stage' that I had requested on my birth plan. Births were routinely induced by drugs at that time and people wanted to know what happened if you left the placenta to its own devices.

What happened was a long wait, during which I crouched naked, holding Frances to my breast. Perhaps 25 minutes later, I felt a mighty contraction and the placenta came out easily.

Half an hour later, I was alone with my baby, a slice of toast and a cup of tea. Frances breastfed with all the instinct she was born with—luckily no one tried to intervene to show us how. Paul arrived on the morning train to find his daughter enjoying a big breakfast. And the trainee midwife came up later to thank me—she said it was the best birth she had witnessed in all her months of training.

Alice: Like most second births, this is a shorter story. Again, it was three weeks before my due date, but by now, we were living in Manchester. We had guests in the house: my mother- and brother-in-law. Braxton Hicks contractions had been cramping my style for a week or more, waking me up at night and keeping me on edge. In the afternoon, I drove Paul's grandmother to the station and had to stop for contractions. A couple of hours later, I was getting into a great rhythm and we phoned to alert the midwife.

Having given birth once, the fear had gone out of it. I had decided to have this baby at home. It wasn't so much the birth I was thinking about, but the aftermath—I particularly wanted to cuddle up with my new baby in my own bed, without any interruptions. At home, there are no sleep police patrolling the ward and telling you to put your baby back into the cot. And after all, if there should be a crisis, we lived opposite the maternity hospital.

Everyone else went out for a meal and my midwife arrived—a friendly face I had met at a Michel Odent talk. She suggested I get into the bath and I recall the frisson of pleasure as I sat in my attic bathroom, knowing my baby was coming and looking out into the electric storm that raged that night. Then everything happened very quickly.

I repeated the affirmations and visualisations...

I got out of the bath and started to repeat the affirmations and visualisations I had been taught by another friend, a trainee hypnotherapist. I really could feel the contractions working in my favour, helping me to open up and my baby to be born. Paul arrived, but he seemed a thousand miles away. I was already completely immersed in waves of sensation. As I sat on the floor with my legs stretched out, watching them shake, I heard a distant voice say, "She's in transition." I thought, "You have to be joking, it takes much longer than this." They tried to help me up to the bed and as I moved forwards, Alice shot out with a yell. Then all was quiet.

Alice was so tiny that, stretched out on her back, she fitted perfectly along the crook of my arm to my fingers. Despite a fast, natural birth, she was a sleepy baby and I had to keep nudging her to remind her to feed. That night, all four of us slept in our low, large family bed and it felt right.

Joseph: Everyone thought Joe's birth would be even faster than Alice's, but it wasn't like that. Four years had passed and now we were living in Bath. My GP was in favour of home birth and all along I planned to have my baby in my bedroom. A friend asked if she could be there to see the birth and I half said 'Yes'. Two weeks before my due date and I already felt as though I was overdue. I was sure it was a girl.

That night, I was serving spaghetti with tomato sauce. I carried my plate along the hall to the dining room and, in my state of pregnant imbalance, managed to drop the lot on the hall carpet. I got down on my hands and knees to mop it up and immediately knew the contractions were starting. "I think the new baby will be born tonight," I told Frances and Alice. I asked Paul to take charge of the girls. I wanted to go into my own cocoon for this birth. When the midwife arrived, she was thrilled to hear that Alice was born in two hours. "That means I shall be able to get home to see my favourite programme," she said. But labour went on for longer than we expected.

I tried getting into a warm bath, but this time the magic didn't work. I kept moving and visualising, but unfortunately, the midwife also kept talking and I didn't have the guts to ask her to keep quiet. I found it impossible to 'let go' while she chatted to me and I felt obliged to smile politely and respond between contractions. Maybe four hours passed and I still felt far too much in control, but I knew it was time for the baby to be born. I decided not to invite my friend to observe after all. Somehow, I felt too observed already. I crouched by the side of the bed and tried to bear down. But it felt as though the baby, far from wanting to come out, was being sucked back inside me. Perhaps she's changed her mind, I thought. After a while, I could hear the panic in the midwife's voice. I was at the top of three flights of stairs, we lived a good 20 minutes' drive from the hospital and contractions seemed to have stopped. I felt very frightened. So I pushed with all the strength I could muster. No contraction, but I pushed my baby out. And out the baby came, screaming with annoyance at having been disturbed. This baby was bigger than the girls, but still tiny compared to 4-year-old and 7-year-old sisters. And the biggest surprise was yet to come: it was a boy.

Deborah Jackson

Where does it all leave us?

It's particularly important to *remember* this 'Do not disturb' principle and to *assert yourself* so that other people remember it too. Only if you take responsibility for ensuring that your own pregnancy, labour and birth remain undisturbed can you reasonably expect to experience a safe, healthy, *optimal* birth yourself. It's only by taking responsibility and taking action that you will be able to maximise your own chances of having the best possible birthing experience, involving minimal pain and discomfort and maximal satisfaction for both yourself and your baby. In other words, it's important to 'care about care' and 'prepare and assert'... We shall consider these two steps soon. But first, let's remember there's a real, live baby in there!

7... HELP YOUR BABY

In this chapter we'll think about your baby's perspective both during pregnancy and during the birth itself.

Pregnancy

Obviously, you need to be careful about what you put into your body when you're pregnant. Eat well and drink plenty of water. Include plenty of good quality protein in your diet, along with loads of fruit and veg. I also recommend you take an Omega-3 fish oil supplement in the third trimester, as I've said, so as to help your little one's brain develop.[1]

Things to avoid include paté, soft cheese, raw fish, raw eggs and liver, as well as the more obvious things, such as alcohol and cigarette smoke.[2] Also, stay away from caffeine because it's a powerful stimulant, which is bound to affect your baby. Finally, as we've already noted, you mustn't use drugs or medicines unless there is a very good reason to do so. Check and re-check safety by doing your own research.

Two more points gleaned from research... One is that hot baths and bright light could be either dangerous or unpleasant for your baby. The other, which I've already mentioned briefly, is that liquorice has been shown to trigger premature labour—so it's best avoided.

Finally, I would suggest you avoid any artificial 'antenatal programs'—the kind of thing where you try and 'teach' the baby as he or she is growing in your womb. Just leave your baby to develop in peace, both physically and psychologically.

Beyond that, the best way to help your growing baby is to find out about him or her and follow his or her progress week by week. Being aware of what's going on inside you will automatically make you want to make the best choices...[3]

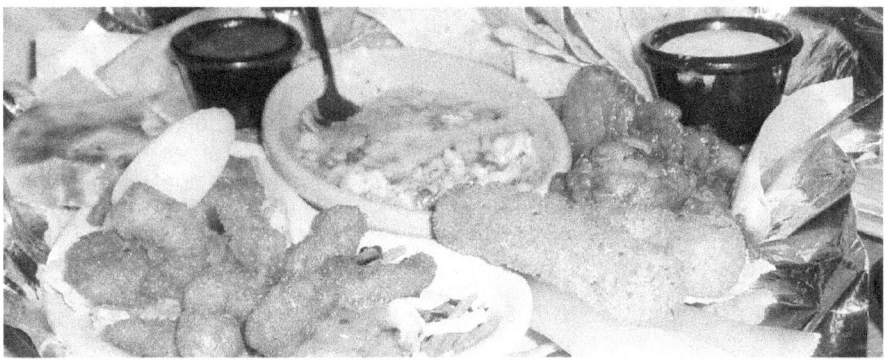

Make wise choices while you're eating—especially informally with other people

THE FIRST TRIMESTER

The first trimester is very important because this is when all your new baby's organs and bones are being formed.

Weeks 1 & 2

During these first two weeks one or more ova (eggs) mature inside one of your ovaries. Meanwhile, your endometrium (the lining of your womb) builds up so as to provide a suitable place for the ovum to nestle in, after it's been fertilised. This will happen after your ovum is released from one of your ovaries and one of your partner's sperm comes up to meet it. (In previous months when no ovum was fertilised, the endometrium was eventually released in the form of a menstrual period.)

When the sperm has fused with the ovum, half your developing baby's chromosomes will be from your partner, and half from you.

Week 3

Conception takes place either at the beginning of this week or later if you usually have a long cycle. (When women ovulate later, their due date is also later because it takes a baby around 266 days—or 38 weeks—to develop.) If, like most women, you're growing just one baby, only one of a possible 200 million sperm fertilises your ovum in this third week so all the sperm released into your vagina when your partner had an orgasm were in competition with each other. It takes about 45 minutes for the sperm to reach your newly released ovum and some people believe that lying down for half an hour after sex helps this process. It's helpful to already be taking folic acid supplements (400mg) by this stage because this is a nutrient many of us are deficient in.

During the process of conception the pronucleus of the sperm which unites with your ovum is drawn into the ovum itself. Very quickly, the cell membrane which surrounds the ovum closes to seal out all the other sperm. Only 40% of the time when sperm and ovum meet is this process successful so this month is an especially fortuitous month!

Within 24 hours the newly fertilised cell, which is called a zygote, divides into two (a process called 'cleavage'!) and becomes a 'morula'. As the morula develops and fluid enters the mass of cells it becomes a 'blastocyst', which continues dividing so that after nine months it will consist of several hundred billion cells. The one fertilised cell manages to transform and differentiate itself so as to make a new human being, thanks to the DNA inside the genes in the ovum and sperm.

After nine months there will be several hundred billion cells!

Being on the safe side...

If you're hoping to get pregnant, keep a record of when your period starts each month. This is the date of your 'LMP'—your 'last menstrual period'—which you will need in order to predict when your baby will be born.

If you make love less than daily, it's also worth recording each occasion when you have sex, because this might help you to predict the precise date of the birth. Use a simple system: an asterisk in your calendar on the appropriate page can mean your period is due; an asterisk circled can mean the day when your period actually started; a small circle could indicate a day when you made love.

All this record-keeping might not seem terribly important before you are pregnant, but it could save you a lot of trouble once you are. It might significantly affect your antenatal care, as well as the kind of treatment you are offered (if any) before and after you go into labour.

This may seem strange, but it's quite simple really. If you know how old your baby is while he or she is still in the womb, you and your caregivers will be confident about stages of development and appropriate courses of action if ever there's a problem. Also, if you know when your baby was conceived you will be able to be very confident about his or her due date. This will mean you are more likely to avoid any pressure to be induced, which—as we've already seen—can seriously disrupt the healthy processes.

So knowing your precise LMP and the probable date of your baby's conception might help you to remain undisturbed and unpressurised while you give birth.

If you understand a little about the process of conception, you can maximise your chances of starting a new life—even if it does take away a little of the romance! Yes, it's very possible that conception is a mysterious spiritual process over which we have little control (or only subconsciously)... but it's also a process which can be understood scientifically. Understanding on this very ordinary level may well help you to get pregnant.

So how does conception occur in scientific terms? It can only occur when you have released an egg and when live sperm are swimming around inside you. As you probably already know, the best way to get sperm inside you is for your partner to experience an orgasm while thrusting his erect penis into you. If one of your partner's tiny sperm manages to swim up to meet and fuse with an egg you have just released, then conception will occur and a viable pregnancy may well result.

It's such a complex process that sometimes everything goes smoothly, sometimes it doesn't. If you want to help you partner's sperm to reach your egg—or eggs!—remain lying down on your back for 30 minutes or so after making love; as we've already noted, this may give the sperm a better chance of swimming up to the right place.

Maximising your baby's chances of existence...

The key, of course, is to know when you produce an egg each month and to make love around that time because each egg only survives for 12-24 hours after it's been released. Sperm survive a little longer, so if they're 'in there' before you release an egg, that's OK too. Interestingly enough, sperm which produce female babies can survive for up to three days in the womb, whereas the ones which end up producing little boys can only survive for 24 hours. Whether this means you should make love more or less often if you want a child of a particular sex is an unanswered question really. Although theories abound, there is no real evidence to suggest you really can control whether you conceive a girl or a boy—so it's not really worth trying. Perhaps it's better to believe the idea that we get 'what we need'—in order to balance out our relationships and achieve our purpose in life!

Anyway, what about that all-important question: when do you release eggs? Normally the answer is 14 days before the first day of your next monthly period. (It's best to count backwards like this, because some women have long cycles.) Just before ovulation occurs, you might notice a change in your vaginal discharge—from milky white to clear jelly. If you see the jelly when you wipe yourself after going to the toilet, it probably means you're highly fertile, or were the day before. Make love anyway! Another, less convenient way of checking your fertility is to feel inside yourself to check your cervix: if it seems hard and low down (a bit like a nose) you aren't fertile. On the other hand, if it seems to have risen up inside you and feels soft (like lips) you're likely to be fertile. There are other methods, of course, and test kits to determine ovulation are constantly being marketed. These methods are probably best avoided, though, unless you really have been trying to get pregnant for over a year. After that point ovulation kits are only one option and searching the Internet (using key words like 'conception', 'ovulation', 'natural fertility awareness', etc.) will eventually reveal many more. Of course, doctors and other medical professionals can also offer help. If you consider a less natural method like IVF, it's also important to consider how you feel about unneeded embryos being destroyed. Look for methods which you feel in tune with in all respects.

If you're not overly anxious to conceive immediately or if you prefer to be less analytical, just 'go with the flow' for a few months. Making love with your partner every second day throughout your cycle would cover all possibilities. Making love whenever you and your partner feel like it is probably also enough for most couples because, for some strange reason, men seem to find women more attractive sexually when they are fertile and women themselves are likely to feel more in the mood for lovemaking at that time too.

Whichever approach you take, it's very possible you'll conceive quickly, without any specialised knowledge. So enjoy! This may be the last time for quite a while that you can enjoy relaxed, unscheduled and uninterrupted lovemaking. You don't even need to use contraception...

Week 4

On the 10th or 11th day after fertilisation, having successfully travelled along one of your fallopian tubes, the blastocyst implants itself into the lining of your womb. From this point onwards your tiny baby is called an 'embryo'. It is nourished by tiny blood vessels called chorionic villi in the lining of your womb. These villi were produced by the embryo itself, even though it is still only the size of a pinhead.

If you have by now conceived identical twins or triplets (or more!) the single blastocyst would have already divided up to form two, three or more separate embryos by the end of this week. If you are expecting non-identical twins or triplets, etc, more than one egg would have been released, fertilised and implanted two weeks ago.

Week 5

By the end of this week many women realise they are pregnant and confirm this using one of the widely available home pregnancy tests. It's useful to do a test early because if you know for sure that you're pregnant, you're likely to be motivated to do everything you can for the good of your developing baby. If your test originally gives a negative result but your period still hasn't started, note that you may still be pregnant. It's possible the negative result is simply due to low levels of hCG—human chorionic gonadotrophin, the hormone manufactured by the blastocyst, which the test tries to detect. Levels may be low if you ovulated late in your cycle. Do another test in a few days' time and again after a week or so, if you still think you may be pregnant.

Taking at least 400mg of folic acid per day is particularly important this week and over the next few weeks. This is because folic acid is crucial in ensuring healthy development of the neural tube, which eventually becomes the spinal column and brain. It's also vital to drink enough water. Requirements vary according to height, weight, activity levels, climate, etc, so I won't give any precise recommendations. However, note that you should drink much more than when you're not pregnant. Make sure you check any bottled water for sodium levels—only drink it if the level is lower than 10mg per litre. (Note that levels in carbonated water tend to be dramatically higher, so it's probably best to drink mainly still water.) Your growing baby's brain already has two separate lobes. In appearance, your baby is a bit like a grey, jelly-like, translucent tadpole, with a head and a tail. It's only a few millimetres long—perhaps as long as a grain of rice. It swims around in a miniature yolk sac and amniotic sac which both protect your tiny embryo from harm.

Your future baby is already connected to you by a miniature umbilical cord and cells are beginning to differentiate so as to form your baby's skin, intestines, a primitive nervous system and bones.

Wondering whether you're pregnant…

When you suspect you may be pregnant, it's important to confirm your pregnancy as soon as possible. That way, you'll be able to do everything possible to optimise conditions for your new baby.

But how will you know you're pregnant? Will you feel different? It's possible that you won't notice conception taking place and it is also possible that you won't realise you're pregnant at first even when your period is delayed, because some early pregnancy symptoms can be mistaken for the imminent onset of a period. A few women, however, do notice a slight ache or pain in one side of their abdomen as they ovulate. Other women have also reported different states of consciousness or dreams which have made them feel that they have conceived. Still others notice some of the early signs of pregnancy, so begin to suspect they might be pregnant long before they have confirmed their pregnancy through a test. A few highly-sensitive individuals report simply 'feeling different'. Only you can, of course, tell what it feels like for you, in your particular life, when you experience it. Whatever the experience is like for you, here are a few common early signs to be on the alert for:

- ♥ a strong aversion to certain foods, drinks or smells which you normally like or accept readily, e.g. coffee, alcohol, cigarette smoke
- ♥ a craving for certain foods or different tastes
- ♥ nausea and/or vomiting, either after eating or after a period of not eating
- ♥ a metallic taste in your mouth
- ♥ a feeling which is almost similar to pre-menstrual tension, i.e. an increased tendency to be emotional, because of hormonal changes in your body
- ♥ a feeling of faintness or dizziness
- ♥ an increased need to pass urine
- ♥ an increase in vaginal discharge
- ♥ an absent period—the more you go overdue, the more likely it is that you are pregnant
- ♥ a very light period—yes, this is possible!
- ♥ sensitive breasts, especially around the nipple area, which may suddenly feel sore if you are breastfeeding another baby
- ♥ unexplained tiredness at any time of the day or evening
- ♥ an increased tendency to have vivid dreams

If you have experienced some of the above symptoms, check to see if you are pregnant. You don't need to go to any public place to do this. Nowadays, chemists and even supermarkets sell pregnancy test kits which are affordable, easy and quick to use at home. The most common type of test involves testing a little of your own urine for the presence of hCG (human chorionic gonadotrophin)—the hormone which your body starts to produce when you are pregnant. You simply collect a little urine in a pot and then dip a stick into it, or go through some similar procedure. (There are lots of versions of the same test—simply follow the directions on the packet.) After a few moments or minutes, you will have your answer… your own private secret.

If the test is negative perhaps you've done the test too early

If the result is negative, this could mean one of two things. Perhaps you have performed the test too early for sufficient hCG to be present, as we've mentioned—which means you are pregnant but can't confirm it yet. (You may have ovulated extremely late in your cycle, for whatever reason.) Or perhaps you are not pregnant and your period is about to start. This could be because you have imagined some symptoms simply because of your desire to get pregnant, or it could mean that you were pregnant a day or two ago, but that your body decided not to sustain the pregnancy. If you experience a miscarriage, try to not to get too upset—after all, some fertilised eggs are rejected from the womb for very good reasons. Stay open to the idea of becoming pregnant again soon, though, and focus on other things. The wait might seem difficult and long, but it will certainly be worthwhile.

Checking your due date

When you find you're definitely pregnant, you can calculate your baby's likely arrival using the chart on page 148. Simply find your LMP (the date of the first day of your last period) on one of the dark grey lines of the chart, then look at the date below it. This is your baby's estimated date of birth. (Caregivers call this the EDD, i.e. the estimated date of delivery.) Note that your due date will be later than indicated in the chart if your cycle is longer than 28 days, e.g. two days later if you have a 30-day cycle, and that it is still only an *estimate* of when your baby is likely to arrive. He or she may be born two weeks before or after this date, or even before or after that. (See 'due dates' in the Index.)

Calculate your own due date

Calculate your own due date by taking into account the length of your monthly cycle and your estimated date of ovulation—as well as the actual length of any other pregnancies. That way, you're much more likely to have an accurate EDD. Some women give their LMP as being a few days or a week or so later than it actually was in cases where they regularly have a longer cycle than 28 days. They do this so as to ensure that they will not be put under undue pressure to be induced after their '28-day cycle' due date has come and gone, before there *actual* due date arrives. This is not as dishonest as it sounds. Women do it because they want a more accurate estimated birth date for their baby to be put in their medical notes. For example, if their normal menstrual cycle is 33 days, rather than 28, they give their LMP as being five days later than it actually was because it's very likely their baby will spontaneously be born five days after the 'due date' that's calculated with the chart, which is based on a 28-day cycle. See www.redbabybook.com for an online calculator.

If your cycle is 5 days longer, your due date is really 5 days later

Sharing your news

It's important to think carefully about when and how you tell other people you're pregnant. Firstly, both false positives and false negatives are possible when you do a pregnancy test, so reconfirming your result with another home test kit a week or two after the positive test result may be a good idea.[4] Secondly, even when you are sure you're pregnant, the impact of sharing your news may not always be what you expect. It's therefore a good idea to think carefully about when to release your news to family and friends.

Your partner

You'll probably want to tell your partner immediately. Sharing the process of conception is extremely important, whatever the experience is like for you. After all, it takes two to make a baby! However, a woman who is repeatedly having miscarriages might want to rethink this.

Your mother and other relatives

It's probably a good idea to wait a little longer before you tell other members of your family because miscarriage is very common in the early weeks. I would suggest it's a good idea to wait until you're at least 14 weeks pregnant because it's not until about 12 weeks after conception that the risk of miscarriage declines dramatically and a pregnancy becomes well-established. A woman who repeatedly has early miscarriages after telling other people about her pregnancies very early on each time is likely to feel under pressure to sustain a subsequent pregnancy. This isn't helpful, because psychological factors seem to be important in maintaining a pregnancy. Another reason for keeping your news a secret for a while is so as to keep yourself away from well-meaning but perhaps unhelpful comments or advice. Blood relatives can also have a very powerful (and sometimes destructive) effect on a woman's mind so this is one time when it's best to keep things private. The impatience that relatives may feel—for the pregnancy to come to an end and result in a baby—may also mean that a pregnant woman feels under pressure to 'deliver' towards the end of her pregnancy, before her baby is really ready to be born. So you might be doing yourself a favour if you keep your new pregnancy to yourself in the early weeks, no matter how close you feel to your mother, sisters or other relatives.

Close friends and acquaintances

Again, it's best to wait. Friends are even more likely to make comments and give out unsolicited advice than relatives. If you remain silent for a while, you will give yourself time to read, learn and think at your own pace. You will also give yourself a chance to adjust to your new status in your own way.

Your colleagues and employers

People you work with can be told even later than everyone else, perhaps at the five- or six-month mark. This is quite simply because your work situation and promotion prospects can be affected when other people know you're pregnant. Instead of advertising your new pregnancy, focus on showing colleagues and bosses that you are a reliable and valuable worker. (You'll have to suffer any minor discomforts in private.) This way, you can maximise your chances of sustaining your career throughout this and other pregnancies into the future, or at least ensure you get a good reference when you eventually leave to have your baby. It is sensible to keep work options open during your childbearing years because having children is not a cheap option and financial difficulties are extremely common. You will, of course, also have the option of putting your career on a 'back burner' for a few years so that you can focus on bringing up your child (or children) yourself.

Your doctor

It might well be an idea to delay going to your GP until you're 14 weeks' pregnant. See the next chapter, 'Care about care', to understand why.

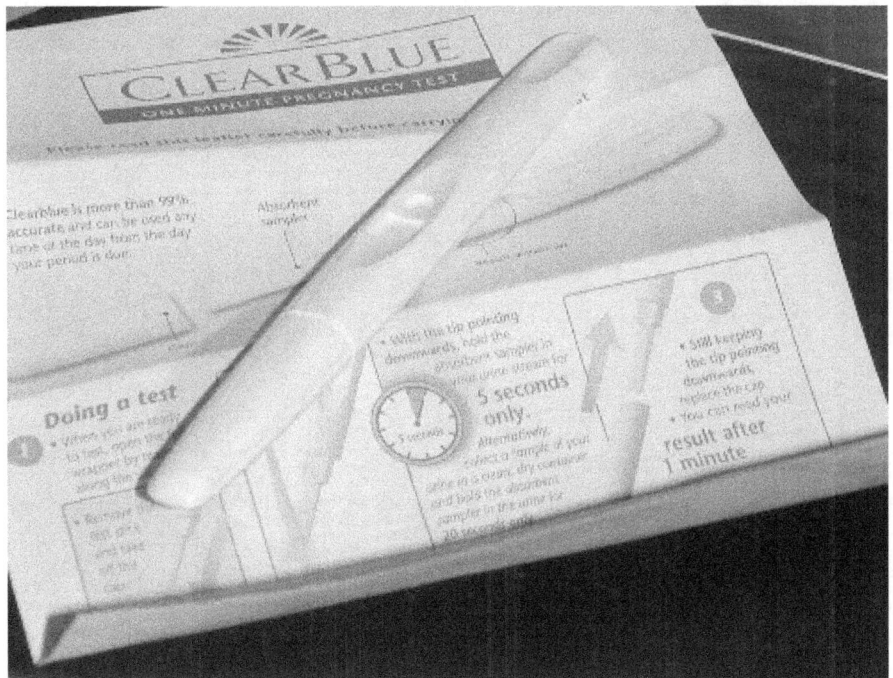

When the test is positive, make sure you don't blurt out news of your pregnancy at your local supermarket! Focus on buying healthy food instead.

148 birth: countdown to optimal

Jan	1	2	3	4	5	6	7	8	9	10	11	12	13	14	15	16	17	18	19	20	21	22	23	24	25	26	27	28	29	30	31
Oct	8	9	10	11	12	13	14	15	16	17	18	19	20	21	22	23	24	25	26	27	28	29	30	31	1	2	3	4	5	6	7
Feb	1	2	3	4	5	6	7	8	9	10	11	12	13	14	15	16	17	18	19	20	21	22	23	24	25	26	27	28			
Nov	8	9	10	11	12	13	14	15	16	17	18	19	20	21	22	23	24	25	26	27	28	29	30	1	2	3	4	5			
Mar	1	2	3	4	5	6	7	8	9	10	11	12	13	14	15	16	17	18	19	20	21	22	23	24	25	26	27	28	29	30	31
Dec	6	7	8	9	10	11	12	13	14	15	16	17	18	19	20	21	22	23	24	25	26	27	28	29	30	31	1	2	3	4	5
April	1	2	3	4	5	6	7	8	9	10	11	12	13	14	15	16	17	18	19	20	21	22	23	24	25	26	27	28	29	30	
Jan	6	7	8	9	10	11	12	13	14	15	16	17	18	19	20	21	22	23	24	25	26	27	28	29	30	31	1	2	3	4	
May	1	2	3	4	5	6	7	8	9	10	11	12	13	14	15	16	17	18	19	20	21	22	23	24	25	26	27	28	29	30	31
Feb	5	6	7	8	9	10	11	12	13	14	15	16	17	18	19	20	21	22	23	24	25	26	27	28	1	2	3	4	5	6	7
June	1	2	3	4	5	6	7	8	9	10	11	12	13	14	15	16	17	18	19	20	21	22	23	24	25	26	27	28	29	30	
Mar	8	9	10	11	12	13	14	15	16	17	18	19	20	21	22	23	24	25	26	27	28	29	30	31	1	2	3	4	5	6	
July	1	2	3	4	5	6	7	8	9	10	11	12	13	14	15	16	17	18	19	20	21	22	23	24	25	26	27	28	29	30	31
April	7	8	9	10	11	12	13	14	15	16	17	18	19	20	21	22	23	24	25	26	27	28	29	30	1	2	3	4	5	6	7
Aug	1	2	3	4	5	6	7	8	9	10	11	12	13	14	15	16	17	18	19	20	21	22	23	24	25	26	27	28	29	30	31
May	8	9	10	11	12	13	14	15	16	17	18	19	20	21	22	23	24	25	26	27	28	29	30	31	1	2	3	4	5	6	7
Sept	1	2	3	4	5	6	7	8	9	10	11	12	13	14	15	16	17	18	19	20	21	22	23	24	25	26	27	28	29	30	
June	8	9	10	11	12	13	14	15	16	17	18	19	20	21	22	23	24	25	26	27	28	29	30	1	2	3	4	5	6	7	
Oct	1	2	3	4	5	6	7	8	9	10	11	12	13	14	15	16	17	18	19	20	21	22	23	24	25	26	27	28	29	30	31
July	8	9	10	11	12	13	14	15	16	17	18	19	20	21	22	23	24	25	26	27	28	29	30	31	1	2	3	4	5	6	7
Nov	1	2	3	4	5	6	7	8	9	10	11	12	13	14	15	16	17	18	19	20	21	22	23	24	25	26	27	28	29	30	
Aug	8	9	10	11	12	13	14	15	16	17	18	19	20	21	22	23	24	25	26	27	28	29	30	31	1	2	3	4	5	6	
Dec	1	2	3	4	5	6	7	8	9	10	11	12	13	14	15	16	17	18	19	20	21	22	23	24	25	26	27	28	29	30	31
Sept	7	8	9	10	11	12	13	14	15	16	17	18	19	20	21	22	23	24	25	26	27	28	29	30	1	2	3	4	5	6	7

A chart for calculating approximately when your baby is due. Find the first day of your last period on a dark grey line, and read your due date underneath.

A Canadian nurse I met was happy to go three or four weeks after her due date. Amazingly, she managed to get her caregivers to agree to this. As it happened, her baby was born perfectly healthy exactly three weeks after her due date. See 'due dates' and 'ultrasound' in the Index for more information and comments on this issue.

> " I had two miscarriages—one in 1998 and one in 1999. Very sad occasions. We were trying for a baby and I already had a 7-year-old at the time so thought it would go OK. We were given no reason why these miscarriages happened.

Week 6

Several crucial developments take place this week. By the end of the week, the umbilical cord, digestive tract, kidneys, liver, heart and bloodstream are already forming and beginning to function—the heart will start beating during this week—and all these organs and systems are helping your new baby to get and use food from the rich lining of your womb. The mouth and jaw are also developing now and 10 discrete dental buds are growing in each jaw. The four shallow pits which have already appeared on your little baby's head will later develop into eyes and ears. The most important development this week sounds unimpressive but is actually crucial. A groove appears down your little baby's body; this will soon form the spinal cord and the brain. If you were wondering why you need to take folic acid until approximately 12 weeks after conception, this is the reason. You need to make sure the development of this neural tube proceeds smoothly. This one tube consists of 125,000 cells, which is amazing when you consider that your baby is still only the size of a pea.

Week 7

Your little baby is still developing at a phenomenal rate. To get an idea just how fast this is, consider that while your baby's limb buds will have developed by the 30th day after conception, by the 31st day (which is in the middle of this week) these same buds will have become subdivided into hands, arms and shoulders. The brain will be 25% bigger than it was just two days earlier.

By the end of this week, your baby is the size of a small grape, growing at a rate of 1mm a day. If you could see it, you might think its head looked big in relation to its body, but this is normal. Already a face is forming, with tightly closed eyelids over dark-looking eyes. Your little one also has rudimentary arms and legs and is making its first movements. At the end of each limb small indentations which will later become fingers and toes are already discernible. Bone cells are also appearing.

The development of your future baby's lungs, intestines, liver and kidneys continues and sex organs begin to form. (To honour this last important change, we shall now refer to your baby as a 'she'—even though you must always remember that you may well be expecting a boy.) The pancreas and thyroid are already in place. Your baby's heart, which recently started beating, is currently beginning to form its four separate chambers.

Your baby's nervous system is almost completely formed

The nervous system, including your baby's spinal cord and brain, is almost completely formed. In about a week's time (41 days after conception) the complex structure of the mature brain will already be in evidence, albeit in miniature. Your baby is becoming so complex, she will soon no longer be called an embryo.

Week 8

By the end of this week (six weeks after conception), your growing baby starts being called a fetus, which means 'little one'. She is no longer dependent on a yolk sac for nourishment, so this has already disappeared.

Your little baby's face is continuing to form: her nose is now pointed and already has nostrils; her eyes and ears are growing; and the two sides of her jaw will have joined together to make a mouth. Inside her mouth, there is a tiny tongue and taste buds will begin to appear on it in two weeks' time. (The palate will also begin to form at that time.) Since the inner parts of her ears are developing your baby will soon have a sense of balance. This is useful because your little one is already moving around a lot in her sac, even though you won't be able to feel this yet.

Your baby's tiny skeleton is now fully formed out of soft cartilage; this will later develop into bone. All the internal organs are in evidence, even though they are not yet fully developed or in their final positions. The arms and legs have grown longer in the last week and if only you could take a peek, you would be able to discern shoulders, elbows, hips and knees. Even fingers and toes are beginning to form, although they are joined by webs of skin for the time being.

There is already evidence that your little one's brain is working because electrical activity can now be measured. By the end of this week your growing baby will be around 2½cm long.

Your little one's brain is already working

Week 9

Your baby's limbs are continuing to develop rapidly and her fingers and toes are becoming more clearly defined.

Movements which were initially merely floating are gradually becoming a form of exercise for newly forming muscles. Movements will increasingly synchronise with your own movements as your baby's vestibular system (which is concerned with gravity and balance in space) starts to develop. Periods of activity will alternate with periods of rest from now on until the birth, when a pattern of nighttime rest and daytime activity will eventually become established. Your baby's brain, which coordinates all this movement, is continuing to develop: by now her brainstem (the lower portion of the brain) will be fully developed and her midbrain and forebrain (a little higher up) will start to expand. The wrinkles on the outer surface of her forebrain (the cerebral cortex), which are so characteristic of human beings and which allow us to accommodate vastly more brain cells than other species, are now also beginning to appear. Oxygen is being pumped round your baby's tiny body in red blood cells, which are already being produced by the liver. Beta-endorphins are already detectable in this blood, which suggests your little one can already experience pleasure.

Your baby's face, eyes, nose, lips and tongue would be clearly visible to you... if only you had a little window flap in your abdomen! The first signs of teeth and bone would also be seen. By the end of this week urogenital development begins for both sexes. If your baby is to be a boy, a penis would now also probably be visible. All this is happening in miniature because the little being inside you still only weighs little more than a grape.

Week 10

Just eight weeks after your baby was conceived, tactile sensitivity has developed in the face. If the cheeks were to be stroked gently with a hair, your baby would move her head away, bend her trunk and pelvis and extend her arms and shoulders enough to push the hair away. (Don't ask me how researchers know this, but they claim that they do.) Sensitivity on other areas of skin will develop gradually over the next few weeks. Chest movements, which are now detectable to researchers, might well be practice exercises for breathing after birth. Inside your baby's chest, the heart has finished dividing into four chambers and each is connected to the others by tiny valves. The placenta, to which your baby is already attached, begins to produce progesterone around this time. Your baby is still being nourished entirely by the so-called corpus luteum but this will soon change. Fingers, hands, wrists, toes and ankles are well-defined and the face is even more recognisably human. Your little one is now roughly the size of a large strawberry.

Week 11

Either by now or in a few days' time (depending on when you conceived), all your baby's major body organs will have finished forming. Even miniature ovaries and testicles will have finished forming and your baby's circulation will be functioning properly. This all means the most critical period of development is over. For some reason, this means the risk of miscarriage also decreases sharply around this time.

Birthframe 32

The first time I found out I was pregnant, we were on an Easter holiday above the Arctic Circle in Finland. My first noticeable sign of pregnancy was terrible insomnia. I crept outdoors at 4.00am, as a pink spring dawn broke over a wide, flat snowscape. I felt overwhelmed with the knowledge that I was not alone. Although still only a microscopic ball of cells, my future offspring was already with me. What would this dawn of a new life be like, for me and for this child?

Three months later, my husband and I took the ferry to Bruges in Belgium for the weekend. As our wake churned behind us toward Dover's chalk cliffs, I thought about how this point in my life was a metaphysical departure, too, towards a time in my life when I would come to know the new human beings who would enter my life through my own womb.

I never stop wondering at the journey that begins with a particular event of copulation—perhaps specifically remembered, perhaps not—into a single cell, into 10 billion cells born months later as a fully-formed human baby.

Nina Klose

Week 12

The tiny baby within you, who continues to be called a fetus, is beginning to look more and more human. Her head is becoming more rounded, even though it would still look rather large in proportion to her body. Her eyelids are now formed, but are closed over her eyes, and her external ears even have earlobes.

By the end of this week your baby will be getting all her nourishment via the placenta, which should now be fully functioning. The blood vessels in the umbilical cord carry food and oxygen to your baby and then take carbon dioxide back out again. Your little one can now open and shut her mouth and swallow; she uses this new skill to continuously take in amniotic fluid. Doing this will help her lungs develop, so that they are ready for breathing, as soon as she's born.

The amniotic fluid is changed once every 24 hours

The kidneys now are beginning to function, which means your baby will urinate into the amniotic fluid. Don't worry about this—your womb constantly replaces this fluid so your baby's environment stays fresh. Amazing as it might seem, a complete change of amniotic fluid is effected once every 24 hours. (This rate will even gradually increase over the next few weeks.) Any waste products in the urine from your baby will be automatically dealt with by your own kidneys; other waste products which do not come out in the baby's urine are stored in the baby's intestines, ready to be excreted soon after birth as meconium, which will be your baby's first 'poo'. This early poo is different from normal poos, incidentally, in that its tar-like consistency actually acts to block your baby's bowel before birth; only if a baby becomes distressed while in the womb is this secreted into the amniotic fluid.

Your baby's muscles, having further developed over the last couple of weeks, now allow for much more vigorous movement. In experiments, babies have been observed rolling from side to side, extending and then flexing their backs and necks, waving their arms and kicking their legs—straight into the side wall of the amniotic sac! The usually graceful and apparently voluntary and spontaneous movements your baby now makes are thought by some to be an early example of initiative and self-expression. Such creative gymnastics seem to demonstrate quite sophisticated brain activity, which only a few decades ago would have been considered impossible. Movements of the face—frowns, pursing the lips, opening and closing the mouth—all seem to indicate an emotional response to whatever's going on, given that the pituitary started producing pleasurable beta-endorphins a few weeks ago.

Various experiments have suggested great sensitivity and emotional responses by this stage of pregnancy

Fetuses at this age who have had their genitals stroked under experimental conditions (accidentally, I hope) have shown a clear response, which suggests a high level of sensitivity. Small, well-coordinated movements of tiny fingers and toes (which are both growing miniature finger- and toenails) suggest further sensitivity and emotional response.

Your miniature miracle now weighs about 14g and is perhaps 7 or 8cm long. Clearly, a lot more growth and development is needed before this little being can survive independently, outside the safety of the womb, but she is at least now a little less susceptible to harm from infection or chemicals circulating around your own body.

THE SECOND TRIMESTER

When you enter this second period of development your baby will be much more of a being in her own right and her support system, the placenta, should be functioning effectively, thanks to the production of progesterone. This means that if you suffered from nausea or vomiting in the first trimester, it's likely to disappear now or at least fade very soon.

Week 13

Your baby now begins to do more and more things which seem more recognisably 'human'. She might suck her thumb, for example, extend her fingers, or even yawn when she's tired. Tiredness is perhaps understandable given that her periods of movement are extremely frequent, with rest periods extending no longer than 15 minutes until around Week 20. Your baby's neck is also longer, which makes her look much more human.

Being completely formed, your baby is now focusing on growing (at an even faster rate than before), so good nutrition with plenty of protein is extremely important.

Her skin sensitivity is increasing to the point where even the palms of her hands would respond to strokes; her arms and legs would certainly be sensitive to hair strokes. Some primitive reflexes are also either already present or will develop over the next four weeks.

Some people believe that personality is also beginning to develop at this stage because at least two research projects have concluded that exposure to influenza during the second trimester (between the fourth and seventh months of pregnancy) results in increased susceptibility to schizophrenia, so avoiding people who are snuffly might be especially important over the next few months.

Week 14

Almost three months since conception, your baby will now be approximately 9cm long and will definitely be receiving all her nourishment from 'her' placenta, which some young children have referred to as a kind of friend in the womb. It looks like a large, liver-like organ and it will be born separately, just after your baby.

Your little one's eyes have now moved away from the side of her head to the front, and her ears have moved up from the neck to their proper position on the head, but they're still fused shut for the time being. Your baby has eyebrows now, as well as a small amount of hair on her head. The basic parts of the spinal cord and brain are in place, and your baby's respiratory tract, which starts at the nose and branches again and again on the way to the lungs, is now ready for your baby's first breathing movements. As for other movements, your baby may now start moving her arms and legs rhythmically. Increased skin sensitivity means that if it were possible to stroke her very gently on the cheek, you would see her turn her head and start searching for something, probably a nipple to suckle from!

The next four weeks are a period of rapid skeletal development. We know this because some researchers have tracked it on X-rays.

Week 15

It is in this week that your baby's sex organs will mature. Her nose will also be better formed and her head and eyebrow hair will gradually start to become coarser. If your baby has a gene for black hair, the pigment cells of the hair follicles are now beginning to produce black pigment.

It seems likely that taste buds are also functioning by now. We know for certain that no essential changes take place in taste receptors after this point, except for the fact that they multiply and spread themselves more widely. This means that your baby will be having taste experiences based on what you yourself eat and drink from now until her birth. It's possible that these experiences may affect her preferences in childhood and possibly also beyond—I've certainly observed this in my own children and other people have commented on it too! Based on the contents of amniotic fluid which has been tested, we know that your baby will be tasting glucose, fructose, lactic, pyruvic and citric acid, fatty acids, phospholipids, creatinine, urea, uric acid, amino acids, polypeptides, proteins and salts, amongst other things. It doesn't sound very appetising but it certainly indicates that she's having a wide range of gustatory experience. As well as sucking her thumb, your baby may also suck her fingers, hands and toes and hold her umbilical cord by this stage.

Week 16

By now, your baby will weigh about 75g and will be about 11½cm long. If you could look at her, you would see transparent skin, with fine networks of blood vessels underneath.

Hard bones are beginning to develop and your baby's legs will have become longer. Both arms and legs will now have joints. She already has well-formed fingernails and toenails and her fingers would already produce a unique fingerprint. She can now coordinate all her movements and she will be moving around energetically, although you probably won't be able to feel this just yet.

Your baby can now coordinate all his or her movements

Even though your baby's ears are not yet fully formed, she is already responding to sound, probably because of feeling vibrations through her skin. Her eyes are now open and quite expressive. During invasive procedures, expressions such as squinting and sneering have been filmed at this stage of pregnancy. Researchers who observed these expressions felt certain they represented meaningful reactions to what was happening.

Your baby's eyebrows and eyelashes are growing and your baby will already have fine downy hair ('lanugo') on both her face and body. This lanugo usually disappears by the time of the birth, but it can still be seen on premature babies.

Although your baby's major organs are now fully developed, she will continue to grow rapidly this month and in the rest of your pregnancy so that she will be capable of independent life. Already, she will be making breathing movements, which are practice movements for after the birth.

Week 17

By now, your baby will measure about 15cm, which is approximately the length of a pen. She will weigh about 175g. These are landmark measurements because for the first time, your baby weighs more than her support system, the placenta. She is still becoming increasingly sensitive... babies' abdomens and buttocks have responded to hair strokes in experiments at this stage and different responses have been recorded when babies were exposed to different kinds of music: Beethoven, Brahms and hard-rock music made babies restless, while Vivaldi and Mozart calmed them down. Perhaps this is worth bearing in mind when you decide what kind of music you're going to listen to, although your own tastes are also important.

Week 18

Your baby may now be as long as 20cm and you may soon notice her moving around inside you. By the end of this week, a midwife would be able to hear your baby's heartbeat with an ordinary fetal stethoscope (a Pinard), i.e. one which doesn't use ultrasound in any way.

Your baby will be drinking amniotic fluid through a perfectly formed mouth and lips. This is a practice exercise so that breathing takes place without undue effort or fatigue after the birth. Sometimes this exercise will make your baby develop hiccups, which you might notice as a jerking of your abdomen. Your little one will also be practising sucking, maybe using her thumb, which is obviously preparation for feeding after birth. Your baby may also be making other sounds quite voluntarily by now, which is perhaps the first step in language learning. Bones are still continuing to form rapidly and your baby's nasal septum will now have fused with her palate.

Birthframe 33

Here's an account from a Christian friend about how she believes praying affected her growing baby. If you don't pray yourself, you can at the very least visualise positive things for your baby. It's a way of making sure your fears don't overwhelm you. Also, since feelings and thoughts have a physical effect on the body (e.g. fear results in muscular tension and other biological changes), any positive visualisations may well be beneficial for your baby. If you do have any spiritual faith, asking for support is an obvious thing to do.

> Our third child received prayer along with me from two intercessors from about the fourth month of pregnancy. Neither of us was ill, but I was too busy and stressed to focus on my growing baby the way I felt was necessary.
>
> It was a wonderful birth. Our daughter knew precisely how to be born and the midwife remarked that she must have been here before. Also, several people commented on her confidence as a newborn and her ability to communicate. When I mentioned this to the prayer group coordinator, she said that this was the case with most 'prayer babies' she had known. To this day, this child is determined, confident and strongly connected to the world and to other people.

Week 19

This week, buds for permanent teeth are forming behind those which have already formed for the milk teeth. Your baby's sense of touch is also still developing: she would now respond if touched almost anywhere on her body.

She will now be making stronger and better coordinated movements, which might even include back flips, rolls and little punches. These gymnastics are only possible because your little one's nervous system is now much more sophisticated. By the way, don't simulate pain in any way in order to practise for labour. Nowadays it's been well-established that hormones (which are affected by our emotions) pass across the placenta—so our own nervousness, tension, pain or fear is likely to be shared with our developing baby.

Week 20

Your baby has been growing fast, so by now her body will have reached its correct relative proportions. She is now about half as tall as she will be at birth; she will only weigh about 340g, though—about the weight of a grapefruit. Ear development is continuing, with myelin insulation taking place in the ear nerve (the cochlear nerve). This no doubt means your baby is hearing even more sounds—those of your body as well as a muffled version of any you can hear yourself. Your own voice and that of your partner are likely to be a particular focus...

The parts of the system which allow a person to register head and body motion and the pull of gravity are all fully grown by now. This means your baby will probably already be aware of her own movements. For some reason it is common for babies to have a quiet period at this stage, in terms of bodily movements.

Hair could probably be seen on your baby's head, and sebum from sebaceous glands mixes with skin cells so as to begin to form 'vernix caseosa'. (This is the greasy covering over the lanugo which protects your baby's skin while she's in the womb.) Your baby can now reach out with her hand for a source of light (such as a torch beam panned slowly across your tummy), even though her eyes are fused shut. It's possible that from now on protective substances may pass through your blood, through the placenta to your baby, so as to help your baby resist disease in the first few weeks.

Week 21

Your baby now weighs about 450g. Hair growth is a prominent feature of the next four weeks. It is also over this period that your baby's permanent teeth buds finish forming and that she will develop so-called 'brown fat', which is an important source of heat and energy for the newborn. She will also begin to make crying motions over the next few weeks and will continue to practise sucking.

You should by now feel very definite strong kicks sometimes high up in your tummy and sometimes low down near your pubic hair.

Week 22

At 22 weeks, your baby will be about 30cm long but will still be very red and wrinkled in appearance. The gradually increasing levels of fat in her body should be noticeable to you through your increasingly rounded form!

You may by now be able to feel the differences between different parts of her body as she kicks, jumps and turns around. Sometimes you may feel a hand, sometimes a foot, the head or the buttocks. These movements may actually usually take place when you yourself are trying to rest because your baby is likely to be at her most active then. (Perhaps she finds the movement of your body soothing and sleep-inducing.) Your partner will also be able to become more aware of your baby this week because if he puts his ear to your abdomen, he should hear a distinct baby heartbeat.

If your partner puts his ear to your abdomen he should hear a distinct baby heartbeat

Over the next four weeks, most organs will become capable of functioning. By this early stage of gestation, your baby will also have started renewing her own skin cells. Your growing baby's eyelids and eyebrows will be well-formed, even though her eyes will still be fused shut, and her face will be even more expressive. In experiments, puckering of the lips, scowling and muscle tension around the eyes have all been associated with audible crying at this stage of pregnancy. (The sounds can actually be heard by the mother and researchers under certain experimental conditions.) These appropriate facial expressions are interesting in that they suggest that your baby has developed clear links between body and brain.

Also, only 20 weeks after conception, research has revealed that hearing and memory are becoming increasingly acute. Researchers have shown that newborn babies remember voices and music which they heard in the womb at this stage of pregnancy. This means that any lullaby you sing and any music you play from now on may have a noticeably calming effect on your newborn later on. The same applies to your partner's voice so it's a good idea to encourage him to speak to your growing baby.

Week 23

Your baby's arms and legs are now well developed. She can now grip with her hands... scans have clearly shown this by this stage of pregnancy. The fine hair (the lanugo) which covers your baby's body is beginning to darken. Braxton Hicks contractions (painless tightenings of your womb which began around Week 6), may now become more pronounced, meaning that your baby is regularly getting practice hugs and massage sessions! If you make love with your partner, your body's own response may also have an effect on your baby. Research experiments focusing on this period of pregnancy have demonstrated that an unborn baby's heart rate either shoots up or slows down when the mother has an orgasm.

Week 24

Your baby will now probably weigh over half a kilo and will be about 33cm long. You can imagine her curled up in your womb, cushioned by the bag of waters that surrounds her and totally dependent on the placenta for food and oxygen, as well as the disposal of her waste products. Everything you might ingest (food, drink, drugs, other chemicals, air, smoke, etc.) would still cross the placenta and would be shared with your baby, so continue to be aware of this.

Since the amniotic fluid is now changed every four hours, it makes sense to drink lots and lots of water. Amniotic fluid is very important because not only does it provide important liquid for your baby's digestion (enabling her to wee), it also regulates her temperature and protects her from infection and any sudden bumps you may experience.

160 birth: countdown to optimal

By now your baby will actually look and behave much the same as a baby at birth. She is continuing to make breathing movements (practising for life outside the womb) and she coughs spontaneously whenever she needs to. She continues to kick and punch and even turn somersaults, so as to build up her muscles for life outside the womb. She might also sometimes make a fist, which indicates that she is developing her grasping reflex, which would be useful if we carried our babies round on our backs—without back-carriers!—like chimpanzees. Your baby is unlike a newborn in that her eyes are still a bit bulgy (because of her thin face) and they are still sealed shut.

Your baby is making great progress in other respects too: her skin is getting thicker; her sweat glands (so important for temperature control) are forming in the skin; and her responses to her environment are becoming even more obvious. Awareness of sounds may have increased to such an extent that any sudden noise makes your baby jump and she is likely to react to sounds she finds unpleasant by moving in different ways. Loud music is likely to wake her up, if she's asleep. Your baby may continue to suck her thumb in an apparent attempt to comfort herself. Over the next four weeks, the part of your baby's brain concerned with personality and intelligence is becoming much more complex so we can guess that her personality may be developing over this period too.

In some countries your baby is already considered legally 'viable' by the end of this week, even though her lungs are not yet sufficiently developed for independent survival outside your womb. Premature baby care is developing and some remarkable babies already survive.

Resting while you're pregnant

It's worth being careful about how you rest from now on. I'm going to explain this in pictures, I'm afraid, so as to be absolutely clear...

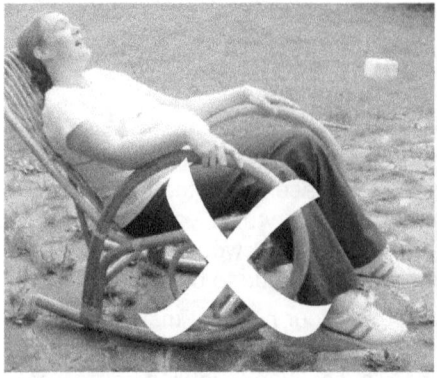 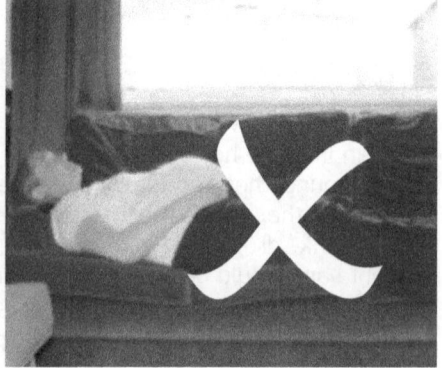

This is what not to do... see why on the next page!

7... HELP YOUR BABY 161

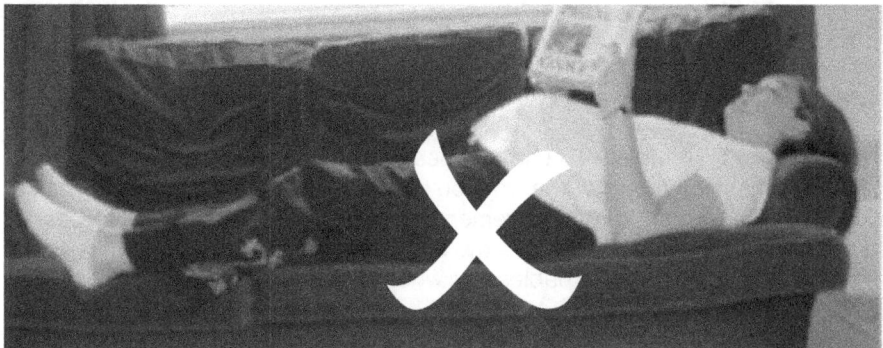

If you lie back while you're pregnant, your baby is likely to be deprived of oxygen because the main vein, the 'vena cava', which takes blood from the placenta, and therefore the baby, gets compressed. Lying back also does nothing to help the baby get into a good position for the birth. Remember not to lie back in the bath either. You can still have a bath, but sit up and lean forward. If this doesn't sound like fun, stick to showers while you're pregnant. Better in any case for baby not to have hot water round him or her for long.

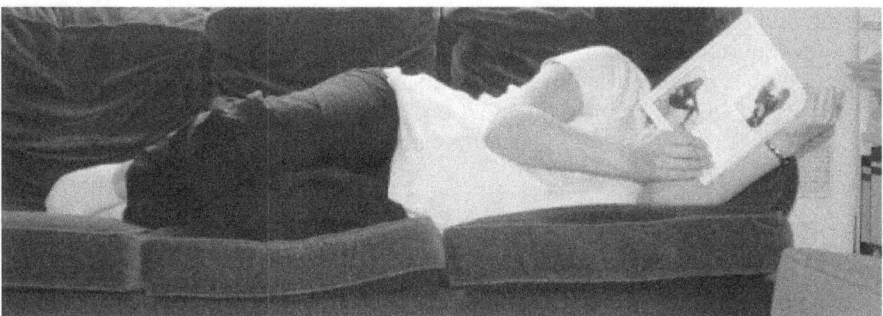

Here's a position to use for relaxation. Note that lying on your left side is much, much better for the baby (from the point of view of getting enough oxygen) than lying on your right side. It will also lower your own risk of getting high blood pressure. Lying on your left side, you can read, sleep, read to children (they're usually more than happy to climb around you), chat to friends... or even watch TV. But stick to gentle comedy or romantic movies. Beware of distressing the baby! I've heard of more than one labour that started after over-strenuous laughter or something noisy or frightening happening nearby. Beyond an awareness of these risks, enjoy yourself. You deserve a rest! Don't put your feet up in the normal manner, though. It makes me so angry when I see photos of pregnant women leaning back, relaxing... To make matters worse, loads of people literally say: "Put your feet up and relax while you have the chance". Not only is leaning back bad for the mother's birth prospects and blood pressure, it's also likely to mean the baby is in the least healthy position—from the point of view of getting enough oxygen. (Is this a minor point or what? Aaargh!)

Lying on your left side is much better for the baby

Week 25

Over the next month, your baby's eyes begin to open and shut, she gets significantly longer and puts on a substantial amount of weight. Her ears are now structurally complete so she can hear your voice clearly. This means you should perhaps be aware of the way you talk about her while she's living inside you, and afterwards too. Always remember that she's a person who needs to be treated with respect and sensitivity. If you question this, just think for a moment about how easily babies cry when a person is around who seems unsympathetic to them.

Your baby's reactions to loud noises may still be quite dramatic: you will simply feel a sudden jolt. Some sounds will be less alarming to your baby because she will be used to hearing many of them, e.g. the continuous sloshing and squelching of your stomach and bowels. Apparently, noises from these places peak at 85 decibels, which is really quite loud. (One researcher found it was the volume which his vacuum cleaner made at his ears when he was vacuuming a carpeted floor.) Sounds which are heard at around 55 decibels include the constant rumble of your blood in the arteries which supply the uterus and placenta, which move in synchrony with your heart. (To give you an idea how loud this is, normal speech is usually about 60 decibels.) As a result of your baby's development in hearing ability, some experts believe it's a good idea to sing to your baby from now on, as well as talk to her. On a more physical level, your baby's bone centres begin to harden this week.

Week 26

Your baby is now growing at a rate of 1cm a week and every extra centimeter is making her stronger. By now, she will weigh almost a kilo. The ongoing increase in length means that your baby's positioning in the womb needs to change. She will find herself either the right way up, or upside down in the womb, depending on how she flexes or extends her knees. These movements must require an enormous amount of brain-to-body coordination and it's interesting that they won't be possible outside the womb until 2-3 weeks after birth.

Other changes are taking place this week. Firstly, your baby's skin, which was previously paper-thin, is now becoming thicker and opaque. Secondly her eyelashes are lengthening. Thirdly, the number of her tastebuds is increasing. Research from as far back as 1937 shows that if something sweet is introduced into the amniotic fluid, a baby will swallow more rapidly. This of course means that you need to consider carefully whether or not both you and your baby really need that chocolate bar or ice cream, before you demolish it... How about a salad, some eggs or some salmon instead?!

By the end of this week, your baby's chance of survival outside your womb would be much higher, although every extra week spent inside you helps to prepare her for the outside world. Nature did not intend babies to be born at this early stage of gestation, but if your baby is born prematurely, don't panic... Read Birthframe 50 (and possibly also Birthframe 49), while remembering that Einstein was also a premature baby!

Week 27

Your baby is still growing very fast and will probably weigh just over a kilo by now. Her eyes are now open and will have blue irises (slate grey, in fact—the colour of muscle), but this colour may change after the birth. The nostrils are open and your baby is practising breathing.

If you want to try and visualise her, you need to include a very wrinkled skin, coated in creamy vernix. The wrinkling is no doubt due to the watery nature of your baby's present home. Her creamy white covering is there for her own protection. It's a bit like staying in the bath for much too long, covered in nourishing, protective moisturising cream so as to prevent your skin from becoming waterlogged. Your baby's heart will now be beating at a rate of 120-140 beats per minute, which is double the speed of an adult's heart rate.

Week 28

Most countries consider a baby legally viable by the end of this week, which means her birth would need to be registered if it should happen to take place prematurely. Paediatricians are optimistic about a premature baby's survival by this stage of development—some even put it at 95%. Assuming you personally are going to carry your baby to term (38-40 weeks), you're now well on your way to having a full-term birth as long as you avoid liquorice, shocks and inadequate diets! The third trimester (which officially starts next week) is your 'home run', so to speak. Enjoy the last few months of being pregnant so that your baby can have a happy emotional environment to swim around in!

Your baby's length and weight will have increased even more. The variety of birth weights and lengths make measurements increasingly difficult to generalise, which is why I shall not mention them from now on. Your baby's ever-increasing size means she is nearing the end of the time when she can lie stretched out. Perhaps because of an increasing lack of space, the volume of amniotic fluid in your womb will reach a peak between now and Week 32. As a result of this increase in size and a decrease in the amount of liquid to move about in, your baby will find it more and more of a challenge to find a position that feels comfortable over the next few weeks... so you will not be the only one who is shifting and twisting about in an effort to find the ideal position for a peaceful sleep!

Your baby is definitely listening to your speech patterns very carefully now. A study as long ago as 1975 which analysed the cries of premature babies born at 28 weeks clearly showed that babies were copying their mothers' basic speech patterns. This requires a sophisticated level of filtering on your baby's part. As well as screening out your body's squelching and gurgling, your baby will also be filtering out louder ambient sounds in order to focus on your voice. Obviously, this is another important stage of language development.

> Your baby is listening to your speech patterns now.
> This is an important stage of development.

Your baby will also be appreciating tastes more, as she gets used to differentiating between whatever you provide. Research has shown that babies can already respond to sweet, sour and bitter tastes. Your baby will actually have more taste buds at this stage in her development than she will have at birth, so her palate really might be quite discerning. Think before you eat!

Difficult as it might be to believe, your baby will probably also start having another range of new experiences around this time: sexual feelings. Quite by accident, some American researchers observed male babies having an erection while analysing a series of sonograms; in fact, six babies at about this stage of gestation were observed in this state! These erections doubtless prove that the appropriate nerve pathways are working by this time and they probably also indicate that unborn babies experience some of the feelings that adult men experience along with an erection. We can guess this because all six fetuses who were having erections were also thumb-sucking—which is almost certainly a pleasure-seeking pastime.

> By now your baby can experience pain and
> respond much the same as a full-term baby.

On a more general level, the thinking part of your baby's brain has now become much bigger and more complex. By now, it is possible for fetuses to feel pain and they respond in much the same way as full-term babies. Muscles in your baby's body are also becoming even stronger, which you will notice in the form of assertive kicks from within! Your partner will almost certainly be able to feel your baby move too, if he puts his hand on your bump. It may even be possible for you both to watch the shape of a foot or a bottom travel across your middle, as your little one changes position.

Finally, from this time onwards, your baby will be laying down fat underneath her skin in preparation for after her birth.

THE THIRD TRIMESTER

Different books mark this trimester as beginning at different points. Assuming it begins at the beginning of Week 29, you are now entering the last phase of your baby's development. The main focus now is on growth and lung maturation, so that your baby can breathe well when she's born. Effective growth over the next few weeks is very important as heavier babies tend to be stronger and healthier. That explains why it really is vital that you eat well over the next few weeks—even if you do feel huge!

Also be careful about your own stress levels. Many mothers I've heard from seem to make a connection between a stressful third trimester and a difficult birth. And while some women find it stressful having to continue working, others have reported stress caused from boredom and having too much time to think. While a house move is too stressful for some women, for others it signals a joyous new beginning. The key is probably self-awareness: make sure that whatever you do, you don't cause yourself too much negative stress. Part of this—whatever your approach to rest, work and leisure activities—is to try to maintain harmony around you so you're in a good state of mind when your due date approaches. Instead of getting embroiled in a disagreement, consider either stepping down with dignity, or asserting yourself amicably and respectfully. If you're still working, you'll need to be particularly careful you don't allow the stresses of the job to affect you. Do what you can in a methodical way, remembering that nobody is indispensable. You have a much more important project on the go! However, if something really is upsetting you, get it sorted so your mind is at rest. In other words, 'Know Thyself' and take action accordingly.

Week 29

By now your baby may already have quite an impressive head of hair and her brain will have become more sophisticated. The two halves of the brain have developed a degree of asymmetry, the left side being stronger. Of course, this is the hemisphere that controls the right side of the body, which is why most people are right-handed. A lot of other things are happening around now... The fat deposits which are being laid down between now and the end of Week 32 are smoothing your baby's body contours, although her skin will still be covered with thick white vernix. Rhythmic breathing motions continue as practice for breathing after the birth.

Be careful about your own stress levels. Many mothers make a connection between a stressful third trimester and a difficult birth. Work, or stay at home—whatever works best for you.

Your baby is also still growing fast, thanks to the nutrients which pass across the placenta and the amount of amniotic fluid your baby is drinking. We know from studies which have used radioactive tracers that babies drink from 15 to 40 milliliters of amniotic fluid every hour from now on until they're born. This nourishment adds up to 40 calories a day when a baby is swallowing normally and is supplemented by the nourishment which is provided via the placenta. Large, well-nourished babies swallow at a higher rate than small, grossly malnourished babies. This is why you need to avoid smoking, alcohol, junk food and bitter tastes, such as coffee. After all, studies have shown that when a bitter-tasting substance is injected into the amniotic fluid, babies suddenly stop drinking it. In the same studies, when saccharine was injected, some babies even doubled their rate of swallowing. (No, this does not mean you can eat loads of cakes and candy! Your baby needs you to provide a balanced diet.) Persuade your baby to swallow fast by providing her with lots of good quality, tasty food. That way, she'll get into a good pattern of growth in the last few weeks before her birth.

Week 30

Your baby's facial features will now be well-developed. Other aspects of her appearance are also continuing to change this week: the lanugo (the fine layer of hair on her skin) is disappearing from her face and her skin is becoming paler and less wrinkled. This is mainly because of the fat which is continuing to build up underneath her skin and which will help keep her warm after she's born. As well as storing fat, your baby is now also storing up iron reserves for after the birth. Finally, male babies' testes will descend into the scrotum during this week.

Your baby's experience of the physical world is probably becoming much more intense. A startle reaction would already be recordable to researchers. It's also very likely that your baby will be aware of any Braxton Hicks contractions you are spontaneously having. Perhaps the experience of these intermittent tightenings in the womb is what gives us a liking for cuddles in later life—who knows? Your baby may also be becoming increasingly aware of her restricted environment. I remember one of my own children recalling her time in my womb, saying, "It got very crowded in there at the end." (Comments from young children about their 'wombhood'—their time *in utero*—have been reported by quite a few mothers. It's obviously not possible to ascertain whether these are 'real' memories or only imagined ones, but some children do give the impression of being able to remember their pre-birth experience up to the age of 2.) Perhaps the strong kicks you now feel are kicks of frustration as well as attempts at exercise. The constant wriggling you will be aware of is almost certainly a sign that your baby is trying to get comfortable.

Getting your baby well-positioned for the birth

In my opinion it's helpful to use certain positions in your pregnancy so as to help your baby get into a good position in your womb. I say 'in my opinion', incidentally, because this advice, unlike advice given elsewhere in the book, is based only on my own views and those of optimal fetal positioning experts Jean Sutton and Pauline Scott (who co-authored a book entitled: *Optimal Foetal Positioning*, published by Birth Concepts in New Zealand in 1996). Research has not yet backed up the idea that adopting different positions will change the way a baby lies... but common sense, my own experience and that of numerous other mothers do suggest it does.

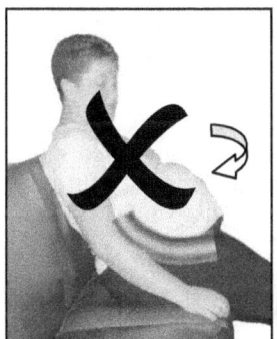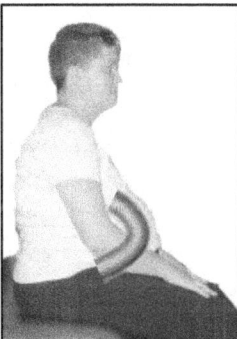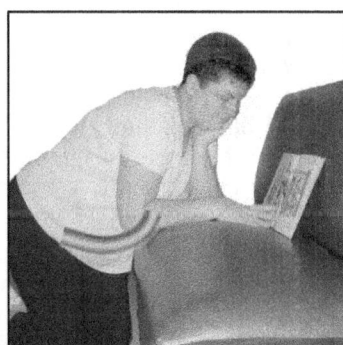

See below for an explanation

If you imagine the stripy dark line being the baby's back, you can easily see how lying back is not helpful in the last few weeks of pregnancy. The baby's back will tend to flip down because of the pull of gravity. This would result in a posterior labour, which would probably be more painful for you.

Kneel down as much as possible, for 10-15 minutes at a time, at least three times a day, especially in the last six weeks of your pregnancy. Make sure that when you do this you keep your back straight. (If anything, arch your back, but whatever you do, don't let it sag.) Think of things you can do in this position. Pick things up off the floor, vacuum clean using the hand attachment, wash the floor, help a child with a jigsaw... the list goes on!

When you're standing up, imagine yourself bouncing from the knees. This will help you to carry your weight well and avoid strain to your back. Your baby is also likely to stay in a good position for the birth.

In this more upright sitting position, the baby's back is more likely to stay round your front. With any type of chair, it's best to sit on the edge. Yes, it is worth it! You'll have a better birth. Alternatively, get a pregnancy rocker—see page 377 and contact details for Back In Action in the Useful contacts.

If you feel like relaxing, consider kneeling down by the sofa and reading a book or magazine which you've propped up. This is also a great position to use when you're reading stories to a toddler.

Week 31

Little by little, your baby will be getting plumper. She should now have gained around 50g of fat, which represents 3.5% of her total body weight. By the time she's born, body fat will account for 15% of her total body weight. (The percentage for an average-sized woman is around 27%.) The additional accumulated fat means it would no longer be possible to see the blood vessels beneath your baby's skin—if only you could take a peek. The shadowy images which represent your baby's growing bones would also no longer be visible now.

Little by little , your baby will be getting plumper

By this stage in your pregnancy you may occasionally feel very breathless, but rest assured that your baby is getting plenty of oxygen from you, thanks to the flow of blood through the placenta, along the umbilical cord. Of course, this oxygen is essential for your baby's survival and brain development so make sure you do nothing to compromise it. This means should continue to avoid smokers (and smoking) and should not lie on your back unless you're asked to at an antenatal appointment!

Week 32

By the end of this week your baby will be completely formed and her body will be in perfect proportion, taking into account the fact that the proportions will be that of a baby, i.e. large head and skinny limbs! She will be building up her immune system, taking antibodies from you so as to fight off disease and infection. She will also have beautifully formed miniature eyelashes and eyebrows, so must look very cute.

Your baby is continuing to gain weight... In fact, from now on until the time when your baby is born, she will gain at a rate of about 250g a week. This means it's more important than ever that you continue to eat well.

By now, she will have curled up into the well-known fetal position. Her head will probably already be pointing downwards, simply because the head is the heaviest part and gravity is likely to draw it downwards. If this isn't the case, don't panic. Before 32 weeks, at any given time, 50% of babies will be in a breech position but as these babies' heads become heavier than their bottoms, they usually spontaneously turn into a head down position around now, or at least by the 36th week of pregnancy. Even if a baby stays breech, a normal, optimal birth is still possible, so keep an open mind.

From now on until the time when your baby is born he or she will gain weight at a rate of about 250g a week

Week 33

As your baby continues to become chubbier, her skin smoothes out even more. If she has turned to a head down position by now, she will probably stay like that now until her birth. After all, she no longer has the luxury of being able to perform somersaults.

She will be going through some important development during the next few weeks. Her lungs will begin to produce surfactant (a substance similar to detergent), which will help them to expand and withstand pressure. It will also prevent your baby's lungs from collapsing at birth. Your baby's brain will also develop some new abilities. According to French research, a baby in the womb at this stage of gestation can be taught to recognise a nursery rhyme or simple piece of music and respond to it after the birth, as long as it's played daily for a month. Mozart and Vivaldi were the composers babies responded to best. I don't recommend you attempt any artificial exercises like these yourself, though, as I've already said. Doing what you spontaneously want to do is probably the best thing for your baby, who will benefit most from having a contented and healthy mother and an uncontrived environment. Babies can have interesting tastes in music, in my experience.

Week 34

This week your baby is becoming more rounded. The lanugo, the fine covering of hair all over her body, begins to disappear and your baby's skin will be getting pinker. Her ear cartilage is still soft, though, and the so-called plantar creases—creases on the soles of the feet—are still visible. Over the next four weeks, the hair on your baby's head will get longer and her nails will grow long enough to reach the tips of her fingers.

The movements you are now feeling will probably be much gentler than a few weeks ago. The increasing lack of space which we've already mentioned makes those vigorous kicks and punches you felt before a near impossibility. Don't worry about this apparent decrease in movement but do continue to be aware of how and when your baby is moving about. If there is a change of pattern or a long absence of any movement, contact your midwife and ask her to check your baby's OK with her Pinard stethoscope.

Avoid any potentially stressful over-stimulating events, such as carnivals, theatre performances, violent films or sports events. I have heard several stories about women who have gone into labour prematurely, perhaps because the babies have suffered great shocks. Loud music, overly prolonged and hearty laughter and energetic dancing are also things you should be careful of. If you are at a concert or play (or other event) and you suddenly feel your baby moving around vigorously in response to some of the sound effects or music, leave immediately or at least move to a seat at the back of the hall or theatre. Your little one might be truly upset.

Putting theory into practice...

Although convinced that the way I stood, sat and lay could have an effect on my baby's positioning, I still hadn't taken any action by the time I was 38 weeks' pregnant. It was only when my midwife told me my baby was ROA (which I knew could easily 'flip' into a posterior ROP as I went into labour) that I took any notice.

Two days later, having still made no significant changes, I realised the only way I would persuade myself to turn my baby to a firm LOA position was to get down on my hands and knees for 10-15 minutes, at least three times a day, using a chart to record that I had done so. It was definitely worth doing this because my baby soon turned to LOA and I had a very straightforward two-hour labour afterwards.

10-15 minutes on hands and knees	Mon 3/10	Tue 4/10	Wed 5/10	Thu 6/10	Fri 7/10	Sat 8/10	Sun 9/10
1 tick per time	✓✓✓	✓✓✓	✓				

A tracking chart for ensuring you really do get down on your hands and knees!

Week 35

If, for whatever reason, your baby were to be born now—anything from 34 weeks and 2 days' gestation onwards—she would not be considered premature and she would have an excellent chance of survival.

During her last few weeks in your womb your baby is now doing an impressive amount of weeing... a remarkable 600ml every day. The wee initially goes into the amniotic fluid, of course, and then the waste products are filtered through the placenta into your own bloodstream. Eventually, your baby's waste products are dealt with by your kidneys, along with your own waste. Since your kidneys need to function very efficiently in order to deal with all this waste, it's very important for you to continue to drink plenty of good quality drinking water.

As well as weeing, your baby will be doing a lot of sucking practice now. If she is sucking her thumb or her hands (which is likely), she may even already have some sucking blisters! Developing a strong suck now and in the weeks to come is, of course, extremely important because it's necessary for successful breastfeeding.

As your baby sucks and moves about carefully inside you, she will carry on trying to decipher sounds coming from outside her little world and will continue responding to tastes and changes in light.

Week 36

If you are one of the 1 in 80 pregnant women carrying twins you will probably know about this by now. (A midwife would usually detect two fetuses when feeling your bump.) If you are under pressure to have your babies early, consider your options carefully. (Check the Birthframes index for twin and triplet birthframes.) Whether or not you are carrying twins, it's interesting to know that babies at this stage of gestation have been filmed hugging, stroking and patting things in the womb. This leads me to guess that babies may have emotional needs at this stage of development, so tenderly stroking your growing bump may well be reassuring for the baby inside you. Remember too that you can talk to your baby with the expectation that she will be listening, and possibly even understanding... who knows? In normal circumstances, you can imagine your baby gaining about 14g of fat a day at this stage. Note, though that this rises to about 28g a day during the last four weeks of gestation. Your baby is doing this so as to be able to cope with the lower temperatures outside the womb, after her birth. Keep eating substantial quantities of good, healthy food. Your baby is almost fully mature now, even in terms of lung maturation. (Obviously, this is important because your baby must be able to breathe when she's born). She may have quite long hair—it may be up to 5cm long. If your 'she' is a boy, his testicles should have already descended. In any case, ideally your baby's head should be directed downwards by now and her back should be round at your own front, preferably on the left side of your bump. This position is called LOA (left occiput anterior). Ask your midwife or consultant to tell you what position your baby's in, if he or she hasn't already done so. If your baby turns out to be in another position (ROA, LOP, ROP or one of the breech positions) consider how you are using your body during the day and at night. For ideal positioning I believe sleeping on your left side and avoiding leaning back is best. This will facilitate an anterior, rather a posterior position, and will result in LOA, rather than ROA. ROA is not ideal because ROA babies are reported to often flip round into a posterior position at the last minute. This happened to me, so I believe it! As for leaning forward and avoiding lying on your back in bed, this is all so as to make sure your baby's hotline to your oxygen supply does not get squashed, and therefore partially blocked off. Apart from your baby's need for oxygen, the reason for taking such an interest in your baby's position is so as to give your baby the best possible chance of an easy birth and also to make your own experience of labour as easy as possible. With anterior positioning you get 100% painfree breaks between contractions. With posterior positioning there are no breaks—just varying degrees of intensity. If a baby who is initially posterior doesn't 'turn' to an anterior position by the time the mother reaches second stage, the birth is much, much more painful. If the baby is anterior, this stage can be completely painfree, apart from that famous 'ring of fire'. From my own experience, I can only urge you to take this positioning issue seriously.

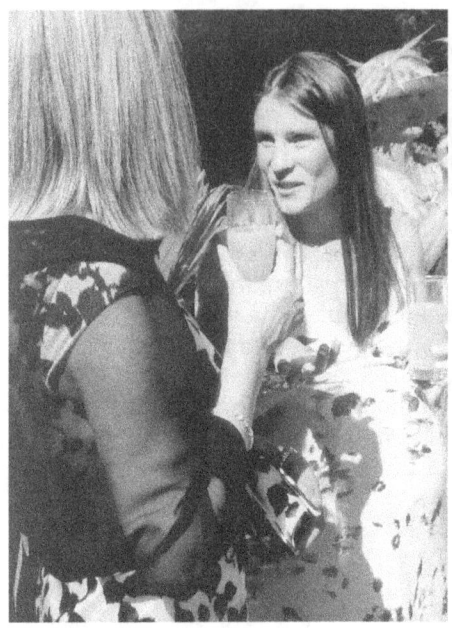
Talk to people, but don't take on other people's fears...

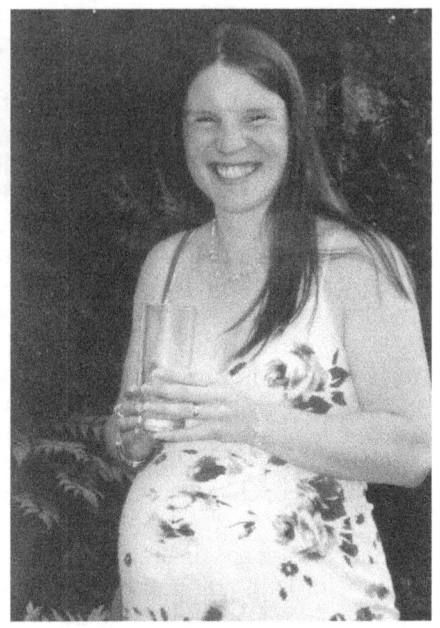
Smile and enjoy the end of your pregnancy...

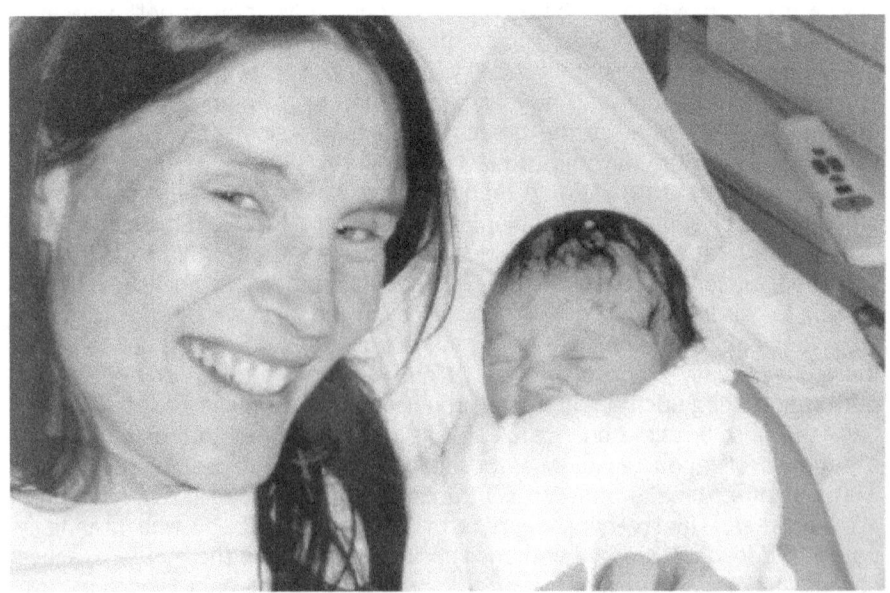
Soon, like Sarah Cave—first-time mother who had an optimal birth at her local hospital—you'll have crossed the divide...

Birthframe 34

I can't quite remember how I got talking to Sarah, but I met her several times at our local church. At first, I just knew her as a breastfeeding mother... but then one day she happened to mention that she'd had a completely natural birth. As you'll see, she somehow knew what was best for her labour and birth quite intuitively—and she was right, of course.

I gave birth the day after those wedding photos were taken. I'm 36 and Alice is my first baby—she's now 19 weeks old. I had a fabulous pregnancy. Loved all of it, even though I had slight morning sickness between Weeks 4 and 12. I was never actually sick—I just felt queasy and sensitive to smells. Amazingly, I also went off coffee and chocolate! Looking ahead to the birth, I decided I wanted to do without painkillers if I could because I felt it would be the best thing for the baby. And it was a fantastic birth. Not painless exactly, but really, really good.

My labour started when I walked in my front door, after I got back from that wedding! My waters seemed to be going. I felt wet and thought, "Surely that's not my waters breaking?" All night long I had contractions and I spent a lot of the time in bed, sort of asleep, but I kept on getting up for the contractions too. My husband wanted to keep me company and massage me, or whatever, but I just told him to go back to bed. "Just let me be. I just want to do this on my own," I told him.

We eventually went into the hospital at about 8.00 the next morning. When we got there, a midwife examined me. "I'll just go and get someone else to have a look at you," she said. "I'm not sure if my fingers are long enough." The second midwife said that, yes, I was definitely 10cm dilated. She asked me why we hadn't come in sooner. "I just wanted to be at home," I said, "just wanted to be quiet." They thought they'd better get me to the delivery room and suggested I get in a wheelchair. "Oh, I'll walk!" I said. Of course, I was naked by this time and one of the midwives tried to hold a towel or something round me, but I told them not to bother. I really couldn't care less who saw me by that stage! The midwife was fantastic—very calm. It was like having Mum at the birth. She looked after me and didn't let the doctors in. It was just me, my husband and the midwife. It was a really intimate and relaxed atmosphere. At one point, the midwife offered me gas and air but I thought, "No, I'll just keep going and see if I can manage," remembering it would be the best thing for the baby if I could. And of course, I did. Somehow, the time just went past.

Alice is an 'angel baby'. She's feeding and sleeping well. She's very contented. The only blip was getting mastitis on four occasions from the second week after the birth until last week. I'd never heard of the condition until it happened. My biggest mistake was leaving the mastitis on the first occasion for over a week *before* going to the doctor's—and it was too late by then. So my advice to other new mums would be to get help any time you feel pain in the breast. Apart from that, I'd say enjoy every day! Don't give up on breastfeeding. I didn't and it's going great now. Alice has nearly doubled her birth weight and she's not even 6 months old yet! Good stuff, breastmilk.

Sarah Cave

Week 37

Many professionals prefer a mother to have reached 37 weeks before they will consider supporting a home birth—so by the end of this week, you will have reached another milestone.

Your baby's vernix (the thick creamy coating covering her body) is disappearing now and she may have almost reached her birth weight, whatever that's going to be. You can imagine your baby with a thicker neck and with eyelids that open and close easily. She will continue to rehearse breathing movements—even though no air will be going into her lungs as yet—and the repeated hiccups you may be aware of coming from your bump are still ongoing proof of this. (It's a sign that amniotic fluid has passed into the baby's trachea.)

If you have been told your baby is lying in a breech position, it's still possible she may turn round spontaneously before the birth so, as well as researching your options for the birth, don't give up hope of having a head-down birth. (See 'breech birth' in the Index if you want to find out more.)

If this is your first baby, and your baby is lying head-down, her head will probably drop into your pelvis very soon, ready for the birth. (When it does this, it's said to be 'engaged'.) If it's your second or subsequent baby she will probably descend just as you're going into labour.

Week 38

At the end of this week, some professionals consider your baby 'at term', i.e. fully developed. A baby is considered at term when she is anywhere between 38 and 42 weeks' gestation. Your baby's contours are now very well-rounded and her skull is firm. Her size will be very close to what she will be when she is born. She is now spending as much as 60% of her time asleep and her sleep is now falling into clearly detectable patterns. Now your baby even dreams like you or I do. We know this because of the rapid eye movement (REM) associated with the dreaming state, which has been observed in babies in the womb at this stage of gestation. (REM sleep has been recorded from as early as 23 weeks' gestation.) Since it is thought that dreaming encourages brain development, we can guess that your baby is continuing to develop in terms of emotions and general intelligence. Measurement of brain waves increasingly shows more organisation, steadier activity, and greater synchrony between the left and right halves of the brain. Research has also shown that your baby is by now uttering a much more definite cry (only audible in research conditions). Since crying is an essential means of communication for babies, this isn't bad news. If she couldn't cry when she was born, how else would she be able to get your attention? Of course, she needs to fit in a little crying practice before she is born.

Birthframe 35

Here's an account which shows how one woman and her husband focused on doing everything they could to help their babies. Although the use of ultrasound is not generally recommended in this book, here the couple used it to ensure that it was safe for a home birth to take place. Some of the advice given in the Russian antenatal classes is also obviously at odds with what you might hear advised in other countries. However, in this case the classes clearly served to inspire the couple to focus on their future babies' welfare and to give them confidence to continue with their natural birth plans, even in unexpected circumstances.

I was 34 when my husband and I decided to have a second child. We were much more careful about everything than with the first. Two years before I conceived, my husband entirely gave up alcohol—even wine and beer—because he wanted to have a healthy baby. I went to my obstetrician for a check-up, and tried to stay healthy too.

When we discovered the baby was on the way, I started collecting information about the best way to go about things. I found out about a number of childbirth preparation schools, and signed up for a course with a midwife and teacher at a local 'family centre'. The atmosphere there was so wonderful. There was an almost magical warmth in the classes. At the end of each class I left feeling full of love for the entire world. One of the most important things the teacher did, I think, was prepare the mother to love her baby. I mean, of course you love your baby, that's natural. But she made you view the whole process as a joint effort, as something special. She made me think about helping the baby, not just helping myself. I began to want the birth to go well for the baby, too.

Usually women think of the future birth as a trial not only for them, but for the child, too. Most women think about themselves, and getting through the birth—whether to have painkillers or not, whether they might end up with a caesarean or not. This teacher helped us to see that the birth is a powerful and challenging experience for the child, too.

When we found out we were having twins, I expected I would have the babies in hospital. But then I saw a video about a woman who had twins at home, in a birthing pool. I certainly didn't expect to have a home birth, but the more I learnt, the more I found out it would be best for both me and the babies. I wanted them to be able to be with me from their first minutes. I so much wanted their first moments after birth to be good and happy for them. So I started planning a home birth.

I also visited a lot of birth centres. A month before they were born, I did a second scan. My doctor saw that they were both head-down, with no sign of the cords around their necks, with a fairly good weight and no visible pathology. So everything seemed fine. On the other hand, during the last month I found it very difficult to walk because of the pressure of their heads in my pelvis. Maybe because I have a narrow pelvis, I felt shooting pains in my legs every time I stood up. So the last month or even two months I spent nearly all my time in bed.

My obstetrician told me that since it was twins, they might be born prematurely, so we thought about what to do. But I knew that if I went to hospital, most likely the babies would be taken to the special care nursery at first. I suddenly began to feel very confident that I should try to have them at home. I made plans with my midwife. The babies came three weeks early.

Sometime around midnight, or maybe a bit after, my waters broke. I began to feel mild contractions. I called the midwife, and she asked me to check how far dilated I was. At around 4:00am, my husband, who had got the car ready, went to pick up the midwife. The contractions were becoming stronger and more frequent. I coped with the pain using the natural methods we learned in the birth classes: breathing, moving around, massage. My mother started cleaning the bath and getting some sea salt to put in the water. [Russian birth classes recommend adding sea salt to the water in a birthing pool or bath. The iodine in the sea salt is thought to kill germs; the salt is thought to be healthy for the baby to be born into]. My older son, who was 9 at the time, was home, too, but he was very nervous. He went into the other room and closed the door. We didn't bother him.

The labour progressed very quickly, and at a certain point I realised that I was about to give birth alone, without my midwife. I felt, not so much panic, but utter loneliness, realising that I was going to have to give birth on my own. And then I summoned my strength. I realised, "Everything is going to be OK." I pulled myself together and began to think about what I needed to do. Thanks to everything I had learnt in the birth class, I knew I would find the strength in myself.

I started feeling that I had to push. My mother hadn't even had time to get the bath ready or fill it. So I went over and lay down on the bed. I lay on my back, because it felt more comfortable. It was purely an instinctive thing. I didn't think what I should do or what I needed. Nature dictated how I should behave. My mother was right there. The first head appeared. I told my mother, "Don't touch the baby. Wait until the shoulders are born, then you can pull the baby out." The obstetrician had told me from the scan that we were having two boys. My mother, who is a paediatrician, caught the first baby. She put him on my tummy. I don't remember it, but she tells me that she saw him crawl up my chest to find the breast. He latched on and began to breastfeed. We didn't clean him off, as we had been told in the birth classes, just let the amniotic fluid soak in. Soon his skin turned pink and glowing.

About 20 minutes later, the second birth began. It was probably harder for the first one, since he had to open the path, so to speak. The second one came out very quickly. The contractions were quite strong and painful. I've heard of women giving birth with no pain, but it certainly wasn't like that for me. My mother put the second baby on my tummy. I wasn't looking at the baby carefully, I was just concentrating on her beginning. "I don't think it's a boy!" my mother said. My daughter had trouble breathing at first and sucking wasn't easy for her. The midwife arrived and looked at the babies. She said we must cut the cord for the girl right away. About three hours later, my husband cut our son's cord himself. He was so proud!

The babies were born with two placentas; each child had had its own sac. The midwife checked the condition of the placentas. We weighed the babies with one of those spring scales you use for weighing vegetables at the market. Liza weighed 3.1 kg, Dmitry weighed 2.9 kg. Of course, it wasn't 100% accurate, but pretty close. Later that week, my husband bought some electronic weighing scales. By that point their weight had stabilised, and they began gaining steadily. From the very first day, we bathed them daily and did baby massage with them.

During the first three weeks, the babies stayed with me all the time. I held them on my chest to keep them warm. I was very weak at first. I lost 5kg relative to my weight before the birth, 55 kg. I gained about 15 kg during the pregnancy. Once a week, I followed the fasting diet recommended in the birth classes: for breakfast, only juices and fresh salads, then juices only for the rest of the day. Because of the inspiring birth preparation classes, I found I didn't even feel like eating sweets. You understand that healthy food is best, and want to eat those things. I think I needed this kind of regimen to get to full term. It's not necessary to gain masses of weight. With a smaller weight gain, the child still takes what it needs. It's better to have natural foods than to take extra, artificial vitamins.

I breastfed exclusively for five or six months—no juices or water, just breast-milk. They breastfed until about a year and three months. We did lots of exercises with them and baby massage and took long walks in the fresh air. In the early days, I was nothing but a milk machine! I hardly had time for anything else. I would just get one fed, when it'd be time to feed the other one again. Now they are 3 years, 2 months old, and weigh 15kg.

Tanya Kudryashova

Tanya's comment when she checked the draft:

I very much want the book to help women who are expecting a child to have faith in their own strength, in feminine intuition and natural instinct during labour. I would hope that a spiritual bond would develop between mother and child from the very first moment of the child's life, which would last throughout their lives. I feel that my birth story sounds optimistic and convincing, so I don't need to change anything.

I realise that various aspects of this last birthframe may have been shocking to you, particularly because Tanya chose a home birth. Some people would say it was irresponsible of Tanya to do so, knowing that she was going to have twins. However, she clearly took this decision because she thought it would be the best thing *for the babies*. Personally, I can understand this, particularly since she'd arranged midwifery care. What surprised me most, actually, was that Tanya spontaneously chose to lie on her back to give birth. Of course, the point is to use a position which feels best for you and your baby—or babies!

Accidental unassisted birth

There are other reasons why you may be rather shocked by this last birthframe. I nearly didn't include it! However, I wanted to introduce the idea that it's possible for someone to give birth before 'help' arrives. You've almost certainly read about women in newspapers or magazines who were 'delivered' by the postman, by their husband, or by a two-year-old toddler. (Sounds like they're Royal Mail parcels or something from DHL... Have you noticed how I haven't been using the word 'deliver' in this book? Who's doing what and to whom?) Of course, the implication behind all these stories is that these women were in a desperate situation and that they were miraculously rescued. Emotions reported range from 'horrified' and 'terrified' to 'relieved' and 'so grateful'. But have you noticed how the same stories always end with the miracle of both mother and baby being fine? Is it just that I've never come across a story like this with a negative ending?

What I'm basically trying to suggest to you is that a fast birth is actually pretty good news. As you already know if you've read Birthframe 2, my second labour lasted two hours in total and the second stage lasted a few minutes at the most. The third stage was completed seconds after my baby's birth. Hmmm... We need to stop thinking in terms of ourselves as patients, in desperate need of 'help' from professionals and remember that giving birth is a natural process (like sex!) which mostly takes place entirely safely and smoothly, provided it's not disturbed. (Sex can also be fast and smooth, with no interruptions...)

One woman, who I met and spoke to for several hours—Heba Zaphiriou-Zarifi—had arranged a home birth, but she somehow gave birth before the midwives arrived. She wasn't actually particularly shocked by the experience—she seemed completely blissed out!—perhaps because she'd thought through the possibility in advance.

Heba told me she'd actually had a kind of precognition that something like this might happen, although she clearly didn't intend to give birth unassisted. During her antenatal classes, the antenatal teacher had asked the class what their worst-case scenarios would be. One participant had said it would be if the baby arrived before the midwives. When Heba heard this, she said she thought, "Hmm... What a fascinating experience that could be, if it actually happened in a way that maybe you didn't have time to have anyone around." When she went into labour, as planned Heba phoned the midwives... and phoned, and phoned, and phoned. Neither she nor her husband managed to get through to anyone at the hospital. Later they found out that the hospital's phone system had broken down that night and she was later informed of this in writing! Life is sometimes stranger than fiction...

Life is sometimes stranger than fiction...

What if it happens to you?

Michel says that in his experience a fast birth is always an easy birth. Here are a few quick-reference practical tips:

- ♥ Don't panic—a *naturally* fast birth is a safe one.
- ♥ Keep yourself and your new baby warm, using anything to hand. Hold your baby against your own warm skin.[5]
- ♥ Don't worry about cutting the cord—it's better to wait.
- ♥ Breastfeed your baby, if he or she wants to feed.
- ♥ Ask anybody who is with you to phone for help.
- ♥ If you can't phone, wait for help to arrive but *stay warm*.
- ♥ Talk or sing to your baby! Do whatever comes naturally.

How far will you go?

Often it's not easy to make decisions with the baby's best interests in mind. My own home vs hospital decision was especially difficult when I was pregnant with my third daughter. At that time—in fact until I was 30 weeks' pregnant— we were living and working in Oman in the Middle East and home birth was illegal there. However, through contact with other women who'd lived in Oman longer than us, I gradually became aware how interventionist the hospitals were, so I didn't want to go to one!

Often it's not easy to make decisions. Options may seem limited.

One woman I met at the swimming pool of the nearby five-star hotel had had various drugs and interventions while she was in labour and giving birth and she and her baby were very ill for a long time after the birth. Another woman had travelled to Muscat, the capital, two weeks before her due date so that she could give birth in a private hospital which had agreed to 'let' her have a natural birth, undisturbed by unnecessary interventions. She stayed with a friend there until she went into labour and then her husband —who must have done the three-hour drive at the last minute—acted as a guard, literally keeping all the nurses and doctors out of the private room in which my friend was labouring! Personally, my options seemed extremely limited because I didn't have a friend to stay with in Muscat, I had two other children to look after and in any case my second labour had only been two hours long in total so it was unlikely my husband would be able to dash to join me at the last moment. Until my husband had confirmation of a job offer in England I felt pretty desperate and was wondering whether I would need to give birth 'accidentally' at home or in the desert somewhere! Of course, I was uncomfortable with this idea because I really do believe that birth supported by midwifery care is optimal. Often our choices for pregnancy and birth are not simple ones.

Week 39

Your baby's rate of growth is slowing down, which is just as well because there is very little room left in your womb. Phenomenal development has taken place over the last 37 weeks (from conception onwards, remembering that your baby only really started growing from Week 3). The original fertilised cell has become a well-organised bundle of two hundred million cells and these cells now weigh approximately six billion times more than the original fertilised egg!

The amniotic fluid around your little one is being renewed every three hours, so keep drinking water. If your baby remains undistressed, the amniotic fluid will remain clear because the waste products which aren't released in her wee will remain in her bowel. The sticky greeny-black substance which results from the storage of these waste products, which as we've already mentioned is called meconium, is a mixture of excretions from your baby's alimentary glands, bile pigment, lanugo and cells from her bowel wall. When this original gestational waste has been cleared in the first few nappies, your baby's poos will become an interesting and pleasant-smelling orange colour if you breastfeed her. (Bottle-fed babies' poos are browner and have a much stronger odour.)

Whether or not your baby is ready to be born this week or next will depend not only on individual variation but also on the precise date your baby was conceived. (When did you ovulate in the month you conceived?) I would encourage you to resist any advice to hurry your baby along at this stage... Nature can cope very well without our interference; in fact, as we've seen, disturbance usually results in worse outcomes, not better ones. You will go into labour and give birth spontaneously when your baby is sufficiently mature and when your body has prepared precisely the correct balance of hormones to make the birth possible.

Enjoy these last few days of life without a tiny baby to care for. Babies are much easier to look after when they're inside us! Relax, walk, dance, paint, write, sing, bake cakes, contemplate the beauty of nature... If you're happy and contented, your baby's likely to be relaxed and happy too—because she is sharing your hormonal environment. Virtually everything crosses the placenta. True intimacy.

However, while focusing on your own well-being do also spend some time preparing for your baby's arrival. Do you have everything you need? Think of things like soft towels, receiving blankets, baby clothes and whatever else you think you will need in your particular situation.

Enjoy these last few days of life without a tiny baby...
Babies are much easier to look after when they're inside!

Week 40

If you haven't already done so, you may now be nearing the time of your labour. On the other hand, since only 3% of babies arrive on their due date you may still have a fair wait. 80% of babies are born within 14 days of their due date, either before or after. The rest are born either earlier or later than 42 weeks—perhaps because they were conceived at the end of a very long menstrual cycle.

If your baby has now been growing inside you for a full 38 weeks, she will already be as heavy as she is to be at the time of her birth, and as long. Her fingernails may be so sharp that she scratches herself with them.

Although most of her lanugo (fine hair) and vernix will have disappeared by now, at birth you may still notice a little lanugo over your baby's shoulders, back, arms and legs and some traces of vernix (cream) in her skin folds.

The temporal lobe of her brain—the part to which the ear sends its data—will by now be fully myelinated. Other parts of her brain and nervous system will only be partially insulated at birth, so it's clear that your baby's hearing is given full priority. It's worth remembering that under hypnosis in later life, people can often recall comments which are made around the time of their birth which have affected them in some way.

Your baby's nose is also fairly well-developed now, meaning that she will display a decided preference for certain smells as soon as she's born. It's interesting that your newborn will express these preferences even with no practice or experience. The smell of your own breasts—and armpits, actually!—will be particularly attractive to your newborn baby. So whatever you do, don't worry about body odour around this time.

The part of your baby which is to be born first—her 'presenting part'—will probably be in the lower segment of your womb, pressing through your already softened, partially opened cervix. If this baby is your second or subsequent baby, she is likely to engage as you go into labour. Obviously, the timing of engagement varies.

If indeed your baby is ready to be born, she will send a hormonal signal to your body calling for an end to the pregnancy. (This is a signal scientists would like to know more about.) Your body will respond by releasing oxytocin (the 'hormone of love') to make your uterus contract. The irregular and then regular contractions which follow are an inevitable part of your labour—so try and view them very positively. They are there to help your baby exit your womb, descend through your pelvis and enter this world...

Of course, it's a dramatic business coming into this world from your baby's point of view. The journey itself will involve travelling down a long, narrow and unfamiliar passageway. Don't worry about your baby getting damaged, though. Her body will now be very flexible, thanks to fluid intervertebral disks and joints which can fold neatly into tight places. Even the head plates which guard your baby's brain will yield to pressure by overlapping, which may result in a pointed head or 'pixie' look at birth. (Don't worry! These plates do gradually reposition themselves again afterwards.) Your baby's arrival into this world will be a shock from various points of view: she will no longer have the reassuring hug of your womb, temperatures will no longer be constant, and supplies of food and drink will no longer be continuously on tap. She will need all your tender love and care.

> I knew that the way in which due dates are calculated in England is about two weeks shorter than elsewhere in Europe, and medics get twitchy and start wanting to induce births here, when in Sweden they wouldn't consider it at the same point. Plus first babies are routinely late—probably because the calculations are wrong. My dates could not be accurate as I'd not known I was pregnant in the first place, but anxieties always seem to grow in the last two months. My way of avoiding them was to keep working and keep to a minimum contact with the world of pregnancy.

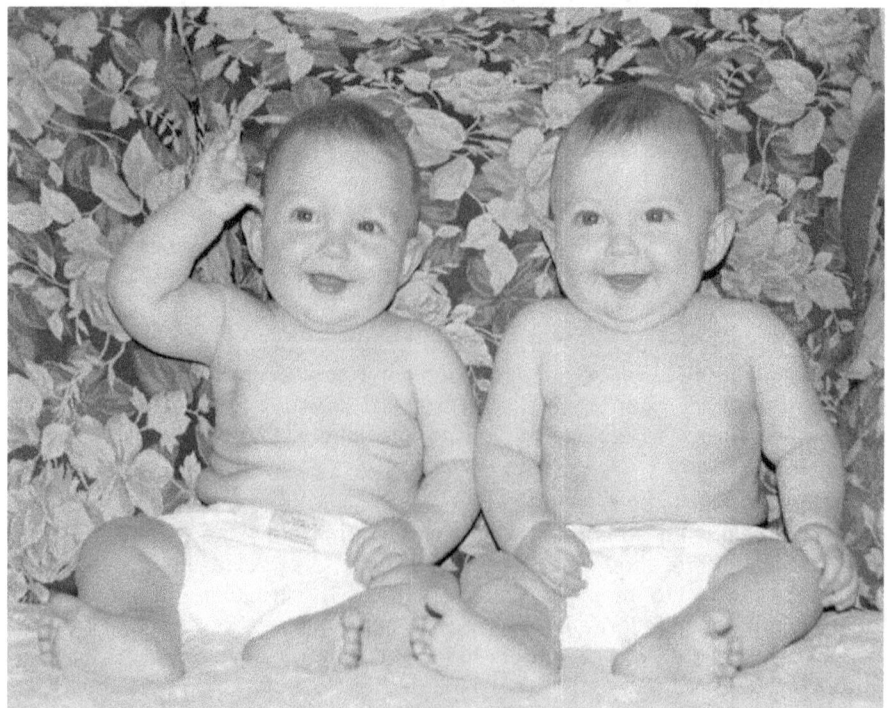

The optimally-birthed Mellor twins at 7 months old (see Birthframe 14)

For your baby it's a dramatic business coming into the world

Week 41

It's worth noting, if you've reached this point in this week-by-week tracker that only a baby born after 41 weeks and 6 days is technically overdue—that's 293 days—since human gestation can be anything from 38-42 weeks.

This means if you still have a proper bump at this stage, you really have no need to worry. Reconsider the precise date of conception if you haven't already done so, taking into account the length of your normal monthly cycle and of course also your sexual activity around the time you think you conceived. When you're not pregnant, does your period always arrive exactly 28 days after the last one began? If, in the past, it usually didn't turn up until Day 33, you can expect your baby to be born five days after your due date—because it's likely your body actually tends to ovulate five days later than in the official charts (which would be near the end of this 41st week). Also, was your partner away on business at any time in the month you got pregnant? You could only have become pregnant when you made love! Unless, of course, yours was another immaculate conception... Actually, I think they should all be considered immaculate. After all, aren't our bodies amazing, managing to conceive a baby, get it grown and then born too? It's a process which takes place with very little help from us. All we need to do is wait and keep faith in the physiological processes. They're working every second of every day and will continue to do so, providing you let nobody disturb them in any way at any crucial moment. Keep going! Tune into your baby and talk to her too. And prepare yourself for the fact that this 'she' we've been talking about may well turn out to be a 'he'!

While you're waiting, it's a good idea to keep thinking about your baby and imagine what he or she might be like. It's not possible to calculate how heavy or tall he or she will be, no matter how large or compact you are, but it might interest you to know a few facts about babies' weights and heights around the time of their birth...

- ♥ A typical birth weight is 3½ kilos. (That's 7½ pounds, if metric means nothing to you).
- ♥ Only 5% of babies weigh less than 2½ kilos or more than 4¼ kilos.
- ♥ If you're expecting a boy, it's likely he will weigh about 200 grams (½lb) more than if it's a girl.
- ♥ Whatever your newborn's weight, it will decrease in the first three days after the birth. This is nothing to worry about—it really is perfectly normal as your new baby adjusts to life outside your body.
- ♥ By about 10 days after the birth, your baby should have regained his or her birth weight and the long-term process of growth will have re-established itself.
- ♥ Your newborn's height will be just under a third of that of a typical adult, i.e. 51cm (or 20in).
- ♥ 95% of babies fall within the range of 46-56cm.

Here are a few more interesting facts to keep your mind off your wait…

- ♥ A newborn's body is made up of approximately 70% water, 16% fat, 11% protein and 1% carbohydrate.
- ♥ Your new baby's heart will weigh less than 30g at birth but your baby's pulse rate will be about 180 beats per minute during the actual birth and will then average 140 beats per minute in the first few weeks. During the first year of your baby's life, the rate will gradually decrease to 115 beats per minute, by which time your baby will not even have doubled in weight.
- ♥ Your new baby's eyesight will already be fairly well-developed at birth: your baby will be able to focus over the distance from your breast to your face and it's likely he or she will be attracted to your face, rather than to less complex, less curvaceous, less mobile, inanimate objects.
- ♥ At birth, your baby will be ideally predisposed to bond with you, provided of course there are no drugs in his or her system. If you yourself were to have any drugs in your system that would also be a disappointment for your baby, because your face would be less responsive. Research into the behaviour of babies just after birth has revealed that babies typically spend up to an hour staring intently at their mother's face, if given the chance, before they fall asleep for the first time outside the womb. This is a first exchange to look forward to and cherish and is one of the reasons why it's best to opt for an optimal birth, i.e. a birth which involves an absolute minimum of intervention and no drugs whatsoever. The aim is to make your baby's birth as gentle and as trauma-free as possible so that you can both have a good start to your relationship.

Week 42

Don't worry. Really! You probably ovulated later than you think. Perhaps that particular month when you conceived was a strange one in terms of your normal cycle. Your baby is developing as he or she should. He or she is probably soon going to start off the birth process. Health professionals who are monitoring your pregnancy may well be putting you under pressure by now to be induced. If you were to succumb to this pressure the optimal birth you've been preparing for would not happen… and the induction would probably prove to have been unnecessary. (Only 1% of babies who are thought antenatally to be 'postmature' actually turn out to be so when they are born. The other 99% show no signs of postmaturity and clearly weren't yet ready to be born.)

What you can do at this time is monitor your baby's movements yourself. You can even keep a kick chart if you want to—this may well reassure you and impress your caregivers![6] If all seems to be well, consider your options carefully before intervening in the natural processes, remembering that the process of labour and birth often begins very suddenly. Strange and wonderful things are happening within your body. Help your baby to get born by remaining trusting of his or her ability to do this. Carry on talking to your little one, maybe even asking him or her to hurry up! You're going to meet properly soon.

Week 43

If you're still reading this, it's useful to note that female babies spend on average one day longer inside their mother's bodies than males. And white babies on average spend five days longer inside the womb than black babies. Apparently, these differences are purely racial and have nothing to do with individual size variations, wealth or indeed poverty. Until now, nobody has been able to explain why these variations occur. In any case, if you're still pregnant now, you probably just miscalculated your LMP (last menstrual period), or maybe you ovulated very late in the month you got pregnant. Don't worry! If you find you are worrying, it's a good idea to focus on this feeling and try and work out why... Are there any psychological issues you need to resolve before you give birth? Do you need to make any other preparations? Are you happy with the arrangements you've made with birth attendants, friends and family? Also, consider whether you really, intuitively, feel there's something wrong. If you feel pretty confident everything's basically OK with both you and your baby, consider what's been happening lately... Has there been any diarrhoea? Any loss of appetite? Any increased sexual desire? Any impatience or a deep need to tidy rooms and organise things? These are all signs of imminent labour, so relax if the answer is 'Yes!' to any of these questions. And when you go into labour, continue to imagine what your baby might be experiencing. This is the beginning of your new life together.[7]

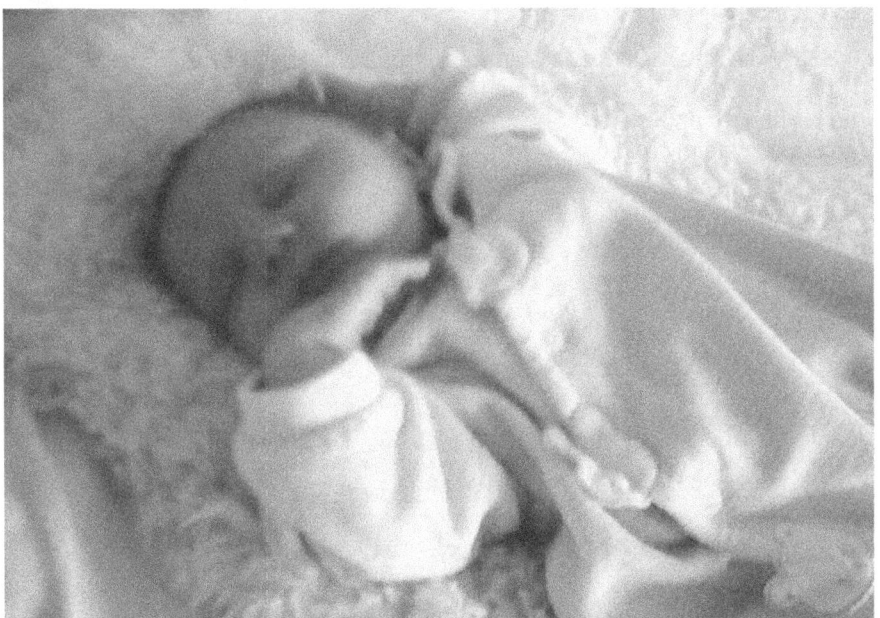

Newborn Jumeira Jeannetta, a few hours after her birth   Next page: *Her birthplace*

Birthframe 36

When Jumeira my third daughter was born (at our new home in England), she seemed very much at peace with herself. She was quiet, alert, and interested in what was going on around her. When she slept she seemed totally calm and restful. When she awoke, she simply murmured or grunted a little to let me know she'd like a bit more milk now, please.

Her own experience of the birth seemed to have been positive. This notion was confirmed by her interesting reaction to both the music I'd played in the early stages of labour and to seeing the bathroom again, where she'd been born. When I put the CD on again, she immediately looked round with interest and surprise, a smile almost playing on her lips. She looked deep into my eyes and seemed very calm and happy. When I took her into the bathroom for the first few times she again seemed astonished but very pleased to be back there again. She looked all around, and especially at the ceiling (which she must have seen first) and out the window (which, again, would have been directly in her field of vision at the time of her birth). Her look suggested she was thinking, "So it was here! This was the place!! Look, Mummy! It was here!" And I couldn't help saying, "Yes, yes. This is where it was. It was a good place to be born, wasn't it?" I often took her into the bathroom with me—clearly, she liked that room enormously. I liked it too, because it reminded me of the joy of her birth, of the accomplishment and wonder of it all.

She was a very calm and alert baby and didn't sleep very much. She took a great interest in her surroundings—especially in her new sisters and her new mummy and daddy. She immediately seemed 'at home' in her new home, outside my womb.

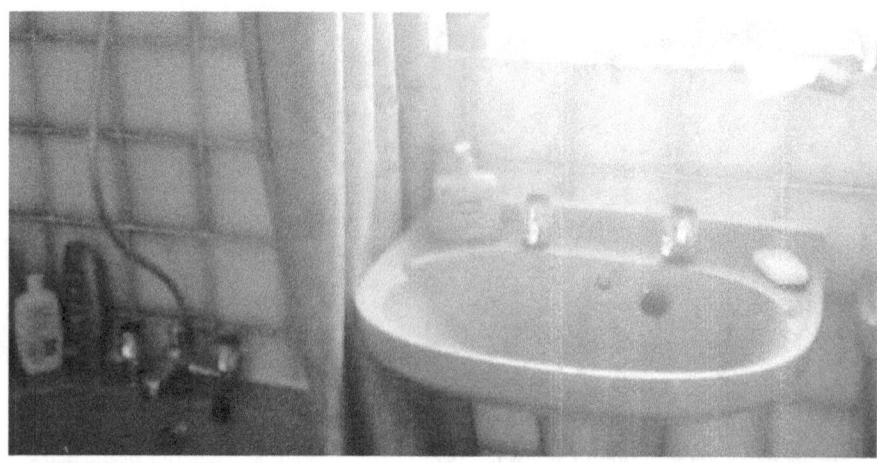

The birth

The baby's perspective is often forgotten when childbirth is under discussion. Do we really need to take care not to disturb our babies' experience of birth?

Years ago, the baby was often regarded as being an insensitive, unfeeling part of the equation of childbirth. Discussion has always taken place as to when a fetus or baby becomes a truly sentient person, with sensations, thoughts and emotions. This debate still continues but research is increasingly providing evidence that our estimate of a person's development of consciousness should be placed earlier, rather than later, perhaps even at a few weeks of gestation, if not before!

Whatever people's conclusions, from the 1920s on, several European psychologists and clinicians researched the effect of birth experiences on human growth and development. Otto Rank's contention in 1923 that adult psychological problems might stem from birth separation anxiety, implying the primacy of the *mother*-infant relationship (over that of the child's relationship with his or her father) was seen (by Freud in particular) as an extreme and unacceptable claim. Today, of course, it is accepted without question, especially as a result of the work by Marshall Klaus et al (first published in 1976) on bonding.

Frederick Leboyer, a French obstetrician (born in 1918), certainly felt that a baby was completely sentient at birth and that he or she could be affected by birth experiences. He successfully raised many people's awareness of what he saw as the baby's perspective through his book *Birth Without Violence* (Inner Traditions Bear and Company 2002), which was first published in 1974. To do this, he used a poetic approach, not one based on hard data, and his book spawned a gentle birthing approach which involved subdued lighting and gentle touch, as well as bathing the baby in lukewarm water after the birth.[8]

David Chamberlain, a psychotherapist based in North America, also came to believe that birth experiences are crucially important to babies, after hypnotising adults and attempting to gain access to their birth experiences. Along with Thomas Verny, he co-founded the Pre and Perinatal Psychology Association. In his book *Babies Remember Birth* (Ballantine Books 1990) David Chamberlain details some of the hypnotherapy sessions he conducted, which seemed to suggest that babies are even sensitive to comments people make at the time of their birth. His research through psychotherapy also led him to conclude that babies became frightened when things go wrong at birth, for example when they have difficulty breathing, when they are suddenly subjected to bright lights or when they are taken away from their mothers.

The idea that babies can be scarred by words and actions at their birth might seem extreme to some. But some people feel they actually have a responsibility to give their children a natural birth because of the potential lifelong physical and emotional after-effects of a traumatic birth.

One example of some more 'solid' research data is that a group of researchers found that obstetric complications were associated with a higher incidence of childhood asthma.[9] (As we've seen, these complications often occur after a cascade of interventions, beginning with one unnecessary one.) Children who experienced certain procedures at birth, i.e. caesarean section, vacuum extraction, the use of forceps, or who were literally pulled out by a caregiver manually, were the ones who had a higher incidence of asthma. Rates amongst children who were birthed normally were significantly lower. Many other studies have shown links between a baby's birth experiences and his or her late experiences or health in life. Michel reports:

Recently, there has been an accumulation of hard data confirming the lifelong consequences of the antenatal environment and also of the way we are born. In other words, the branch of epidemiology I have called 'primal health research' (since 1986) has developed dramatically. It developed at such a pace that in 1997 we found it necessary to establish and to continuously update a Primal Health Research Data Bank so that everybody can refer to this data. [See www.primalhealthresearch.com, www.wombecology.com or www.birthworks.org/primalhealth]

Today the databank contains hundreds of abstracts of articles published in authoritative scientific and medical journals. All of them show correlations between what happened during the 'primal period' (from conception until the first birthday) and what happens later on in life in terms of health and behaviour. It is not easy to detect such articles because they do not fit into the current classifications. This is the main reason for trying to bring them together.

From an overview of the bank we see immediately that, in all fields of medicine, there have been studies detecting correlations between an adult disease and what happened when the mother was pregnant. It is even possible to conclude that our health is to a great extent shaped in the womb. There are many studies confirming that the emotional states of pregnant women may have lifelong effects on their children. This might lead us to conclude that the first duty of health professionals should be to deal tactfully with the emotional state of mums-to-be. This is not easy in the framework of industrialised childbirth, which implies a certain style of antenatal care, constantly focusing on potential problems. Health professionals need to avoid the common mistake of doing more harm than good by interfering with the imagination and belief system of the person they are taking care of.

Through the data provided by primal health research, we are in a position to try to forecast what sort of disaster might be induced by the industrialisation of childbirth [i.e. excessive intervention]. The data indicates there might be more violent young criminals, more teenage suicides, more drug-addicted adults, more anorexic girls, more autistic children... All these conditions have never been as frequent as they are today. We don't know why this is the case. But, for all of them, the Primal Health Research Databank reveals studies detecting risk factors in the period surrounding birth.

Today we know much more than we did a few decades ago about the behavioural effects of all the hormones that fluctuate in the period surrounding birth. And this knowledge should lead us to reevaluate why and how we intervene, if indeed this is necessary in any one pregnancy or birth.

Here are a few examples of research reported in the Primal Health Research databank:

- ♥ Anorexia nervosa has been found to be more common in girls who have had difficult births, i.e. births with a great deal of intervention.[10] Girls were found to have been more at risk for anorexia nervosa after having a cephal-hemotoma (which is a marker of a highly traumatic birth) or a vaginal instrumental delivery, i.e. forceps or vacuum. Interestingly, the fact of having had a caesarean birth did not predispose girls to anorexia.
- ♥ Adults who have committed suicide using asphyxiation were usually babies who had breathing difficulties at birth.[11] (These difficulties are more likely when babies have drugs in their system at birth.)
- ♥ Adults who have committed suicide by violent mechanical means usually had some kind of mechanical birth trauma caused, for example, by the use of forceps.[12]
- ♥ Autism has been associated with various aspects of the period surrounding birth: induction of labour, 'deep forceps' delivery, birth under anaesthesia and resuscitation at birth.[13] Babies born in certain hospitals where induction of labour and the use of a mixture of sedatives, anaesthesia agents and analgesics during labour were routine were particularly at risk.[14]
- ♥ A marked increase in the incidence of schizophrenia was shown in adults whose birth showed an excess of complications of both pregnancy and delivery.[15] Although pre-eclampsia (which the mother can perhaps do nothing about) was associated with schizophrenia, other complications would certainly have resulted from inappropriate or excessive interventions during labour and birth.[16]
- ♥ One study showed a clear link between left-handedness (which is often associated with behavioural disorders) and complications either during pregnancy or birth.[17] Again, complications at birth might well have been caused or exacerbated by inappropriate or excessive intervention.
- ♥ Babies born under the influence of nitrous oxide (a component of Entonox, i.e. gas and air) have been found to be more susceptible to amphetamine addiction later in life. The use of opiates or barbiturates (or both), alongside nitrous oxide, has been associated with opiate or other drug addiction (e.g. amphetamines) in offspring later in life. Researchers think that the clear link established could be the result of 'imprinting' during labour. I wonder if there's any link between the widespread use of ecstasy and cocaine in nightclubs and the way the same young people were born...[18]

Adults who committed suicide using asphyxiation were usually babies who had breathing difficulties at birth. These difficulties are more likely when newborns have drugs inside them.

A lot more research needs to be done to explore possible links between birth experiences and behaviour in later life. But these early studies certainly raise worrying questions.

In case you're still sceptical, let's go back to the idea of considering the birth entirely from the baby's perspective. Imagine for one moment what it must be like to be born under pressure, with artificially-induced contractions (which are stronger and which often compromise the baby's oxygen supply), in an unfamiliar drugged state, with an electrode pierced through your head or suctioned to it. Consider what it must feel like to be confronted by an unresponsive, dopey or merely passive mother, after hearing her lively voice for weeks, and indeed months in the womb. What must it be like to be born into a noisy, overly bright room, full of clanky metallic instruments and uncaring faces? Imagine the reality of having difficulty establishing breathing because of a hurriedly severed umbilical cord or an excess of drugs in your system. Imagine what it must feel like to have unnecessary difficulties with your circulation or with basic temperature regulation. And how do babies feel when they have something thrust up their nose, when something is put into their eyes at the moment of birth, or when they are immediately laid on their backs so as to be weighed on cold, hard scales? How must babies feel when they are taken away from their mothers so as to be washed and examined? What might they feel when they are put to their mother's breast and find they can't suck, again because of drugs in their system affecting their instinctive sucking reflex? Can they possibly feel any panic, confusion, sadness, pain or distress?

Parents are clearly attuned to their babies' movements, and right after birth a kind of entrainment is established that probably sets up behavioural patterns and language—and yet women are still medicated during the birth process, leaving them incapable of responding to the cues of their newborns, while babies are left in rooms to cry for the expected touch of parental skin. Why are cultures so intrusive? Why do we not follow what should be a very normal path of parental care?

Here's a midwife's comment:
> I'm familiar with fetal scalp monitoring from my training but in my unit we only use it extremely rarely (myself, never) and seem to manage perfectly well without. I'm sure little thought is given to the baby and what it must be like to have a pin through your scalp. Fetal blood sampling has recently been introduced here and is an equally invasive procedure to the baby—I've yet to see a direct improvement in infant morbidity/labour outcomes.

And also a comment from a mother:
> Fetal scalp monitoring... My first twin was monitored this way. We were advised that this would not affect the baby at all, but he had a bump for two to three weeks. The doctors could not say why this had happened. He seems OK, but at the time it was a little worrying as they checked him daily.[19]

What about your baby's capacity to love?

Why do some caregivers dismiss the idea that the baby's state of mind at birth is important? (Perhaps they don't even think about it.) Interventions or drugs are surely highly likely to affect a baby's feelings and perception of the world. If contractions were artificially accelerated, they were probably more stressful for the baby so he or she is likely to be more tense or tired. If forceps were used, a headache at birth is a probability. If drugs were used for pain relief, the baby is likely to feel drowsy, woozy, sleepy or nauseous and anaesthesia of any kind may well desensitise a baby for up to a month after the birth. Not a very nice way to start life really.

Imagine, for a moment, the alternative, which is actually the default setting as far as nature is concerned—a fresh, alert, happy sort of feeling, with a usefully strong suck; heightened sensitivity to your mum's soft, responsive arms, in a room full of kindness, dimmed lights and subdued sounds. Consider for a moment your baby's first experience of looking up into your eyes... Consider your baby's first attempt to suck at your breast—it's likely to be fulfilling if no drugs are affecting your baby's innate ability to suck. Consider the relief at having completed a journey which might perhaps have been a little frightening and physically tiring... Consider this very different transition from life in the womb to life outside it. It seems pretty obvious that your baby—let's imagine it's a little boy now—will be at an advantage at this important time if he does not have any drugs in his system, if he has not been traumatised by any obstetric procedures or even comments and if he has been 'allowed' to remain with you. In his completely natural state of consciousness, he will be able to experience the world in its authentic state and have a true first impression of you, his new mother. He is even likely to be less tired because undisturbed labours are usually much gentler than those which have involved interventions and, consequently, disturbance. He won't be as stressed out as a baby who's been hurried along in a managed labour.

And what about your new son's capacity to love? Michel has explored the ramifications of disturbing the natural birthing process in his book *The Scientification of Love* (Free Association Books 1999). All his hypotheses are backed up by research data, drawn from a wide range of sources. He is of the opinion that even a baby's lifelong capacity to love might be affected by an interventionist birth involving drugs and alienating procedures which disrupt the natural production of hormones in both mother and baby. It's easy to understand how. In a fully undisturbed labour, a woman produces various hormones which may 'imprint' on the baby's mind as he or she is being born. These hormones—oxytocin and prolactin, in particular—produce loving, mothering behaviour in the mother, and they may well also prepare the newborn for a new loving relationship and for relationships in the future. Makes sense somehow.

192 **birth:** countdown to optimal

Photo © Jill Furmanovsky

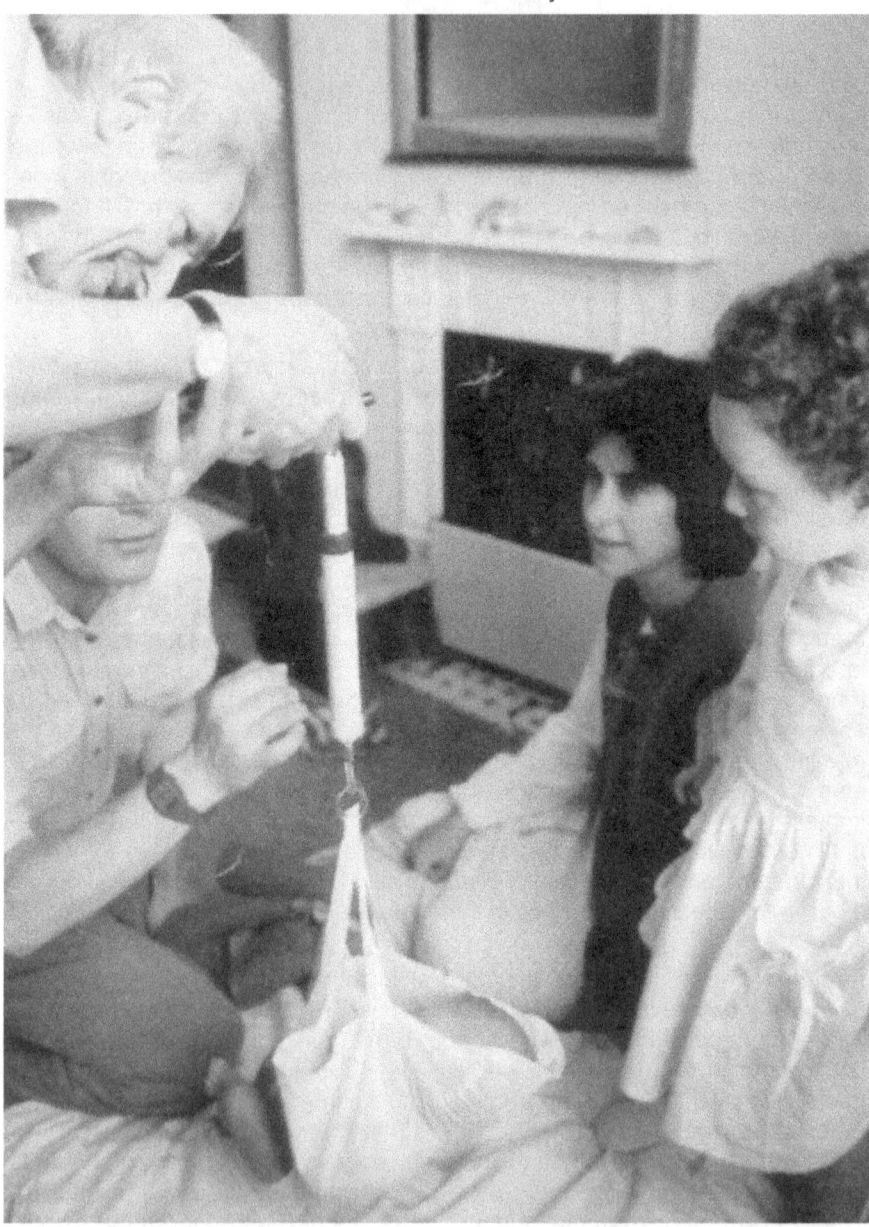

Michel weighing Liliana's baby soon after the birth (see Birthframe 91)
Of course, there's no hurry to weigh your baby—he or she is unlikely to change weight
in the first few hours after birth. It's more important for you to spend time together.

7... HELP YOUR BABY   193

Photo © Jill Furmanovsky

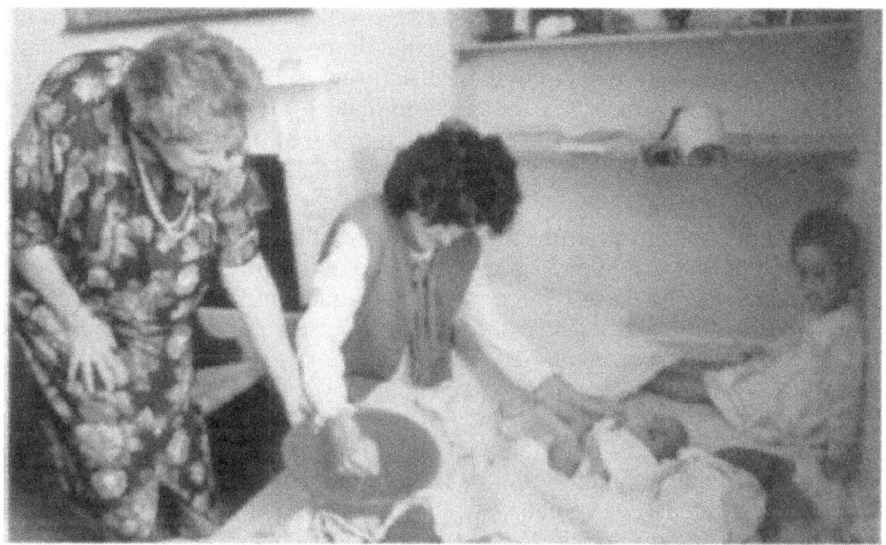

Liliana bathing her newborn baby (see Birthframe 91)

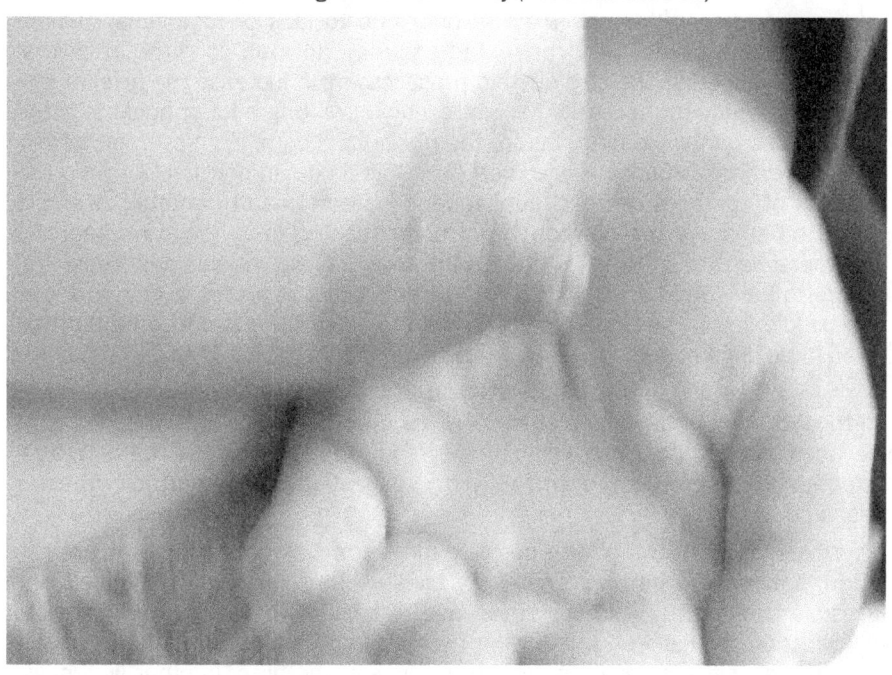

*Milk's come in... But is baby able to suck?...
or does he have drugs in his system which make it impossible?*

If these ideas seem extreme, at least allow them to stay at the back of your mind for a while. I remember my own reaction when my obstetrician in Sri Lanka wrote some comments in a letter to me after the birth of my first daughter. "For a long time," he wrote, "and this is no exaggeration, I have wondered if violence at birth contributes to making a violent society." I must admit, it seemed an almost ridiculous notion to me at the time. But the more I think about it and the more I study the research data, the more I feel inclined to think a link may not be so outlandish after all.

If you are about to interrupt me to say that babies born in the developing world don't always grow up to be gentle and peace-loving, do note that these countries may be the places where most intervention and disturbance is going on. I only started realising this through living in Sri Lanka and Oman and through extensive travel elsewhere. In Sri Lanka, in a very rural place called Ella—a tiny mountain hamlet seven hours by train from Kandy—I was astonished to hear from the landlady of the guest house that all women in Ella travel to their local hospital to give birth. (Apparently, it was only eight miles away.) Gradually, I realised that in highly undeveloped places technology and 'Western' ideas are sometimes almost worshipped as gods. In a World Health Organization presentation I attended at that time in Colombo (the capital) the caesarean rate was announced as being 25% in Sri Lanka.

In other places, hygiene may be poor due to lack of resources, climate and lack of training, and these factors may all lead to difficult births. Traditional superstitions also sustain practices which increase the level of risk and the subsequent necessity for intervention. Creating a lot of noise to scare off evil spirits after the birth, before the placenta is born, is an example of this because any disturbance to the mother at this time can dramatically increase the risk of haemorrhage and consequent maternal death. Another example would be stopping the newborn from breastfeeding for a few days because of superstitions associated with the early 'milk', colostrum; this might result in failure to breastfeed at all. All these problems occur in places (e.g. in Africa or the Middle East) where female circumcision is very common, making birth an even more difficult and dangerous undertaking.

It would be good if researchers could continue to study any links between birth and later behaviour or health more systematically over the next few decades and beyond. Links which have already been established between birth experiences and later life certainly do suggest it's an important area for research.

Whatever our views on the possible long-term side-effects of interventions during labour and birth, we can only be sure that we have minimised any possible long-term effects if we give our own babies the smoothest possible introduction to this world, involving no drugs or unnecessary interventions, and no insensitive comments around the time of the birth. In other words, we can only relax if we really have given our own babies optimally optimal births.

6... CARE ABOUT CARE

"What a stupid thing to say! Of course, I care," I can hear you saying. But do you care enough to take action?

In this chapter, I'm talking about antenatal care—antenatal tests, monitoring and classes—as well as care during labour and the birth itself.

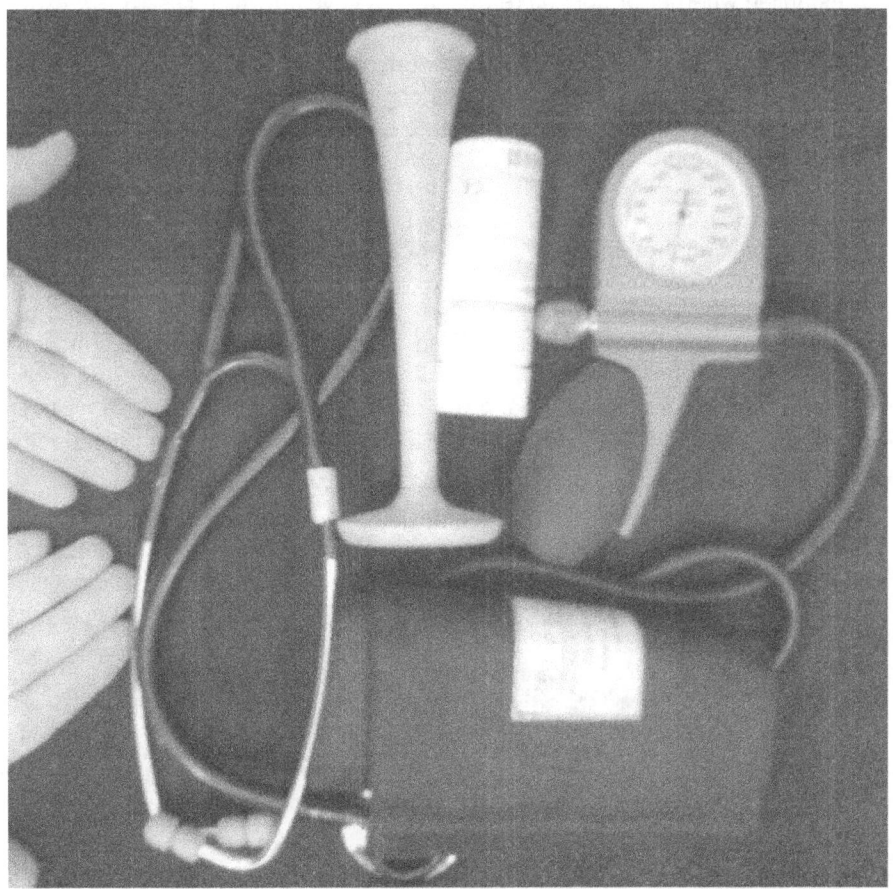

As you can see from the photo above, a surprisingly little amount of equipment is needed for optimal antenatal care—but note that hands need to be kept in the picture! The Pinard stethoscope (in the middle) can be made of wood, as here, or stainless steel, for example.

Surprisingly little equipment is needed for normal antenatal care. As a result it can be carried out at home or in the hospital.

Why worry about antenatal care?

First, so as to put it all in perspective, let's consider a few basic questions... During the antenatal period, generally speaking, caregivers aim to:

- ♥ Confirm your pregnancy and estimate when you're likely to give birth
- ♥ Encourage you to take folic acid supplements in the first trimester
- ♥ Talk about diet, i.e. encourage you to eat healthily and avoid certain foods
- ♥ Confirm your blood group in case a blood transfusion is needed later, and establish whether or not you're Rhesus negative, in which case a few extra procedures would be recommended
- ♥ Offer you various checks to look for abnormalities and subsequently offer an abortion if any are found or suspected
- ♥ Offer you scans to monitor your baby's size and positioning in the womb, to check for multiple babies and to check the position of the placenta and any fibroids
- ♥ Screen for rubella immunity, sexually transmitted diseases, diabetes and gestational diabetes, as well as genetic disorders (if there is a family history)
- ♥ Track your blood pressure and urine in case hypertension develops or protein appears in the urine, so as to detect pre-eclampsia and ward off eclampsia
- ♥ Track the baby's positioning and the quantity of amniotic fluid, as well as your little one's growth through ongoing manual 'palpation' (i.e. feeling with the hands).

If we and our caregivers were machines and pregnancy, labour and birth proceeded in a mechanical way, there would be little scope for problems and those that arose could be solved easily. Since we're extremely subjective, emotional and political beings there is lots of scope, unfortunately!

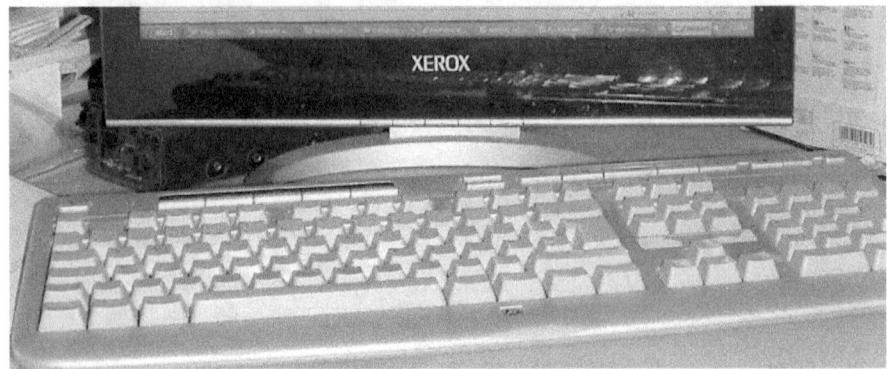

Although we're at a disadvantage because we're not machines who can be dealt with objectively, we're at an advantage if we use machines to help us... e.g. to do research

Birthframe 37

I had worked for a publishing company that specialised in some parenting and childcare books, and had published several on active birth, breastfeeding, taking part in one's own care, etc, so I felt happily enlightened. I went to my first antenatal check-up thinking I would know what questions to ask, that I would be an informed patient. I was relieved to see that the head of the 'Normal Obstetrics' department was a woman, a Certified Nurse Midwife (CNM). That sounded proper and competent. Hoping to ask lots of questions, I actually could not get a word in edgeways.

The usual first questions: age, marital status; blood pressure taken, weighed, measured; the pelvic exam. She listened to my heart, then with a shocked look, she said, "Did you know you have a heart murmur?!" "Well, no," I said. "I have had regular medical care my whole life and no one has ever found any heart irregularities." She looked at me in disbelief. I was wondering what the hell she was talking about and was afraid that it might hurt the baby. Later on, another practitioner told me that it is very common for women to develop a mild heart murmur in pregnancy, and it isn't anything to worry about.

Then we had the following conversation:
Midwife: Was this a planned pregnancy?
Me: (ready to laugh and joke about our spontaneity)
Well, ha, not exactly, but...
Midwife: What birth control were you using?
Me: Uh, condoms.
Midwife: Did the condom break?
Me: Uh, no ... We weren't using one.
Midwife: Well, why not?! Surely you knew what could happen!

I had no response. I was shocked, I think. I just looked at her. I was wondering what about me had given her the impression that I was so young and ignorant, or unworthy of respect. I had come straight from work, was dressed and groomed respectably, she knew I was married. I had no idea. She told me that she had something that could make the pregnancy 'more real for people like you'. I thought: People Like Me? Exactly what category was that? Middle Class Working Married People in Their Mid-Twenties Who Dare to Be Happy When They are Pregnant? I had a feeling instead I had been put in the Irresponsible Idiots category, which was distinctly shameful. Suddenly, I was 6 years old, caught drawing on the walls.

She wheeled a machine on a little trolley into the room and told me to lie down. I was uneasy and didn't like the situation at all any more, but I was also not going to stand up for myself. I had to be a good patient. I was not a troublemaker. The machine was a brand new portable scanner, which she had been 'wanting to try out'. I was instructed to look at the little screen, to see the baby, to make it 'real' for me.

I was instructed to look at the screen to make it 'real'

> She didn't know anything about me, hadn't asked me anything about myself or my feelings, yet she seemed certain that I was in denial and this experience wasn't sinking in for me. Looking at the nondescript image on a small greyish-green screen, I thought that my changing body and swelling, tender uterus, my nausea and cravings, were certainly more real than anything she had shown me. I then got a lecture about nutrition, even though she didn't seem even vaguely interested in my personal diet or knowledge of the topic, and was sent on my way with an order to make my next appointment at reception on my way out. The whole thing took about 20 minutes and this was my 'long, personal, initial interview'.
>
> I was on the verge of tears all the way back to work. I was suddenly not so excited about this pregnancy and felt ashamed of myself, both for letting her use ultrasound on me and my baby for no good reason (even though I didn't know at the time that there were any risks associated with it) and for being so 'irresponsible' as to get pregnant without 'trying'.
>
> I tried to remember why I had been so cheerful on my way in.

It's easy to see from this account how easily we can become discouraged, fearful and dependent after antenatal appointments. Even the best caregivers are in danger of making us feel anxious simply by wanting to check for so many potential problems. And anxiety could well mean that many more tests or interventions are offered and accepted than are necessary or desirable for optimal outcomes. So we need to take antenatal care seriously—we need to care about the care we receive so much that we take action, if necessary. Antenatal care is not just a question of having a few 'harmless checks' to make sure that you and the baby are OK. It's part of a process which may have profound psychological consequences and very real physical ones. In fact, because of the chain of interventions it triggers and the fear it inculcates antenatal care may prevent many women from having an optimal birth.

What kind of antenatal care do you need?

Your choice of care may depend on your geographical situation, your finances, personal recommendations, as well as on your intuitive feelings and rational conclusions. You can choose your local GP practice, midwifery practice or hospital, a private clinic or an independent midwife not attached to any particular institution.[1] You can also choose to have a minimum level of antenatal care. The reason most people don't do this is because in the research this is usually associated with poor outcomes in terms of mother and baby health and safety. This may be mostly because it is economic, psychological or lifestyle factors that keep many women away from experts, rather than choice. In other words, lack of money, depression, shame or even drug addiction may stop some women from going for antenatal care. Of course, these women are not typical of the normal, healthy population, who eat well and get regular medical attention, whenever necessary.

Here's an extract from one of Michel's articles:

In many countries about 10 antenatal visits is routine. Each visit offers an opportunity for a battery of tests. These traditional patterns of medical care are based on the belief that more antenatal visits mean better outcomes. They are not based on scientific data.

Studies made in the UK failed to find any association between late enrolment in antenatal care (after 28 weeks' gestation) and either adverse maternal or neonatal outcomes[2] or between the number of visits and the onset of eclampsia.[3] This casts doubts on the efficacy of such protocols.

I asked Michel for more specific comments...

What advice would you give someone who's just discovered she's pregnant?

I rarely give advice. It's not in my nature. Hmmm. I suppose I'd say, if you know that you are pregnant and if you know when you have conceived your baby and you think that everything's OK, doctors can probably do nothing for you. Women need to realise that the role of medicine in pregnancy is very limited. Really, if a woman feels she's in good shape, the only thing doctors can do is to detect a gross abnormality and offer an abortion. That's all. And even then, there are false positives. What's important is for a pregnant woman to be happy, to eat well, to adapt her lifestyle to her pregnancy, to do whatever she likes to do. If a woman has a passion for her job, perhaps it's better for her to go on working... I think that's what we have to explain to women. They have to realise that doctors have very limited power.[4]

Shouldn't we worry about things going wrong?

A lot of people feel care is vital because of the number of problems experienced in poorer countries, where 'natural' is the norm. These people conclude that leaving things to progress naturally means leaving things to go wrong. In fact, if our basic living conditions are good and we are enjoying a normal level of health, leaving things well alone is the best course of action.

Photo: © Jenny Matthews/CARE

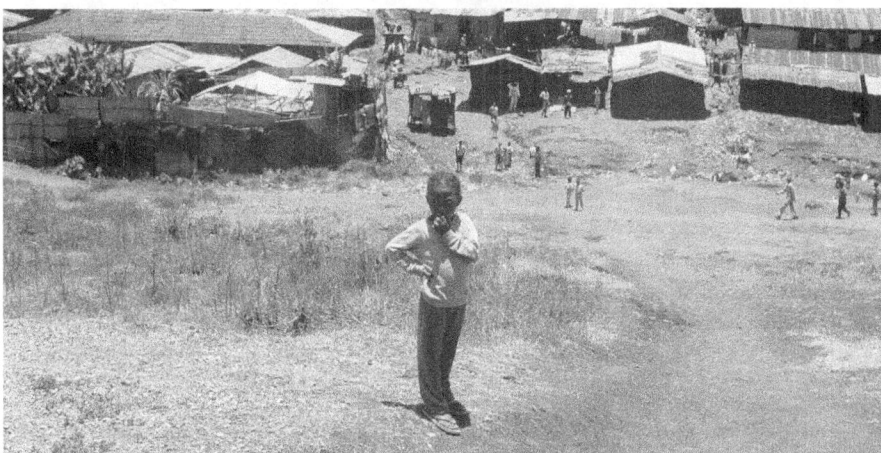

Is our lifestyle so very similar to that of people living in a place such as Kiberia?

A PARTICULAR STARTING POINT FOR BIRTH…

Unlike these women, you probably have clean water and a good diet. You probably live in a climate which is much less conducive to disease. If you live in an urban area, as most people do, you probably have quick access to high quality, health care if ever anything should go wrong—and I reckon you don't travel by bullock cart. Even if you're not wealthy, the chances are you have access to the NHS or can manage to pay for health care. What's more, unlike many other women, the chances are, you probably haven't been circumcised, incised or infibulated—i.e. your genitals have not been ritually damaged in any way—and your healthy diet in childhood means that you body grew properly….

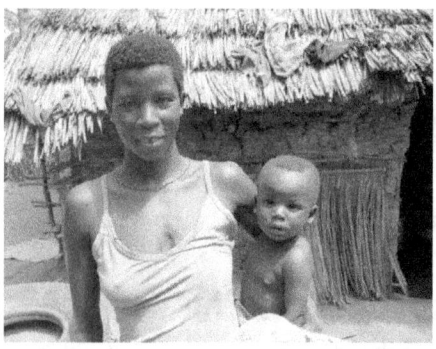

As you can see from the background, this Kenyan woman's living conditions are quite different from your own

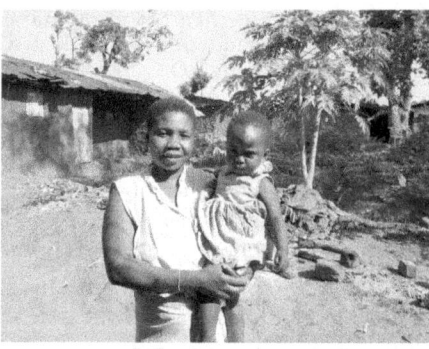

Uganda is battling HIV, AIDS, TB & Malaria. In 2009 there were 1.2 million AIDS orphans and 940,000 people live with HIV or AIDS.

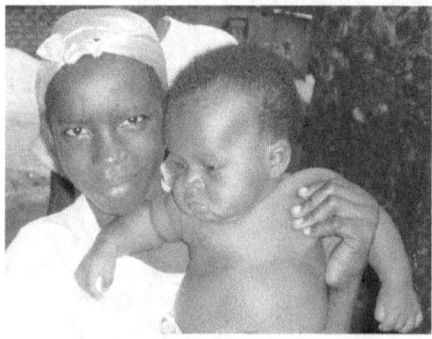

Consider the experience of this woman from Angola. She may or may not be one of the lucky 30% of people who have access to government health care facilities, which were severely damaged during the Civil War up to 2002. Apart from difficulties getting treatment, she and her children will also be in danger of dying from malaria or other diseases.

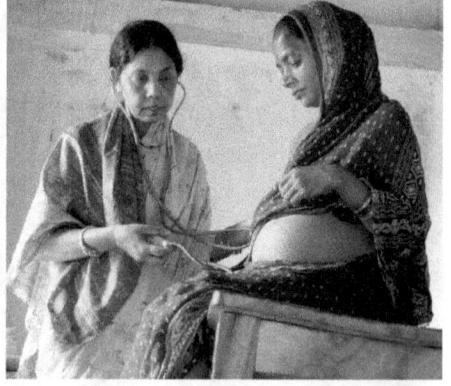

Many women in India and other South Asian countries have arranged marriages (when they're as young as 12 years old) and might be having their 5th child by the age of 30. What's more, few of them have access to clinics because of transport problems or financial difficulties.

As I've already suggested, there are all kinds of reasons for the 500,000 maternal deaths which took place in 2005 in developing countries. (This figure was reported by the UN Department of Public Information in 2005.) Deaths and other problems are caused by various issues, which don't affect us in Britain...

Early marriage

In certain regions of the world, especially sub-Saharan Africa and South Asia, adolescent marriages are very common. This is a particular problem because with insufficiently grown bodies, girls aged 15-20 who get pregnant are twice as likely to die in childbirth as those in their 20s. Girls under the age of 15 (who are also married off in many countries) are five times as likely to die in childbirth. Young girls who survive pregnancy and childbirth often suffer another problem because of their size—they are often left with a fistula. In case you don't know, this is a rupture in the birth canal which occurs during prolonged, obstructed labour, which leaves the girl incontinent and ostracised from her community—for obvious reasons. Although 9 out of 10 fistulas can be successfully repaired surgically in Britain and other developed countries, repairs rarely occur in developing countries simply because of a lack of funds and trained surgeons. (The UNFPA-led Campaign to End Fistula is working in 40 countries to rectify this situation.)

Disasters, shortages, political upheaval and war

Maternity services may be dramatically affected by natural disasters (such as earthquakes, tsunamis, floods, etc), accidents (fires, burst pipes, traffic problems), terrorism (which often affects civilians), shortages (of all kinds, including medicine and equipment), politics and war... These problems are extremely prevalent in most poorer countries and reconstruction work is slow.

Preventable medical causes

According to UNICEF, the UN Population Fund (UNFPA) and the World Health Organization (WHO), more than 80% of maternal deaths take place as a result of medical problems which could be solved through additional funding. These preventable causes include haemorrhage, sepsis, unsafe abortion, obstructed labour and hypertensive disease in pregnancy. Haemorrhage alone, which may well often be caused as a result of ritual disturbance occurring before the third stage of labour, accounts for 21% of the 500,000 deaths occurring each year. Although this and other problems can be treated in Britain—e.g. by the use of oxytocics, blood transfusions and other skilled midwifery or obstetric care—treatment is rarely available in some countries because of a lack of skilled personnel (especially midwives), a lack of roads, clinics and blood banks, etc.

Lack of expertise

Without skilled professionals teaching family planning, attending births and acting when problems occur during labour, any problems which do arise quickly result in deaths. Those who qualify often want to work abroad to earn more...

Consider in detail how different your lifestyle is—in terms of hygiene and health—from that of a woman in Africa. Bill Bryson, the travel writer, reported on the conditions that many women experience in his book *African Diary* (Doubleday 2002), which was commissioned by the charity CARE International.

To step into Kibera is to be lost at once in a random, seemingly endless warren of rank, narrow passages wandering between rows of frail, dirt-floored hovels made of tin and mud and twigs and holes. Each shanty, on average, is 10 feet by 10 and home to five or six people. Down the centre of each lane runs a shallow trench filled with a trickle of water and things you don't want to see or step in. There are no services in Kibera—no running water, no rubbish collection, virtually no electricity, not a single flush toilet. In one section of Kibera called Laini Saba until recently there were just 10 pit latrines for 40,000 people. Especially at night when it is unsafe to venture out, many residents rely on what are known as 'flying toilets', which is to say they go into a plastic bag, then open their door and throw it as far as possible. In the rainy season, the whole place becomes a liquid ooze. In the dry season it has the charm and healthfulness of a rubbish tip. In all seasons it smells of rot. It's a little like wandering through a privy. Whatever is the most awful place you have ever experienced, Kibera is worse. Kibera is only one of about a hundred slums in Nairobi, and it is by no means the worst. Altogether more than half of Nairobi's three million people are packed into these immensely squalid zones, which together occupy only about 1.5 per cent of the city's land. In wonder I asked David Sanderson what made Kibera superior. [David is CARE International's regional manager for southern and western Africa.] "There are a lot of factories around here," he said, "so there's work, though nearly all of it is casual. If you're lucky you might make a few dollars a day, enough to buy a little food and a jerry can of water and to put something aside for your rent."

"How much is rent?" "Oh, not much. $10 or $12 a month. But the average annual income in Kenya is $280, so $120 or $140 in rent every year is a big slice of your income. And nearly everything else is expensive here, too, even water. The average person in a slum like Kibera pays five times what people in the developed world pay for the same volume of water piped to their homes."

"That's amazing," I said. He nodded. "Every time you flush a toilet you use more water than the average person in the developing world has for all purposes in a day—cooking, cleaning drinking, everything. It's very tough. For a lot of people Kibera is essentially a life sentence. Unless you are exceptionally lucky with employment, it's very, very difficult to get ahead."

Every day around the world 180,000 people fetch up in or are born into cities like Nairobi, mostly into slums like Kibera. 90% of the world's population growth in the 21st century will be in cities.

Bill Bryson

Is it surprising, given this environment, that the developing world has such poor birth statistics? With your lifestyle in Britain your need for antenatal care is altogether different. In fact, as Michel explained, you probably need very little.

Photo © Jenny Matthews/CARE

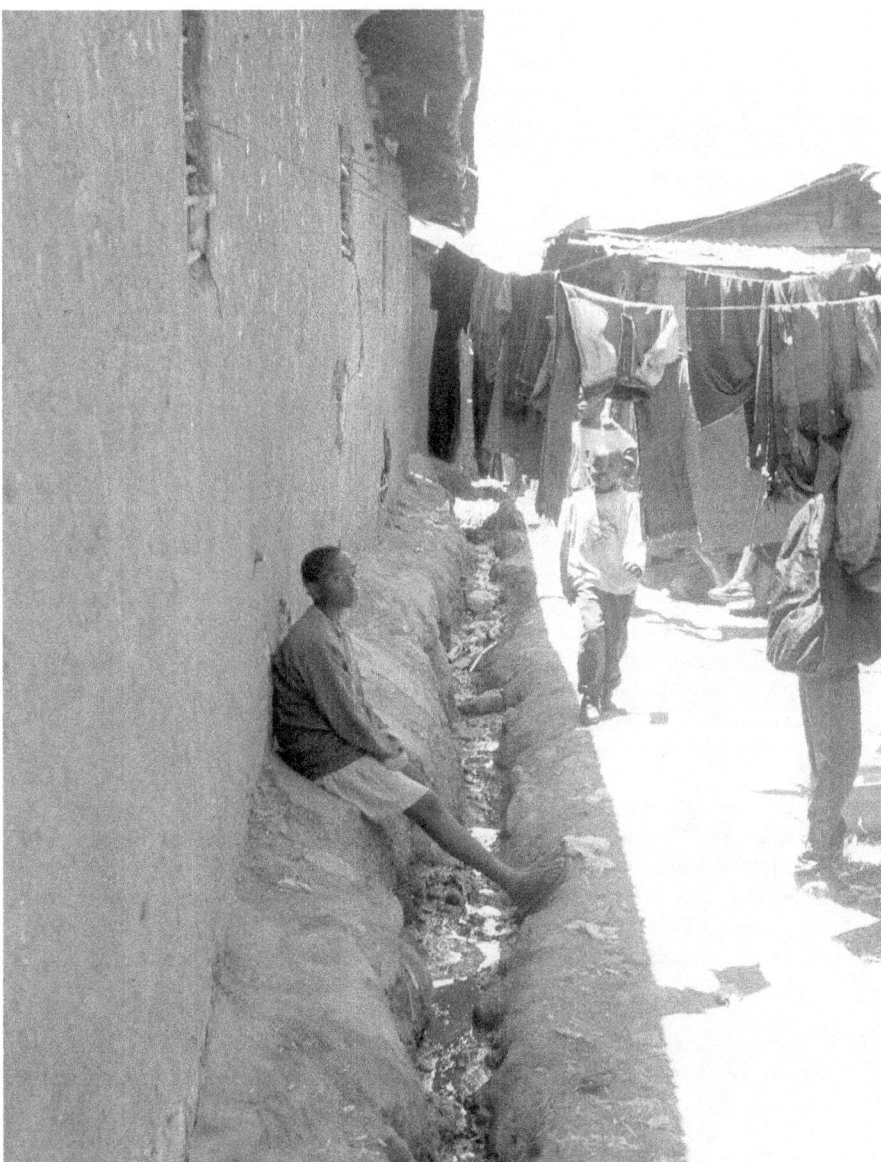

Over 700,000 people live in Kibera, Nairobi in Kenya, the largest slum in Africa. Open drains and poor sanitation are an everyday problem, which has clear implications for safety when women give birth. if you would like to support the work to improve living conditions for people in places like this, go to www.careinternational.org.uk

What can we do constructively?

Although you no doubt appreciate how different your situation is here in Britain, you're probably also aware that problems do sometimes arise during pregnancy or birth for a small minority of women. So how can you make sure that it doesn't happen to you? How can you make sure you don't disturb the physiological processes while also making sure that everything's going OK? How can you enjoy the best of what the British system has to offer?

One option is to register for care well after the first trimester is over, i.e. when you are 14 weeks' pregnant, or later. Note that in many places, in order to be considered 'low risk' you need to have registered by the time you are 20 weeks' pregnant. If you register at say 18 or 19 weeks' pregnant you will be ensuring that your growing baby remains as undisturbed as possible during the first, crucial weeks of development. (In any case, 1 in 4 women has a miscarriage by the end of the first trimester.) You will also be giving yourself time to adjust to your new pregnancy and develop positive emotions towards your new baby. If you register early, you might be pressurised into having tests which could be harmful to your growing baby.

A comment from a mother of three born 1967-72, and grandmother of seven, born between 1984 and 2006):

❝ It seems there's a lot more worry involved in being pregnant for women nowadays. Pregnancy was an awful lot simpler in our day without all the antenatal testing. There was a lot less worry. Since there weren't any tests, we just had to trust that everything would be fine. You can always find people who will tell you horror stories about what can go wrong, but you just have to block them out and believe that the best will happen. Most of the time, it does.

❝ I was 36 and didn't want a lot of medical intervention so I didn't go to the doctor until at least 14 weeks were up, just in case the fetus dropped out beforehand. I used to be a nurse and had delivered babies in developing countries, and knew that the medical system in the UK is not very good at reducing stress in the mother. In fact I knew that lots of trips to the hospital, clinics or even antenatal yoga classes would make me more anxious. Pregnant women are forever being told what to do and not do, there are loads of prohibitions on what we must eat, drink, smoke, work at, etc and we're treated as if we are to blame for everything that might go wrong. I figured that if it was so hard to have a healthy baby there wouldn't be an over-population problem in the world, although most first-time mothers are a lot younger than I was.

Whether you register earlier or later, what else do you need to do so as to maximise your chances of having an optimal birth?

How can you maximise your chances of having an optimal birth?

CHECK YOUR OWN DUE DATE

We talked about this in the last chapter. Have you done it? Rethink your dates carefully while you can still remember details. Calculating a more reliable due date, based on when you probably actually conceived, is a good idea because menstrual cycles do not all function like clockwork and timing of love-making is obviously also important. Was your partner away when you were supposed to have conceived? Are you sure when your last period was?

MAINTAIN GOOD RELATIONS WITH YOUR CAREGIVERS

This may seem obvious, but it really is essential. You need to keep a delicate balance between friendliness and firmness. With a good relationship you will more easily be able to assert your wishes when the need arises. You will also feel more comfortable asking questions when unfamiliar terms are used. If at any time you feel you really cannot develop a good relationship with a particular caregiver, find another one.

> I remember how small I felt when my consultant told me that although he might reconsider the necessity of performing an episiotomy, he would have to insist on 'EFM'. ("What's that?!" I silently wondered.) In as 'grown-up' a voice as I could manage, I said that I would come back to him on EFM at my next appointment, after I'd read up a bit more on the subject... but could he please, in the meantime, just tell me what it stood for? Needless to say, it was rather difficult for me to maintain my own sense of dignity. However, I looked it all up later and managed to refuse EFM too in the end... under a different consultant.

Whenever any difficult issue arises, it's obviously a good idea to write down any key words, checking spelling if necessary, so you can do your own research later. Look up key words in the Glossary and Index in this book, in books on obstetrics or midwifery in your local libraries or bookshops, and/or search the Internet. Focus proactively on finding out about anything relating to your own situation, so you can anticipate any suggestions from caregivers. Also, take care to evaluate sources as you go because not all information published is accurate. If you are interested in finding out about advice from Michel and experienced midwives on specific topics, go to: www.mothering.com/experts

BE CLEAR ABOUT YOUR VIEW ON TESTS AND ABORTION

If you want an optimal birth, it's best to avoid tests for abnormalities because they almost always carry risks and a 'positive' result would result in the advice to have an abortion. If you're very keen to be tested, read up on individual tests in other pregnancy books, or research them on the Internet. Accept that any invasive test is an intervention in your pregnancy, so may well disturb it, and also realise that opinions differ as to what constitutes an 'invasive test'. A completely non-invasive test (e.g. a blood test for Down's, which is currently in development) is only a good idea if you are ready later to have an abortion.

Michel advises us not to overreact to a 'positive' test result:

> Think about what a screening test really is. When you go into the airport, you go via the metal detector. In some cases it rings but it doesn't mean you have a weapon in your pocket; it may just be a piece of wire. So if a test is positive, it simply means a risk which is more than 1 in 200, for example. That means there is an almost 99.5% chance that there's no problem.

Here's a comment from a woman who ended up with an unnecessary section:

> Almost every visit I was given some test for something that I was at 'very low risk' for, but that I should have the test 'just in case'. They would say it was my choice, but it was obvious that they really thought I should take the test, so I would do it. I was a good patient. I was afraid, both of being seen as irresponsible or a troublemaker, and of the serious diseases and situations I was supposedly being tested for. I would wait with anxiety for the test results.

And a couple of comments from other women...

> As I was nearing 40 when pregnant with my fourth baby, we read about amniocentesis and decided to have it done. The information we read had informed us that the positioning of the needle was carefully monitored by ultrasound. We were both very surprised when staff identified what they considered to be a pool of amniotic fluid then switched the scanner off before inserting the needle. Our baby was very active at this stage and could easily have changed position during the time taken to prepare the needle and insert it—a risk we would not have taken had we been given ALL the information.

> The medics told me my bloods were wrong and I needed amniocentesis to check for Down's syndrome, but I declined, saying I'd rather have another scan or check my blood for fetal blood cells to check its chromosomes. My partner didn't agree, but I decided that at this late stage (five months) I wouldn't have an abortion anyway, so what was the point in giving the fetus a headache or worse? Every trip to the clinic made me feel worried as they found 'inconsistencies' so I stopped going—I felt absolutely wonderful, the fetus was growing and moving, if I was out of their standard ranges then what of it? Although I understood how the system worked, it was extremely hard to withstand the pressure that the community places on you. You are so vulnerable when pregnant and it's hard to go against the flow.

In *Birth Reborn* (Souvenir Press 1994), Michel mentioned the view the staff had of amniocentesis at Pithiviers. Apparently, they only recommended the test to women in cases where there was a history of genetic disease in the pregnant woman's family (because then, the test might put the woman's fears to rest). Michel points out that the test is only useful if the woman would be prepared to have an abortion (in the case of a positive test result) and also that the risk of miscarriage (which researchers put at anywhere from 0.5-2%) needs to be taken into account.

In this commentary from *Birth Reborn* Michel also mentions that some studies suggest a higher incidence of respiratory difficulties for the newborn baby and that others also link amniocentesis carried out in the second trimester of pregnancy with orthopaedic malformations. His recommendation is to suggest that mums-to-be consider their risk for Down's syndrome (Trisomy 21) and other abnormalities in a positive framework. In other words, instead of thinking about the 1 in 94 women aged 40 who are at risk of having a child with Down's syndrome, they should think about the 93 out of 94 40-year-olds who have a perfectly normal baby. Finally, Michel reminds us that the widely-believed increased risks of fetal abnormalities for women over 35 may be misguided if the abnormalities are in fact connected to an increased exposure to radiation, with increased age, rather than age itself. It's up to you to decide!

In any case it's perhaps also important to consider your baby's perspective. Researchers have noted a range of reactions from unborn babies, including an accelerated heart rate, staying motionless for two minutes after insertion of the needle and even slower breathing movements for up to two days after the amniocentesis test. One fetus who was accidentally hit by a needle was filmed twisting away and then repeatedly striking out at the needle barrel.[5] Another retracted a limb and turned a somersault when accidentally hit by the needle and one even knocked the needle away with its tiny hand.[6] One scientist even found that the catecholamine levels of a fetus whose mother had amniocentesis rose after the test—indicating that the growing baby felt under stress.[7]

What if you refuse most antenatal tests? Do you then have to worry about having an 'imperfect' child? Although many parents initially feel shocked, disappointed and angry if they are the 1 in a 1,000 who have a baby with Down's syndrome, they do often change their minds later on. This is because having a child with Down's is not necessarily the negative experience they had expected. After all, people with Down's syndrome have all kinds of personalities and widely differing capabilities.

Richard Bailey, himself the father of a girl with Down's, travelled the UK taking photos of children with Down's syndrome in an effort to challenge people's misconceptions. Here are some of the photos he took...

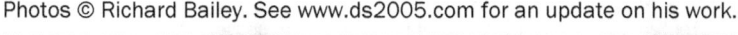
Photos © Richard Bailey. See www.ds2005.com for an update on his work.

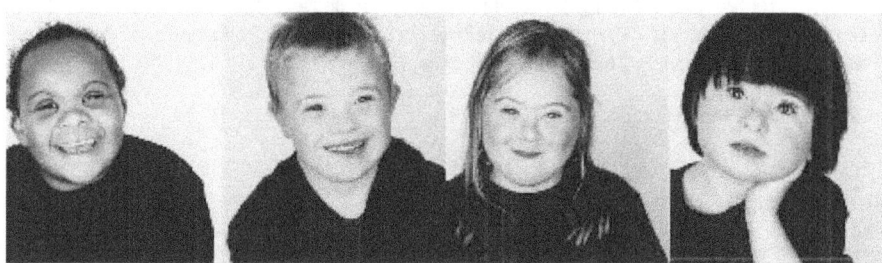

A few children with Down's syndrome

Birthframe 38

Sometimes Down's syndrome does not mean a person is unremarkable and merely a drain on people and resources. As the following account shows, some individuals with Down's syndrome make an enormous contribution to the world.

Sally Johnson was born with Down's syndrome and a rare heart condition which threatened to kill her at any moment. Sheila and Ken, her parents, were told that the best they could do with their daughter was put her in a home and forget all about her. Today, almost 30 years after she heard those harsh words, Sheila is still deeply hurt.

"They'll stay with me for ever," she says. "One doctor even said, 'She will grow up to be the village idiot.'"

The birth of baby Sally seemed to be the icing on the cake for Ken and Sheila, who met and fell in love through their mutual passion for art.

"Ken had a little art gallery. I loved painting and happened to be visiting the area and called in. We hit it off immediately," recalls Sheila.

After they married, the couple moved into the picturesque cottage in Thornton-le-Dale, where Sheila still lives. Their happiness was complete when Sheila gave birth to Sally.

"Sally was beautiful," says Sheila. "My first impression was that she had a face just like a flower. I fell in love with her in an instant."

But Sheila's elation was shattered by a comment made by a hospital doctor. "He asked me, quite coldly, if I noticed anything different about Sally and said, 'She's a Mongol.' Back then, that was the brutal term everyone used."

Worse was to come. A local GP immediately advised them to give Sally up. "He said, 'You won't want to keep her. You'll walk down the street and she'll be dribbling and drooling. You'll be ashamed of her,'" says Sheila. "I was furious and it made me all the more determined to keep her, protect her and love her. I saw a little fighter in Sally from Day 1."

But the couple faced hostility, even from some villagers. "It was awful," recalls Sheila. "No one would look at her in her pram, and people would hide in shop doorways if they saw me coming."

Sheila had resigned herself to a difficult and lonely future for the family—but she hadn't banked on Sally's resilience.

"She started to sit up in her buggie and beam at passers-by," says Sheila. "People couldn't help but smile. She was so affectionate, she began to draw people to her. It was as if she was saying 'I'm here, you can't ignore me!'"

A local GP said: "You'll be ashamed of her."
I was furious and it made me more determined..."

> She was reading at 3 and went to school.
> At 15 she proved how talented she was.

Despite her heart condition, Sally went from strength to strength. She was reading at 3 and went to mainstream school. But it wasn't until the age of 15 that she proved how exceptionally talented she was.

"We bought her a paintbox for Christmas and she became absorbed by watercolours," says Sheila. "I thought I was just being a proud mum, but one of the teachers saw her first painting and asked if she could buy it. Sally sold it for £5!"

Ken and Sheila were even more impressed when Sally announced she wanted to sell more pictures, so that she could give the money to charity. But they had no idea how influential and prolific their daughter's work was to become. Over the next nine years she painted more than 2,500 original watercolours, selling every one and raising over £250,000 for charity.

"Someone once said, 'Do you realise she has painted more pictures than Van Gogh?'" says Sheila, now 69. "That put it all in perspective. But the best thing was seeing Sally happy in her work. She used to say, 'There's a lot of things I can't do very well, but I can do this.'"

Word soon spread about Sally's talents. She was asked to design Christmas cards and calendars for the National Down's Syndrome Association. Her work was advertised at London tube stations—the former Prime Minister, John Major, even hung one of her pictures in Downing Street.

"He wrote to tell Sally that the painting expressed the peace and tranquility missing from his busy life," says Sheila.

On average, Sally painted five originals a week and sold them instantly. An exhibition of her work in a North Yorkshire gallery attracted buyers from all over the UK and sold out in a weekend.

"Sally just said, 'Right I'll have to paint some more,'" says Sheila.

Not only that, when Sally wasn't busy at her easel, she managed to complete a Duke of Edinburgh's Bronze award, followed by the coveted Silver and Gold Awards in the Mencap Gateway Challenge.

Sadly, despite Sally's successes and achievements, Sheila knew they were living on borrowed time.

"From the day she was born I'd been told her heart condition could kill her at any moment," says Sheila. "It made every day with her very precious."

Seven years after her husband's death, Sheila's fears came true.

"Doctors told me Sally didn't have long at all, so I decided to make the most of the time she did have left," she recalls. "We took off to all the places she loved in Yorkshire and Scotland. I have such precious memories of that trip."

Gradually Sally became so ill she could no longer leave the house. Despite being in constant pain, Sheila says her daughter's sunny nature shone through.

210 birth: countdown to optimal

I won't hear her lively chatter and laughter again...

"Our last day together, I cuddled her and said, 'I wish I could bear the pain for you.' But she just smiled and said, 'You can't, but you can help me bear it. Let's have a game of dominoes.' So we played a game. Eventually she made her way to bed, but collapsed on the stairs. She looked up at me and whispered, 'I just can't cope any more.'"

Sally died in Sheila's arms, aged just 25. Four years on, Sheila's heartbreak is still evident.

"I can't get used to the fact I won't hear her lively chatter and laughter again," she says.

But, thanks to the paintings and the letters from people who still write to say how much Sally inspired and touched their lives, Sheila knows she has been left with a very special legacy.

"Sally gave hope to so many people," she says. "I'd give anything to have her back, but her short life was so fulfilled. Single-handedly, she changed attitudes to Down's syndrome and had a life full of purpose and love. And she filled my life with joy."

Adapted extract from *Sally, Face Like a Flower* by Bill Anderson (Dent Dale Publishing 2004). A slightly longer version of this extract first appeared in *Woman's Weekly* on 21 September 2004.

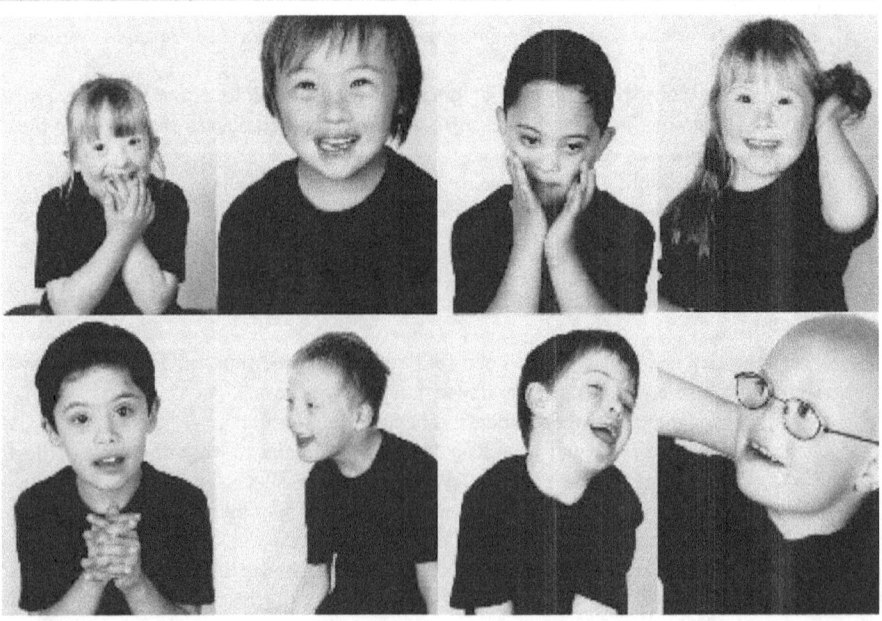

Here are a few more of Richard Bailey's photos of children with Down's syndrome.

CONSIDER YOUR VIEW ON ULTRASOUND

At your very first appointment a midwife is likely to use a Doppler Sonicaid to listen to your baby's heartbeat. While this may be exciting, it's also worth remembering that this involves the use of ultrasound and that there is a non-ultrasound alternative: a Pinard stethoscope. Soon after this first appointment, you may also automatically be booked in for a scan, which you can cancel if you wish. So very early on, you do need to decide on what you feel about ultrasound.

Here's an adapted extract from one of Michel's articles:

Routine scans in pregnancy have become the symbol of modern antenatal care. They are also its most expensive component. A series of studies compared the effects on birth outcomes of routine ultrasound screening versus the selective use of scans. One of these randomised trials, published in the *New England Journal of Medicine*, involved 15,151 pregnant women.[8] The last sentence of the article is unequivocal: "Whatever the explanation proposed for its lack of effect, the findings of this study clearly indicate that ultrasound screening does not improve perinatal outcome in current US practice". ['Perinatal outcome' is to do with the baby's health—or otherwise—at or within 10 days of the birth.]

Around the same time, an article in the *British Medical Journal* assembled data from four other comparable randomised trials.[9] The authors concluded: "Routine ultrasound scans do not improve the outcome of pregnancy in terms of an increased number of live births or of reduced perinatal morbidity. Routine ultrasound scanning may be effective and useful as a screening for malformation. Its use for this purpose, however, should be made explicit and take into account the risk of false positive diagnosis in addition to ethical issues". ['False positive diagnosis' is when a person is told a growing baby has a problem, when in fact he or she doesn't.]

It is possible that in the future a new generation of studies will cast doubts on the absolute safety of repeated exposure to ultrasound during fetal life. One of the effects of this might be to reduce dramatically the number of scans, particularly in the vulnerable phase of early pregnancy.

Even in a high risk population of pregnant women, scans are not as useful as is commonly believed. Evidence from randomised controlled trials suggests that sonographic identification of fetal growth retardation does not improve outcome despite increased medical surveillance.[10] In diabetic pregnancies it has been demonstrated that ultrasound measurements are not more accurate than clinical examination to identify high birthweight babies.[11]

> I am appalled at the practice of renting hand Dopplers out to expectant mothers, some of whom are listening to their babies several times a day. Talk about exposure! Also, if a woman isn't really trained at using one correctly, I would assume that every time she can't find the heartbeat it causes undue distress.

> I have a currently pregnant friend who has had Weeks 8-20 of her pregnancy completely ruined by a false positive scan which gave her all sorts of alarming 'news', none of which has now been found to be true.

What is ultrasound, though? Sarah Buckley explains:

Originally, it was a technique developed during WWII to detect enemy submarines, and it was subsequently used in the steel industry. In July 1955 a Glaswegian surgeon, Ian Donald, experimented with it on abdominal tumours (removed from his patients). He discovered that different tissues gave different patterns of 'echo', so realised that ultrasound offered a new way of looking into the previously mysterious world of the growing baby.[12] Apparently, the new technology spread rapidly into clinical obstetrics. Commercial machines became available in 1963[13] and by the late 1970s ultrasound had become a routine part of obstetric care.[14]

During an ultrasound ultra-high frequency soundwaves travel at 10 to 20 million cycles per second—which is very fast, considering audible sound only travels at 10 to 20 thousand cycles per second.[15] These waves are emitted by a transducer (the part of the machine that is put onto the body), and a picture of the underlying tissues is built up from the pattern of 'echo' waves which return. Hard surfaces such as bone will return a stronger echo than soft tissue or fluids, giving the bony skeleton a white appearance on the screen.

Ordinary scans use pulses of ultrasound which last only a fraction of a second, with the interval between waves being used by the machine to interpret the echo that returns. In contrast, Doppler techniques, which are used in specialised scans, fetal monitors and hand-held fetal stethoscopes (Sonicaids) feature continuous waves, giving longer exposure than 'pulsed' ultrasound. Many women do not realise that the small machines used to listen to their baby's heartbeat are actually using Doppler ultrasound, although using a lower dose.

Sarah reports that more recently, ultrasonographers have been using vaginal ultrasound, especially in early pregnancy since better pictures can be obtained this way. Here the transducer is placed high in the vagina, much closer to the developing baby. The problem is that when ultrasound is used vaginally, there is little tissue to shield the baby, who is at a vulnerable stage of development, so exposure levels will be higher. Having a vaginal scan is also not a pleasant procedure for the woman; the term 'diagnostic rape' was coined to describe how some women experience vaginal scans.

And what information can be obtained from a scan of any kind? Although ultrasound is used when there's bleeding in early pregnancy to detect whether or not a miscarriage is inevitable, this would obviously be discovered soon afterwards anyway. Generally speaking, it seems that ultrasound is only really useful for confirming whether or not a woman is expecting more than one baby, for determining whether or not a baby is breech, very close to 40 weeks, and for checking for placenta praevia. However, the midwife's hands can usually check for both breech babies and multiples. Furthermore, in 19 out of 20 cases placenta praevia is misdiagnosed because it's checked for too early: the placenta will effectively move up later in the pregnancy and will not cause problems at the birth. In any case, a study conducted in 1990 concluded that detection of placenta praevia by ultrasound is not safer than detection in labour.[16] Research shows that dating by ultrasound may be inaccurate, especially for ultrasounds later in pregnancy.[17] Using scans to check fetal growth also seems unnecessary.

Performing scans for abnormalities is also widespread even though it seems to be unreliable. Apparently, only between 17% and 85% of the 1 in 50 babies that have major abnormalities at birth are identified.[18] A recent study from Brisbane showed that ultrasound at a major women's hospital missed around 40% of abnormalities,[19] and major causes of intellectual disability such as cerebral palsy and Down's syndrome are unlikely to be picked up on a routine scan, as are heart and kidney abnormalities.[20]

You also need to remember the possibility of a 'false positive', where the ultrasound diagnosis is wrong. A UK survey showed that, for 1 in 200 babies aborted for major abnormalities, the diagnosis on autopsy was less severe than predicted by ultrasound and the termination was probably unjustified. In this survey, 2.4% of the babies diagnosed with major malformations, but not aborted, had conditions that were significantly over or under-diagnosed.[21] There are also many cases of error with more minor abnormalities, which can cause anxiety and repeated scans, and there are some conditions which have been seen to spontaneously resolve.

As well as false positives, there are also uncertain cases where the ultrasound findings cannot be easily interpreted and the outcome for the baby is not known. In one study involving women at high risk, almost 10% of scans gave uncertain results.[22] This can create immense anxiety for the woman and her family, and the worry may not be allayed by the birth of a normal baby. In the same study, mothers with 'questionable' diagnoses still had this anxiety three months after the birth of their baby.

In 1975 a study of scans on unborn babies using Doppler ultrasound was published in the *British Medical Journal*. The researchers didn't tell the mothers whether the ultrasound machine was switched on, but when it was the fetuses were found to move about much more. In the UK in 1993, the Association for Improvement in Midwifery Services' journal, the *AIMS Quarterly*, published a selection of comments from mothers about their babies' responses to having scans.[24] They included:

> The baby was moving around so much the technician could not take any measurements...

> It had both hands up to its ears, fist fashion.

> The consultant got very frustrated because he could not get a clear picture because she (the baby) would not sit still. At first she would move to a totally different part of my womb, then when she was bigger, turn around and around.

> She (the baby) was extremely active when we wanted a picture of her. Then she put her head as low as possible in my pelvis where the ultrasound seemed to have difficulty getting a clear picture.

Here are some personal comments from Sarah Buckley:

When I was pregnant with my first baby in 1990, I decided against having a scan. This was a rather unusual decision, as my partner and I are both doctors and had even done pregnancy scans ourselves—rather ineptly, but sometimes usefully—while training in General Practice Obstetrics a few years earlier.

What influenced me the most was my feeling that I would lose something important as a mother if I allowed someone to test my baby. I knew that if a minor or uncertain problem showed up (this is not uncommon), I would be obliged to return again and again, and that after a while, it would feel as if my baby belonged to the system, and not to me.

In the years since then I have had three more babies who had no scans, and have read many articles and research papers about ultrasound. Nothing I have read has made me reconsider my decision. Although ultrasound may sometimes be useful when specific problems are suspected, my conclusion is that it is at best ineffective and at worse dangerous when used as a 'screening tool' for every pregnant woman and her baby.

And what of the known effects of ultrasound? Sarah tells us that ultrasound waves are known to affect tissues in two main ways. Firstly, the sonar beam causes heating of the highlighted area by about 1 degree Celsius. (Apparently, this is presumed to be non-significant, based on whole-body heating in pregnancy, which seems to be safe up to 2.5 degrees Celsius above normal.)[25] Secondly, ultrasound apparently causes 'cavitation'. This is where the small pockets of gas (which exist within mammalian tissue) vibrate and then collapse. In this situation, according to the American Institute of Ultrasound Medicine Bioeffects Report (1988) "temperatures of many thousands of degrees Celsius in the gas create a wide range of chemical products, some of which are potentially toxic. These violent processes may be produced by micro-second pulses of the kind which are used in medical diagnosis..." The significance of cavitation effects in human tissue is unknown.[26]

A number of studies have indeed suggested cause for concern. Studies not involving humans have shown that cell abnormalities persist for several generations,[27] that the myelin that covers nerves is damaged[28] and that rates of cell division are reduced, while 'aptosis' (programmed cell death of the small intestine) happen two times as often.[29]

Studies on humans exposed to ultrasound have shown that possible adverse effects include premature ovulation,[30] preterm labour or miscarriage,[31] low birth weight,[32] poorer condition at birth,[33] perinatal death,[34] dyslexia,[35] delayed speech development[36] and less right-handedness.[37] (Non right-handedness is, in other circumstances, seen as a marker of damage to the developing brain.)[38] One Australian study showed that babies exposed to five or more Doppler ultrasound scans were 30% more likely to develop intrauterine growth retardation— a condition that ultrasound is often used to detect.[39]

For Sarah Buckley (who provided most of the information in this section), ultrasound represents yet another way in which the deep internal knowledge that a mother has of her body and her baby is made secondary to technological information that comes from an 'expert' using a machine. She says this is how the 'cult of the expert' is imprinted from the earliest weeks of life. She feels that by treating the baby as a separate being, ultrasound artificially splits mother from baby well before this is a physiological or psychic reality.

For these reasons, Sarah urges all pregnant women to think deeply before they choose to have a routine scan. It is not compulsory, despite what some doctors say, and the risks, benefits and implications of ultrasound need to be considered for each mother and baby, according to their specific situation. She says if you do choose to have a scan, you should have it done by an operator with a high level of skill and experience and you should say that you want the shortest scan possible. If an abnormality is found, she says you should ask for counselling and a second opinion as soon as is practical... remembering that it's your baby, your body and your choice.

Here are two commentaries to give us more insight into the experience...

> At around 19 weeks, I chose to have one scan. Based on measurements of my baby's body at that time, the sonographer's program computed that my baby's head was 19 weeks and 5 days gestation, but his body was only 18 weeks and 6 days. So much for the accuracy of ultrasound dating! I pointed out to the ultrasound operator that I am broad, Graham is tall, and we both have big heads. Ultrasound dating software doesn't take account of variables like this. After about 14 weeks' gestation, ultrasound dating is notoriously inaccurate. If all babies were born at exactly the same gestation, with exactly the same length, weight, and head circumference, then ultrasound dating would be accurate. As things are, it's just a computer's guess.

I had plenty of scans during my first two pregnancies. I'm not sure now it was such a great idea. During each pregnancy, I had a false positive for a serious defect! Not only did these false positives cause endless extra anxiety, which can only have been bad for the fetus, they also probably contributed to an unnecessary caesarean section for my son.

During my first pregnancy, the 'triple test' for neural tube defects showed an 'abnormally high' AFP level, which is supposed to indicate a higher likelihood of spina bifida. I was rushed in for an extra scan the next day, at 18 weeks. The scan indicated no sign of any problem. "The best way to explain why the AFP level was high is that your baby is actually older than we thought," the doctors said. Even though I was certain I knew the date of conception, I agreed to let the doctors re-date the pregnancy based on the first (12-week) scan, giving me a due date two weeks earlier. Later, I went 'overdue' past the new, earlier due date. I got nervous I would be induced. I tried to bring on labour. Things went awry. The rest is history: my waters broke, the baby passed meconium, I ended up in hospital: induction, epidural, caesarean, the classic sequence.

They decided 12 weeks was too early to tell...

The second time around, the 12-week scan showed choroid plexus cysts, according to the doctors. Apparently, cpc's—which appear in the scan as flower-like empty spaces in the developing brain—are a normal stage of fetal brain development. However, they're 'supposed' to disappear by 12 weeks. If they are still visible at 12 weeks, they can be 'associated' with Trisomy 18, a very rare, fatal genetic disorder. "We can't see the fetus too well, but it looks as though there could be something unusual in the brain. Do you mind if we use a vaginal scanner?" Next, I had the pleasure of a roomful of male doctors stuffing a dildo-shaped scanner up my vagina while they searched for evidence of my baby's ostensible abnormality. (My husband was abroad, so I went to the scan alone, expecting it to be entirely routine.)

They decided 12 weeks was too early to tell conclusively if there was a problem. "Don't worry," they said, "you have only a very small chance of having a baby with T-18. Just go home, relax, and come back in three weeks for another scan, at which point we'll be able to tell more clearly if there's any problem. Meanwhile, don't let this spoil your early pregnancy." Giving me no more information than this to go on—not even the spelling of 'choroid plexus cyst,' or any statistics on the occurrence of cpc's and their link to Trisomy-18, I was sent home to panic alone.

I researched cpc's and learned that the chance of any problem really was very low, at most only 1-3%. I trusted my intuition that everything was fine and calmed down. Not surprisingly, the next scan indicated that everything was fine, and we soon forgot all about it. Why did we put ourselves through such an ordeal in the first place? It was all in the interests of our child's future health, or so we thought. But what did we gain by it?

Even though I felt doubtful about ultrasound by the time I got pregnant for the third time, when it came to it I just couldn't withstand the pressure! I felt that a third pregnancy was an even bigger responsibility than a first or second, because now I already had three other people (husband and two kids) involved. I wasn't 100% sure I would decide to carry a Down's baby to term. I wanted to be able to demonstrate to myself and my partner that I had been responsible in trying to have a healthy baby. I decided against amnio, which was routinely offered at 38, in favour of the 'integrated test', which includes one scan and two blood tests. I decided to do the scan because it was less invasive than amnio. So I made compromises, accepting some tests and declining others. A funny approach? Perhaps.

A baby is so much a gift from God. No matter how many tests you do, there's only so much you can know in advance. There are plenty of other things that can go wrong either before, during or after birth that can't be measured or tested for. Does it really make sense to put the baby on trial? Isn't it better to have faith that things will go well, to love the baby and let it develop as it's meant to?

Nina Klose

In my own third pregnancy, it was a bit of a battle at the local hospital in Oman, but I did manage to come home without having had a scan. When the midwife smeared gel on my bump and turned on a Doppler unit, I immediately said, "No! I don't want that. I said I didn't want any ultrasound." Amazingly enough, she was completely unaware that the unit had anything to do with ultrasound—she initially denied it completely—and was only persuaded not to turn the thing on again when I used the term Pinard and agreed that it would be no use yet because she probably wouldn't be able to hear the fetal heart until 18 weeks. I said, "Anyway, don't worry. There's definitely somebody in there—he or she occasionally gives me polite kicks." Using a couple of obstetric terms certainly helped... although she did insist I see her boss, and *her* boss, and *his* boss too.

I asked Michel about the value of using ultrasound for multiple pregnancies...

What do you think about repeated scans during twin pregnancies? Surely the only justification could be if the consultant ordering the scans was prepared to 'order' an induction with the rationale that the baby might be 'better out than in'? What other treatment could be given? Presumably none, so aren't these scans more or less useless?

I used to consider a twin birth a 'normal birth' and do nothing. I have never seen a huge discrepancy between the weight of two twins. Had it happened, my hands would have found that there was something strange.

In *Birth Reborn* (Souvenir Press 1994), Michel further explains how he used scans at his maternity hospital in Pithiviers, which aimed to be as non-interventionist as possible:

1. **Detection of twin pregnancies** Michel did not usually use ultrasound to diagnose twin pregnancies for the simple reason that there was little practical point in doing so. In his view, either only one of the two fetuses will continue to develop anyway, or the mum-to-be could wait until the eighth or ninth month of the pregnancy to find out about her imminent twins! A discovery would be made during the routine antenatal checks.
2. **Detection of neural tube malformations** Michel agrees that scans can sometimes detect these (e.g. anencephaly or spina bifida) but he reminds us that this information is only useful a) if the malformation is detected early enough for an abortion to be possible, and b) if the woman is prepared to have one. Michel feels there is little point in putting pregnant women through tests and decisions about abortions because in most cases fetuses with malformations die in utero or shortly after they are born anyway.
3. **Confirmation of the date of conception** Michel preferred to determine this through careful questioning and examinations early on in the pregnancy.

Michel's overall conclusion, then, is that scans should only be performed if the information they might provide would *change* decisions made about the pregnancy—in terms of treatment given by the caregiver, or action taken by the pregnant woman.[40]

DECIDE HOW YOU FEEL ABOUT MONITORING

Monitoring is another aspect of antenatal care which you need to take seriously because it can lead to additional tests, interventions and radically different birthing experiences.

But what is 'monitoring', how is it done and why? I prefer a broad definition... Broadly speaking, it can be anything from a few questions, to feeling your bump, to the use of ultrasound or other technology so as to detect and check the fetal heartbeat. The idea is to track both mother and baby's progress so as to ensure a positive outcome. The following forms of monitoring are carried out at each antenatal appointment:

- **Blood pressure and urine check** Your blood pressure is recorded and a sample of urine is tested. This is mainly so as to check for symptoms of pre-eclampsia and the life-threatening condition eclampsia, which very occasionally follows it. Pre-eclampsia is diagnosed when high blood pressure is accompanied by protein in the urine and—if found—does need to be monitored closely. High blood pressure alone is not necessarily a problem, though, because research shows that a woman's blood pressure is *supposed* to rise later on in pregnancy.[41] It's actually associated with good outcomes! However, high blood pressure can also be associated with poor fetal growth so that's another reason it's monitored.
- **Palpation** The woman's belly is felt and usually also measured because this should help the caregiver get an idea of how well the baby is growing, how it is positioned in the womb and also how much amniotic fluid is around him or her. If a baby isn't growing well, it could be an indication of some medical condition which needs attention (probably hypertension), or it could simply mean that the mother needs to either eat more or stop smoking, for example. The baby's position in the womb is of particular interest later on in pregnancy because it is always hoped that a baby will go into an ideal 'head down' position, preferably with its back facing forward, on the left side of the woman's abdomen. (As we've already noted, this position is officially termed LOA—left occiput anterior). When this doesn't happen, the birth can be more difficult and in some cases a caesarean is even necessary. Having too much or too little amniotic fluid is a sign that there are problems with the baby, and this would initially be noticed through palpation (feeling the baby belly). Risks are associated with this problem and further investigations would be recommended, although it's worth mentioning that research has shown that drinking more water seems to help and that 40-50% of problem cases sort themselves out within a few days, without any hospital intervention.
- **Auscultation** A Sonicaid or Doppler unit (different words for the same thing), or another type of fetal stethoscope, such as the Pinard (which does not use ultrasound) is used to check the fetal heartbeat.

The idea is that babies can sometimes be saved in time (with a speedy emergency caesarean) when the baby sounds poorly, although it must be said that this is unlikely. After all, auscultation—as it's called—is only carried out once a month or once a week later on in most pregnancies—so the chances of detecting problems in time are minimal. In cases where the baby actually dies in utero, the woman will spontaneously go into labour a few days later. So checking the fetal heartbeat is really just a reassuring thing for the mother to have done.

It's easy to see why the ultrasound device (the Sonicaid or Doppler) has become so popular... Firstly, it's easier for the caregiver to use (than a Pinard) and secondly, it allows the mother to hear the amplified heartbeat herself. However, the Pinard does offer the option of having the same check without the use of any ultrasound, so it's worth holding out for, just in case ultrasound is harmful in any way. If your midwife doesn't have one, ask for this check to be carried out at the next visit. I asked Michel about the usefulness of checking the fetal heartbeat (auscultation):

Why is auscultation a routine part of antenatal care? Obviously, it's to listen to the fetal heartbeat... but why? A dead fetus would be detected, but the woman would have found out a few days later anyway, since presumably she would go into labour if that were the case. Since auscultation is carried out only once a month/once every two weeks/once a week (depending on the stage of pregnancy), the chances of catching a fetus while in distress, but early enough to carry out an emergency caesarean, seems remote. So what's really the reason for auscultation? I can understand it better in labour—but even then, a minimum of disturbance to the labouring woman seems ideal—hence your preference for the Sonicaid, of course, which allows more discrete auscultation.

Sylvie, you are right. Antenatal auscultation is not a very useful ritual and cannot change outcomes. [Michel then provided a list of studies on monitoring, with commentary.][42] None of these studies could detect any effect on birth statistics.

Cynics would say that other types of routine monitoring are also merely ritualistic. They give caregivers clear tasks and help them look authoritative but the usefulness of the actual monitoring may be highly questionable. In some cases it can simply make the pregnant woman unnecessarily fearful. For example, if palpation reveals that a baby is lying in a breech position early on in pregnancy it may make her worry about labour. In a few cases, though, monitoring can be life-saving or it can provide information (e.g. about the fetal position late in pregnancy), which can be a useful springboard for discussion and advice. So it certainly isn't something we need to dismiss out of hand.

How much monitoring you allow in your own pregnancy is a question only you can answer, based on what you know about your own health levels. Whatever you decide, remember that if you are not 100% happy with the idea of having any test, you can refuse it.

CONSIDER YOUR VIEW ON OTHER TESTS

There are two other commonly performed tests which need to be mentioned. Since you may well be offered these, they're well worth thinking over...

- **Anaemia check** The amount of red blood cells pigment (the haemoglobin concentration) is usually routinely measured in pregnancy. This is because there is a widespread belief that this test can effectively detect anaemia and iron deficiency. In fact, it cannot diagnose iron deficiency because the blood volume of pregnant women is *supposed* to increase dramatically. The haemoglobin concentration indicates primarily the degree of blood dilution, which is an effect of placental activity. In fact, a large British study, involving 153,602 pregnancies,[43] found that the highest average birth weight (which is good) was in the group of women who had a haemoglobin concentration between 8.5 and 9.5. These are the women who would normally be called 'anaemic'! Michel says that although caregivers tell women they are at risk of anaemia unless their haemoglobin concentration is above 10.5, when the haemoglobin concentration *fails* to fall below 10.5 research shows there is an increased risk of low birth weight, preterm birth and pre-eclampsia! He says it is a regrettable consequence of routine evaluation of haemoglobin concentration that women are told they are anaemic—when they aren't—and are given iron supplements. There is a tendency both to overlook the side effects of iron (constipation, diarrhoea, heartburn, etc) and also to forget that iron inhibits the absorption of such an important growth factor as zinc.[44] Research has shown that iron supplementation can also exacerbate lipid peroxidation (a process which leads to the development of free radicals, which is bad news) and it can even increase the risk of pre-eclampsia![45]

- **Gestational diabetes check** Another routine test given in some practices is for so-called gestational diabetes. Michel says that diagnosing gestational diabetes is useless because it merely leads to simple recommendations that should be given to all pregnant women, i.e. avoid sugar (including carbonated drinks, etc.), choose complex carbohydrates (brown pasta, bread, rice, etc) and make sure you get enough physical exercise. A huge Canadian study showed that the only effect of routine glucose tolerance screening was to inform 2.7% of women that they have gestational diabetes, a diagnosis which doesn't change birth outcomes.[46]

This all leads us to a very important question: what can a health professional do in order to influence outcomes? Over to Michel again...

Since prematurity is a major preoccupation, let's focus on what medical care can offer in order to reduce the incidence of preterm births. Recently, considerable research has focused on how useful antibiotics might be to prevent this. A large multi-centre randomised controlled trial involving 6,295 women did not support the use of antibiotics.[47] Another study concluded that the treatment of vaginal infection in early pregnancy does not decrease the incidence of preterm delivery.[48] Cerclage of the cervix, although widely used to reduce the risk of premature birth, has now also been called into question: research into this technique is inconsistent but has shown that the risk of postpartum fever is doubled as a result.[49] Medical interventions also do not reduce the risk of having a small-for-dates baby. Finally, even bedrest restrictions have been shown to be useless and even harmful.[50]

From the point of view of the expectant mother, the primary question should be: "What can the doctor do for me and my baby, since I already know I am pregnant and I can feel the baby growing?" The doctor should answer with humility: "Not a lot, apart from detecting a gross abnormality and offering an abortion."

We should not conclude that there is no need at all for medical visits in pregnancy: we cannot make a comprehensive list of all the reasons why women might need the advice or the help of a qualified health professional before giving birth. It is the word 'routine' that should be discarded. It is easy to explain why current habits are a waste of time and money; it is also easy to explain why they are potentially dangerous. It is dangerous to misinterpret the results of a routine test and to tell a healthy mum-to-be that she is anaemic and that she needs iron supplements. It is dangerous to present an isolated increased blood pressure measurement as bad news. It is dangerous to tell a pregnant woman that she has 'gestational diabetes'. In general, it is the very style of medicalised antenatal care, constantly focusing on potential problems, which causes problems by making pregnant women worry.[51]

The decline of routine medicalised antenatal care should take place alongside a rediscovery of the basic needs of pregnant women. I well remember the atmosphere of happiness that accumulated at singing evenings in the maternity unit at the Pithiviers hospital, in France. These singing sessions probably had a more positive effect on the development of babies in the womb than a series of scans. Mums-to-be need to socialise and share their experiences. It is easy to create occasions for this: swimming, yoga, antenatal exercise sessions... Let us dream of the potential of specialised restaurants for parents-to-be!

THINK CAREFULLY ABOUT ANTENATAL CLASSES

Returning to our list of things we can do to show we care about antenatal care, we also need to think about antenatal classes. There is a common assumption they are a 'must' for every first-time mother. This is not true. (Perhaps the fact that I had three optimal births has something to do with the fact that I've never attended a single class?)[52] As a non-expert on classes, here's what I suggest:

- ♥ Only attend classes if you find some run by a teacher who you like the sound of.
- ♥ Only continue to attend classes if you have a positive feeling about your antenatal teacher when you first meet him or her. Trust your intuition.
- ♥ Opt out of a series of classes at any point—even during a class, if necessary—if you feel that your natural suggestibility during pregnancy is making you receive unhelpful messages. Also opt out if you feel uncomfortable for any other reason.

People assume classes are a 'must' for a first-time mother

Birthframe 40

Very often, the classes run by a particular hospital or clinic only prepare women for the protocols and preferences of that particular institution. This extract from a letter to a Head of Midwifery Services illustrates this. The writer of the letter—a first-time mother at that time—subsequently had a successful home birth over an intact perineum (see Birthframes 64 and 65). Presumably, the teachers running the antenatal classes mentioned in this letter would have been surprised that it was possible for a first-time mother not to require stitches and to give birth in such low-tech surroundings.

> Dear Miss...
>
> We met briefly on Tuesday, 20 June regarding my request for a home confinement. I would like to thank you again for being so helpful and for opening my eyes to the 'birthing suite', which you so kindly showed my husband and I.
>
> I believe I expressed my surprise at the time at it not being used more often. I have since discovered why. Nobody—out of nine expectant mothers, including two second-time mothers—who attended your clinic's parentcraft classes had any idea of its existence! I mentioned to you that we were given a tour of the hospital and this room was not included or even spoken of.
>
> Today I asked our teacher and tour guide why this was so. Firstly, I was told we had seen it, but after several other women backed me up on this, it was dismissed as being no different to the delivery rooms, apart from there being carpet on the floor, which apparently causes problems anyway. After several other women expressed an interest, we were told that this room was unsuitable for first-time mothers as the low-style bed is not suitable for stitching and we would just end up being moved again anyway. I was not aware that routine episiotomies were given at your hospital and had been informed by the other midwives that they were rarely used.
>
> I strongly disagree that this room is not a very welcome alternative to the delivery suites. Many women find the cold clinical atmosphere of the delivery room off-putting and not a little frightening. I, for one, would feel very much more comfortable and at ease, should the need arise for me to be admitted.
>
> I realise that not everyone shares my views but I feel that everyone should know the options and make their own choices. At today's class (which I subsequently left halfway through) I was ridiculed in front of the class for my ideas on having an upright labour. I quote: "It'll be very interesting to find out who feels like running around the room during labour." I resent being spoken to like an idiot and belittled in this manner, simply because our views differ.
>
> Yours sincerely,
>
> *Karen Low*
>
> For more on 'upright', active labour see Birthframes 81 and 83.

Here are some comments from other contributors:

> I found the exercises in the class [in the UK] to be 'permission-giving', supporting me to use whatever worked for me. A far cry from the hospital-based antenatal classes here in the US. We didn't attend one, but I have heard from others that the classes mostly prepare couples for all the interventions that will be done to them in the hospital and give info on the various pain medications available. Yuck!

> One day I saw a colleague standing behind her desk at work, looking more radiant than usual. She was excitedly telling a friend about her antenatal class the previous evening. "She revved me up so much—I feel I could do it right now!" she said, flinging her arms in the air. Later that day, prematurely, she gave birth to a tiny, 4lb baby boy. I'm not sure what that antenatal teacher did or said, but I'm glad I didn't attend her antenatal classes myself.

> There's lots to say about antenatal classes. The main thing is, I really don't think the classes were thorough enough, or cynical enough. In my case, there were a few very simple, specific things that no one ever told me in the birth classes. They didn't tell me, "Distrust the NHS! Distrust hospitals, because they will do their best to get involved and mess things up." Classes should really be taught by home birth midwives, I think, not by some lady who's had a couple of kids and likes babies.

Obviously, there are some excellent classes around, organised by all kinds of hospitals, birth centres and educational centres. Look out in particular for:

- ♥ **Active Birth classes** These classes are based on the yoga system developed by Janet Balaskas, the founder of the Active Birth Centre in London (see Birthframe 83). Janet says that although the starting point is physical, the exercises may unlock a transformation in consciousness too.
- ♥ **NCT (National Childbirth Trust) classes** These interactive classes provide research-based information and support. See www.nct.org.uk for more info.
- ♥ **Classes run from a midwifery-led unit or birthing centre** Unlike some of the hospital-based classes (which might emphasise drug-based pain relief and hospital protocols), these classes may be inspiring and informative. They may be run by some of the many midwives who are enthusiastic about supporting normal, healthy birth—who may, in fact, attend you in labour.
- ♥ **Aquanatal classes** These classes offer another approach and are based simply on the idea of encouraging pregnant women to take some safe non-weight-bearing exercise during pregnancy.
- ♥ **Singing groups** It was Frederick Leboyer who first suggested the link between open mouths and open vaginas/cervixes. Michel later took up this idea in Pithiviers, when he used to sing with mums-to-be and new mothers. Look for—or start up!—a similar group and invite your caregivers along too.

If you want to explore your options you can obviously do the usual Google searches or you might also consider asking one of your midwife or consultant for advice, explaining to them first that you want to do everything possible to prepare yourself to have a normal, healthy birth.

I asked Michel about antenatal preparation...

Do you think that first-time mothers need to be 'prepared' for childbirth? I can almost imagine your shock, your disgust and your astonishment as you think of an answer to this! I imagine you will say that if a woman is left undisturbed and goes 'to another planet' she will automatically know how to give birth. The reason I'm questioning this idea is because I've just read a book of birth stories. In it, repeatedly, the idea comes through that it's necessary for a woman to be 'trained' if she's to have a pleasant experience of giving birth. Mention is made of women in earlier decades of the twentieth century who writhed around in pain while giving birth because they were 'untrained'. Teenage pregnancies are also mentioned and in these cases the young girls gave birth ineffectively, in great pain and distress—again reportedly because they were 'untrained'. So let me rephrase the question... What kind of preparation do you think a pregnant woman needs if she is going to be capable of 'going to another planet' successfully while she's in labour?

Knowing too much is a handicap during labour. It is easier to forget everything if you don't know too much. A woman obstetrician does not give birth more easily than a young lady whose job is to sell flowers round the corner. Teenage girls can give birth very easily, sometimes at home in the bathroom. But they are very vulnerable if they have a lack of privacy. Your question makes me think of my first visit to the US in 1980. I was participating in a panel about preparation for childbirth. Before it was my turn to speak we heard childbirth educators saying, "I use the Lamaze method" or "I use a modified Lamaze method" or "I use the Bradley method", etc. Then I said, "In our hospital in France we meet around the piano on Tuesday evening and sing together." I explained all the implications of these singing sessions, that it was a way for pregnant women to become familiar with the place and with the people—midwives, cleaning ladies, the secretary, etc—and therefore a way to make the birth easier.

This view of Michel's was recently confirmed to me... Quite by chance, I met a woman who happens to provide educational and pastoral support to teenage mothers. During the conversation, I breezily asked her what kind of experience the teenage mothers usually had—whether their labours were short, long, easy, difficult. "Almost always short and easy," she immediately replied.

What about the older ones among us? Perhaps you will find a class that suits you, or perhaps you won't. Really, the most important thing is to find a class (if you feel you 'need' one), which will help you develop positive feelings towards your body, your baby and your upcoming labour. If the class can also help you to develop rapport with your caregivers, so much the better, and if it takes place in your future birthplace, that's great. If it helps to prepare you for the time immediately after the birth when suddenly you will be responsible for a new human being, that would also be perfect.

If you can't find a class which you feel suits you—or if you don't want to try—don't worry! Your body and your mind will still know what to do.

Finally, so as to optimise your use of the antenatal period...

PREPARE A CARE GUIDE AND GET IT ACCEPTED

This is easier said than done, but it does need to be done. Preparing a care guide (another phrase for 'birth plan') will help you to identify what is important to you when you go into labour and give birth—because you'll be confirming your preferences on paper. Getting your care guide accepted will then help you to establish whether or not the caregiver you are already receiving antenatal care from is supportive of your wishes. If he or she isn't, you will need to search for someone else! There are many midwives, GPs and consultants who will support your desire for an optimal birth—you just need to find them. Remember you can search face-to-face, by phone, by letter and on the Internet. Note that in the UK we are actually allowed to register with any doctor or midwifery practice for antenatal care and we are free to change midway through a pregnancy, if we like. We can also pay to hire an independent midwife (who you may find is more open to the idea of an optimal birth) or go to a private clinic or birth centre. You have many options, but it may take a bit of effort to search them out and actually identify a place and a person you are happy with.

The practicalities of preparing the care guide itself are considered in the next chapter. (After that, we will also be discussing how to 'Choose who' and 'Choose where'.) These are all ways in which you can ensure best outcomes.

Why worry about care when you're in labour?

The 'care' you receive while you're in labour and giving birth may actually be mostly intervention and it may not always be necessary medical intervention from a safety point of view... Although intervention may indeed be life-saving for either the mother or the baby, nowadays women are increasingly complaining that interventions they experienced were unnecessary. In addition, research is revealing more and more clearly just how harmful many unnecessary interventions can be to the mother, the baby, or the family as a whole.

Birthframe 41

Here's an account to give us some intuitive insight into the reasons for avoiding the alternatives to normal, physiological birth if at all possible. This account came in very late, accompanied by the following note:

Dear Sylvie,

At last I have managed to find the report and your address at the same time! I am so sorry to have taken so long—I am really ashamed of myself! I do hope this will be of some use to you. I hadn't read it for some time and it really brought tears to my eyes. Rosie's birth really was a magical experience and I so much wish I could have repeated it.

Pauline

I sat down to write about the wonder of Rosie's birth at home, but felt it all started over two years ago with Sean's birth in hospital, which affected both myself and my family so much that we were determined our next baby's introduction to our world would be a happier and easier event. So, firstly, I am writing about the birth of Sean Henry on 17 October 1986.

I attended excellent NCT antenatal classes, which helped me to look forward with excitement to my baby's arrival, instead of with the fear of childbirth which I'd always held. I had hoped for a natural and gentle birth but due to slightly raised blood pressure following a family crisis, at 36 weeks I found myself on the local hospital baby extraction line. Although I instinctively and intellectually felt that all the intervention was unnecessary, and indeed dangerous, and that the baby was the best judge of when he would be 'better out than in' (the antenatal ward catchphrase), I did not have the confidence to totally resist the daily pressure from the doctors during my two weeks on the ward. Being told I was killing my baby did not help the situation—or my blood pressure!—although some of the midwives were very kind and supportive and were obviously concerned at the number of inductions being performed. However, I did have the knowledge and courage to decline their frequent offers to break my waters (at 1cm dilation) and 'pop' me down to the theatre for a nice, convenient, planned caesarean.

Unfortunately, due to the constant harassment and worry, my blood pressure rose even higher and I finally agreed to prostaglandin pessaries and had seven inserted over seven days. Sean still showed no sign of budging, which simply meant that he was not ready for the outside world. (All my other tests on urine and placenta, etc were perfectly normal.) I was then a Failed Induction and subjected to the full panoply of modern obstetrics: waters broken, numerous drips (including syntocinon), gas and air, and meptid. I didn't really know what was going on during 15 hours of labour, except that everything stopped at one point—not surprising with that cocktail of drugs, which made me quite unable to stray from the bed.

The resultant birth was a 'normal delivery' with a bullying, insensitive midwife who took Sean away immediately (despite my written and oral requests to the contrary) and returned him to me clean and swaddled, so that I couldn't even get to see or touch his fingers. I didn't have a chance to put him to the breast for four hours, despite frequent requests for help, and Sean and I had great difficulty with feeding for ages afterwards. He was sleepy for a few days due to the drugs he received through me, and I was in such a state trying to fend off the bottles from the night staff, it is amazing we ever got the hang of breastfeeding! Needless to say, it took me nearly a year to get over the trauma of those three weeks, so when Mike and I found we were expecting another baby, we realised that we could not risk the same things happening again, especially as I would have to be on top form to cope with a baby and our extremely boisterous 2-year-old.

We realised we could not risk the same again

> My request for a home birth made all
> the medical professionals very twitchy.

The reactions of the medical profession to my request for a home birth could take me through several paragraphs. Suffice to say, it made everyone very twitchy. Tactics used to dissuade me ranged from coercion to disbelief ("There is no such thing as a home birth in this country") and from the usual threats ("What if something should go wrong?") to the sudden discovery of a problem with my antibodies which meant the baby should be checked by a paediatrician at birth!... none of which, of course, were valid.

I pursued every avenue imaginable and pestered all sorts of people in my determination to ensure that this time my baby and I would not start off our relationship emotionally battered. Time was running out when I read an article in the newspaper about Michel Odent. It appeared that he had attended some home births, so I attempted to contact him via his publisher. A few days later I answered the phone to a gentle French accent—I couldn't believe my luck. Much to our amazement, Michel was willing to attend our baby's birth if possible (he refused to use the word 'deliver'). From then on we just hoped that baby would have the good sense to be born out of rush hour times as we knew that, with Michel, we would be able to truly get to know our new baby during that very sensitive period immediately after the birth and she would be treated with gentleness and respect.

I wake up on 9 October feeling that this would be a good day to have a baby—the sun is shining and I feel well and reasonably energetic for a change. Baby due today, though, so I'm sure nothing will happen. Cathy and daughter Emily (aged 2) are coming to have lunch and spend the afternoon with us.

Around mid morning I feel very mild period-type pains but I had them Friday night so I take no notice. About 1.30pm I have to stop for a moment through the quickening—I couldn't really describe it as a pain—but manage to prepare a simple lunch quite easily. We sit down to lunch about 2.00pm and I finally tell Cathy that I am having 'pains' but think it is probably a false alarm. About an hour later Mike comes in from painting the gates outside to have lunch and I tell him about the 'pains'. He says he'll finish the gates but I tell him I'd rather he didn't risk welcoming our baby into the world covered in black gloss. It then registers that something might really be happening so he looks a bit panicky and rushes about in confusion.

4.00pm: I still can't be convinced I'm definitely in labour as I'm not really in pain and I don't want to call Michel unless I'm sure, so we start writing down times. Contractions seem to be about three minutes apart. Mike gets electric fires and polythene sheets (the only special equipment needed) and looks agitated. I keep laughing because I can't believe this is the real thing. Everything is so normal and Sean is rushing about terrorising Emily, as usual.

4.40pm: Mike decides it's time to call Michel—he's getting worried about being 'in charge', I think. Luck is with us and he is at home and says he will be right over. Cathy sits reading a book with Sean and Emily and I join in, but have to stop suddenly to lean on the back of the chair. Emily asks, "What's Auntie Pauline doing?" "Having a baby, darling". We both can't stop laughing, which is a bit tricky during a contraction. My own sensitive little angel hasn't noticed a thing!

5.30pm: Cathy prepares food for the children as Mike is not capable in present state of agitation. I go upstairs to change but keep getting delayed by a contraction. It's cool and peaceful upstairs and contractions seem stronger.

5.40pm: Mike is looking out of the window and announces Michel's arrival with great relief. I greet him with a smile then wish I hadn't as he tells me I don't look like a woman in labour. We show him our list of times of contractions but he isn't interested. (Michel told us that he can tell if labour is normal and how it is progressing simply by listening to the noises an uninhibited woman makes and I remember clearly how I could not stop myself from making different noises as labour got stronger.)

5.50pm: I go upstairs with Michel and he checks baby's heart and my blood pressure as I tell him it has been raised... in fact to the same level as when I was admitted with Sean. It's now the lowest it's been for two weeks.

6.00pm: Children having tea with Cathy. Michel joins them to chat to Cathy and asks about their bedtime. (He had previously told us that it is best not to have anyone else around for the birth as the number of people present is directly proportional to the length of labour, and the longer the labour the more likely complications occur.) Mike orders pizzas for himself and Michel due to vivid recollection of no food or drink for 12 hours before Sean's birth, and we feel it will be a long night.

6.45pm: Cathy and Emily leave. Mike takes Sean up to bed—skips the bath today! Pizzas arrive.

7.00pm: Sean asleep in record time. Contractions getting stronger now. I try out the newly acquired bean bag but it radiates heat back at me so I kneel in front of the sofa with my head on my arms, leaning on the seat, swaying my hips through contractions. I had intended to wear my 'Singapore happy coat' for the birth but don't feel like moving now! It is incredible how the contractions have taken off now it is quiet and there are no distractions. Mike has organised our birthing music—Irish harp and music from a band called 'Clannad', which is very soothing.

7.15pm: Contractions stronger so I start moaning through them. Mike and Michel chomping away on pizzas at the other end of the room. Mike comes over to see how I am and reminds me to 'breathe', which I had forgotten! He gets me a pillow to lean on which is lovely and cool. I ask him to hurry and finish his pizza as I'm in pain!

> I ask him to hurry and finish his pizza as I'm in pain!

7.25pm: Making a lot of noise now as contractions really hurt, and I'm worried about coping for hours like this. I hear Mike make a move to get up but Michel whispers that I am best left 'in my own world'. Any outside interference will delay things.

7.30pm: Mike now joins me. He is very calm and reassuring and I hold him through contractions.

7.45pm: I feel I want to go to the toilet. I remember this feeling before Sean was born but don't allow myself to possibly imagine baby is coming as I couldn't bear the disappointment if it's a false alarm. Mike helps me upstairs between contractions. I sit on the toilet and feel very constipated and confused. Waters break. Maybe baby is coming... I put my hand down thinking I might feel the head and find blood on my hand. Michel comes upstairs and tells Mike to get the electric fires on at the bathroom door—we have a very small bathroom!—so we know this must be IT. Mike helps me off the toilet and they pull my clothes off and Michel tells him to hold me from behind in the supported squat. I feel my uterus push and a burning sensation and give a little cry as (at 7.55pm) baby's head is born. Then my uterus pushes again. Mike and I are still standing in suspended animation as Michel tells us to look down at our baby daughter lying in his hands! We can't believe she has arrived so quickly and easily. Michel hands her to me and I cradle our beautiful daughter in my arms, her lovely virgin skin touching mine. The wonder and joy of that moment, to be holding my newborn babe so close and feeling her perfect little body next to mine, I can never describe. I kept saying to Mike, "We have a little girl!" and his face was alight with happiness.

I sat in the bathroom amidst the goo and mess for about 30 minutes while Michel and Mike sorted things out. I was blissfully unaware of what was going on, having eyes only for my baby. I remember Michel tying the cord after about 10 minutes and Mike cut it and found it quite tough! Then Mike took Rose Eleanor while I went to lie on the bed.

About 9.00pm Michel felt my stomach and said the placenta had separated. He massaged my stomach and the placenta came away with a contraction. Mike was trying to clear up the bathroom and was pleased the birth hadn't been on a carpet! Michel left about 10.00pm, and we sat in bed marvelling at our new baby daughter. She was very alert and never cried, although she gave the occasional whimper. We had the lights very low for her all the time. She didn't want to suck immediately after the birth but kept nuzzling my breast and looking around. Mike opened a bottle of champagne but I didn't like to drink more than a glass so I contented myself with two packets of Mintolas! We sat and caressed our little miracle and talked over and over about her birth, we were both so excited. About 2.00am I thought we should get some sleep and maybe Rose Eleanor was tired, so we all snuggled up in our bed. It was incredible that Sean had slept through all this but at 5.00am he woke and came into our bed. His little face was a picture when he heard Rosie stirring and he laughed and said, "Baby sister!"—he was so happy to see her.

Pauline Farrance

The father's tale...

I began to realise that the medical profession was perhaps, after all, just as horrified as I at having the responsibility for the birth

Whenever there was a choice I have always opted for nature's way in areas such as food, environment and general health. However, this had never extended to having a baby and I preferred to abdicate the responsibility to the medical profession, who appeared more than willing to take over.

I attended the NCT classes and that's when doubts began to creep in, especially as I learnt of all the medical hardware, paraphernalia and drugs that were deemed essential nowadays for giving birth. I began to realise that the medical profession was perhaps, after all, just as horrified as I at having the responsibility for the birth.

However, we went ahead with the hospital birth of our firstborn as it was decided by a hospital screening process that Pauline's blood pressure was outside the norm, for which she was immediately admitted. Sean was eventually extracted in a very workmanlike manner, some two and a half weeks of protestations, seven pessaries, two gas tanks, two doses of chemicals, 10 yards of graph paper, one cup of tea and 15 hours of narcotic trance later. It would be an understatement to say it was a very traumatic time for all of us and I was disappointed at not experiencing the joy one has heard about as the father in attendance at the birth of his first child. It was more a sense of overwhelming relief that the whole episode was over with and all three parties (physically) healthy and alive.

16 months later we found we were expecting our second baby and this time we were determined from the outset that this baby would be born at home so that we could have more control and responsibility. Our GP reluctantly agreed to cover the birth but opposition grew from all quarters of the medical profession and eventually no doctor would agree to cover the birth at home. This again I would attribute to their horror at having the responsibility for the birth. However, in desperation and clutching at any possible straw, Pauline managed to meet Michel Odent, who agreed to be present at the birth, if he was available.

The day of the birth thankfully arrived on a Sunday. Although we had read every possible piece of literature on the subject, I was filled with dread and my heart began to palpitate. I thought I might possibly have to deliver the baby myself if Michel was held up in the traffic... I began to race around looking for textbooks, plastic sheets and the bucket. (The requirement for the bucket had somehow lodged in my mind from the NCT course.)

I was filled with dread and my heart began to palpitate

I was greatly relieved when a French-registered Renault pulled up outside and the calming presence of Michel entered the house. I had by this time got my act together and put on some soothing music. Later, we turned the lights down very low and Michel told me to let Pauline get into her own world, and we chatted casually as we ate the enormous home delivery pizzas while Pauline got on with the business of having a baby, leaning on the sofa with her head in a pillow. For some reason I was convinced it would be a long night and I was building up my reserves of energy in anticipation! Minutes after finishing the pizzas we were all in our tiny bathroom with me holding Pauline in the supported squat and Michel holding a beautiful baby girl in his hands. She gave what seemed to be an obligatory whimper to let us know she was OK and settled blissfully into her mother's arms and there they stayed for about half an hour. I was totally dumbstruck by the ease and beauty of the birth and just gazed in disbelief. After coming back down to Earth, I began clearing up operations and gave thanks for lino tiles instead of carpet in the bathroom, but wished I had not eaten the pizza! Michel's presence was quite unobtrusive throughout his visit, but it was his confidence and experience in allowing nature to take its course without any unnecessary interference which made the birth such a trouble-free and memorable event, and gave us so much joy and confidence during the weeks that followed.

Michael White

And afterwards...

We have obviously talked endlessly about the birth and were so happy and grateful that everything had gone so well, but we felt so sad for the vast majority of mothers (and fathers) who are denied the joy of such a precious and unique experience in our so-called civilised society today. It is widely accepted that about 90% of women are able to give birth normally, without complications, so why don't we keep the costly expertise and machinery for those who really need it? Of course, many men and women are happier in the hospital environment, and we would never try and dissuade them from this as the labour will always be prolonged by fear and anxiety. But the present day fear of complications during childbirth is largely unfounded and we should look at the event in perspective as a part of family life.

We were so excited by Rosie's birth that we were on a high for at least a week and had loads of energy to carry us through the sleepless nights, etc. Added benefits of the birth at home include much less disruption and confusion for older brothers and sisters, and it meant so much to my parents to be able to hold their second grandchild so soon after she was born—a privilege not allowed after Sean's birth. In addition, the baby will not succumb to any of the infections which abound in hospital.

To put it all in a nutshell, three days after Rosie's birth we were feeling a little down because we had enjoyed the birth so much. We wanted the clock to turn back to Sunday so that we could do it all again!

Pauline Farrance and Michael White

We wanted to turn the clock back so we could do it all again!

Why is there a tendency to be interventionist?
Of course, there is only a problem when interventions are unnecessary. In order to consider why we now have a climate of high intervention in most hospitals, here's a brief historical overview of what's been happening over the last few decades in the developed world. This historical perspective should help us to see modern-day intervention in perspective.

From the birth of time...
Hundreds (and thousands) of years ago interventions were initiated when women were in difficulty and it seemed likely that the mother was about to die in labour, or that the fetus was already dead, or having difficulty getting itself born. Caesareans were performed from very early times (although they usually followed the death of the mother). Extraction of a fetus in distress by other means initially meant its own death, but the invention of forceps in 1600 (which remained a family secret until 1734) meant that intervention by doctors soon became a valued, life-saving procedure in an important minority of cases.

Other interventions were very common and culture-specific (as is confirmed by anthropological research (carried out by Sheila Kitzinger, Jacqueline Vincent Priya and others). These interventions came about as a result of certain beliefs, which were often not based on any facts. The beliefs themselves affected the ways in which birth was facilitated or unintentionally hindered. For example, women may have been isolated or, alternatively, surrounded by people, perhaps given a shock or kept away from all stress and there was often the belief that the pre-milk 'colostrum' was bad for the baby. (Of course, research has now shown us how wonderfully beneficial it is.)

Finally, interventions became necessary as a result of the use of pain relief, which usually created problems which then needed to be dealt with.

1800-1900
One midwife's diary suggests that doctors were already using laudanum for pain relief or anaesthesia early in the 19th century, although opium and other forms of pain relief may have been used centuries before. Ether (diethyl ether, to be precise) seems to have been first used in January 1847 in Edinburgh and in April or May of the same year in North America. As we've already noted, Queen Victoria set a new trend in 1853 when she decided to use chloroform for the birth of her eighth child.

Other kinds of intervention were also being advocated by doctors as soon as they started taking over from midwives as the usual birth attendants. This takeover took place naturally since it was the literate doctors who wrote the texts on childbirth, which were used in midwifery schools. Of course, since these 'writer' doctors had primarily witnessed difficult births (since that was the only time they were called in to help), their approach was interventionist.

Interventions of any kind also became more possible when 'lying-in hospitals' were established and when they became popular in places such as France, Ireland and Australia. This all led to intervention coming to be seen as 'normal'.

By the late 1800s, intervention had also become routine in some American hospitals. At one hospital in Philadelphia it was routine to administer quinine (as it induces uterine contractions), as well as drugs for constipation, sleeplessness and headaches; at the onset of labour women were given an enema and bath, the amniotic sac was ruptured and at birth forceps were applied; the third stage was helped along by the use of ergot (ostensibly so as to minimise blood loss) with the attendant pressing down on the woman's abdomen. Awareness of the need for cleanliness and sterility was emerging, thanks to Ignaz Semmelweis's thoughts about causes of puerperal fever in Vienna, Austria.

1900s and 1910s

By the early 1900s in both America and Britain, midwives were really losing their power, partly because they were becoming associated with uneducated, illiterate women. (First hand experience was seen as being inferior to the institutionalised study of obstetrics, which meant that educated, wealthier women tended to avoid midwives.) Up until the 1920s, maternal mortality was still a major problem since 1 in 250 women died in childbirth. According to *Obstetrics by Ten Teachers* (Hodder Arnold 2000), this was because the modern pharmacological treatments for postpartum haemorrhage and sepsis (which caused many deaths) were unavailable. Research was being conducted in Germany in the early 1910s into new forms of pain relief. The result—a mixture of morphine and scopolamine, which induced a condition known as 'twilight sleep', followed by the use of ether or chloroform—was so exciting to one group of American women that they actively promoted it as a form of liberation. The attitude of these women is not surprising, given the 'obstetric management' promoted by obstetricians just a few years before, which must have *caused* a great deal of pain, emotional trauma and disempowerment.

The 1920s and 1930s

In 1920, an American professor of obstetrics, Joseph DeLee—a popular speaker, textbook writer and the inventor or modifier of many obstetric tools—gave a seminal speech to fellow obstetricians, recommending that forceps and episiotomy be routine for every birth, that women should be sedated, that ether should be administered as soon as the fetus entered the birth canal and that ergot or a similar drug should be used to speed up delivery of the placenta. These practices, known as 'prophylactic obstetrics', soon became routine in most US hospitals. From 1928 onwards active steps were taken in the UK and the US to reduce risks through better education, although antenatal care itself was a fairly haphazard process until the 1940s, undertaken only by doctors. In 1937 the antibiotics sulphonamides were discovered and penicillin came soon after. These discoveries quickly reduced the rates of puerperal sepsis.

The 1940s

Before WWII more than 90% of women in the UK gave birth at home under the care of a midwife, and only occasionally with a GP in attendance as well. The increased experimentation with different forms of pain relief from the 1940s onwards meant that hospitalised childbirth became preferable from both a choice and a safety point of view—since more was likely to go wrong when drugs and other interventions were involved. At that time, morphine was widely used, often alongside other drugs. In the USA, it was usually used while women were in 'twilight sleep'. In France the morphine was part of a mixture called 'spasmalgine'. In the UK, ether and chloroform were still widely used. It was in this decade that the so-called 'natural childbirth movement' developed in the USA and with it the concept of the husband as 'labour coach'. It was also the time when blood transfusions became safe and when it was discovered that ergometrine could treat and prevent postpartum haemorrhage.

The 1950s

Induction and augmentation of labour now became more of a focus so intramuscular injections of artificial oxytocin (syntonicin and pitocin) became popular, used alongside different painkillers. Since the effects of intramuscular artificial oxytocin were uncontrollable (since nothing can be done to 'take the drug back' after an injection), drips soon became common. With a drip in place, if the effect of the artificial oxytocin already given was too strong and therefore dangerous (i.e. causing too intense and continuous uterine contractions) it was possible to slow down or stop the drip altogether. It was in fact during this decade that drips became safe because the original rubber tubes—which often caused intense allergic reactions—were replaced by plastic tubes. It was also the time when the vacuum extractor (ventouse) was invented in Sweden. This device appeared to present a good alternative to forceps, which had been in use since the 16th century because it seemed to offer less trauma to both mother and baby. Ultrasound was also first adapted for obstetric use in the late 1950s. By the late 1970s and 80s it had become available in most hospitals. Techniques and treatments which we now take for granted (relating to anaesthetics, antibiotics and blood transfusion) were also further developed.

The 1960s

In the 1960s drips of artificial oxytocin continued to be used widely as a means of inducing and augmenting labour. The main painkiller used was pethidine (a synthetic morphine, which is an analgesic and anti-spasmodic). Caesareans, which had until this time been unpopular, suddenly became more appealing to women, thanks to the new use of the 'bikini line' incision (instead of the vertical incision which had been used until then), which was originally proposed by Muro-Kerr in the 1920s. This technique, which was developed in the 1950s, now became widely used, not only because of its increased popularity with women but also because surgically trained obstetricians were now available.

The 1970s
The fast development of electronic fetal monitoring (first invented in 1957) radically changed the atmosphere of delivery rooms. Caesarean rates started to increase dramatically, partly because of the use of electronic fetal monitoring (EFM).[53] Drips of pitocin and pethidine were still used. The growing public confidence in the technology and pain relief options offered by hospitals resulted in a rapid increase in the number of births taking place in hospitals. In the UK between 1960 and 1979 the use of drug-based pain relief increased from 25% to 99%. (Thanks to awareness of risks associated with attempts at pain management, there has since been a drop in the number of women using these forms of intervention.) Perhaps people's preference for technical management of birth was also linked to the increasingly technical nature of our lifestyle generally and to the drift towards an urban lifestyle, which may have made people wrongly associate physiological birth with old-fashioned methods.

The 1980s and 1990s
In the 1980s the conventional technique of epidural anaesthesia became available in large departments of obstetrics. So as to facilitate the administration of epidurals, which many women saw as extremely appealing, large well-equipped maternity units were built in the 1990s. Size mattered because it was only economics of scale that made it possible to provide anaesthetists and paediatricians 24 hours a day. Protocols to support the large numbers of interventions now carried out had become necessary, perhaps because the enormous increase in interventions made risks increase too. Of course, insurance companies had (and continue to have) an influence on the number of protocols too, because premiums payable are sometimes based on the level of autonomy and discretion given to individual health care providers—cheaper premiums being payable when more protocols are in place. Incidentally, the injection of an oxytocic agent for the delivery of the placenta had also become routine and women wanting a physiological third stage were often seen as being unusual. Episiotomy was still routine in many hospitals.

What kinds of intervention take place now?
In the 21st century there seems to be the implicit assumption that intervention only takes place to save lives. This is far from true since the use of drug-based pain relief still constitutes one of the main forms of intervention in modern childbirth and, as we've seen, pain relief usually necessitates other forms of intervention. Here's a brief summary of practices which are still common in some parts of the world, looking at what takes place before any one pregnancy and birth, during it and afterwards. It's necessary to take this broad view because interventions taken at any stage can affect what occurs later on. I've taken an international perspective because we do, of course, live in a very multi-cultural society, with plenty of movement from country to country.

INTERVENTION BEFORE THE BIRTH TAKES PLACE

Many women experience intervention before pregnancy or during pregnancy. This may affect the health of their baby and how successful they can be in giving birth.

Before a woman becomes pregnant numerous old interventions might influence her ability to give birth and her baby's ability to get itself born easily, safely and smoothly. Episiotomies performed in previous labours which have not healed well, old forceps trauma and abortion injuries (especially those inflicted by unqualified surgeons) can all affect a woman's muscular control and comfort when subsequently giving birth. Circumcision is another practice which constitutes a pre-pregnancy intervention which can affect a woman's subsequent experiences. In the notes accompanying the novel *Possessing the Secret of Joy* (Walker 1993), it is reported that an estimated 90 to 100 million women and girls living today in African, Far Eastern and Middle Eastern countries have been genitally mutilated. The author also states that recent articles in the media have reported on the growing practice of 'female circumcision' in the United States and Europe among immigrants from countries where it is part of the culture. This means a significant number of women begin pregnancy with a compromised physical starting point.

During pregnancy all kinds of screening and diagnostic tests are offered, as well as routine antenatal checks, which I regard as interventions because they must in some way affect either the woman or the baby. They include blood tests, repeated use of ultrasound with a Sonicaid or Doppler machine, maternal serum screening (the alpha-fetoprotein test, the triple screen test or the quad-screen test), ultrasounds, chorionic villus sampling, nuchal translucency testing and amniocentesis.

Psychological interventions might also have an influence either before or during any one particular pregnancy... After all, almost all women are seeing an enormous number of fear-inducing images relating to labour and birth on TV or in magazines and newspapers before they even become pregnant. Perhaps the negative images prevail because they are considered by planners to constitute more exciting viewing than the positive, natural alternatives, which many people wrongly associate with alternative lifestyles or primitive cultures. The prevailing fear of childbirth and tendency to leave responsibility to 'the professionals' mean that many women feel disempowered and incapable of giving birth successfully. A negative mindset is created well before women even begin to actively explore real-life facts and figures, or read about other women's experiences with a view to forming their own opinions. In other words, modern myths about pregnancy and childbirth often replace the reality in people's minds and create a psychological environment of fear and foreboding. Antenatal appointments filled with fear-inducing 'routine checks' reinforce this negative mindset.

INTERVENTIONS DURING LABOUR AND BIRTH

In Britain in 2008, induction rates ranged from 9.7% to 34.6%, depending on the hospital and area.[54] Of 3,000 women in the UK who responded to a *Mother and Baby* magazine survey in 2002, 94% used some form of pain relief involving drugs. The caesarean rate varies enormously from 6 or 10% (amongst independent midwives) or 11.1% (in one hospital) to 34.7% in another hospital (in 2008). Instrumental delivery rates (i.e. forceps or ventouse) ranged from 2.3% to 18.8%. From my own experience I know that the use of syntometrine in the third stage of labour to speed up delivery of the placenta is usually routine.

In the US induction rates are high and seem to be rising. 22.1% of women had their labours induced in 2004. While in labour, as many as 60-70% of women have some sort of anaesthesia (according to research conducted in 2005)[55] and epidural usage is high—it's estimated that epidurals are used in around 50% of births. Around 31.8% of births were caesareans in 2004. In 2002, when the 'Listening to Mothers' survey[56] was conducted, the overall intervention rate was more than 99%.[57] In Latin America, there is also a tendency for high intervention. The caesarean rate is the most impressive statistic... In some private hospitals in large cities, it can reach 90%! In poor areas it is much, much lower.

There is also a great deal of intervention in Australia. In 2001 the Australian Institute of Health and Welfare reported that 25% of women had their labour induced and another 20% had it augmented. In Israel according to Wendy Blumfield (author of *Life After Birth,* Element Books 1992), an estimated 30% of first-time mothers and 40% of multiparas [women who've had children before] opt to give birth without pain relief. (Of course, this means that 60-70% of women do use pain relief.) Induction is apparently a common intervention. Episiotomies were routine for first births up to 10 years ago. Now they are done according to need. Forceps are little used, but together with ventouse, are used in about 4% of births. This figure is increasing along with increasing use of epidurals, which give women less control over the pushing stage of labour. Caesareans are performed in about 16% of births and are on the rise.

In most other countries—in particular in the developing world—health professionals are highly interventionist and drug-based pain relief is widely used. I was surprised to discover this to be true in both Sri Lanka and Oman when I was pregnant with my first and third babies. It seemed odd that so much intervention and so many drugs should be used in cultures which in many ways still seemed in tune with their cultural traditions. The Western model from a few decades ago (which was *not* evidence-based) is being copied, despite growing evidence that it is causing huge problems. In China intervention has become so common that— according to one eminent source— 70% of all babies are now born by caesarean section and the figure is 90% in some urban hospitals. In these places, given the high rates of intervention, it really does seem that women are in danger of losing the art of giving birth.

Sometimes intervention is necessary for the safety of either mothers or babies. At other times, one intervention—to induce labour or use so-called 'pain relief', for example—leads to all kinds of other interventions, which would not otherwise have been necessary. Here, we see some life-saving intervention, carried out for the sake of a baby who was born prematurely, who would not have survived without it. See Birthframe 50 for the full story.

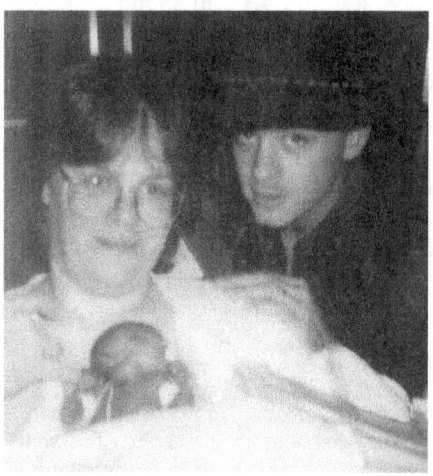

"No alarms. Yippee!" The new mum's first time holding her baby at 4 days old. In this case a loving, low-tech intervention, kangaroo care, was combined with high tech ones so that the baby thrived.

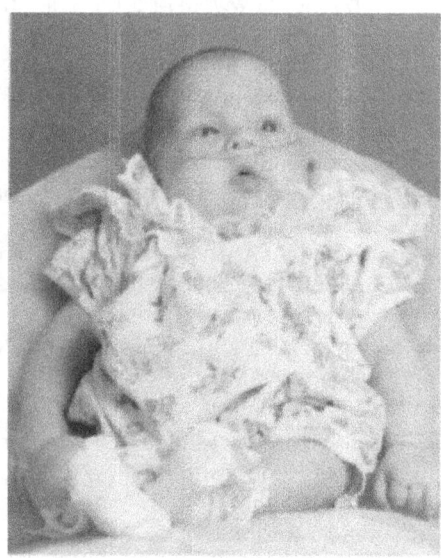

At 4 months old this little girl still needed intervention to help with her breathing.

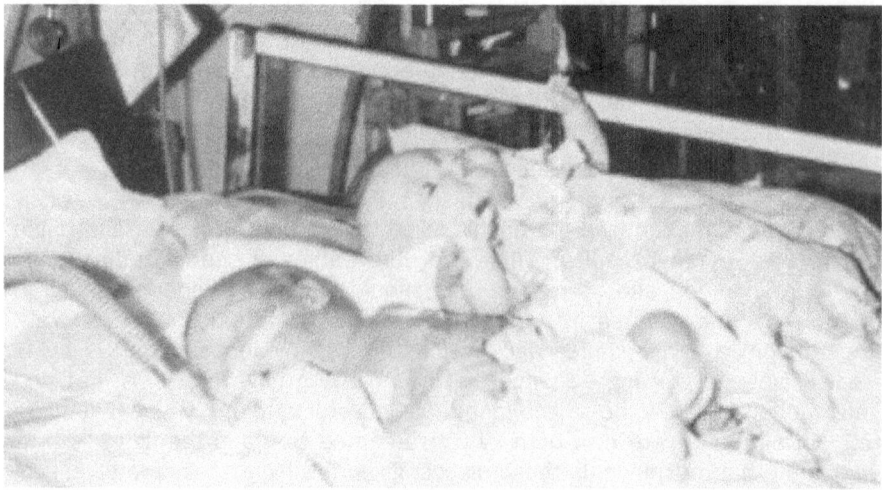

At 8 weeks old, Kaia, the baby, weighed just 2½lb. Here she's lying next to a small doll.

I think people generally believe that intervention is all life-saving like this... One former WHO director, Marsden Wagner, carried out an overview of how practice in US hospitals (which is not unlike that in the UK in some cases) differs from research recommendations. The table below is an adaptation of his findings, included in his book *Born in the USA* (Uni of California Press 2006).

The theory...	In practice in the USA today	The research says:
Women should have one caregiver for the whole of their labour and birth (rather than a series of caregivers on different shifts, with different duties)	Less than 10% of the time they do	Women should always have continuity of care
Midwives should be the routine caregivers, not obstetricians, because birth is a normal physiological process, which is usually healthy	They are in only 5% of cases	This should happen in 80% of cases, i.e. usually
Women should not have food or drink in labour	86% don't	It's fine to do so
EFM should be carried out routinely on all women	93% have it	It doesn't help
A drip should be set up routinely for all women	86% have it	They shouldn't
Women should stay in bed for their labour	69% do	None should
Women should lie back in bed and give birth with their legs in stirrups (in the lithotomy position)	Almost all women do	None should. They should be upright
An episiotomy should be carried out routinely so as to widen the outlet for the baby being born	35% of the time it is	Less than 20% of women need one
Women should have labour induced with drugs	44% do	Only 10% should
Labour should be accelerated with drugs too	53% of labours are	Only 10% of labours need to be
Women need ventouse or forceps to get babies out of their bodies	13% appear to need these	Less than 10% should, in fact
Caesareans should be carried out because nobody wants a vaginal birth any more, do they?	27% of births are sections	Only 10-15% of births should be
The new mother should hold her baby during the routine examination of her newborn	She almost never does	Well, she should. It's more humane.

The data about real-life practices was sourced from that national survey of obstetric practices in the USA which took place in 2002, called 'Listening to Mothers'. (The survey, published by the Maternity Center Association, is available at www.maternitywise.org.) The data from research come from the Cochrane Library (www.cochrane.org)—an excellent place to go for further info.

So as to be very clear, here are details of practices which I personally consider to be interventions. Some were mentioned on the table on the previous page...

- **Induction or acceleration of labour by any means** Both 'natural' and artificial means are sometimes used to induce or speed up labour. Friends, relatives and even caregivers might suggest ingesting various substances (e.g. curries or cod liver oil), or they might encourage excessive exercise or laughter. Professionals try to intervene and trigger a woman's labour by administering prostaglandins (by pessary) or syntocinon (intravenously); alternatively, they might break a woman's waters (i.e. perform an amniotomy) or 'sweep her membranes'—with or without her consent. When a labouring woman has a drip inserted in her arm, it is possible that syntocinon may be added to the original glucose mixture to accelerate contractions; again, this might be done without the woman's consent.[58]

- **Prepping** Hospitals and birthing centres always used to 'prepare' women for labour in some way, but now—hopefully—all or most of these routines have disappeared from most institutions. So-called preparation can include asking the woman to put on a hospital gown, shaving off her pubic hair, administering an enema and setting up a drip ('just in case' it's needed later), or slipping in a heparin lock for the same reason. (A heparin lock is basically a small tube connected to a catheter, which is inserted into a vein in the arm so that a drip can later be quickly inserted.) All these practices constitute interventions because they can disturb the woman. Firstly, they might inhibit her physical movement. Secondly, they might make her fearful and make her feel like a patient who is sick and in need of treatment.

- **Electronic fetal monitoring (EFM)** This is often part of the routine admission procedures so may be considered a type of 'prepping'. Whether it takes place for 20 minutes when the woman first arrives at hospital or at any other stage of labour or birth, EFM is certainly an intervention which immobilises the labouring woman either completely or partially. EFM usually forces her to lie down (rather than lean forward, for example) and it's also likely to create a feeling of anxiety, which will inhibit production of oxytocin.[59]

- **Dietary controls** Women are often told not to eat or drink during labour in case a general anaesthetic is required later. Stopping a woman from following her natural impulses interferes with her normal ability to regulate her intake of food and drink. Appropriate levels of hydration and the absence of ketones (which start being produced when a woman has not eaten for a while) are both important if labour is to progress well. In any case, research has not shown fasting to be helpful even when a general anaesthetic is used.

- **Directed activity** Women are often told to take a bath because it will 'help them relax'. (In fact, it's more likely to slow down contractions, which is unhelpful.) Women may also be encouraged to walk up and down hospital corridors or take a walk in the hospital grounds. Any time a woman is told to do something in this way, an intervention is taking place because the suggestion is likely to distract the woman from tuning into her instinctual knowledge of how to labour and give birth. The only non-intrusive kind of 'direction' anyone could give a woman would be, "Do whatever you feel like doing." This would simply remind the woman that she can be confident in her own ability to choose appropriate activities and physical positions.

> The nursing staff wanted me to stay on the trolley, to keep an eye on the monitors, but I put the equipment on a little table and got my mother to push them along while I walked up and down 'to the toilet'.

- **Physical constraint** Even when no EFM is used, women are often told to lie down or stop walking around, or their movements are constricted indirectly through the use of some other medical procedure. Even stopping a woman from making noises is a form of intervention because it is a way of stopping a woman from releasing tension in a way which might help the normal, healthy processes to progress. Obviously, insisting that a woman give birth with her legs in lithotomy stirrups is also a form of physical constraint and an intervention, because it makes it impossible for a woman to use her natural ability to find a physical position which is helpful for both herself and her baby. Left to her own devices, a woman is likely to want to work with gravity, not against it, so will usually spontaneously choose a standing, kneeling or squatting position. Many women who have given birth with their feet in stirrups have complained that it was difficult 'pushing uphill'.

- **Any communication verbal or nonverbal** People often fail to see the role of comments or eye contact in disturbing a woman who is in labour or actually giving birth. Because any comment or communication (including a glance or eye contact) can disturb the woman or distract her, it constitutes an intervention. Giving a woman instructions on how to push her baby out into the world is an obvious form of communicative intervention—but by no means the only one. Merely mentioning within earshot of a labouring woman that something negative or frightening might be necessary is a form of intervention, again because it is a way of disturbing the woman's state of mind as she moves through labour and birth. Negative or frightening possibilities which are often mentioned include breaking a woman's waters, using drugs for pain relief and the so-called 'probable' need for an episiotomy, forceps or a caesarean.

- **The use of analgesia or anaesthesia** The use of any drugs to alleviate pain constitutes an intervention.

- **Techniques for relieving pain** The use of any technique might disturb the normal course of a labour and birth so must be considered an intervention. This includes breathing exercises, TENS machines, acupuncture, shiatsu, aromatherapy and any other complementary therapy.

- **The use of a fetal scalp electrode** This is often done in order to make the EFM more reliable—which is considered necessary because EFM has been widely reported in research studies to be ineffective.
- **Episiotomy** Obviously, cutting a woman's sexual parts while she is giving birth is an intervention.
- **The use of forceps or ventouse** Large metal 'salad tongs' are used to pull out a baby who appears to have got stuck. In the case of ventouse, a suction pad is attached to the baby's head and he or she is sucked out by a vacuum pump.

How much intervention really is necessary from a health and safety point of view? How much of it is used because protocols are in place, because it is expected, because it impresses the client or because it's part of a cascade of intervention? How many lives are saved or endangered by all this intervention?

Of course, this is the $64 million dollar question. Nobody knows the answer. We have drifted so far away from the normal, undisturbed physiological processes of pregnancy, labour and birth that it's impossible to have a clear answer. We have never really allowed the healthy processes to take place on a large scale within the safety net of our modern expertise and technology. Unfortunately, for psychological reasons, as well as humanitarian ones, it would be impossible to conduct a randomised control trial.

There are indeed a small number of women who need help from caregivers when they conceive, gestate a baby or give birth. These are the women who—years ago—would have remained childless, who would have had dangerous pregnancies, who would have died in childbirth. There are also babies who genuinely need rescuing, who would otherwise be born dead or brain damaged.

Let's take one case where intervention is sometimes helpful. There are actually times when an episiotomy really is a life-saving procedure (for babies). In the case of breech births, it can speed the delivery of the baby's head, which might mean that breathing can start more quickly. This means that lack of oxygen could not cause brain damage.

> First they decided to wait for the contractions to start up again and see if I could push Ben out. When they did start I was told to push, so I pushed... and out came Ben's feet! Pushed again and out popped his legs! Pushed again and out popped his shoulders! But his head was stuck and we could hear him crying while his head was still inside. (Probably why Ben cries really loud now!) So then I had to have an episiotomy. Ben was born within four minutes. He weighed in at 7lb 8oz..

An episiotomy is also performed in another situation...

> The next bit was the worst; something that I had really wanted to avoid was an episiotomy, I am so glad that I couldn't feel it (it sounded bad enough). It was necessary so that forceps could be placed around his head.

Whether or not intervention of this kind was necessary in this second case is debatable... because some professionals (including Michel) would argue that forceps themselves should never be used. Ventouse or a caesarean would be better alternatives for both mother and baby and of course, they would not necessitate what has been called 'the unkindest cut'.

There are other grey areas, of course, and professionals hotly debate what should be considered an 'acceptable' episiotomy rate in any one hospital. According to the Royal College of Obstetricians and Gynaecologists, in the year 2000 the episiotomy rate was 8% in Holland, 14% in England, 50% in the USA, but still an incredible 99% in Eastern Europe. (Of course, the wild inconsistency of these statistics raises important questions.) While Michel was working at Pithiviers in the 1970s, he and his staff felt that episiotomies were only needed in 7% of births which took place there—despite the fact that the rate in most other modern French hospitals was then 95%. In *Birth Reborn* (Souvenir Press 1994) he explains that episiotomies were only used when the baby's physical state was a cause for concern, e.g. when it was lying breech. Performing an episiotomy then helped the baby avoid the stress of the last few contractions and enabled it to be born more quickly. I wonder what reasons other caregivers would give for their rates for induction, drug use and caesareans? (The fact that some consultants only do inductions on Fridays prompts me to think too...)

The kind of discrepancy between hospitals that we see in the case of episiotomy and in others mentioned earlier (between countries) makes it clear that while interventions are sometimes life-saving, they must also often be over-used because of fear, misjudgement or inappropriate protocols.

Birthframe 42

Sometimes, as we've seen in earlier birthframes, medical intervention really is necessary. In the next account we see how it made it possible for a couple to have another child against the odds. This is a clear case of medical support being life-saving for both mother and child.

Having had one fairly straightforward birth, it came as a shock when I realised things can go wrong in pregnancy. My second pregnancy was ectopic so at nine weeks I had emergency surgery. Luckily, I did not lose the fallopian tubes but they did end up damaged. So, in order to have any future children the only option was to go through a lengthy, costly IVF programme. We were extremely lucky to be successful on the first attempt, where I became pregnant with twins. However, fairly early on I developed hyper-stimulation (painful swelling) and one of the twins died by the 10-week scan. (A lot of early scans are performed with IVF to detect ectopic pregnancies and check that everything is developing normally.)

The only option was to go through an IVF program

As I had lost one of the babies I was told to expect some minor bleeding. They also mentioned that bleeding can be a response to all the vaginal scans... So when I had some small bleeds before the 13-week scan I was not surprised, but a little worried. At the 13-week scan I was told I had placenta praevia, which was fairly low down, but was told that for most women by the mid-term scan and certainly by 28 weeks, the placenta moves sideways and away from the cervix, along with the growth of the baby. I continued to get small bleeds and was up and down to the hospital like a yoyo. At the mid-term scan (20 weeks) I was told that I had major placenta praevia, being classed as Grade 4+ (1 being minor and 4+ being serious). This meant that the placenta would not be able to move away from the cervix as it was completely covering the os, and in some places was adhered to the cervix. I was told I would not be able to give birth normally and would have to have a caesarean.

At 25 weeks I started to have a fairly heavy bleed and was admitted for the duration of my pregnancy. Luckily, I stopped bleeding but had to keep a cannula in [a device for a drip] just in case I started to haemorrhage. I was allowed home occasionally as long as someone was with me 24 hours a day and I was within 10 minutes of the hospital. This is because I would have to be on the operating table within 20 minutes if I started to haemorrhage, as the worst-case scenario is death of both mother and child. At my 28-week scan the earlier diagnosis was confirmed—there was no way I was getting away with a normal birth.

I started to have contractions at 32 weeks, which caused problems as I was not allowed to go into labour. (This is because the cervix dilates in labour and this would mean the placenta would rip, causing a major haemorrhage.) After being monitored on the labour ward to see the strength and frequency of contractions I had an emergency caesarean under general anaesthetic.

[It was necessary to have a general anaesthetic in this case for the sake of speed. An epidural takes much longer to set up and sometimes doesn't become effective the first time it is administered—which then means needing to try again.]

I was extremely poorly after the caesarean because I did end up having a haemorrhage, as well as some sort of reaction to the anaesthetic. My daughter spent a short time on the special baby ward before being whisked into the Neonatal Unit as she was having breathing difficulties. Mother and baby are now both fine—and the 'baby' is now 3 years old!

In general, I would definitely be on the pro 'normal birth' side of things, wherever possible. My pregnancy was clinical and from the outset not only was it a traumatic experience, I was unable to hold my baby for nearly two weeks after she was born. I was not aware I had had a baby until four hours after the birth.

Caesareans as a birth option are ridiculous

Caesareans as a birth option are ridiculous. Mothers 'opting' to have an elective caesarean when it is not a necessity are totally nuts! I did not recover properly until four months after the birth. It is major abdominal surgery.

Birthframe 43

Here's another example... In this case, the problem was ongoing nausea and vomiting in pregnancy which became totally debilitating. What could be done?

You've probably heard of the drug 'thalidomide', which eventually became known as a teratogen (i.e. harmful to the growing baby). It was originally prescribed to pregnant women in the late 1950s to treat morning sickness, but it eventually became clear that it caused gross deformities when taken within a certain period during the first trimester of pregnancy. As a result, health care professionals are now usually more careful about any interventions or prescriptions during the first trimester because the after-effects in pregnancy or during birth are still unknown in most cases, or unconfirmed. However, experimental intervention does sometimes seem necessary or desirable in certain cases, such as the one described here...

I was having difficulty keeping even sips of water down

It was December 2001 and I was delighted to find out that I was expecting our second child, if a little apprehensive following a miscarriage earlier in the year. With our first child I had started feeling sick at about Week 8. This sickness had then rapidly intensified until I was vomiting up to six times a day.

A sympathetic doctor diagnosed hyperemesis and allowed me time off from my full-time teaching job. After three months of this sickness level and some anti-emetic drugs, I gradually felt better and the pregnancy continued uneventfully until the birth of our healthy first son in the May of 1999. The memories of this were still fresh two and a half years later when we decided to try for our second child. I had not really researched the condition of hyperemesis and naively believed the many comments I had heard about every pregnancy being different and the unlikely event of this level of sickness returning.

In the fifth week of this pregnancy I was understandably anxious when I started to bleed again. After two scans, however, the hospital were able to reassure me as far as they could and told me to come back in Week 8 for a further scan to see if they could detect a heartbeat. Then, on the Saturday commencing my sixth week of pregnancy I woke up feeling weak, battered and extremely sick. The vomiting started on the Sunday, and by the Monday—which was Christmas Eve—I could hardly get off the sofa and was wondering how I was going to manage to get through the celebrations of Christmas Day. At first I felt cross with myself and kept repeating that it was only morning sickness, even if it did last all day. But by the following week I was having difficulty keeping even sips of water down and New Year's Eve was spent lying dehydrated on the sofa until my partner arrived home smelling of wine, which immediately sent me rushing for the toilet again. I could not tolerate the smell of anything and started to sleep on my own. Even the smell of the sheets on my bed would make me retch uncontrollably.

Two days later and despite having a hospital appointment for a scan the following day I felt I could not wait and went to see the doctor. By this stage my partner had to practically carry me in and out of the car. The doctor asked me to give her a urine sample but, as I explained, I couldn't because I had not really had anything properly to drink for days. She took some blood and explained that although it was unlikely, if the results were abnormal, she would contact me the following day. She did contact me the following day and left a message on the answering machine. I never heard it as I had already been admitted to hospital.

My appointment on the next day appeared to go well. I had been having some bleeding and I was reassured to see a healthy heartbeat. After the scan, my partner and I were unclear about whether we should wait again to see a doctor or go straight home. I wanted to go home because of the terrible way that I was feeling, but we waited anyway to have the results of the scan confirmed by a doctor.

I was sick again while we were waiting and heard a nurse say, "What's the matter with her?"

"Oh, just morning sickness", came the reply.

The doctor confirmed the pleasing results of the scan but said that it was obvious that I was suffering. She explained that high levels of ketones had been found in my urine, that I would need to come into the hospital to have some anti-emetic drugs and a drip, and that I would feel a lot better after about 24 hours. I had not known about the existence of ketones, or that it was possible to be hospitalised for hyperemesis. I also felt frightened as, apart from the birth of my son, I had been lucky enough not to be hospitalised before. Little did I know then this was to be the first of seven hospitalisations and the beginning of six really difficult months for our small family.

The attitudes of the nurses in hospital varied. Some were sympathetic, others appeared to think that I was wasting a valuable bed—despite repeated vomiting and fainting every morning when I was forced to get up to allow the bed to be changed. (I later found out that low blood pressure is one of the symptoms of this condition.) There were other difficult aspects to being in hospital with this condition—for example, sometimes I was placed in wards with women suffering from miscarriages, and I was forced to smell the food at mealtimes.

There were other side effects of the illness that I did not know, or that nobody explained to me. As I previously mentioned, my blood pressure was very low and I passed out daily, which was both unpleasant and frightening. After a few months of the sickness, apart from the weight loss, my skin started to look yellow, I was constantly cold and shivering, my hair started to fall out and I started to vomit small amounts of bile and blood. The latter, I was reassured, was normal and simply caused by small tears in the stomach. It was intensely painful and started to create a fear of being sick any more. I was constantly cajoled in hospital to drink more if I wanted to get better, when every sip made my sore stomach retch. I found the cajoling patronising and felt that it showed a lack of understanding, with the implication that I was not helping myself.

I was also given a variety of anti-emetic drugs which did not work for me, and this was echoed by other women that I talked to with this condition. The pattern followed that after being on a drip for two or three days, the ketones would be gone, I would be sent home feeling only marginally better (because of not being dehydrated any more) and within 24 hours I would be back in the same state again. After two or three hospital visits, I was given some ketone sticks with which I could measure the levels of ketones myself at home. For the first four months of the pregnancy I had constant ketones and would only go back to the hospital when I really felt that I could not stand it at home any longer.

Being in hospital did provide the invaluable opportunity to chat with other women suffering from this condition, and we talked about how even the smell of our children and partners would make us retch. I also discovered some Internet sites where other women who had similarly suffered had written their stories and I found this really supportive in the times when I thought I must be going mad.

My son, who was $2\frac{1}{2}$ at the time, appeared to take it all in his stride—that his mummy had simply stopped looking after him and spent the whole time sleeping and being sick. My partner and I had a bedroom in the attic and when he left for work I would be too weak to get out of bed and climb down the ladder, so I simply stayed in bed the whole day, vomiting and retching into a bucket. He would arrive home and I would attempt to get up, but even this effort would send me into more retching and vomiting fits. Without his unceasing sympathetic support I would not have got through this pregnancy.

We moved house when I was 12 weeks' pregnant as the sale had already gone so far along. Three days later, I was back in hospital again, dehydrated. My partner had a wonderful boss who was supportive whenever he took time off to take me to hospital or to take care of our small son on the days when the nursery had no space. Before the pregnancy, I had been studying and working part-time as a supply teacher. I suspended the study at 20 weeks and, of course, received no pay for the supply teaching as I was only casually employed. That was the financial effect of the hyperemesis.

At about four months, in desperation I started to research the condition and I found one particular study linking the use of antibiotics to curing hyperemesis, so I went to persuade my doctor to give this a try. This was my own doctor, who I had not seen since the start of the pregnancy. She was shocked at my condition and despite having no ketones in my urine, she sent me in an ambulance straight to the hospital. There, after I broke down in tears, they readmitted me and I persuaded a sympathetic doctor to try out the antibiotic theory. He did, but it didn't work and the pain of taking the antibiotics was difficult with such a sore stomach. He suggested, however, that there was one last solution: a high dose of steroids with about a 1 in 5 chance that they would affect the adrenal glands of the baby. I was desperate, so immediately agreed to take them.

I persuaded a doctor to try out the antibiotic theory

After about three days, the effect was remarkable. The constant nausea and retching had gone and I was finally able to slowly start living a more normal life again. The high dosage made me agitated and unable to sit still, but this seemed a small price to pay. I was ecstatic and could not stop moving about and eating, after months of enforced starvation.

A follow-up appointment a week later with the consultant led to the immediate question as to who had given me these and why. The consultant explained that I had to come off them as soon as possible, which has to be done gradually with steroids. This took about five weeks and as the dose started to diminish I could feel the nauseous sensation starting to return and then gradually I started to actually be sick again. After coming off them completely, I ended up in hospital again, but this time for the last time. After about 25 weeks, the sickness was no longer so severe that I needed to be hospitalised, but it did continue 5-6 times daily until the last 6 weeks, when it was just once or twice a day.

The controversy of the steroid treatment led to a close monitoring of the rest of the pregnancy, with numerous growth scans and blood tests, etc. The heart of this controversy appeared to be that this was not a conventional treatment for this condition and I was informed that there was a 1 in 5 chance of the baby's adrenal glands being affected. I did feel that the steroids relieved the symptoms of hyperemesis, but also that the hyperemesis probably reduced in severity on its own by about seven months.

At almost two weeks' overdue and following an induced birth, I had our second whopping 9lb 8oz son. He is 11 weeks old now and completely gorgeous. When I hold him, I cannot believe how placid and gentle he is, and how lucky I am to have him.[60]

Tina C from the UK

Very often a woman is not in a clear-cut situation...

Grey areas

Often a woman does not find herself in a clear-cut situation for other reasons...

Birthframe 44

While I was living in Sri Lanka a few years ago, feeling very isolated, out of the blue a letter arrived, which had been forwarded by my mother. I began to read... Hey, it was from Jeannette Cockell!—sorry, Clark—the person I studied German with. It turned out she was arranging a class reunion. Of course, I couldn't attend, but I did send a synopsis of my life so far for inclusion in the newsletter that was to accompany the reunion. I left out various bits of 'potential' information, not wanting to tempt fate or show off, including the fact that I was pregnant with my first child at the age of 37.

When I returned to the UK, hoping that Jeannette might arrange another reunion and also wanting to say hello to her, I contacted her again. This time, since I had a certain amount of evidence, I mentioned the fact that I now had three children, aged 4, 2 and 2 weeks. A few weeks later I read Jeannette's reply, not expecting to be upstaged. Lo and behold, in her letter she calmly announced that she'd *also* had three babies since we'd last corresponded ... but all at once! Here's her story. As you'll see, she clearly feels that the medical intervention and support she received was helpful in all respects.

Having waited a long time to conceive I found out that I was pregnant very early on. We were delighted to learn that we had found the goal first time, but we had to wait a few more weeks to discover that we had scored a hat trick. An early blood test showed hormone levels off the end of the Richter scale, so we had psyched ourselves up for twins, but we were not geared up for triplets. Our initial reaction to seeing three little heartbeats on the screen was a mixture of delight, excitement, terror and worry whether all the babies would make it.

Our reaction was a mixture of delight, excitement, terror...

We decided against any invasive tests for abnormalities and opted instead for the nuchal fold scan at King's College, London. It was most reassuring (and morale-boosting) to know that I had the same chances of carrying a healthy baby as a woman 10 years younger than myself. We received wonderful scan pictures, which helped to make the pregnancy 'real' for us.

My antenatal care was shared between the hospital and my GP, so I had a lot more check-ups than most other mothers-to-be. I was on first name terms with the antenatal and ultrasound staff and Gordon and I became minor celebrities at the parents-to-be sessions at the doctor's surgery. I was extremely pleased with the quality of my antenatal care, even though I could have done with some special information sessions for multiples.

Apart from the usual minor ailments which seemed to affect every orifice and cause extreme breathlessness from 17 weeks onwards, I had a trouble-free pregnancy. I did not even suffer from morning sickness. As a precaution I was given steroid injections to help the babies' lungs develop, should they arrive early. Towards the end I became very uncomfortable and was desperate to have the babies delivered, but managed to stagger on to almost 36 weeks before the C-section was scheduled. Originally, the babies were to have been delivered on 1 April, but we insisted on changing the date for obvious reasons—April Fools' Day!

The planning for my hospital stay resembled a military operation: hospital pre-visited and route planned, bags packed at 32 weeks, mobile phone charged up, draft birth announcement cards and address labels ready on the PC, baby equipment on standby. But the best-laid plans...

I was looked after by extremely busy but wonderful staff

Having taken nil by mouth and suffering from a raging thirst, I checked in at the hospital at the crack of dawn, as requested. When I announced myself as 'the triplet caesarean' a rather panic-stricken look revealed that my booking had not made its way to the Maternity Ward diary. I was allowed to suck on ice cubes whilst the staff gallantly summoned up every colleague who was not actually out of the country so that the operation could take place later that day. When I was eventually wheeled into theatre there were 17 people present and tickets were for standing room only. There was a great party atmosphere and the morning's problems were quickly forgotten.

I had opted for a spinal/epidural anaesthetic so that I could be awake for the delivery. Gordon was present and kept up near the top end of proceedings for fear of seeing anything remotely unsavoury. The only painful part was the initial siting of the needle, but by the time I had mouthed the S-word the pain had gone. There was a lot of rummaging around and then within minutes Ryan, Lawrence and Amelia made their noisy entry into the world. Two boys and a girl, just as predicted. The babies were taken to the Special Care Baby Unit (SCBU) weighing in at 4lb 12oz, 5lb and 4lb 2oz respectively. Ryan was delivered by forceps and had a bit of a headache, and Amelia needed warming up in an incubator, but within a day they were pronounced fighting fit. In the meantime I stayed in a single side room by the ward and was looked after by extremely busy but wonderful staff.

The next day getting out of bed was pretty excruciating, but I was wheeled to SCBU to see my little treasures and to feed them. I recovered quite quickly from the operation and the only real problem was getting enough sleep, which was good practice anyway for what was to follow. After two days the babies were ready to leave SCBU but I managed to negotiate an extended stay of two more days to enable me to get fitter to care for them. On Day 8 we all left the hospital wearing our L-plates.

Jeannette Clark

Post scriptum by Jeannette:
I had this account published in a TAMBA [Twins and Multiple Births Association] magazine some time ago. The reaction was mixed: some readers complained that I had painted an overly rosy picture, especially considering the problems with many multiple birth babies, and pointed out that even the nuchal fold test could not guarantee against abnormalities. On the other hand, some people were heartened to have a positive story. Anyway, I hope it's of interest.

Comment from me:
There are several other positive stories of multiple births elsewhere in this book, along with a few negative ones. Check the entries for 'twins' or 'triplets' in the Index if you'd like to find them quickly.

But grey areas do not always need to mean a managed pregnancy and birth... As we've already seen earlier in this book, in many cases women who are categorised as high risk do manage to avoid intervention, while still getting the care they need to ensure safe outcomes. Here's a case of a woman who did...

Birthframe 45

Thanks to careful preparation, Debbie Brindley—a midwife working within the NHS—managed to arrange a very natural water birth for the birth of her twins. (For her first baby, she'd had a water birth at home.) When I wrote to her to ask her a few questions, I discovered that even during her pregnancy, Debbie really did 'care about care'...

What's your view on the use of ultrasound in pregnancy?

Our unit policy is for regular serial scans. However, it only appears to be safe, doesn't it? Research is not conclusive so I feel it should be used as with all medical intervention and technology—when it's needed and not routinely. Following this philosophy, I chose to have two scans: an anomaly scan at 20 weeks and one further scan at 34 weeks to check presentation (they were both cephalic)—so I could then plan how to manage my labour. Growth was diagnosed clinically on palpation.

> Our unit policy is for regular serial scans. However, it only appears to be safe, doesn't it? Research is not conclusive.

But, presumably, the midwives who looked after you while you were pregnant used a Sonicaid to check the fetal heartbeats at each appointment?

Carole, my community midwife, did all my antenatal care (at home—I'm so lucky) and she agreed to listen to the fetal hearts with a Pinard instead of a Sonicaid [which uses ultrasound]. They always had good movements so we were both happy with this.

And how were the fetal heartbeats checked while you were in labour?

I was happy to have the heart rates checked with the Sonicaid, as the Pinard's awkward in labour because the labouring woman may have to lie down for it to be used effectively. I had a 10-minute CTG [cardiotocograph], i.e. electronic fetal monitoring, which the student midwife held on, while the pool was running. Beforehand I had agreed to a short CTG of the second twin when the first had been born but in the event, it turned out there was no time!

> I was happy to have the heart rates checked

Did you make any special requests of your birth attendants for your labour? I mean, did you want them to behave in any particular way?

I wanted as much privacy as I would have had if I'd been at home and I didn't want people 'popping in' or coming for a look. (Not that any of my colleagues would dare!) I believe in needing a quiet, relaxing environment so as to raise endorphins and lower adrenaline. I agreed to Carole's student witnessing, though, as Carole had been so kind to me. Otherwise, I wanted midwives only. I wrote a detailed birth plan and then made an appointment with my extremely supportive consultant to discuss it. (I met him twice in all, once early on in my pregnancy and then at 34 weeks in order to discuss my birth plan.) He agreed with most of it, we discussed one or two points regarding monitoring and physiological third stage and then he signed it. In the birth plan, I requested privacy and he and the paediatrician kindly agreed to wait outside in the corridor during the birth. My consultant was there in case I needed any help—even though he wasn't officially on duty. He's a very special man.

What was the room like where you gave birth in hospital? Did you make any requests about this in advance?

It is common to deliver twins in an operating room—large and clinical, usually with a drip, epidural and in the lithotomy position [lying on your back]. I definitely didn't want this, so asked to use the small standard delivery room connected to the pool room. The room was reasonably but not fantastically homely, but at 9cm dilated on admission I didn't care. It was night, so it was dark and warm and it was down the quiet end of the corridor.

Under what circumstances would you have accepted intervention?

I trusted my midwife implicitly and if she had voiced any concerns I would have accepted any interventions necessary. I strongly believe in the importance of a positive birth experience but my babies' welfare was always more important. I wouldn't have accepted any interventions unless I had thought they were for the direct benefit of my twins. I wouldn't have accepted a routine intervention.

Presumably, you had syntometrine for the third stage?

No, I didn't have syntometrine for my third stage. I'd had a physiological third stage with my first baby and had wanted to keep this labour normal too. I discussed this with my midwife and we agreed to have something ready in case I needed it, in which case I would have happily accepted it. Actually, this was syntocinon, rather than syntometrine because it has less side effects because it includes no ergometrine. Syntometrine is a combination of ergometrine (which is rapid-acting) and syntocinon—i.e. oxytocin (which has sustained action). Ergometrine's side effects can be raised blood pressure and vomiting, dizziness, headaches... so syntocinon (oxytocin) alone can help avoid these.

Anyway, I felt if I had strong labour contractions then the chances are that my uterus would effectively expel the placenta. And I had no complications. The placenta was expelled within a few minutes and blood loss was minimal. Of course, having a physiological stage means that the cord can be cut later and I think the transition to extra-uterine life is more gentle with delayed cord-cutting. Cutting the cord later, babies receive their intended extra bonus of blood.

The transition is gentler with delayed cord-cutting

Intervention all women may experience without realising it

It's very likely that many caregivers you come across during your labour (and also in your pregnancy beforehand) will use language carelessly, without considering the effect it may have on you and even on the optimality of your birth. After all, words don't just have clear-cut meanings, they also convey feelings and judgements. And the meanings that words or comments suggest may not be helpful. Let's consider a few examples relating to labour and birth…

- **Pain:** Caregivers often talk to women about *pain,* even though not all women would consider it that way if just left to float off into their own world. The mere assumption that sensations are painful leads many caregivers to repeatedly talk to women in gloomy tones and offer them drugs of various kinds, most (if not all) of which are likely to have an effect on the baby, making him or her sleepy at birth and unable to suck. (Needless to say, this has a dramatic effect on the first hour the new mother spends with her baby.) They might offer pethidine (which many women report doesn't take away the pain, but makes them feel unpleasantly drunk and out of control); they may offer diamorphine (which is actually just another word for heroin). They may present an epidural as being the answer to the labouring woman's 'problem' although it's highly likely to slow down labour and trigger further interventions, quite apart from the immediate 'medicalisation' of birth it immediately involves… and then they may well want the woman to let the epidural wear off just at the point in her labour when the sensations really would suddenly feel painful. All this negative talk occurs completely disregarding any likely postnatal effects of drugs used and the *real* needs of the labouring woman, which are to have emotional support, privacy, dim lighting, silence and a complete lack of disturbance in other respects.
- **Contractions:** Although the cervix is *opening up* during labour there is a tradition of describing the process as involving 'contractions'. Shouldn't it be 'expansions'? Although it's true the woman's uterus is contracting, the more important process taking place is the cervix opening up like a flower.
- **Birth canal:** This is the phrase which is used to describe the soft, fleshy, flexible folds of your vagina. It's a strange choice of words since 'canal' usually refers to something extremely inflexible and hard, which couldn't possibly 'open up'. Couldn't this place be called 'birth folds' or a 'passage'?
- **Delivery:** The birth of a baby is something which will normally occur whether or not other people are around—so nobody really 'delivers' babies, least of all your caregivers. They are born as a result of the processes which both your baby and you are involved with, throughout your labour, all of which happen without the need for any conscious control. In fact, as we've seen, it's actually best if you just 'let things happen', without resisting at all, or trying to control things. The hormonal cascade will move your forward… Neither a FedEx delivery man, an obstetrician with a scalpel, nor a stork are necessary in the vast majority of cases. Your body knows how to give birth.

INTERVENTION AFTER THE BIRTH

Only a few decades ago it was routine practice in hospitals around the world to put eye drops into newborn babies' eyes and to put the babies in a separate nursery from their new mothers—and it still is in some places. The eye drops were a solution of either silver nitrate, or more recently neomycin or chloramphenicol; the idea was to prevent eye infection (followed, potentially, by blindness) from gonorrhoea or chlamydia. The people who introduced these interventions were clearly focused more on worrying about potential, but rare, problems than on promoting bonding and breastfeeding between new mums and their babies—which needs to take place in *every* case.

Still nowadays, a lot of babies spend time in Intensive Care Units (ICUs). If the babies are premature, this intervention may well be life-saving and some full-term babies who are experiencing real difficulties may also need this kind of intensive care. Others who are transferred to ICUs may experience considerable distress unnecessarily. How many babies are affected by this kind of intervention? All premature babies and most multiples are, but in *Immaculate Deception II* (Celestial Arts 1996), Suzanne Arms implies that many singleton babies may also be affected. She writes: "Various studies show that between 15% and 25% of full-term, healthy babies born to healthy mothers are also spending days or weeks in intensive care units." Unfortunately, she doesn't refer us to any specific studies but we can at least guess that the percentage is still high in some hospitals around the world.

Full-term healthy babies born to healthy mothers may be taken off to the ICU if there are any breathing difficulties at birth (which are much more likely after drugs have been used for pain relief). Babies are also taken away if the mother's (and therefore the baby's) temperature is raised, because this could indicate the presence of an infection. The raised temperature is often the result of the mother having an epidural and indicates no problem in the baby but because an infection is *possible*, babies are given what is called a 'septic workup'. This involves repeated blood tests and one or more spinal taps, all of which could be painful and unpleasant for the baby. As with interventions occurring during pregnancy and labour, there is perhaps the tendency amongst caregivers to over-test in order to be sure that no problems need dealing with. (However, in over-testing, they may well be creating new problems.) The long-term effects of separating mothers and babies is apparently not considered and even supplementary compensatory measures, such as kangaroo care (see Birthframe 50) are not used as widely as we might hope in order to be humane.

Whether or not a baby has started life in an ICU, one other significant intervention which many babies are experiencing is bottle-feeding. Programmed to consider breastmilk their birthright, numerous babies are forced to consume formula made from cows' milk for the first few months of their lives. Despite the fact that almost all women would theoretically be able to breastfeed if they tried, many decide to use formula. The negative experience of friends, relatives and health professionals (who have often not breastfed themselves, or who gave up early), as well as the 'scientific' look of

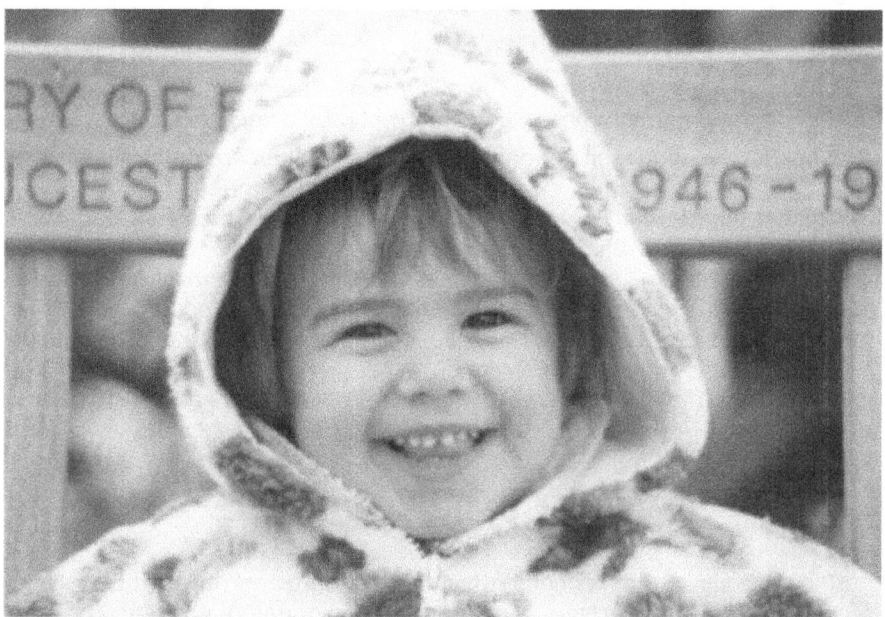

Sophia Zaphiriou-Zarifi experienced a birth with absolutely no interventions quite simply because her mother gave birth before the midwives arrived. (For the full story and guidelines on what to do in that situation see Birthframe 97.)

formula, make many feel they are succumbing to the inevitable. Aggressive promotional advertising by the major formula milk companies was widespread until very recently. Even without it, interventions which take place during labour and birth have an impact on the hormones a new mother does or doesn't produce as she is giving birth and therefore affect whether or not she will spontaneously breastfeed. Fortunately, worldwide awareness of the benefits of breastfeeding is triggering another kind of more positive intervention: various schemes and promotional campaigns are being set up worldwide to encourage mothers to breastfeed, even if they appear to have no desire to do so. This kind of intervention is necessary for mothers who have had a medicated birth because the natural processes have been so badly disturbed that new mothers are unlikely to spontaneously put their newborn babies to their breast.

Finally, writers and researchers such as myself are trying to intervene to create a new awareness of childbirth in the 21st century. Some are angry mothers who have had bad experiences themselves; some are midwives who are disenchanted with practices and outcomes they have witnessed; some are researchers who have uncovered disturbing new data which put old practices into a new perspective.

In order to prepare for your labor and birth you need to understand what constitutes an intervention. If you are aware of what might disturb your labor, you will be in a better position to avoid it.[61]

Good reason to be careful...

In conclusion, there does seem to be a lot of unnecessary intervention around, but there are clearly also cases where intervention is a necessary part of care.

When intervention is inappropriate, it is as if health care professionals are intervening out of fear and a desire to control. Their interference in what are essentially very delicate processes often leads to more problems and more risk. Michel supports this view in one of his books—*Birth Reborn* (Souvenir Press 1994). He says that a lot of medical intervention (involving artificial hormones for inductions, anaesthesia and caesareans) introduces new risks, rather than reduces them. He also makes the point that the emphasis on high-risk cases poorly serves the interests of women who have healthy pregnancies and births, who make up the great majority of pregnant women.

> Perhaps caregivers sometimes intervene too readily
> because experimentation has become standard

The cascade of interventions, which so many women have written about, results in more caesareans and the more frequent use of forceps and ventouse. Women who would otherwise have had a normal, healthy, uneventful birthing experience end up having an extremely managed, artificial birth—often all because they accepted one small intervention. As a result, risks increase and the safety of both mother and baby is undermined.

Refusing interventions in cases where there is a choice is in no way irresponsible. In fact, it is the opposite because it is respecting something which is enormously complex and easily disturbed. Refusing drug-based pain relief or treatments to apparently ease pain is also wise because you're likely to have less pain in the long run. Physical and emotional damage caused by episiotomies, forceps bruising and damage, caesareans, catheterisation and disappearing babies (who are whisked away 'for observation' or treatment) can last for years. We need to remember the advantages of having full alertness, privacy and dignity as we meet our new babies... and they meet us too!

Perhaps caregivers sometimes intervene too readily because experimentation has become the standard approach over the last couple of centuries. Experimental procedures have become routine before research has confirmed they are safe or even helpful. Electronic fetal monitoring and ultrasound are just two examples of practices which have continued despite research showing possible risks and drawbacks.

> Experimental procedures have become routine
> *before* research has confirmed they are safe or even helpful

Another problem with intervention is that it often takes place without the informed consent of the woman giving birth. Although there are times when a woman is taken by surprise during labour, a woman should really be able to inform herself about all possible interventions in advance because nowadays information can be accessed from the Internet, either using a computer at home or at a local library or Internet café. Simply typing in www.google.co.uk allows anybody to search for key words which will lead to information on almost any topic. Most of us are more than capable of evaluating the quality of information we see posted on websites. Sometimes we forget that we have the legal right to participate in decision-making relating to our own bodies while we're pregnant or giving birth. If we feel diffident about acting on knowledge we have collected or feel intuitively, we should perhaps remind ourselves that even experts disagree, especially in the field of childbirth! We need to accept responsibility for our bodies and our babies.

While I was researching this book, I often asked Michel how much intervention had really been necessary, in his opinion, in the case of particular births. Here is one example of an emailed conversation about one of the birth accounts I was sent for possible inclusion in this book.

I attach a twin birth story which is full of interventions, along with detailed questions about each intervention. Was all this intervention really necessary?

You cannot imagine the number of emails and phone calls I have about twins. Midwives practising home birth before 'the industrialisation of childbirth' were not scared by twin births. In general those who know about privacy as a basic need in labour are not scared by this sort of birth. It is the art of doing nothing. First you wait for the first baby. Then you wait for the second baby and finally you wait for the placenta. The point is to make sure that there is not too much excitation around after the birth of the first twin, so that the mother is not distracted and has nothing else to do than look at her baby in a sacred atmosphere. The same after the birth of the second one, while waiting for the placenta. It is important to know that a twin delivery is often less violent, less intense and longer than a singleton delivery. Those who don't know about the importance of privacy are so scared of twin births that they create a cascade of interventions... if they have not chosen the easy way, that is to say a caesarean section. Today many practitioners are right to prefer a caesarean section. Giving birth without any privacy among scared people can be dangerous. This twin story you sent me is one among many others. You know my answers to all your questions.

Michel's response to my questions was usually similar and we were usually in agreement as to the appropriateness (or otherwise) of intervention. However, all his comments are tempered by his overall view (which also coincides with my own) which he expressed in his book, *Birth and Breastfeeding* (Clairview Books 2007):

Should the method of the mammals be inefficient in any particular instance, there must always be teams capable of doing epidurals to compensate for the lack of endorphins; to use drips to compensate for a deficiency of hormones from the posterior pituitary; and to perform caesarean sections to rescue babies in distress.

> Facilitating the normal, healthy processes, i.e. *normality*, not pathology, must become the new focus for caregivers.

That brings us back to the concept of optimal birth... We need to encourage caregivers in modern birthing facilities (or in our homes) to take a new approach to care. Facilitating the normal, healthy processes, i.e. *normality*, not pathology, must become the new focus. Non-invasive tests utilised to identify the tiny minority of women and babies who really do need intervention should be just that—non-invasive. They should not impinge on a pregnant woman's sense of well-being or undermine her confidence in her ability to give birth. Empowering the great majority of women and supporting them unobtrusively as they labour through a completely physiological birth should be the new aim. Only this shift in focus will enable women and babies to experience truly safe births, which are life-enhancing for everyone involved.

Finally, here are some comments from a mother who experienced an undisturbed birth, Fiona Lucy Stoppard:

> The world is a wonderful place and there are some beautiful things. Lovely people. Nature. Art. Poetry and music. Writing. Friendships and love. But, basically, what I feel is that at the core of it all—the one real thing, the crux of it all—is pregnancy, labour and birth... and also breastfeeding and bonding. It's like the sun coming out. It really illuminates everything. I'm not saying that if a woman chooses not to have children, she can't have a wonderful life and do a lot—I don't mean that. But it's just that it's like everything else is pushed away, all these wonderful things. It's like the core of life. When women give birth without drugs, they're really connecting then. It's so subtle, what's going on, and drugs just spoil it. It's like some wonderful beautiful flower that's incredibly delicate and beautiful. It just can't be a production line. A production line's for making bread, for very practical things. This is just the absolute... it all needs to be treated with the greatest of care.
>
> I know there are all sorts of different things happening during pregnancy and labour. It would be wonderful if midwives could just look at a pregnant woman and know exactly what was going on and know just how to deal with it. But so often they say, "Oh, something's not right, we'd better induce you"—and maybe that might not have been the right thing at all. I know there are times when it is true the case is "Quick! Hospital! Get the baby out." Great, that's wonderful—you have a beautiful baby, if that had to happen. But if the woman is healthy and it's a healthy pregnancy then you have to let the baby have the best possible experience.
>
> And it's not just the experience at the time, because it affects the future of the mother and the child.
>
> *Fiona Lucy Stoppard*

> Experience of birth affects the future of both mother and child

5... THINK AHEAD

> As a first pregnancy I assumed I would be told when, where, what I should do. This didn't happen. How can you 'prepare' for what you don't know?

What can happen when people don't prepare?

Here, we're talking about preparation—the kind where you decide what you would do if certain things should happen, how you would react if... etc. We prepare for other things in life, so the idea of preparing for a birthing experience should not be terribly new. Not only do we have to prepare for the unknown, we're actually used to doing it in almost all areas of our lives. We even prepare for something like our first lovemaking experience by talking to friends and reading books or magazines, even though we know it's supposed to 'come naturally'. Childbirth definitely needs preparation too... We need to think through relevant issues, find caregivers who are supportive of our preferences for care, have bookings in place (e.g. with a hospital or birth centre whose protocols we like the sound of)—whether we're planning to give birth at home or in a hospital—and we even need to prepare to have sufficient privacy. If things really do take us by surprise during labour, we can still think things over at the time, unless it's clearly an absolute emergency (e.g. haemorrhaging or severe abdominal pains which are obviously not contractions).

Conduct your own research, make your own decisions and be ready to seek a second opinion in any cases where you're not sure...

Birthframe 46

Here is a scenario which is, unfortunately, very typical. I haven't included many birthframes like this in this book... You'll be able to read plenty of others in pregnancy magazines or books on childbirth, and you'll hear similar stories when you take your new child to playgroups.

I had my first child, Samantha, in January 1985 but what influenced my expectations and hopes was a TV programme I'd watched about four years before. The programme had Miriam Stoppard as its hostess and the subject was Michel Odent and his work in Pithiviers, France as a natural childbirth pioneer. It inspired me to read books about the subject (home births, natural birth—by Sheila Kitzinger and Michel Odent)—and my enthusiasm grew. When I first became pregnant I sought out a doctor who was sympathetic and experienced, who would attend me at home.

The labour started on Saturday morning. The first sign was a little gush of amniotic fluid—but no pain. The doctor examined me, and assessed that I was not dilated at all. He seemed a bit put out that this was happening on a Saturday—he had to visit his sick wife in hospital. I tried the usual tricks to bring the labour on—taking castor oil and scrubbing floors.

We went to the hospital very disappointed and afraid

The doctor said at 3.30pm that we had better go to hospital as some hours had elapsed since the waters had leaked; he said that there was a risk of infection and that the baby could become blind if that happened. We went to the hospital very disappointed and frightened. The house doctor at the hospital read the letter of introduction from my 'home birth doctor' (who had to go to visit his wife). He looked and acted very disdainfully towards me—that I'd hoped for a home birth and now here I was needing professional help after all. I was wired up to a machine to measure contractions... there were none. I'd heard about the method called sweeping the cervix, whereby the doctor uses his fingers to manipulate the cervix into loosening, and maybe rupturing the membranes. I wanted to try this first before resorting to drugs. It was done very painfully and some contractions started.

Over the hours, I was put on a syntocinon drip—the contractions were not strong enough and the baby had to be delivered within 12 hours, according to the hospital's rule, because of the risk of infection. I had the water sac broken so that a monitor could be attached to the baby's head. This was very upsetting and painful. I felt raped. So much water came out—I realised that before it was only a leak and was not as dangerous for infection as the full water emptying. Then I was persuaded to have an epidural because they wanted to increase the syntocinon to speed things up. The baby's pulse was now dropping so low they were worried, so they phoned their top doctor who advised a caesarean. The epidural was wearing off now and I could feel the baby low down in the canal, almost ready to come out. They still went ahead with a general anaesthetic and I woke up to see my husband showing my lovely baby wrapped up tight in a shawl. She was born at 12.30am on Sunday, nine hours after I went to the hospital.

I was so happy to have a lovely baby that I soon forgot about my ordeal. On Samantha's first birthday I relived the humiliating, disappointing and painful time of her birth. I duly wrote a letter to the hospital. I complained about my treatment. I did receive a reply and I was invited to meet the doctors at the hospital for a talk/discussion. I did not go in the end as I felt that I would be out of my depth at the meeting—and it would be me against them. I had already been through a lot of grief with Samantha's health since she was 8 months old. A doctor at the hospital had told me she had a heart murmur. She was also taking a paediatric steroid in tablet form to try to combat the low blood count they had discovered she had because of a rare blood disease called Diamond Blackfan anaemia. I had enough battles to win ahead of me. I discovered that a suggested allergy to wheat could be her problem. We discovered that in fact her blood count went up when she didn't eat wheat or other wheat gluten products. It took me three years to finally wean her off steroids. She's now a healthy young lady, though.

Christina Mansi

Thinking back to the beginning of Christina's account, we can see that believing in and wanting an optimal birth, and reading up on the subject is not enough. We need to take responsibility for ourselves and anticipate and refuse treatments which we believe to be unhelpful or even harmful. It's a shame Christina didn't refuse to have an internal examination because it's well known that internals increase the risk of infection and that was the main danger.[1] It's also a shame she agreed to go into hospital because if she'd relaxed at home, her contractions may well have started more quickly. (She could have checked for signs of infection by taking her own temperature every hour.) Finally, it's a shame she agreed to be induced—both 'sweeping' and the syntocinon drip were intended to start contractions. If she'd behaved differently—less like a 'patient'—the epidural and caesarean would have been much less likely and she may well have had the natural home birth she was hoping for.[2]

Birthframe 47

In case you question my comments on Christina's first birth (in Birthframe 46), read about the same woman's next three births...

My second daughter, Kathryn, was born in February 1988. I made contact with Michel Odent, who was living in London then. I wanted to try again for a home birth and he agreed to help and support me.

Again, the first sign of labour was a gush of amniotic fluid. This time the baby was born after four hours of labour.

The first sign of labour was a gush of amniotic fluid, as before. This was at 8.30pm. The real labour pains came at 10.30pm. Kathryn was born on my bed at 2.30am after four hours of labour. It was painful and I was glad to be on my own in the dark of my bedroom. My husband and Michel Odent were there but kept out of the way and didn't interfere.

At the last moment Michel Odent came over and helped, while my husband supported me under the arms as I gave birth in a supported squat position. She weighed 7lb 2oz. I held Kathryn immediately and put her to my breast. About half an hour later the afterbirth was expelled naturally.

I was in shock for the first half hour after Kathryn's birth and was shivering—but that is apparently normal—so we turned on the electric fan heater. Kathryn did not cry when she was born. She lay on my thighs—skin-to-skin—for a long time, contentedly looking around in the half light. I breastfed Kathryn exclusively (no solids) until she was 6-8 months old. I didn't have my first period until she was 18 months old and carried on feeding her until two months before my third child was born, when she was 2 years 4 months.

My son Anthony was born in August 1990. I had put on more weight with this pregnancy than before. He was overdue by a week or so. We had visitors—relatives—staying in our home at the time. The night that the guests went to spend one night away my labour started at 10.30pm. It was a long and hard labour—six hours. The second stage only really started when I forced myself to get up into a squatting position. Michel Odent, who had been outside the room listening to the progress of my labour, came in as I was starting to push. He helped to deliver Anthony's shoulders. He later said that his shoulders were broad—he was a bigger baby than the others: 8lb 4oz. I recovered quickly again and breastfed him until my second son (my fourth child) Jonathan was born in October '92.

Jonathan was four weeks' overdue. My labour started at 8.30pm and he was born at 10.30pm. I wanted to try a water birth so I was in my extra large bath with lots of lavender oil when the midwife arrived at 9.30pm. (Michel Odent was not in the country at the time.) She didn't think that I was in real labour as I seemed so calm in the water. When I got out of the bath to call her from my bedroom she was surprised. Jonathan was born on the floor of the bathroom, my husband again helping to support me in a squat position. I had no tears, he didn't look overdue and weighed 7lb 14oz. I breastfed him till he was over 3. I felt very emotional when I tried to stop. He was my last baby. He's now 9 years old!

Christina Mansi

Comment from me:

While some forms of lavender oil are good for helping relaxation, as well as easing perineal pain and healing, it should only be used with great caution in early pregnancy as some types can cause vaginal bleeding.[3]

Birthframe 48

I had a similar problem to Christina...

At 38 weeks in my second pregnancy I had a leak of something and I also had the flu. Naturally, I phoned my doctor because I wanted to be checked out. He said it was probably amniotic fluid and that I should go to hospital immediately. I asked him what would be done there. Firstly, he said, a few cells would be scraped from around my cervix to confirm whether or not the leak had been amniotic fluid. After that, I would probably be induced because I was, after all, at 'term'. (Term is considered anything from 38 to 42 weeks.) Knowing that an internal examination would increase my risk of infection (which is the main danger after a leak of amniotic fluid) I said I would rather not go in. The doctor repeated his instruction to me five times and five times I refused! (A letter followed in the post the next day suggesting he wanted to strike me off his list but a well-considered reply from me managed to persuade him against this.)

That afternoon and evening I searched through my pregnancy books. I also phoned an independent midwife as well as Michel himself, who happened to be at home. (Most of the time Michel is travelling round the world lecturing at conferences or setting up research projects. I was lucky that my due date occurred in his Christmas holidays.)

Both the midwife and Michel said the leak could well have been urine—I did, after all have a bad cough so it could have been 'stress incontinence'—or it could have been a leak of hindwaters, which would 'heal' up. I was told one option was to keep taking my temperature to check it didn't rise dangerously and indicate an infection. Both Michel and the midwife agreed my risk of infection would increase if I went into hospital and had an internal examination.

Two and a half weeks later, after recovering from the flu and after attending my Master's graduation ceremony on my official due date (looking extremely large!) I had a very straightforward, two-hour labour. Nina-Jay, my second daughter, was—and still is!—beautiful and very healthy.

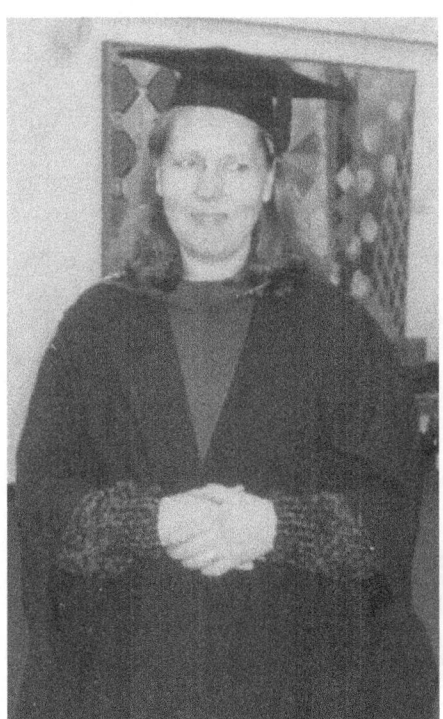
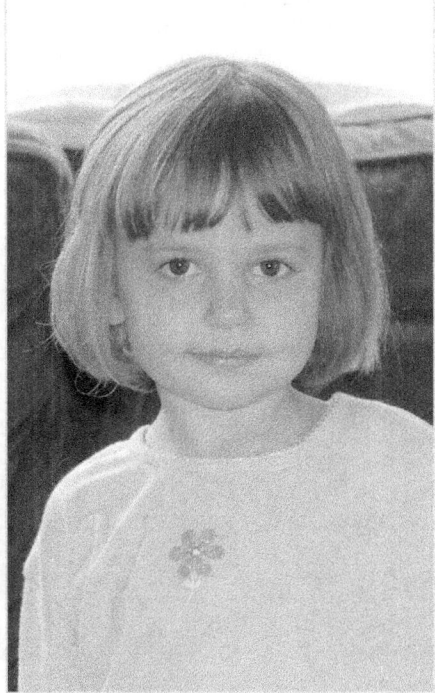

Me, at my Master's graduation ceremony—and the girl who was born two days later...

Proactive planning

Clearly, whether you're expecting one baby or three, you need to consider many questions. Think through these alone, then discuss them with your partner and caregivers, because their support may be crucial to your success.

- ♥ Are there any legal issues relevant to your situation? What are your rights?
- ♥ Are there medical issues which relate specifically to your own pregnancy? What does research say about your situation? Which areas are undisputed and which areas are controversial? What are your options and what are the risks involved? What do you feel is possible on both a rational and an intuitive level? Can you find any professionals who agree with you or who would be prepared to offer you support?
- ♥ Can you make contact with other women who've been in a similar situation?

Next, you need to consider what you, your baby and partner might need. Prepare things well in advance, so you can relax during the last few weeks of your pregnancy.

- ♥ What will you yourself need while you're in labour and after the birth? Think about music, clothes, sanitary towels and easy-to-prepare food.[4]
- ♥ Do you want a birthing pool? When will hire and set-up practice begin?
- ♥ What will you need for your new baby? Buy a few useful items—six bodysuits, six sleepsuits, a couple of hats, nappies, a shawl or two, a breastfeeding cushion, a baby sling and a Moses basket or pram for the baby to sleep in during the day.
- ♥ Which phone numbers might be useful? Prepare a detailed list which is clear enough to be used by other people too. Stick it up by your telephone.

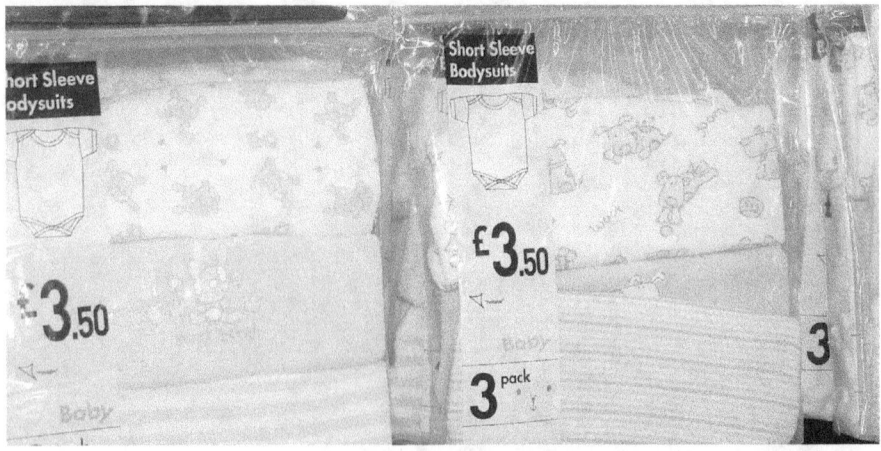

Have you bought a basic stock of baby clothes yet?
Of course, many items can easily be left until later on, when your baby is a bit bigger.
Remember you don't yet even know whether you're having a girl or a boy!

What you could have

... for a hospital birth
- ♥ A hairband to tie your hair back
- ♥ A secret cache of favourite food
- ♥ Your usual cosmetics
- ♥ Ear plugs, so you can rest

... for a home birth
- ♥ A bucket or bowl for being sick or catching the placenta
- ♥ An old bath mat, towel or sheet to stand or kneel on while you're giving birth. Place this on the plastic sheeting (to stop you sliding around) and throw it away afterwards
- ♥ A hair band to tie your hair back
- ♥ Some candles and matches for candlelight
- ♥ Bottles of water to swig
- ♥ Relaxing music

What you need

... for a hospital birth
- ♥ A care guide (see overleaf)
- ♥ Comfortable clothes
- ♥ Disinfectant wipes for bathrooms
- ♥ Money, telephone cards, etc.

... for a home birth
- ♥ A portable heater, with a long lead, so it can be plugged in anywhere. Women often feel shivery just after they've given birth and babies need to be kept warm.
- ♥ Something to protect the floor where you give birth. Depending on the design and size of your home, you might consider using a plastic tablecloth, an incontinence sheet or some plastic groundsheets from your local home and garden store.

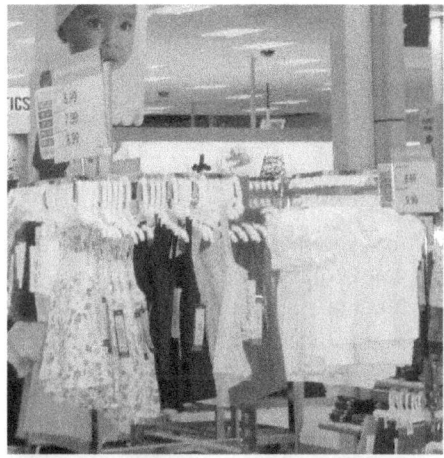

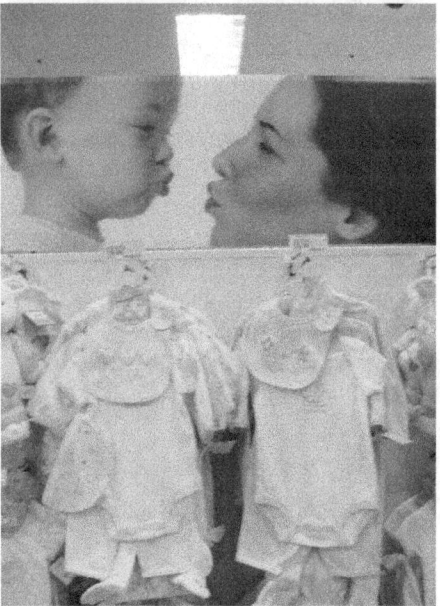

Don't go wild... but now you can perhaps start to explore the baby shops

Prepare wisely, taking into account where you're planning to give birth

What you don't need...

- ♥ **A camera or camcorder** If you let people photograph you while you're in labour or giving birth, you can't possibly feel you're not being observed. They'll be plenty of time after the birth to take photos and make videos. Just be private for the birth and until after you've birthed the placenta.
- ♥ **Special food or drink** Just stock up on what you like. In particular, do not buy in any glucose tablets for use during your labour and birth. Research has shown they lower a woman's pain threshold... and that's definitely not going to be helpful, is it?!
- ♥ **Medical equipment** Cavewomen didn't have any and we still don't need any today. Birth attendants usually bring along whatever supplies they feel they need, including a little emergency equipment.
- ♥ **Drug-based pain relief of any kind** If you're giving birth at home, remember to stipulate in advance that no 'pain relieving' drugs (such as 'gas and air' or narcotics) are to be brought into your house.

For your new baby (or babies!) you will need a soft towel for wiping him or her just after the birth; a nice new receiving blanket for keeping him or her cosy; some nappies (cloth with covers, or disposable ones); a baby bath for after the first week; a soft natural sponge; baby towels; muslin squares for mopping up milk; baby clothes, including hats; a Moses basket; baby-size blankets.

If this is not your first baby think carefully about what you will do with your other child(ren) when you go into labour and give birth. Make arrangements early and have back-up arrangements in place too! Don't rely on the 'Oh, we'll manage somehow' philosophy. You'll manage better if you think ahead.

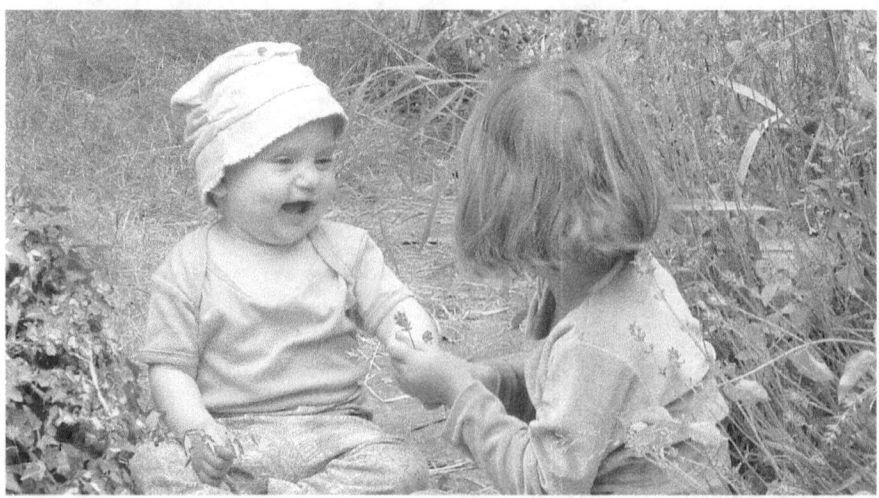

Consider who could look after any other children—they may not stay busy for long!

CARE GUIDES

A care guide is a very important document because it will outline your wishes. This is vitally important if you're planning to give birth in hospital and at the very least extremely helpful if you're planning a home birth. When you're in labour you may not feel able to communicate all your wishes. Yes, I agree it's usually called a birth plan, but I've coined the term 'care guide' because the words 'birth plan' often seem to trigger negativity in caregivers. Midwives and consultants rightly say that birth cannot be predicted or planned to the last detail but they are wrong if they assume that experiences will always be worse than hoped for. They are often much better, or simply different, as we've seen, and will continue to see in various birthframes. While you're pregnant, your care guide will give you a starting point for communication with your caregivers. It may also prompt some discussion and necessitate some negotiating skills on your part! When you go into labour and give birth your care guide will remind your caregivers of your wishes or it will communicate your wishes if you haven't met your birth attendants before. In other words, it will free you up to focus on your labour and birth—although even then you will need to be prepared to remind caregivers of its contents!

Debbie Brindley writing on birth plans from a midwife's perspective...

> Most of what women write is fairly standard, but in these times of fragmented care I think it's important to let your caregivers (who you may be meeting for the first time) know how you would like things to go. My advice would be to keep birth plans relaxed and try not to be too rigid. Having the opportunity to discuss my birth plan in advance of the birth with my consultant was invaluable to me, as he signed it to say he'd read and agreed to it. That gave me the confidence that I wasn't going to come up against any unexpected resistance during labour.

What if your caregiver objects to your care guide?

If you encounter a great deal of negativity from health care professionals when you present your care guide, be prepared to fight or go elsewhere. If you were to accept every objection made to points on your care guide and absorb another person's negativity it's likely you would be setting yourself up for a very different birthing experience—because physiological birth is not something that can be 'half done'. Only compromise if you truly feel another person's objections are valid in medical terms in your particular case. When you are discussing arrangements and approaches also remember that your caregivers may not have much (or any) experience of physiological birth. If this is the case, again it may be better to start looking for another caregiver who either already has experience or who is clearly willing to support your approach.

> *It wasn't really the risk of haemorrhaging, he finally admitted, that was preventing him from agreeing to a completely physiological third stage... He simply didn't want to have to hang around waiting for the placenta for what could be a very long time. Enormously respectful of his honesty, I then tentatively suggested we limit the time to two hours, which he agreed to.*

What if it isn't taken seriously?

Be respectful but gently assertive with your potential caregivers. They may well be stepping into new territory. Help them to develop confidence in both you and the natural physiological processes. Listen to their concerns about risk—they're bound to have some!—but check and double-check the research yourself and present it to them too for discussion, if necessary. Remember, you are collaborating on this for success. Both you and your caregivers will be hoping for positive outcomes.

> Twice I prepared birth plans, and twice my births proceeded as I wished. There were small differences, small unexpected eventualities, but nothing proceeded against my wishes and after each birth I felt strong and satisfied. My midwives were very happy too, although somewhat astonished!

> Stating in my birth plan that I wanted no pain relief meant that none was offered to me while I was clearly in pain. This was important because I would have been more likely to have 'given in' if I had been offered things.

SAMPLE CARE GUIDES

The real-life care guides on the following pages should help you prepare a care guide which is relevant to your own needs. Make sure all key details are included, including the name of your doula, if you plan to use one. This will ensure she has no trouble gaining access to you, wherever you are. (In case you don't already know about them, I'll explain soon about 'doulas'. Check the Index if you want to know now!) Also, if at all possible make your care guide all fit onto one sheet of A4, or two maximum, if you want it to have a chance of it being read.

Horses for courses...

How you write your care guide will depend not only on your personality and preferences but also on your particular situation and what you want your care guide to do for you—and other people! As the first sample guide shows, a care guide can actually help you to visualise a positive outcome, which is a very useful thing for it to do. If you want your care guide to create this kind of positive expectation in your heart and your head, you need to keep the language very positive. Some people feel it's useful to visualise all eventualities in a positive light and to include your wishes in case these eventualities ever arise. Personally, I don't agree, but it's worth thinking about whether or not this would be appropriate for you, given your particular situation.

The positive visualisation on the next page is the guide I prepared for my third baby's birth. (I think the midwife I met for my antenatal care showed it to the other midwives in her practice because they seemed to know about it.) The other care guides aim to achieve different purposes, as you'll see...

Care guide 1: Positive visualisation

> For the birth of this child, I would appreciate minimal intervention on the part of my caregivers. I would prefer any caregivers to stay in a separate room from me while I am labouring and to make every effort not to disturb either me or my baby being born. This includes monitoring, which I would like to be absolutely minimal and only done with a fetal stethoscope (Pinard) periodically. It also includes the second stage of labour, during which I want no disturbance, comments, instructions or 'help'. I do not want a midwife to 'catch' my baby as he or she emerges—I can do this myself. I also do not want an episiotomy or timed second stage.
>
> After the birth, until the placenta is born, I would again ask for no disturbance. It is even preferable if my caregivers stay out of the room in which I've given birth until they're sure that the placenta has been born. This is for the sake of safety because it is clear that disturbing the woman at this stage can slow down expulsion of the placenta. I will say when I would like the umbilical cord to be cut.
>
> To summarise, I hope you can be there in case I need you. I shall call you if I feel that something is wrong, or if there are any worrying symptoms (e.g. early blood loss during labour, meconium-stained amniotic fluid). I would appreciate it, for your part, if you could simply watch very discretely from through a crack in the door, or listen from an adjacent room, to check that all is OK. Expect to hear some noise! I believe that making noises in labour—in a totally spontaneous way—is helpful in working 'through' the pain, if there is any!
>
> I would particularly appreciate it if you could be careful about your choice of words at any stage, if you need to talk to me at all, which you may not need to do. I believe labouring women are very suggestible. This means no implication that I'm in pain, that it must be bad, that anything is taking a long time... just please trust the natural processes. Also, no bright lights, please, no loud noises, no unnecessary talking either to me or between yourselves—do this well out of earshot if you find it necessary—because I believe all this could disturb the physiological processes.
>
> After the birth, I again do not want any unnatural interventions or unnecessary disturbance. This means that the baby must not be taken away from me at birth, there must be no Vitamin K in any form, no eye drops or cream, no shots or tests, no bathing (I can do this myself later on), no immediate weighing or measuring (it can wait a couple of hours or so, or even until the next day), no routine suctioning of the nasal passages, no swaddling, etc. I plan to breastfeed on demand and keep my baby with me, except when I am showering after the birth, when my partner will probably take the baby. Please do not provide dummies or milk/water supplements.
>
> Thank you, in advance, for your help at this special and sensitive period and for helping to make my new baby's entry into the world a pleasant and harmonious one.

Having shown you a very positive approach, it's now necessary to justify using a negative one. If you believe your caregivers are set on certain interventions or if you think there's any possibility they might not understand your meaning, it might be best to state clearly what you *don't* want, if only for the sake of clarity.

Care guide 2: A very clear approach

Here's the care guide I used for my first birth. Note the use of key words in the left-hand column for quick reading. My husband, who has a PhD in Molecular Biology, did his own research and insisted I use the first part, which he wrote!

	Physiological birth has been shown to be the safest way for mothers to give birth and for this reason amongst others I wish to have as few interventions as possible. To this end here are some points which are of fundamental importance to me about the birth.
Support person:	I will be accompanied by my partner, [name]. I would like him to be with me throughout labour at every stage. We wish to have ongoing guidance, information and advice during labour but my wishes must be paramount in any decisions relating to the birth. We have made ourselves well-informed about the most recent research on birth and do not wish to be pressurised into any procedures.
No induction, no intervention:	I do not want any form of induction. I would like my labour to be left to start spontaneously, even if it is up to three weeks late. In other words, I do not want any rupturing of the membranes, I do not want any continuous electronic fetal monitoring, I do not want syntocinon and I do not want anything administered in a drip or in a vaginal gel.
Monitoring:	I would like to be monitored periodically by a fetal stethoscope (a Pinard).
No shaving or enemas, no catheterisation:	I do not want to be shaved and I do not want to have an enema. I also do not want to be catheterised. I want to be free to empty my own bladder, as necessary.
Food and drink:	I want to be free to take food and drink during labour so as to keep up my energy and follow my natural rhythms.
Positions:	I do not want to be confined to bed. It is important to me that I am free to move around as I wish at all stages of labour. I will probably want to deliver the baby in an upright or semi-upright position, or in any other position which seems natural and comfortable to me.
No pain relief:	I do not want to be offered or given any form of pain relief. Instead, I would like people around me to be supportive of whatever efforts I am making and to encourage me gently if I seem discouraged at any time.
No episiotomy:	I do not want to be cut.

Spontaneous pushing:	I would like spontaneous pushing (not commanded pushing) because I want to tune in to what my own body is telling me what to do. I would appreciate it if my caregivers could remain quiet and watchful during this stage of labour, unless there is any urgent medical reason for communication.
No caesarean, no forceps:	I do not wish to have a caesarean birth. I also do not want to have a forceps delivery. I believe there are many ways of preventing both.
No syntometrine:	I do not want syntometrine or any other medication to be used to speed up delivery of the placenta. I want the placenta to be expulsed naturally without the umbilical cord being pulled at all and without any pressure being applied to my abdomen. I am happy if this process of expulsion takes some time, so would appreciate it if my caregivers could remain quiet and watchful during this wait, taking pains not to disturb me, because I feel it is important that I am left undisturbed so as to be able to focus on my new baby.
The umbilical cord:	I would like the umbilical cord to be cut only when it has stopped pulsating.
Immediately after the birth:	I want the baby to stay with me immediately after the birth and to be allowed to suckle if he or she wishes, without disturbance. It is important to me that my partner is able to remain with me at this time and that the baby continues to be with me for the rest of my time in hospital. We want the baby to be treated gently if and when any procedures (e.g. weighing) are necessary (preferably later on) because we want the birth to be as stress-free for the baby as possible. We do not want the baby to be bathed fully for a week or so following the birth, but help cleaning him or her up straight after the birth may be appreciated, if necessary.
Breastfeeding:	Following an initial, uninterrupted period with the baby and my partner after the birth, I plan to feed on demand. Please do not provide any water/breastmilk/formula supplements or dummies since this would affect breastfeeding success.
Rooming in:	I would like the baby to stay with me in the same room.
Routines:	Neither I nor my partner want hospital procedures to stand in the way of our new family relationships.

I will appreciate your cooperation and help in achieving a successful birth, a happy mother and father and a happy, healthy baby. Thank you in advance for your help. Your sensitivity will be much appreciated.

Care guide 3: Another conversational approach

The next care guide was prepared and used by Georgina Taylor, whose comments and birthframes appear elsewhere in this book. It divides comments clearly into the three stages of labour, which is useful in case some of your caregivers only join you at a late stage in your labour.

MY PREFERENCES...
I wish to go into labour naturally and spontaneously, without artificial induction, whatever stage of gestation I reach. I have confidence in my ability to deal with the sensations of labour. Please support me by not suggesting or offering drugs. I wish my labour to proceed at its natural pace, without haste. If I feel like sleeping at any time I wish to be allowed and encouraged to do so. If I need to have my baby in hospital, I wish as few hospital staff as possible to be present at all stages. I do not wish to be visited by trainees or students. Also, I do not want to be monitored continuously.

First stage:
I do not want to be admitted to the first stage room. I do not want an amniotomy. I wish my labour to proceed at a natural rate, without a syntocinon drip. I wish to labour and give birth in an environment with dim lighting, music and with furnishings arranged in a way in which I can feel comfortable.

Second stage:
I do not wish any time limit to be placed on the duration of the second stage of my labour. I do not wish to be monitored, certainly not continuously.
I do not wish a catheter to be used on me. I do not wish forceps to be used to deliver my baby. In an emergency I would prefer the use of ventouse, and in any case I would prefer that when the baby crowns any mechanical device is removed so that I can finish giving birth. Please do not administer syntometrine before the third stage.

Third stage:
I do not wish to be told the sex of my baby. I do not want the baby to be taken away from me for weighing or examination. I do not want the baby to be bathed or washed. I wish the cord to be left uncut until it has stopped pulsating, and possibly until after the placenta is delivered. Please offer me or my partner the opportunity to cut the cord. I wish to deliver the placenta naturally: do not pull it out. I wish to keep the placenta.

After the birth:
I would like to return home as soon as possible after the birth. However, during the time I do spend in hospital... I wish to be left alone after the birth, with lights turned down. I wish to have the baby in bed with me at all times. I want my partner and our first child to be able to stay with me at all times.

Care guide 4: A twin care guide

Here's the care guide the midwife Debbie Brindley used (Birthframe 45 & 67). Of course, it deals with issues specific to twin pregnancies.

If possible, I would like [names] to look after me in labour. I trust and respect their practice and judgement implicitly and will follow their advice and recommendations. The babies' health and safety are of paramount importance and in the event of complications I would be grateful for all the medical technology and expertise available. I feel very positive about the birth. I've been lucky enough to enjoy a problem-free pregnancy and have kept fit in preparation for labour. Both babies are cephalic, the first is 2/5 palpable [i.e. well-engaged]. (If the second baby turns to breech, I'd still prefer to deliver upright, perhaps kneeling, as Mary Cronk suggests, to prevent the baby coming down too quickly.) Both are active and appear to be growing well and are more than 37 weeks' gestation.

The following covers my hopes and wishes, should labour proceed normally:

Privacy I'd appreciate maximum privacy during labour and birth by reducing the number of birth attendants to just two or three midwives. I'd be extremely grateful to have your expertise readily available—perhaps from a room nearby, rather than the same room? If the babies appear to be OK, I'd rather the paediatricians were close by, than present. I'd also like to remain in the labour room to deliver the babies, only transferring to theatre in the event of complications.

Care in labour I'd prefer not to have any continuous fetal monitoring unless indicated at the time, but am more than happy for the twin monitor to be used in place of Sonicaids and Pinards to differentiate between the heart rates and ensure the babies are OK. If palpation of the babies' presentation is not adequate, a quick scan is OK.

Delivery I'd like to use gravity to promote efficient uterine contractions. I'd also like to avoid having an epidural, again so as to make sure contractions are not affected. Instead, for pain relief, I would like to use the pool for the first stage of labour and possibly also for the birth of the first baby. I then plan to get out almost immediately to facilitate palpation and monitoring of the second baby and to remain upright during the interim and for the second birth. Hopefully, there won't be a long delay between the two babies' births but if possible I'd like it to feel unrushed and avoid augmentation and ARM [artificial rupture of the membranes].

Third stage If things have progressed well during the labour and births and my uterine contractions are good, I'd appreciate the opportunity of having a physiological third stage. I understand the complications of a larger placental site (i.e. that I am therefore at a higher risk of having a postpartum haemorrhage) and am happy to follow advice at the time. However, I would like to try and avoid a prophylactic drip and routine oxytocics, only having them if deemed necessary. If an oxytocic is thought necessary, I would prefer to have syntocinon to syntometrine because it avoids unpleasant potential side effects such as nausea and vomiting, a headache and a temporary rise in blood pressure. If a postpartum haemorrhage does occur, syntometrine would be a first-line drug as the ergometrine component has a more rapid effect than using syntocinon on its own. I would also prefer to be left completely undisturbed between the first and second birth and for no one to feel for the cord.

After the birth I would not like my babies to be given Vitamin K in any form.

In summary, the babies' health and safety is the most important thing, but if everything goes well, I'd just like to have a normal delivery, without the medical trimmings!

Care guide 5: A care guide for an elective caesarean

This guide was prepared so as to make a caesarean as personal an experience as possible. A friend used a similar care guide and the outcome was lovely. I visited her in hospital soon after the birth.

> We would like...
> - ♥ surgery to be performed under epidural anaesthesia, not a general anaesthetic
> - ♥ our choice of music in theatre
> - ♥ sutures, not staples please
> - ♥ to be informed of everything that is happening, as it happens
> - ♥ the screen to be lowered so [the mother] can see the baby delivered
> - ♥ to discover the sex of the baby ourselves
> - ♥ to be given the baby to hold straight away, if possible
> - ♥ the baby to be washed, weighed and checked within [the mother]'s view
> - ♥ to see the placenta at the time of delivery and then to have it frozen for us to take home
> - ♥ help offering the baby the breast at the earliest opportunity, if necessary
> - ♥ additional help with offering the breast so that baby gets an opportunity to suckle every hour or so, to help establish breastfeeding as quickly as possible
> - ♥ no other nourishment or fluids to be offered to baby
> - ♥ [the mother] and baby to bed-share as much as possible during our hospital stay, or to sleep in a cot beside the bed
>
> Thank you for helping us to optimise this birthing experience for both mother and baby.

Care guide 6: A more poetic approach...

This last guide, which first appeared in *Midwifery Today*, apparently took words from the dreams of 200 women, 'translated' for hospital staff! The editor/author, Janine DeBaise, has four children herself so she no doubt also included some ideas from her own experience.[5]

> No blue hospital gown. No sterile drapes. When I give birth, I want to be naked. I want my body to choose the colour of its growing.
> No enema. No antiseptic wash. No shaving of pubic hair. If I wanted to shave something, I'd shave my head. Like Jean-Luc Picard. I've always wanted to be captain of a star ship. When I give birth, I explore uncharted territory, I move and writhe into new worlds. I want to go where no man has gone before.
> In 1872, an English doctor named John Braxton Hicks discovered pre-labour contractions. This was sort of like Columbus discovering America. Some people already knew it was there.

No drugs. No epidural. I want to feel the baby moving, his hard head pushing through layers of me. My bones shifting, my uterus contracting. I want to feel birth. I want to know fire.

No episiotomy. No amniotomy. I don't want anything that rhymes with lobotomy. I prefer to stretch slowly, burning in a rim of panting breaths around my baby's head.

The doctor, Pierre Vellay, wrote that mums-to-be must be 'trained in the proper way'. His vision: "Labouring women should be like expert engineers with perfect machines and carefully presented information [who] control, direct and regulate their bodies."

No syntocinon drip. No synthetic hormone to stimulate labour. Let my baby choose his own birthday. My body does not recognise the ticking of the clock on the wall.

I don't want to control my body. I want to surrender. Let the darkness soak through me, drip down my legs. Let the pulse of that unborn voice throb through me.

I don't want a needle stuck in my hand. If labour slows, I'll lie in the sun on a fur quilt and let my husband caress my nipples. I prefer to get my hormones the primitive way.

No electronic fetal monitor. I don't need a machine to tell me how my baby is doing. He kicks, he twists, he somersaults inside of me.

The doctor, Robert Bradley, advocated the idea of the husband as the labour coach. He liked the idea of natural birth, but still he thought that somehow a man had to be in charge.

No bright lights. No noise. No cheerleading cheers. Don't give me instructions. My body knows what to do. Birth is not a team sport. I don't want a coach. I want my husband's presence. His hands to grip. His arms a sling to lean the baby bulk against.

No stupid jokes. No cheerful chatter. No television, please. I want to listen to the moans rising in my throat. I want to hear the child singing in my womb.

In the 1950s a French obstetrician named Ferdinand Lamaze began teaching something he called childbirth without pain. French Catholics were horrified, the Bible said it was supposed to be painful. [Actually, no it didn't!]

No delivery table. I am not a plate of spaghetti. Let me give birth on the bed. A table works fine for conception, but it's way too hard and far too awkward for birth.

"Male science disregards female experiences because it can never share them." Grantly Dick-Read said this in 1933. No one listened to him. I know what I want for my baby.

No nursery. No dummy. No bottles. No cot. No cheerful, white-coated, well-scrubbed, briskly walking, thermometer-wielding nurses, please. Let the baby sleep against my skin, feed from my breast, wrap his wrinkled blue limbs in the heat of my body.

Nothing intrauterine, nothing intravenous.

I prefer to give birth in simple words. Breathe. Push. Touch. Pain. Wet. Stretch. Bum. Birth. Yes. For 50 years, doctors have used these terms: Braxton-Hicks contractions, Bradley birth, Lamaze breathing. But a woman knows. The mystery is too overwhelming. We can never name it.

When the baby's head crowns, I want to touch the wrinkled scalp. I want to cradle the head in my palms while he is still inside of me, his neck stuck in the warm swollen parts of me. My moans will be the guide I need to pull him out of myself.

Hot compresses. Yes. Dim lights, a bath of warm water. Yes. Hands massaging me. Yes. My husband lying next to me, solid to lean against. Yes. The smell and feel of a slippery newborn baby wriggling against my naked skin. Yes. Yes. Yes.

When things don't go well

Preparing for the birth is particularly important because your experiences are likely to affect your future self-image and peace of mind, as well as your new baby's health and happiness. And the arrangements you have in place when you go into labour might well determine the outcome of your birth experience.

> I was concerned when I heard the experiences of two colleagues, who'd had the same consultant, at the same hospital. One had been forcibly held down by midwives during the actual birth, and given an obligatory episiotomy. The other had had a traumatic 'emergency' caesarean which she felt sure afterwards had been unnecessary. She just couldn't stop talking about it—I felt she needed to go for therapy.

Birthframe 49

When women don't think ahead the outcome is often far from ideal, as the next account shows. Sometimes, tragically, life gives us no second chances.

No family history on either side of multiples...
I suppose history has to start somewhere.

No family history on either side of multiples... I suppose history has to start somewhere. I continued to work full-time in a leisure centre on my feet all day. Felt well throughout. A little breathless on dog walks up hills. Sickness always at tea time. I didn't feel I got very big but people tell me otherwise. I would have to roll off the sofa, though!

Hospital appointments—scans took longer to ensure they didn't do the same one twice! I never bothered to learn any doctors' names as I did not see the same person twice. My named consultant was on 'long-term sick', I later discovered. Three heart monitors across my bump was always long-winded. One consultant said it was a waste of time because of interference between them... It didn't stop them doing it.

The local midwife eventually made contact. We had been overlooked. She talked about antenatal classes. I was aware the kids would probably come at around 33-36 weeks. But there seemed no sense of urgency from anyone. I never heard from or saw the midwife again. So a rapport was never made with any professional. We seemed to be continually 'overlooked' or forgotten about.

At 28 weeks (only 10 weeks after finding out I was expecting triplets) I went into premature labour and had an emergency caesarean.

Didn't learn names... never saw the same person twice.
My named consultant was on 'long-term sick'.

I had another week at work before maternity leave started. I had been at work all day. Came home in the evening and couldn't get comfortable. At 10.00pm I noticed a pink tinge going to the toilet and had 'period pains'. Called the hospital for advice and they said, "Come in." The journey was very uncomfortable. John wanted to drive quickly but every bump in the road jarred. Arrived 11.30pm-ish. Heart monitors x3 and internal examination. "You are 4cm dilated. Do you know what an epidural is?" I was then shaved. Very uncomfortable. It all happened very quickly with no suggestion of trying to stop labour. I was wheeled into theatre with John. At 1.49am, 1.50am and 1.51am Friday Triplet 1, 2 and 3 were taken out of me. As far as I'm concerned, I didn't give birth. We were not shown the babies. Not even a quick lift up over the screen to see. Not a "One boy, OK." Nothing. Didn't hear them cry. John saw them four or five hours later. My first look was Polaroid photos in my ward room. Taken down to Intensive Care to see them later Friday afternoon, about 12 hours after having them. They were pointed out to me. It felt like: "That one, that one and that one are yours." 2lb 3oz, 2lb 5oz, 3lb 1oz birth weight. All wires, netting around the heads, feed tubes down the noses. They could have pointed to any incubator in the room and said it was mine. I felt nothing. Which one do you look at first? What are you supposed to do? What are you expected to do? That was the start of three months' hospital care.

I was given a breast pump. Express, bottle, label, fridge. This continued in the hospital and with a double electric pump on loan at home as well. I came home Monday—two nights after having them. The nurses care for them 24 hours a day. In an attempt to involve you, they hold back. How am I supposed to know what they want or need when walking in for only a few hours? An idea of timing for you: April, wedding—May, pregnant—July, found out triplets—15 October, had kids—22 October, moved house—January, kids come home.

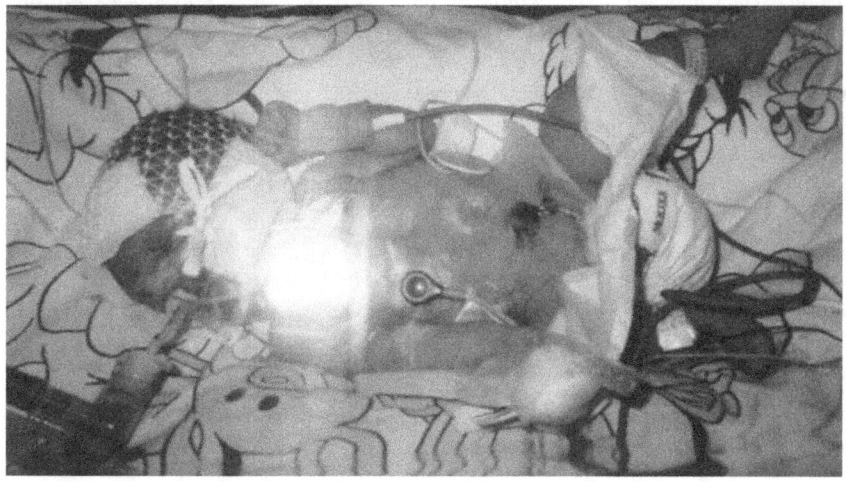

One of the triplets, shortly after the birth

Bill developed hydrocephalis. We were told he was going to have another lumbar puncture—we didn't know he had had the first one! He needed a series of six. This was to reduce pressure and stop the head diameter increasing. If it didn't work, a shunt would be required. He was OK. Nine months later we were told he had cerebral palsy.

As they improved and gained weight, and were able to breathe without help, they were moved from Intensive Care to High Care, then Special Care. We were going through the motions of caring for these kids—learning how to do everything. Still no feeling of bonding or attachment.

The day before bringing them home John and I spent the first night alone—in charge—in control—responsible for our children. Hard work, no sleep, but satisfying. Our departure from the hospital involved being let out one door and being asked to bring the cots back. Not escorted or helped to the door. Three car seats. One three-door car. John in the back, jammed between two babies. Me driving with another alongside. No looking back. (I wouldn't go back 'to visit' if you paid me.) Life can start now. Note: Need another car before our backs give out.

We put a big whiteboard on the wall in our lounge. This kept track of who had been fed and changed and when. No sleep, not eating proper meals, needing help but not wanting it all resulted in postnatal depression. I asked for help from our health visitor three or four months after the kids came home. I was given anti-depressants. For a couple of days I felt dizzy but began to feel more 'myself'. I took one course or packet, but didn't go back for more. I didn't like needing help. I should have kept with them—they really did make a big difference.

Three and a half years on. We still go through the motions of caring for our children. We have a bigger family than we wanted. We have never had a rush of love for them. We still look longingly at parents with singletons, seeing all the things we couldn't, can't and will never be able to do. I feel the whole premature birth and experience described has played a huge part in this lack of emotion.

Things I wish other women pregnant with triplets could do:

- Go and see a Special Care Baby Unit now—just in case. Ask about 'kangaroo care'. It was never mentioned and now I think that skin-to-skin contact with each child may have helped 'connect us' a little. (See Birthframe 50 on the next page.)
- Rest and read as much as possible now. Pregnancy, birth and ideas for later. You won't get time when they arrive.
- Arrange help, especially regular week in, week out (same time, same day). It's a lifeline. Knowing when someone is going to walk in is great.
- Go outside with them. Being stopped and asked questions is much better than being stuck indoors.
- Try and make time to have a bath or shower! Do something for yourself.

Come to terms with the fact you will never be able to sit and chat with other parents in the same way as parents of singletons. You are not rude—just preoccupied!

It's true, things do sometimes go wrong... But is the outcome of an apparent disaster always awful? Can we ever do anything to improve things?

Birthframe 50

In the following account, an American woman Krisanne Collard explains how she came to use a very natural approach to supplement her new daughter's technological support system.

In July 1994, my husband and I moved to the little town of Canon City, Colorado. We had no family in the state—in fact, we had no family within a day's drive. I found out I was pregnant within two weeks of the move. We were ecstatic! We had tried to get pregnant for three years and suffered a miscarriage eight months before. We were finally going to have the baby we had dreamt about for so long.

I had my first antenatal appointment at the end of September when I was 11 weeks pregnant. The doctor asked me to provide a urine sample, confirmed I was pregnant and told me my due date would be 4 March. He sent the rest of my sample off, so the lab could run all of the standard tests for new mums. He told me everything looked wonderful and I would be able to hear the heartbeat at my next appointment. I scheduled my next appointment for a month later and my husband and I left the office overjoyed at the thought everything was fine. We went to Wal-Mart and looked at all of the pretty baby things, dreaming of what our new baby's room would look like.

The doctor called me three days after the appointment and asked to see me in his office later that day. He sat us both down and gave us the bad news. All of the standard tests he had run indicated that I no longer had a viable pregnancy. Our baby was probably no longer alive. He scheduled a scan for Monday—just to be 'sure'. It was then Friday. All weekend we worried and panicked. By Monday afternoon, I had convinced myself that she was indeed dead—that we would have to try again. When I lay down on the table and told the technician why I was there, she had tears in her eyes as she prepared to take a look. For two agonising minutes, all was quiet. Then, she screamed, "Oh my God! Look! Your baby's moving!" Sure enough, there was my little fighter, angry at the world—wiggling and trying to get comfortable. Her heartbeat was strong. My doctor never had an explanation for the incorrect test results.

For the next two months, my pregnancy went by the book. I had some morning sickness and started to get a bump. I felt her move for the first time on my birthday (14 November). We bought baby stuff and started to decorate the baby's room. We were the happiest parents in the world!

Her heartbeat was strong. My doctor never had an explanation for the incorrect test results.

But, on 30 November, 24 weeks into my pregnancy, everything went black. I woke up with a dull ache in my lower back. I didn't think much of it till I started bleeding at about noon. I called my doctor and my husband, who rushed me to the local hospital. I was immediately hooked up to a fetal monitor and checked for dilation. I was already 5cm and her feet were in the birth canal. She was coming breech. Next thing I knew, I was being prepped for an immediate C-section. I was sobbing, screaming and confused. No one had time to talk to me—no one would let me know how the baby was doing. My husband and I were terrified!

When I woke up, I was in the recovery room. All I can remember was asking for a drink of water. I didn't ask about my baby because I thought she was dead. I just started crying—mourning her already. After about half an hour, another nurse came into the room. I asked her, "Was it a boy or a girl?" She smiled at me and said, "You have a beautiful little girl!" I was confused. She hadn't spoken in the past tense and she was happy. My daughter was still alive!

I was moved into a private room and my doctor came to talk to me. He told me that my daughter had been born weighing only 1lb, 12oz and only $13\frac{1}{2}$ inches long. He said she came out kicking and screaming, angry at the world, but she was VERY sick. They were transporting her to a level three NICU (Neonatal Intensive Care Unit) at Memorial Hospital, an hour away, in Colorado Springs. He told me that there was only a 30% chance that she was going to make it through the night. I didn't get to see her before they took her away. As I recovered from the C-section, I called the hospital she was in three times a day to check on her. She had been put on a special oscillating ventilator, I was told, and required maximum oxygen doses to keep her saturation up. They said she had got an infection from me and was very sick. I had a bladder infection I didn't know about (I have always been symptom-less), and she had come early because she was too sick to stay in my womb. They assured me over and over that she was a fighter and was going to be fine. They encouraged me to talk to her over the phone—but I felt silly because I hadn't even met her yet. Since we now felt she was going to make it, we decided on a name—Kaia Michele. A strong Norwegian name for a very brave little girl.

When I was released from my local hospital, four days after her birth, my husband and I immediately went to visit Kaia. When I walked into the NICU, nothing could have prepared me for what I saw. She was the size of two Barbie dolls stuck together. She had the blue bilirubin lights on her and tubes and wires everywhere. Her skin was translucent and her veins showed through her skin. I looked around, hoping to see 'my' baby in another bed. I looked back at Kaia. The nurse urged me closer and turned off the blue lights so I could take a closer look. I was terrified. The nurse urged me to touch her and talk to her—let her know I was there. I hesitated. She looked like she would break if I touched her. I started to talk to her, but it took 15 minutes to finally get up the nerve to touch her. When I did, her alarms went off. I jerked my hand back as the nurse came over. She had to rub her till her heart started again. I couldn't handle it—my baby had rejected me—I left the nursery in tears and went home.

> The next night, as we were eating dinner,
> I burst into tears. My husband led me to the sofa.

The next night, as we were eating dinner, I burst into tears. My husband took my hand and led me to the sofa. He put my shoes on and said, "Let's go—Mummy needs a baby fix." We drove the hour to Memorial Hospital. All the way there, I told my husband that THIS time I was going to be strong. I was going to count her toes and talk to her and let her know how loved she was. I was so excited!

But, when I got to her side and touched her, her alarms sounded again. The nurse had to start her heart yet again. I just sat there for the next 30 minutes and looked at her, crying. Why didn't my baby love me? I wondered. A nurse specialist named Theresa Kledzik (nicknamed 'The Whisper Lady') came over to talk to me. She asked me if I had held my baby yet. I just laughed and said that Kaia couldn't tolerate me touching her—I would kill her if I tried to hold her. Theresa just smiled at me and asked me to follow her into the other room. She gave me a gown, told me to take off my bra and shirt and put the gown on with the opening in the front. I was in shock as I changed.

When I walked back into the nursery, there were three nurses getting Kaia ready to be transferred to my chest. It took about 15 minutes for them to get her ready and I got more and more nervous every second. I changed my mind about 10 times, but the nurses didn't pay me any attention. I sat down in a strange-looking chair. (I learned later that it was specially designed to be used with babies on oscillating ventilators.) They laid Kaia on my chest, on her tummy, skin-to-skin with me. Her head was resting above my heart and her tiny feet were curled up in my hand. The tubes and wires were taped to my gown. I stared at the monitors as she wiggled into a comfortable position. I knew they were going to sound. I held my breath. She calmed down after about five minutes and stopped moving. I thought she was dead. I tried to make sense of the monitors. I called Theresa over and asked if I had killed her. She just laughed and said, "No, she's happy!" I looked down at Kaia and noticed the peaceful look on her face. I looked back up at Theresa and smiled. My daughter had just made me feel like a Mum for the very first time!

I was able to hold Kaia every day for two hours. I couldn't get to the hospital fast enough every day to share that special time with her. Within a few days, I was able to transfer her to my chest all by myself, even with the tubes and wires everywhere. I was always disappointed when our time together came to an end. She responded very well to it, and her oxygen requirements lowered during every session. She never had any episodes where she stopped breathing (apnoeas) or periods where her heart stopped (bradyas) while I held her. She would just go into a deep, healing sleep and actually tolerated my touch when she was on the warming table. The future was looking very promising for her.

When she was two weeks old, she had trouble getting comfortable on my chest. I wound up putting her back after only half an hour. I spent another hour with her, then headed home. When I got there, there was a message on my answering machine telling me to immediately return to the hospital. My husband and I rushed back just in time to say goodbye as they rushed her into theatre. They had no idea what was wrong, and no idea how long we would have to wait. Four hours later, the Neonatal Surgeon came out and told us she was going to be fine. She had had a small perforation at the end of her large intestines and the surgeon had made a colostomy. We got to see her within an hour. She had a huge bandage on her tummy and they had given her paralysing drugs. She looked so little and sick. I cried as I held her hand for the next two hours. The nurses assured me I'd be able to hold her again in a few days. I missed her so much.

I visited her the next morning. She was very uncomfortable and was requiring maximum pain medication doses. She wiggled and cried (silently because of the ventilator tube in her mouth). Finally, after an hour of seeing her suffer, the nurse said, "Hold your baby, she needs you!" I leapt at the chance and got her out of bed myself—making sure not to put too much pressure on her tummy. The nurse came over a few minutes later to check on us. She smiled. Kaia was actually lying on her newly operated-on tummy, sleeping peacefully. I held her for the full two hours and she didn't even need her next dose of pain medicine! I was on top of the world. I had got to hold and comfort my child!

Kaia required another operation, at 3 weeks old, to modify her colostomy. She was moved to the Intermediate Nursery after two months, and came home on oxygen and a heart monitor a month later, on 27 February, two weeks before her due date.

She went back into the NICU two weeks later for an eye operation to correct ROP (retinopathy of prematurity), which is common in preemies who have been on oxygen for long periods of time.

A month after that—she was $4\frac{1}{2}$ months old by this time—she had a fundoplication [an operation in which the top of the stomach is wrapped around the oesophagus, creating a valve] to correct severe reflux. We had to feed her through a tube (called a G-tube) for the next four months.

> I was given strange looks or asked questions.
> We didn't get out much because it was such a hassle.

When she was $8\frac{1}{2}$ months old, she had her final operation to reconnect her colostomy and take out the feeding tube. She remained on oxygen and a heart monitor, continuously till she was a year old. This meant lugging around a 15lb oxygen tank and a 10lb heart monitor everywhere. People were very curious. In the grocery and department stores, I was given strange looks or stopped and asked 100 questions before I could continue my shopping. We didn't get out much because it was such a hassle.

That first year was the most stressful one of my life

That first year of Kaia's life was the most stressful year of my own life. There were so many things to do: doctor appointments, operations, therapy sessions, medications and colostomy bag changes. And so many milestones: first smiles, first words, first steps, first hugs! I was on a roller coaster that didn't seem to have an end in sight. I joined a local playgroup and an online preemie support group when Kaia was 6 months old. Both groups gave me so much love and support. They kept me from going insane. There are MANY premature baby support groups on the Internet and probably one in your own city or town. To find the one that's right for you, join several—don't limit yourself to just one. Every support group is different and unique. Your hospital will be able to tell you if there is a local support group in your area.

At our NICU reunion party in August 1995 Kaia was 9 months old. I ran into the nurse specialist who had encouraged me to hold my daughter the first time, Theresa Kledzik. We talked for almost an hour about 'kangaroo care'. That's what she called the skin-to-skin contact I had with Kaia. I asked her if all babies were able to be kangarooed and she told me that I had been very lucky. Most parents in other hospitals weren't able to kangaroo their babies as soon as I was. Most parents had to wait till their babies were 'stable', off the ventilator or three pounds before they were allowed to hold them. I was shocked! Kaia would have been over two months old if I had had to wait. I couldn't imagine having to wait that long to feel like a Mum.

When I got home, I immediately told my online support group about what I had learnt. Most wrote back asking what kangaroo care was and how they could do it. They had never heard of it before. I searched the Internet and found only one site that even mentioned kangaroo care. I was upset. How many other babies had to suffer without the loving touch of their parents? I emailed Theresa and she sent me all of the literature and research she had on the subject.

There was so much, it took days to go through it all. I was amazed at all I learnt and angry that more hospitals didn't embrace kangaroo care. Here is just a glimpse of the amazing discoveries I made...

- ♥ Kangaroo care—originally called 'kangaroo mother care'—was developed in Bogotá, Colombia in July 1977 by neonatologists Edgar Rey and Hector Martinez. It received worldwide publicity in 1983 when the startling success of the approach became known. The mortality rate for premature babies in Bogotá had been 70% (39% in the US at that time) due to lack of power and reliable equipment (such as ventilators and incubators). After getting mums to carry their babies continuously in slings on their chests, the mortality rate decreased to 30%!

- ♥ Research has shown that mums and babies have a natural thermal synchrony. When Mum thinks her baby is getting too cool, her body heats up in response. When Mum thinks her baby is too hot, she cools down. Sorry, Dad, this only seems to happen with mums.

- ♥ The skin-to-skin contact helps in milk production and milk letdown. It is very important for mothers of premature babies to pump and store their milk for the time when the baby can start eating. The breastmilk of a mother who has given birth prematurely is tolerated by the baby's immature digestive system more easily than formula.
- ♥ Apnoea (interruptions in normal breathing), bradycardia (severe heart rate decreases) and tachycardia (severe heart rate increases) decrease or disappear altogether because kangaroo care regulates breathing and stabilises heart rates. These episodes are VERY common in premature babies and can easily lead to death or lack of oxygen to the brain, which could cause brain damage.
- ♥ Kangaroo care stimulates the baby to gain weight more rapidly and be discharged up to 50% sooner because there are greater periods of deep sleep that enable the preemie's body to heal faster.
- ♥ Kangaroo care can also be done with full-term babies who have colic. Colic is believed by many to be a baby's inability to transition from one sleep-state to another. Kangaroo care allows babies to enter into the deepest sleep state with ease. Most preemies that are kangarooed never suffer with colic. Mine didn't.
- ♥ Preemies who are kangarooed during treatments (such as 'heel sticks' to check the amount of oxygen in the blood—an hourly requirement for preemies on a ventilator) experience far less discomfort and require no extra pain medication during these painful procedures. Kaia didn't even seem to notice the treatments if she was being kangarooed.

After telling my online support group about what I had learnt, I was encouraged to set up a website to educate the world about the wonders of kangaroo care. One of my online friends helped me design the website www.geocities.com/roopage and several preemie mums wrote stories about their first kangaroo care experience. I received so many wonderful stories, I decided to compile them all into a tiny booklet that I could send to NICUs and parents across the world. *Kangarooing Our Little Miracles* lets parents, nurses and doctors share the emotional joy kangaroo care brings to babies and parents. Most parents shared with me that by writing down their emotions, it helped with their healing process. I gave away over 200 booklets within the first year and received at least 15 emails a month from parents, neonatologists and nurses who wanted to implement kangaroo care in their hospitals. It feels wonderful to be an instigator.

In October 1996, I was asked to speak at the First International Congress of Kangaroo Care in Baltimore, MD. I was both flattered and nervous. I blew the minds of several nurses and neonatologists in the audience when I told them about my kangaroo care experience. They couldn't believe that I had been able to hold her on a ventilator (an oscillating one at that), or hold her when she was so unstable. They actually gasped when I told them about her reaction to being kangarooed after tummy surgery. They all cheered at the end of my speech when I told them that all babies deserve to feel their mother's and father's love and all parents deserve the opportunity to be parents, not visitors.

My 'preemie' is now 8 years old and going into 3rd grade. Where has the time gone? She is doing wonderfully in school and has no lasting effects of being born prematurely. She is sweet and kind and funny. She puts a smile on my face every day. The other day, when we were swimming at the local pool, another child asked her why her tummy was all messed up (she insisted on getting a bikini even though her massive scars showed). I held my breath, wondering if I should step in and help her explain. My eyes filled with tears as she said, proudly, "I was born the size of two Barbie dolls. I have these scars to show me how strong I had to be to live." I know that I helped give her that strength. I am so proud of her and thankful to Memorial Hospital of Colorado Springs for giving me the opportunity to be her mum!

We found out I was pregnant again in December 1995. My pregnancy was uncomplicated. My doctor checked me every two weeks for bladder infections. (I was treated for two during my pregnancy.) My doctor informed me that the antenatal pills I took with Kaia might have played a role in her early birth because they contained a high content of iodine, which I am highly allergic to. He switched me to an antenatal vitamin that contained no iodine. With Kaia, whenever I had missed one pill, I spotted. After missing two, I had Kaia. I am still very allergic to iodine and have to watch which multivitamins I take and keep salt out of my diet as much as possible. Even though I showed no signs of premature labour (i.e. contractions or bleeding), my doctor put me on terbulatine (used to stop contractions) at 28 weeks to be sure I wouldn't go into premature labour. I strongly encourage women who have ANY problems with their pregnancy to talk to their consultant. Don't just let it go. Even a small problem could snowball and mean life or death for your baby.

My mum teased me as I went through the summer months uncomfortable and VERY pregnant. Every time I would complain about how miserable I was, she would laugh and say, "YOU are the one who wants to see what it's like to carry a baby to term. You are going the full 40, young lady!"

My doctor left for his first holiday ever on 1 August, a Friday, right after my 36-week appointment. He took me off the terbulatine and told me that I was NOT going to have her till he got back! I just laughed and told him that I wanted to have her that weekend. I did! I started having contractions within 24 hours of discontinuing the terbulatine and Katherine Elsie was born on 4 August, Sunday, weighing a healthy 6lb, $15\frac{1}{2}$oz by C-section. I was able to hold her within a couple of hours after she was born. I unwrapped her, counted her toes and fingers, and held her 'kangaroo care' style for hours as I slept.

She has been perfectly healthy—I was able to actually enjoy her first year. However, Katherine is a real free spirit. The tantrums that child threw! WOW! Kaia tried to imitate her sister when she was about 3 years old. She lay down on the floor, spread her arms wide and said, "Mum, I'm angry!" I just smiled down at her and said, "You forgot to scream." She got up, dusted off her trousers and smiled at me. She never tried it again. I found out later that year that Kaia was short for Katherine in Norwegian. As they get older, I have noticed how ironic this is. They are as close as identical twins, but as different as night and day. Just like their names!

The doctor who delivered Katherine suggested, after she was born, that I shouldn't have any more children. I was heartbroken AND relieved. My husband always wanted eight! He said that I hadn't healed well from my first C-section, and delivering Katherine had been very difficult with all of the scar tissue. It would be nearly impossible for him to deliver another baby safely. I was also told that I would never be able to deliver vaginally because I have a heart-shaped uterus (called a bicornuate uterus), which allows the baby only half the space to grow and no space in which to turn near the end of the pregnancy. (This had no affect on Kaia being born prematurely, incidentally.)

Today, both of my children are healthy and happy. They are the lights of my life. I know I wouldn't be the person I am today without the experiences of having them and bringing them up. They have taught me so much and made me stronger. I am forever grateful. Thank you, baby girls! I love you!

Krisanne Collard

Note: There is some uncertainty as to when 'kangaroo mother care' was first used. In some articles and websites it's given as being 1978.[6] However, in the French translation of the first article by Edgar Rey, it is clearly given as July 1977.[7] I asked Michel about kangaroo care...

In what circumstances would you say it's appropriate to use so-called 'kangaroo care' with premature babies, instead of using conventional incubators?

In Bogotá [Columbia, South America], they have used kangaroo care with babies below 1000g. The prerequisite is that the baby can breathe without any assistance. In Pithiviers we could not be as audacious as in Bogotá. We used this method for babies weighing more than 1700 or 1800 grams (and breathing easily). If a woman wants to use kangaroo care, it is better to start in the birthing room, without interrupting at all the skin-to-skin contact. It is difficult without the enthusiastic cooperation of the health professionals.[8]

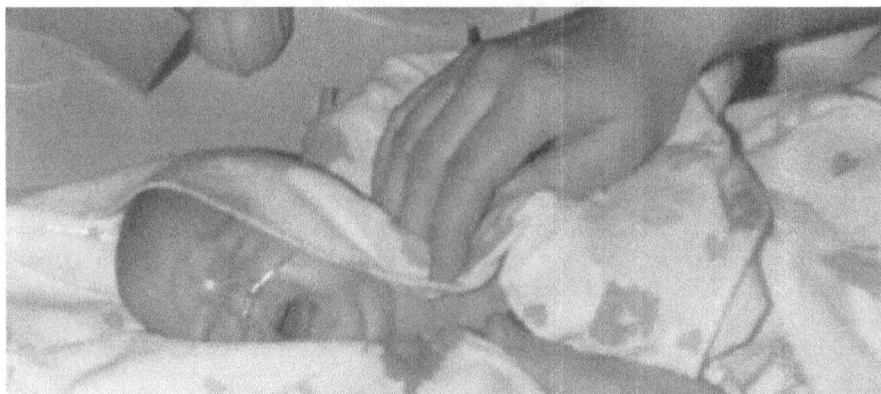

Kaia, 3 months old. First bath at home.

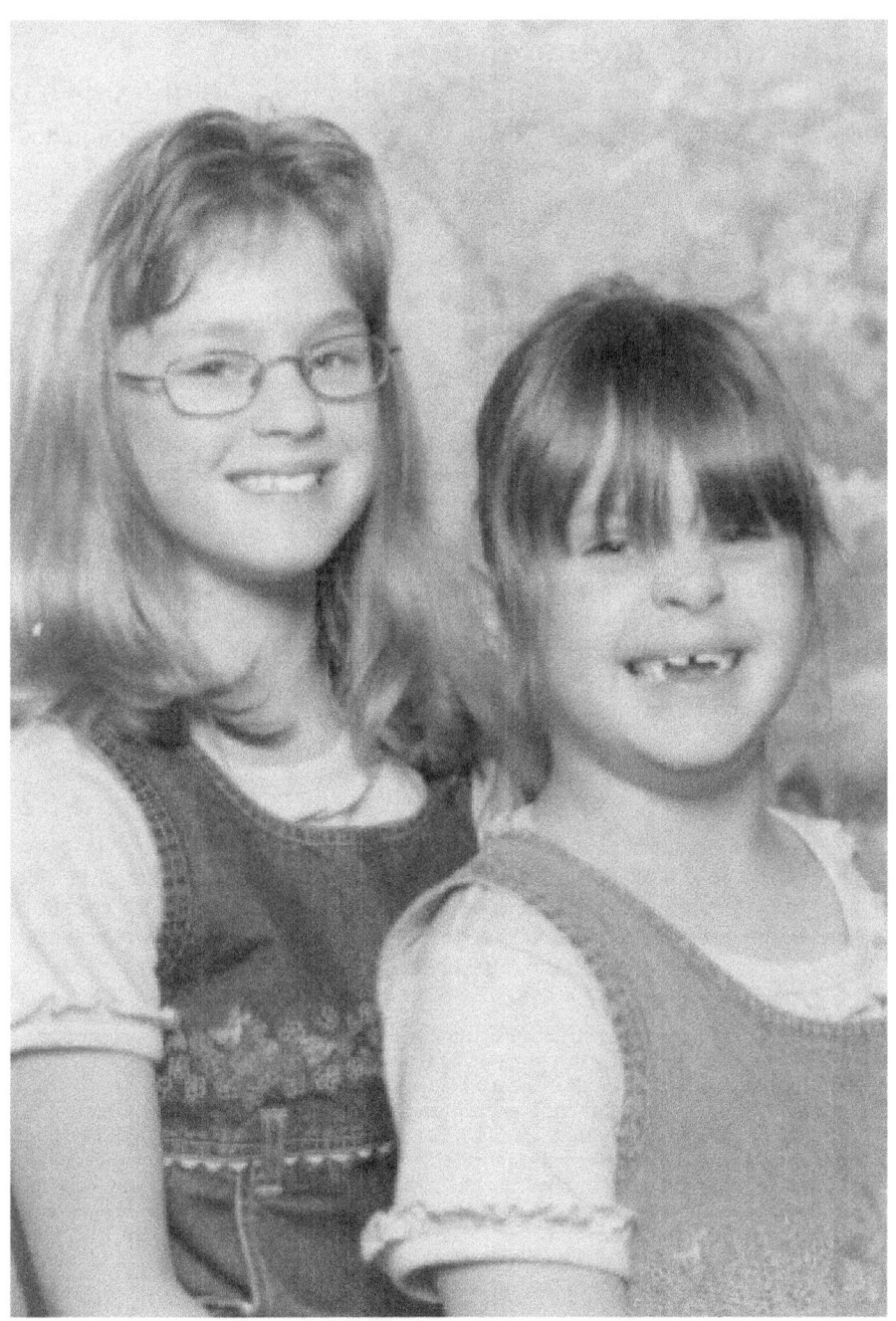
Kaia, aged 8, with her sister Katherine, aged 7

When things go just fine!

Birthframe 51

On a more positive note here's a woman who succeeded in getting the births she wanted through thorough preparation, research and persistence. Without all this her experience would probably have been quite dramatically different. (This is a summary, produced by the contributor, of a much longer account.)

> I am a 40-year-old woman who gave birth to twins normally five months ago in an NHS hospital. It is possible! I did it with a lot of persistence and research, after several meetings with various midwives, consultants and hospital managers and by finding independent midwives and a consultant who supported me in trying for normal deliveries for our babies. With some luck, a very supportive partner and midwives, and a consultant who went beyond the call of duty by being available for me in the labour ward (though by my request, not in the delivery room) when he was not normally on call, I gave birth to the first twin in a birthing pool, and the second on land, without any drugs or intervention at 39 weeks and two days. Both babies were well and weighed in at just over and under 6lb. I would like to encourage other expectant twin mums or those with a high risk pregnancy to inform themselves of what the risks associated with their pregnancy are, what the birth options are with their various pros and cons and to persist in trying to lay the conditions and plans for a natural birth, if that is what they want. Giving birth to our babies is one of the most satisfying, joyous and proud experiences I have had.

Birthframe 52

Here's another account of a potentially difficult birth which was eased through good preparation. After careful planning, this woman, Esther Culpin, gave her fourth baby a completely normal, safe and, as it happened, easy introduction to the world. In the light of her obstetric history, the practical preparations she made seem to have made all the difference.

> At a time when breech presentation is almost synonymous with caesarean section, I find it useful to write up the story of the easiest of my four deliveries. In this case, changing the birth environment absolutely transformed the way I gave birth. I set out to create a new birthing environment this time around, as my previous births, although loosely defined as 'normal', were definitely not. The births of my three sons followed long and traumatic labours and I experienced excessive blood loss immediately afterwards. Overall, birth appeared to be extremely risky and to contemplate it all over again did not seem like a good idea. The solution to my difficult birth experiences could have been an elective caesarean section. Instead, I had the opportunity to look more closely at important issues that might have affected the way my first three births had turned out.

Giving birth at home was a really important factor for me because of the absolute freedom it gave me to do as I wished in labour. I needed to arrange for a midwife to be in attendance who would respect my need for a calm and undisturbed environment. Michel Odent was happy to assume this role and was noticeably unperturbed by my traumatic labour and delivery record!

When, after 30 weeks of pregnancy, my daughter was persistently a breech presentation, I made no change of plan. I was still happy, confident and looking forward to an easier birth in the privacy of my home. At this point technology could have taken over, but all the required information seemed to be available, literally through the midwife's hands. There was never a suggestion that I should undergo an external cephalic version (ECV) and, having experienced that procedure 14 years previously, I did not feel I wished to undergo it again. Although I was still aiming for the birth to be at home, I booked in at the maternity hospital just one mile away, in case admission to hospital and emergency treatment should be required. Local midwives, although acquainted with home birth, indicated their preference not to be involved with a breech birth if it was to be at home.

I went into labour a week after my due date. This time around, as part of a strategy for giving birth easily, I aimed to keep myself rested. This was achieved by not doing too many things in a day so that I would be able to cope with the rigors of labour whenever it started. As the process got underway, I found that being at home had a direct effect on the way I coped and on the optimism I felt. (Remember, the baby was breech, I had never experienced an easy birth before, and I was at home!)

On the domestic front I was assisted by my husband. Again, considering my history of traumas associated with giving birth, he was superb. His responsibilities were wide-ranging, but his priority was to maintain a safe, dark and secure environment for me, so that I should experience no disturbances. A birthing pool in the living room was filled with warm water, in case it should be needed for pain relief. The children went out to breakfast with their grandparents. For this birth, because I badly wanted things to progress easily, I did not wish to have any distractions at all.

For me, labour in any circumstances remains hard, but given that this time I would be able to adopt any position, and there were no outsiders coming in and out of the room (as there could easily be in the hospital setting), I felt that I was on the way to giving birth quickly and easily.

In fact, for the first time in my experience, labour progressed extremely quickly and I found myself trying to slow things down so that I would not give birth before assistance arrived! What was noticeable at this point was the lack of instructions I was given: Michel gathered silently all the information he needed to assess the situation. I was obviously ready to deliver and, because I was not directed in any way, I decided to get into the pool! At the next contraction and whilst standing upright, my baby's body was born. I was assisted out of the pool and supported from behind so I could maintain a standing position. Now there was a long pause while the cord, which was wrapped tightly three times around her neck, was unwound. Her head was deflected by inserting a finger into her mouth before her head was delivered. During these few critical minutes there was no discussion about whether I had a girl or a boy.

For the first time, labour progressed extremely quickly

My daughter lay on the carpet, motionless at first. But, in that situation, I was her life support, just as I had been all along. The fact that I was personally and actively involved in those early moments was of prime importance to me, whatever the outcome would be. I trusted deeply that my daughter would live and I felt that my participation in every way would give her an optimal chance. But, whatever, we were together in this and that's how it should be, whatever the outcome.

The position that I adopted at this point, immediately after her birth, was also extremely advantageous. I was leaning over my daughter, who was lying on the ground. This was the optimal position in the early moments of her life: it aided the natural compression of the uterus, and meant that the baby could be readily gathered up as soon as this became appropriate. There was no cutting of the cord, no touching of my abdomen, and no administration of artificial hormones.

After a little while, I moved on to a nearby sofa and instinctively lay on my side with the baby. The move from floor to sofa was easily undertaken, the cord remaining slack in the process. I was now in that wonderful time following birth but had not experienced any preceding trauma.

Probably within the hour, the placenta separated and by that time the cord was lifeless and could be cut and tied. I really preferred the idea that the cord would not be cut in the early moments following birth, since this would maximise all the benefits to the baby. Blood loss was minimal. I had experienced a totally physiological third stage.[9]

This birth turned out to be easy and untraumatic. Very simple measures were taken to change the factors surrounding birth and these appeared to make a huge difference: I was at home, I had freedom to move around as I wished, I was not watched by anybody (including my husband), and I had faith in 'the midwife'. From my perspective as the mother, the fact that my baby was in a breech position proved to be a secondary consideration.

Esther Culpin

I asked Michel about his approach. Here are his comments...

Esther's daughter was born several years before the publication in *The Lancet* in the year 2000 of the huge randomised multicentre trial that is considered a landmark in the history of breech births.[10] It is easy to summarise what we learnt from this study: we learnt that a breech birth in a conventional hospital and in the presence of an obstetrician is dangerous. The case of Esther's delivery does not belong to this framework. It occurred outside the conventional hospital environment and, in the mind of Esther, I was probably an old friend of the family with an experience of home births and breech births, rather than an obstetrician.

What can we say today to women who want to avoid a caesarean section in spite of a breech presentation at term? Here are the rules that I gradually adopted after supervising about 300 breech births by the vaginal route:

- The best possible environment is usually a place with nobody else around other than an experienced, motherly and low profile midwife who is not scared by a breech birth.
- The first stage of labour is a trial. If it is straightforward, easy and fast, the vaginal route is possible. If the first stage is long and difficult, a caesarean section should be decided without any delay, before a point of no return is reached.

- Because the first stage is a trial, it is important not to make it artificially too easy, either with drugs, or even with water immersion.
- After the point of no return, privacy remains the key word.
- It is permissible to be more audacious with a frank breech than with a footling breech. A cord prolapse outside the hospital environment can be a disaster.

When the worse comes to the worst

Esther hinted at the possibility of something going wrong. Of course, this is everyone's ultimate fear.

What if it really does? I was interested to read Nina Klose's comments on this in one of her emails to me...

> I'm not religious in any formal Christian sense, and there's a lot in Christianity or organised religion that I don't agree with. But when you start talking about pregnancy and birth, you endlessly come up against the utter wonder of so many miracles. To be pregnant is to inhabit a divine state. How is it that I am blessed with such a gift, to carry another spirit?
>
> While pregnant one must face the knowledge that not all pregnancies culminate in a birth. And not all births culminate in a new life. If the Life Spirit brings death in this pregnancy, I must be strong enough to accept it. Accepting pregnancy means accepting potential death, the baby's or even one's own. It is a huge—and potentially painful—gift to be given this risk.
>
> I can hardly imagine what it would be like to experience the loss of a pregnancy through miscarriage or the loss of a child through stillbirth. Even healthy pregnancies contain huge losses. No one ever talks about the mourning we go through as mothers. I fret over my new, fat, just-pregnant self. Does that sound petty? But we are so conditioned to look at ourselves in the mirror, to try to be thin, pretty, desirable. I must relinquish my usual self for the childbearing year and more.
>
> Then I grieve for the end of the pregnancy—for no longer carrying the babe under my heart; and for no longer being a Queen among Women, Bearer of Life, but only a tired, overtaxed new mother. I grieve for the changes in the family—the loss of a bond with my husband through exhaustion and the demands of the new baby. I grieve for the loss of the older children's places as youngest child, or only boy, or only girl. I mourn the passing of the huge drama of birth. I mourn that I can't return and try it again some other way. If the birth didn't go how I longed for, I will mourn the loss forever.
>
> Birth is a huge gift, but so painful.
>
> *Nina Klose*

Accepting pregnancy means accepting potential death, the baby's or even one's own. It is a huge gift to be given this risk.

What if things really do go wrong and it's too late to do anything?

Birthframe 53

This account is about a woman I met when she was 38 weeks pregnant with her third child—her name is Monica Reid. I was 36 weeks pregnant myself at the time and had no idea what significance '38 weeks' had for Monica. We became great friends almost immediately and within four weeks we had both given birth again.

One day when Monica came to visit me with her new baby (while our older children were at school and playgroup), she told me what had happened when she'd been 38 weeks pregnant with her first child. As our two babies sat or breastfed on our laps, the story eventually came tumbling out. (She'd agreed to let me record it.) Monica said when we'd finished that this was the first time she'd told the story in such great detail since the birth.

To make the transcribed interview more readable—and also somewhat shorter!—I first edited the account to turn it into a monologue. Then, as I did with every contributor, I asked Monica to check through and rewrite (if necessary) before giving me permission to use it in this book. Monica has told her story because she would like to give other women who have similar difficult experiences the comfort that comes from knowing that we are never entirely alone in our experiences in life, however awful, and that, yes, there is a light at the end of the tunnel.

It's funny because when people ask me how many children I have I always go to say actually I have three children but I always have to stop myself and say I have two children because I don't always feel comfortable talking about my first child, who we called Marley after the legendary Bob Marley. He was actually called Marley Levi Mandela. We called him after Nelson Mandela, the great civil rights leader of South Africa and Levi after his dad. It's a very powerful name. It's just unfortunate that he wasn't powerful enough to stay on this Earth. On record at the hospital I'm a mother of three but I only have two living children.

Marley was born on 11 August at 7.48 in the evening. I remember everything, It was a very rainy night in 1994. The labour was awful. He was actually born on a Thursday, but I was started off on labour on the Tuesday. And it all started, if I go back to the Monday morning before, when I was 38 weeks pregnant. That weekend before I had him had just been a normal weekend. Looking forward to the baby, going through the baby's things for about the hundredth time. Looking at it all and picking up the little matinee jacket and putting it on my tummy and giggling and getting really excited and then getting scared because, oh God, I knew it was going to kill—all the pain and everything—and then getting excited again. We were going to do so much with this child...

Then on the Monday, I'd come down with very bad flu and was very ill and I'd actually called the doctor. I said that I had a bad cold and felt that there was something that wasn't quite right. I didn't feel quite right within myself. I was actually told by my doctor at the time that I only had a cold and I was pregnant, not to worry about it. He said many women had colds while they were pregnant. But sometimes you know that something's not quite right within your inner self. It was like a little voice in the back of my head telling me that something wasn't right. It was a sudden feeling, an inner voice telling me, "Something's wrong". I don't know whether it was preparing me or something but I just knew that something wasn't quite right. I had a very bad cold but beyond that I just knew that there was something not right, but I just couldn't put my finger on it. So, the rest of the day I actually spent in bed just sipping on honey and lemon and not really eating much.

On the Tuesday morning I woke up feeling a little bit better—not a lot but a little bit better. In the afternoon I had my last antenatal check for the pregnancy. So I got up as usual and ran a bath. I thought it very strange when I ran the bath that there was no response from Marley, because usually he loved the sound of running water, be it a bath or just putting the taps on. I got into the bath anyway and started by putting water over my tummy for a reaction, for kicking, for some kind of movement, and I didn't get anything. And at the back of my mind I kept thinking, "Oh, something's not quite right" again but I dismissed it and carried on with the rest of the day.

And then Levi couldn't make the afternoon appointment at the antenatal clinic so my mum came with me. And we walked there. It was a very nice day that day. It was very sunny. And I remember it all exactly. I was wearing a blue checked maternity dress with blue sandals and I carried my antenatal notes in my hand. And I remember walking up the hill with my mum and we got to the antenatal clinic. Sat and waited for my turn. And then when the woman called me through I knew the first thing she would do was weigh me. When she weighed me, she said, "Oh, you've lost some weight." And I said, "Well, I have had a bad cold." So she took me through to the other room to listen to the baby's heartbeat using a Sonicaid. And she couldn't pick anything up. I know it's a long time ago but it feels like yesterday. I actually said to her, "The baby's dead." It's like God was saying to me, "It's just not meant to be."

When I had walked in there I hadn't thought anything. I didn't think... I just kept thinking there's something, something's not right. Something's not right at all. I didn't say anything to my mum or anything. I said to the midwife, "The baby's... the baby's dead." She said, "Don't be silly. It's probably just... it's gone into a breech position or something." Because sometimes they can't get the heartbeat. So she called for an ambulance and she said, "Look, we're going to send you off to the hospital. We'll take you to the hospital and do you a proper scan to see what's happening." So I waited. My mum's very religious and we sat and prayed that everything would be OK. I kept saying to my mum, "Oh, don't... Everything's going to be OK." I hoped everything was fine and said, "Mum, it's all right" but knowing, knowing that it wasn't OK.

I said, "Mum, it's all right", but knowing that it wasn't OK

So we got to the hospital and I remember the midwife, Mandy, was a really nice girl. She was new to the job and she'd never had to deal with a stillborn baby at all. I was lying down and they put me on a scan and I looked at the scan and he was just lying there as if... with his head to the side. They just said, "We're so sorry. There isn't a heartbeat. We're so sorry." And of course then I just started vomiting and being sick and I don't know why I was just being sick. I couldn't hold any body fluids down. It sounds disgusting but I think my body just went into shock. So the doctors came down and one doctor said to me, "You've got two options. We can either start your labour now, or you can go home and wait for the labour to start yourself," which horrified me. I'd never had a baby before and the thought of being at home when the labour started... and I could have been overdue. I could have been sitting there another four weeks, waiting for it to happen, with a child basically rotting inside. So I said, "Look, you're going to have to start the labour off."

So they took me upstairs and hooked me up onto a drip. It must seem so funny... Before I had Marley I was a smoker but as soon as I found out I was pregnant I packed in smoking. At that moment, I desperately wanted a cigarette just to feel calm. But I wouldn't have one because I kept thinking, "Oh, no, I'm pregnant so I can't I still can't." I hate seeing pregnant women smoking or drinking because I think, "You've got a life inside you and for nine months can't you just... Don't be so selfish. Just give up, just for nine months, just let that living thing come out."

They started putting all the drips in me and explained the procedure of what would happen. They'd got a drug that would start the labour. That was on the Tuesday night at about 4 o'clock.

About 7 o'clock, Levi, my husband, came. He'd been working. I hadn't been able to get hold of him because at the time mobile phones weren't in abundance as they are now. He was very distraught and we were both of us just sitting on the... it was horrible. We were both just sitting there. Sitting there in silence, wondering why, wondering what we had done. To go down this path of fertilising an egg, for it to become a human being, and then for me to deliver a dead baby, which I was going to do. It wasn't going to be alive. It was going to be dead. And that's what we had to keep telling ourselves. That it wasn't going to be a proper birth at all.

I didn't know how to handle the situation

That evening a lot of friends and family were sort of hearing what was going on so they were coming to see me. I was lying in the hospital wanting to be brave, saying, "I'm OK", with everybody coming round. But inside I was breaking up and wanting to just be left alone. I didn't know how to handle the situation, to be honest. It was very difficult having people coming in and saying, "What's happened?" and to sort of go through the story over and over again: "I don't know what's happened, all I know is I went for a scan and there was no heartbeat so now I'm going to have to deliver a..."

I went for a scan and there was no heartbeat

The midwives were absolutely fantastic. But that night I was just getting off to sleep and a midwife came in and woke me up to take a sleeping pill. I remember that really made me laugh. That was the only time I had a really good laugh. Both Levi and I thought, "How ludicrous!" We were laughing. We felt really guilty, but it was so funny because I'd just got off to sleep and she came in and woke me up to say, "Here's a sleeping pill for you." I was still in labour but it was very, very slow. I was just getting to the stage of period pain which is bearable.

The Wednesday morning, the pain started to get worse and they said, "We're going to have to break your waters because nothing's happening and it's too slow." So I had my waters broken. It didn't work the first time so they had to try twice. It was just horrible because I'd always pictured in my mind that I wanted a natural labour. I didn't want all these people coming in and out and peering at me and hoisting my legs up all the time. I just wanted it to be a personal thing between me and Levi. I didn't want people coming in and disturbing us. Anyway, they broke my waters and that Wednesday nothing happened at all. I was in a lot of pain. A tremendous amount of pain. And then I just felt that I was no longer in control. I was basically just a piece of meat and they told me what was going to happen and I'd have to say, "Yes", type of thing. They said, "We're going to have to give you an epidural because you're in so much pain." I said, "But it's going to affect the baby" because I kept thinking, "This is going to be a miracle child. It's going to be in the papers: BABY PRONOUNCED DEAD BUT BORN ALIVE." But I was just kidding myself, I think. I didn't want the epidural because I kept thinking, "Oh, the drugs are going to harm the baby and he's going to come out all floppy." The midwife just said, "Well, Monica, he's dead anyway. The baby's dead anyway." And one minute I'd be crying, then I'd be cooperating with them, then I'd be saying, "No, I don't want you to do it."

So they finally took me down to another ward to be given this epidural. The guy who did the epidural was in so much of a rush to get home, because it was the end of his shift, he didn't do it properly. It came out, so two hours later I had to be taken back down again. There was no anaesthetist at the time because it was about 10.30 at night so they had to call an anaesthetist in from home, so I had to wait for that. I was in a tremendous amount of pain. The gas and air was making me very sick, it just didn't agree with me, so I had another epidural. So now I suffer from a lot of backache because of it, especially at period times.

Then I was taken back up onto the ward. In the meanwhile, my mum had been sitting outside, praying with my dad and there was an Asian woman whose daughter was in the next room. She'd said to my mum, "Why are you crying? It's such a happy time... having a grandchild." And my mother said, "My grandchild's dead" but the Asian woman couldn't understand. I don't know whether it was because of lack of the English language or just... Sometimes when you've got your own happiness to be told that a child has died is not as easy to accept as to be told an adult's died. You can sort of accept that. When an adult has died you can think, "Well OK, they've had a life and they've seen and done things." But he hadn't harmed anybody. He hadn't even got to see that the grass was green or the sky was blue or anything like that.

I felt that things were going a little bit faster than they had been. My mum had set up this prayer ring and people were constantly coming in and out of the room, praying for me and for Levi and for the baby. I wanted the prayers but at the same time I just wanted to be left alone. I wanted to deal with it on my own and not have anybody there, because I just thought it was such a private thing. If it wasn't people from the church coming in it was doctors and paediatricians, and they had a lot of student nurses and doctors in as well to sort of have a look. Not that I was a guinea pig or anything. It was just a case to have a look at. They'd never seen a woman delivering a stillborn baby before. Looking back on it now, if it ever happened again, and touch wood it never will, I'd just ask to please be left alone and to let me deliver alone. When the doctor had come and said, "Do you want to go home?" I was horrified with him, thinking, "How can you allow me to go home?!" But now, looking back it's what I'd do. I'd just wait for nature to take its course.

It's funny because when I gave birth it was just me and Levi in the room. I felt something really pushing, so I went with my feelings and I pushed. And he said, "His head's here. The baby's head's here." He called for a midwife and I asked that only Mandy, the original midwife, come in. I didn't want anybody else in the room. She came and she encouraged me to keep pushing. And he was born at 7.48 that Thursday night. I'd been induced at about 4.30 on the Tuesday afternoon so it had been a long time, mentally as well as physically, because it was my first birth. Because it was my first birth I wasn't aware of what was going to happen. I wasn't aware of anything. And to be told the baby was going to be dead anyway. It was just a shock and horror.

As soon as I'd delivered him it was as if they were waiting, it was like vultures waiting outside the door. Two doctors just walked in and said, "Right do you want an autopsy?" I said, "No" because the thought of them cutting him up... I just said, "No." In hindsight, I should have said "Yes" because it would have helped to establish what was wrong. I have no idea why... They don't know why either. They took some blood and some tissue cells and tried to grow them to see if anything abnormal would come back but nothing did, there was nothing... And they said to me, "Do you want him?" I feel so bad now because I was scared and I said, "No, give him to his dad."

They said it was a boy. I asked what colour hair he had, if he had red hair but they said he hadn't. And they said, "Do you want him on your tummy?" and I said, "No, give him to his dad." I really regret that now, when I look back. I think, how could I have just rejected him? I wish I'd been the first to hold him. It was difficult. It was very difficult because he was cold, he was very cold and I was scared and Levi was trying to give him the breath of life. He was blue but Levi kept saying, "If I breathe in his mouth, he might just come alive." Then he gave him to me and I held him and kissed him and dressed him. I put a little white all-in-one on him and a nappy too. Silly, isn't it? I put a nappy on him and I kept thinking, "Just in case he does a poo." And I talked to him. Then they said they'd have to take him and put him in the mortuary. So they took him off me but I called them back because I hadn't put a hat on his head. I wanted to put a hat on him because he was cold. Silly, isn't it? And that was it. They put him in the mortuary and...

As for me, I went to the special room they have for mothers who give birth to stillborn children. Actually it was a special flat. It was beautiful. It was all pine, all rustic colours, really warm in there. There was a TV and a radio and a private nurse. I could stay in there as long as I wanted and I stayed in there for three nights. While I was there, there were three others on the ward who'd delivered stillborn children. The other two ladies already had children so they were quite happy to go home. I was scared to go home. I was very scared. I remember telling a very close friend of mine at the time to clear the flat out of all the baby stuff. I didn't want the baby stuff there. I didn't want her to throw the stuff away or give it away, but I didn't want to see it. She very kindly kept it all at her house for two years, then I took it back. Once a year, around the time that I lost Marley, I would go through his things. I kept them and Noah got to wear them. He wore all the clothes—he's 3 now—and Isobel has worn them as well. [Noah and Isobel are the two children Monica had a few years later.] I kept trying to think back over what had happened. That weekend before, did I pick anything up awkwardly? Did I rush or did I have a hot sweat or a hot flush? I was trying to think back. Did I have any mucous in my knickers? Was there anything... There wasn't and I kept trying to think. Was I sick? Did I have a headache? And then when you try to think and you start thinking too much, everything just becomes a muddle. That's how it all became in the end. It just became a muddle and I didn't know whether I was coming or going. So I don't know what happened.

When he was inside me, Marley was very active, especially at water time. When I was up in the bath or when I was swimming. I used to swim a lot as well. He was very active around that time. I was at university while I was pregnant and I was doing a drama course. We used to do a lot of dance and he used to become very alert to music. He used to love music and he used to sort of bounce about and kick. And Levi and I used to have a little game where he brought me a little pig and I used to put it on my tummy and the baby would kick the pig and we used to see the pig falling off. It was so much fun, amazing just to watch my stomach grow and to know that there was a little baby inside who was coming out.

And then the hospital priest came. He did the service for when he was buried.

It was just horrible because for the next five years I went to sleep praying that I wouldn't wake up sometimes. Especially, the first year because I kept thinking when I woke up I'd have to relive the nightmare of what I went through. I joined a counselling group of ladies who'd had stillborn children, but the thing is, out of everybody in the group, none of them had experienced it as a first-time mother. They'd all experienced it second or third time. And it's funny because Wolverhampton has the highest rate of stillborn babies in Europe. They don't know whether it's because of the factories and the air or whatever. I think that's why the hospital's got this room set up.

It was just horrible for the next five years...

We were so scared to have another baby, in case it happened again, which—chances are—it wouldn't, which I've proved. I've got two now. I got pregnant five years later. It wasn't planned. I'd had a coil fitted straight away and it was only because the coil got infected that I had to have it taken out. If I hadn't had it taken out, I wouldn't have either of the children now.

But there was the horror of being told that I was pregnant. I was so scared. The pregnancy was fine, I could deal with the pregnancy, that wasn't a problem. It was just when I got to 38 weeks. When I got to 36 weeks I was a nightmare to live with. I was an absolute nightmare, constantly thinking something was wrong and phoning the doctors and going to the hospital. And then from 37 weeks I was literally at the hospital every day. They took scans to see that everything was fine and everything was fine. But they said because of what happened they were scared to let me go full term, so I would have to be started off again at 38 weeks. So, again, I was started off. Waters were broken. Two hours later, I heard the cry. And when I heard the cry I knew that I'd done it. It was a very fast labour. Two hours from start to finish. And he was here. I was relieved. Relieved and... It's silly but it was wonderful just being able to talk to other mothers and saying, "Well, I've done it too."

A friend of mine phoned me a couple of weeks ago and her friend had gone through the same thing. I've never met her but I gave her my number and I've been talking to Bobby now for three or four months. She lost her baby in February. That was a stillbirth as well and she was a first-time mother. We've never met but we talk once a week even now. She's still in the early stages. She cries a lot and questions why. It's 1 in a 100 and it's almost always the boys who die. [Note: This statistic varies from country to country and time to time.][11] When we go to see him in the cemetery it's all boys. It's a special cemetery for babies and children and 9 out of 10 of the babies were boys. It's the odd little girl who gives up the fight. But they say that girls are fighters. If there's something wrong in the womb, the girls fight and they survive, but if it's a boy he'll give up. Boys don't fight. A friend of mine, her sister gave birth at 5 months. And we all expected that there was no way that she would live but she did. She fought and she lived.

Another friend of mine gave birth and everything was fine. She had the baby in the plastic thing they have at the hospital, you know the plastic thing next to your bed. She fell asleep and woke up and the baby had died. That was straight after, which is worse, because she'd held the baby and bonded and put him on the breast. I always say that I'm glad that he was taken then because if I'd built any type of bonding with him I honestly think I would have taken my own life as well, I really do. I know it sounds awful, but I do. But I say to Bobby, "Don't give up and... don't wait five years to have another baby. Don't. It's hard work, but you'd be depriving yourself." Noah's a hard little boy, he really is. He's 3 now. He tries my patience but he brings me so much laughter. When he comes up to me and says, "Oh, Mummy I like you. You're my friend." I think that's lovely. Don't deprive yourself because they're a blessing, they really are living angels. Definitely try again.

Photo © Colin Smith

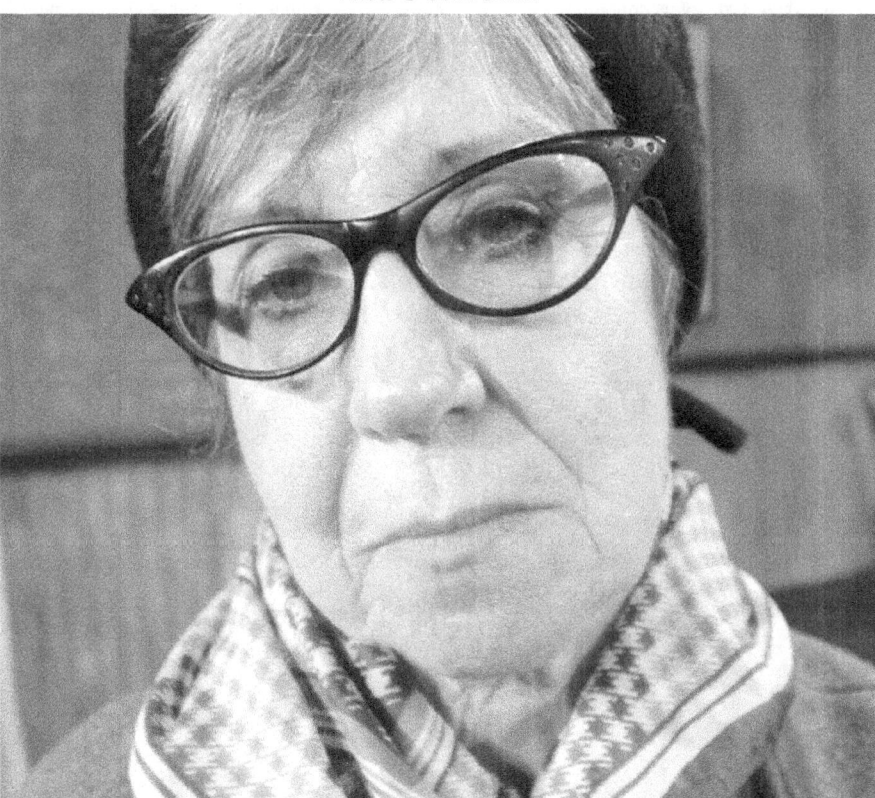

This isn't the woman Monica's talking about but she reminds me of the importance of never pre-judging people we meet. They sometimes have painful memories...

It's ever so funny... I met an old woman yesterday. I was taking Isobel round the park and she stopped me and she said, "Oh. How many babies have you got?" And again, I went to say three but I said, "Two".

And she said to me, "Oh you don't want to be having any more. You should get yourself sterilised." And I just thought, "That is the most horrible thing you could ever say to somebody!" And I said, "Why do you say that?" She said, "They're horrible things, children! You spend all your life looking after them and you get no thanks back, you know!" I said, "You do. Even if it's a smile or a hug. You get it back." What a cantankerous woman! It turned out, though, when I got talking to her that this old woman had lost two babies—a girl and a boy. Both had been stillborn. The boy at 6 months and the girl at 4 months. They'd both died because she'd taken the thalidomide drug while she was pregnant. So she had no living children. Maybe it was that that had made her so bitter. It was her way of coping, I suppose.

If it was to ever happen to anybody reading this, don't let it put you off having other children. Now I just look at it as a chapter in my life. It's something that I went through and it's something horrible that I went through but I can help Bobby who's going through it now. It's just hard sometimes.

Monica Reid

Note: Just to let you know... In June 2003 Bobby had a baby boy too. He's doing fine. I also met up with Monica again a couple of years after she gave me this account and there she was with not just two, but three children. She's since had another beautiful daughter.

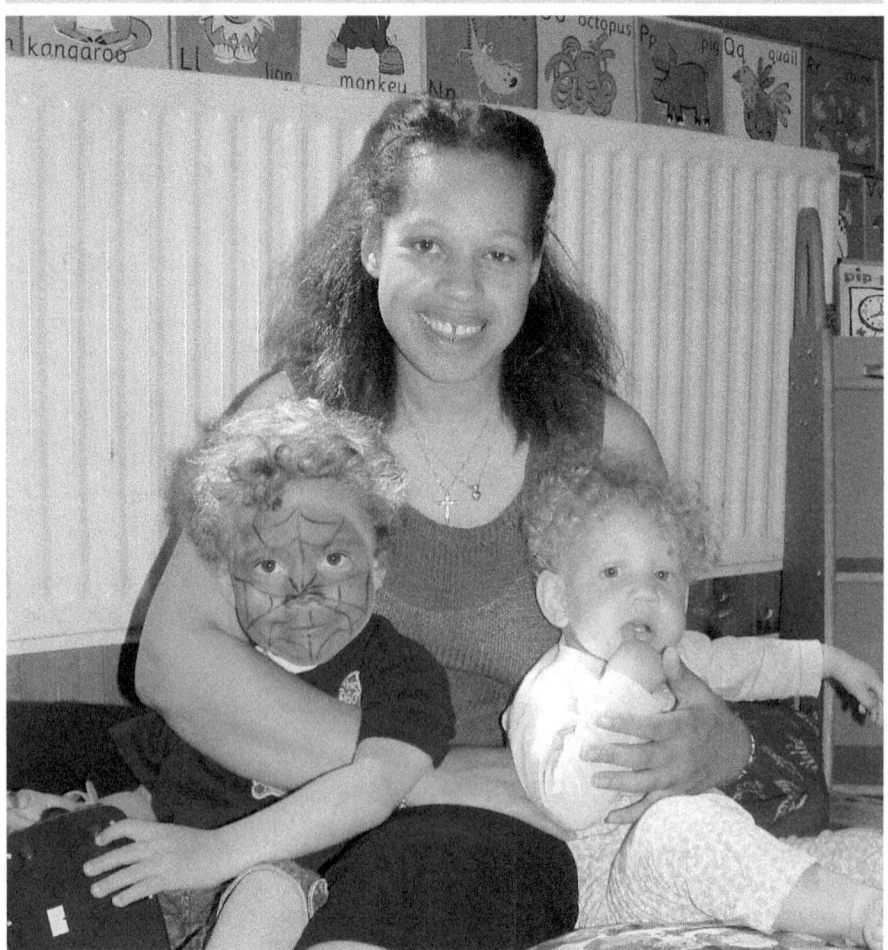

Monica with Noah (almost 4 years old) and Isobel (1 year), who was born in June 2002. (A few years later Monica had another little girl—and she's fine too.)

4... CHOOSE WHO

The importance of having the right caregiver

As you've probably gathered, choosing the right birth attendant can save you a lot of trouble. This is because the way your caregivers behave is likely to affect your own behaviour and, of course, the amount of disturbance or support you receive.[1]

As we've noted, talking of any kind can stop a woman from tuning into her knowledge of how to give birth and switching off the part of the brain that controls speech. Also, an over-directive midwife or obstetrician may well coax an otherwise decisive and confident woman into the role of a patient, making her doubtful of her own research as well as incapable of tuning into her intuitive knowledge. This is why birth attendants have such an enormous influence over birth outcomes... if we let them!

Another reason why you need to think carefully about who might be present when you labour and give birth is because, as Michel has observed, the more people a woman has around, the longer her labour tends to be. If you already have a couple of people in attendance, having just one extra person around for some purpose may have a negative effect. It's no coincidence that women often give birth when people around leave them alone for a few minutes—perhaps to see to other children or go to the shops. Giving birth when no potential danger is present makes evolutionary sense, after all.

In fact, all we need when we give birth, if indeed we need anyone at all, is one well-chosen birth attendant, perhaps with another standing by (behind the scenes) in case of emergency—or more if we're expecting twins or triplets.

Birthframe 54

Do you remember meeting Jenny Sanderson in Birthframe 10? Here she is again, with some information on how she came to have Michel in attendance—with another photo too!

When I was pregnant with my first child, and in a state of almost total ignorance about childbirth, my husband Tim and I attended Active Birth antenatal classes. I retained very little of the information we were given but will never forget the assertiveness role-play we did. It seemed that a hospital birth would involve countless interventions that had to be resisted—and I knew that I would not be able to resist them.

Then a friend told me about a lecture by Michel Odent that she had attended and suggested I phone him; he lived in London and delivered babies at home. So as not to disappoint her, rather than anything else, I called and made an appointment.

It was all very straightforward—my pregnancy was normal, he was available around the time I was due and, almost before I realised it, we had arranged for him to deliver me at home.

My Active Birth teacher, surprisingly, was concerned. How would I cope just with my husband, Tim, as a labour companion? Did I know that Michel would pretty well leave us to it? This didn't seem like a problem to me compared with the treatment I seemed certain to get and the battles we'd have to fight in hospital. And it was the right choice for me. Rebecca was born in January 1988 after a straightforward if not an easy labour. Rosamund was born the following year, also at home with Michel. Two (and by 1995 that would be four) natural births. No continuous monitoring, no vaginal examinations, no episiotomies, no tears, no syntometrine, no hospital food...

Michel's calm confidence in the labour process and in the labouring woman encouraged me, and his extensive experience reassured me that everything was normal. I knew that he would know at once if there was a problem. If he wasn't in the room with me, he was within earshot and very much aware of what was happening— although he left me mostly to find my own way.

Jenny Sanderson

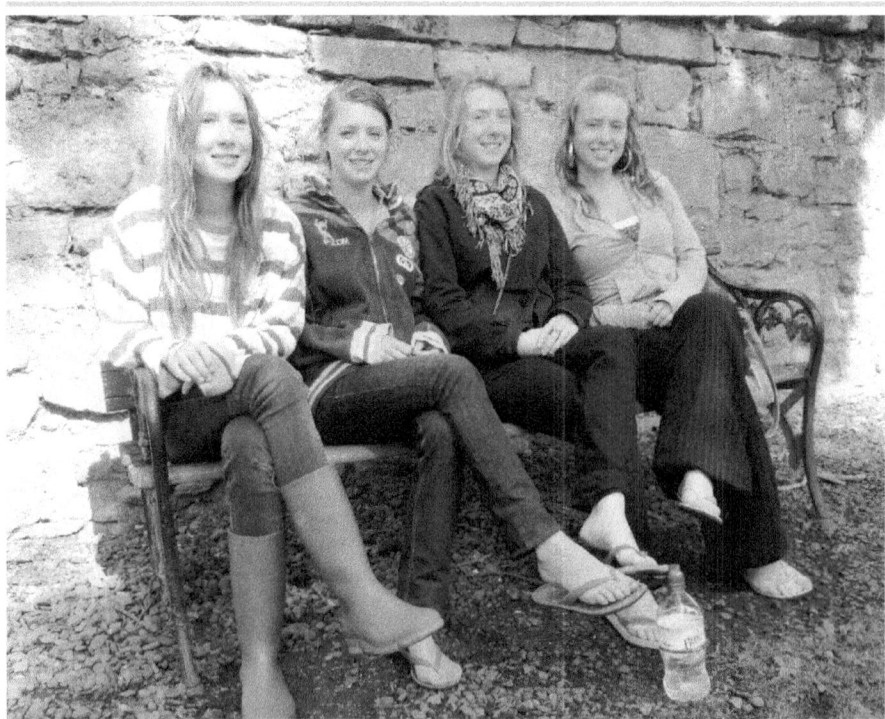

*A recent photo of the Sanderson girls, out in the garden
(also see Birthframe 10)*

Variations in quality of care

Can it really be true that other women's experiences can be so different? What kind of negative experiences do some people have? For obvious reasons, most of the contributors to this section preferred to remain anonymous.

Birthframe 55

I met this woman by chance, in an Internet chat room... Here's her account.

I am coming to terms with my anger and bitterness. They eat at me and paralyse my body, while those I am angry and bitter at go blissfully about their work. I believe that the people I entrusted with my care believed that they were doing their best, that they were doing their job. I also believe that in the circumstances under which it was performed my caesarean was necessary. I also certainly believe that those circumstances were, for the most part, caused by my caregivers and were completely preventable. I was caught up in a system that has it all WRONG.

> I realise how little REAL information I got

When I realise how much fear I carried with me throughout the pregnancy, how many things I did because of fear and how little REAL information I got, it makes me heartsick. I had a cascade of interventions leading, finally, to the caesarean. When my baby was taken out, he showed absolutely no signs of the postmaturity that I had been threatened with, along with insinuations that I was an irresponsible ignoramus for simply wanting to let him come when he was ready. I was so tense and/or terrified for the last three weeks of my pregnancy, it's no wonder that my body would not allow the baby to come. My body knew that babies should not be born where it is not safe. No mammal will give birth in a dangerous place.

I am free to seek expert opinions, but no one else has our interests at heart like I do. I am now a doubter, never taking any statement at face value and now, I trust myself more. I may never learn to trust myself completely, as I have been taught from my earliest moments, like most of us, that the authorities know best. At least I know now that I am worthy of trust.

I have learnt that just because a doctor or organisation of doctors says something or holds a belief it does not mean that it has a root in hard science. I have also learnt that when something has been discounted as 'never scientifically proven', it may simply mean that no one has yet bothered to do, or been able to get funding for, the research. I have learned that science doesn't have all the answers. I have learned that most statistics can be cleverly twisted to anyone's end. I have learnt that people are lied to by people who have been lied to themselves, ad infinitum, until they really believe the lie to be true. I have given up the naive belief that a woman practitioner or midwife, because she is a woman, will be a sympathetic and knowledgeable advocate.

This woman had a hard time asserting her wishes... **Birthframe 56**

I was expecting twins, having already had two children by normal vaginal delivery with gas and air for pain relief.

At 34 weeks I discussed with my consultant the need for an epidural, i.e. I told him I didn't want one. He said that it was my choice, since the first twin was head down and the second was breech. However, he said that I had to realise that if I had to have an emergency caesarean, then it would be done under general anaesthetic: I wouldn't be aware of the birth, my husband wouldn't be able to be present and a general anaesthetic would be more risky for me. I decided that I still would not have an epidural and accepted the downsides, should they occur. At 37 weeks I saw the registrar who, in discussing my being induced, indicated that he expected that I would have an epidural. I repeated the discussion that I'd had with the consultant but the registrar said that if he was delivering he would want me to have an epidural and I'd have to discuss it with whoever was on duty when I came into the hospital. I was very upset, having thought it was all agreed that I wouldn't have to have one.

> I decided that I would not have an epidural...
> Then the registrar expected me to have an epidural.
> I repeated the discussion I'd had before. I was upset.

At 38½ weeks I was induced. I arrived at the hospital at 6.00am and went into labour at about 12.30pm. I had a birth plan which said that I wanted to discuss the possibility of having an epidural with the registrar. At some point in the afternoon, having been taken down to the delivery room and while I was on gas and air, the registrar on duty came to discuss an epidural. I felt this very unfair as at that point I was in no state to rationally discuss anything, whereas the hospital had had all morning to talk to me. Fortunately for me, he was then called out to an emergency and when he returned I was too close to delivery.

My first twin was born at 5.45pm. Unfortunately, the cord came down for the second twin and the registrar called for the anaesthetist to come immediately. However, I pushed like mad, the registrar pulled the second twin by a leg... and he came out! So a caesarean was avoided! The registrar made the comment, "I told you you should have had an epidural."

During my time in labour the babies' heartbeats were monitored continuously, which meant me lying down on my back. I had learnt from my previous labours that contractions were a lot less painful sitting, crouching or standing, but having to lie down made these positions impossible. I was originally concerned about the lack of privacy with males being present but, in the event, was too engrossed with getting the babies out to be concerned about it.

My first two labours—at a unit run by midwives—were special experiences: my choice of music was being played, it was a nicely decorated room and I had the feeling the midwife was just there to help me. The twin labour felt very much more like a hospital procedure: there was no music, I was in a much more clinical-looking room and there was a very busy midwife who just popped in to monitor things. I'm not blaming the staff—it was obvious they were very busy. I am just pleased that the twins were my third and not first experience of labour and that I had the opportunity to have my first two in the midwifery-led unit.

Looking back on it all, I found it very upsetting for the consultant and registrars to have different policies. Obviously, professionals will have slightly differing views, but there should be broad agreement of policy, within which the mother's wishes and, if not strong, then the registrar's preferences should be taken into account. Of course, such policies should be backed up by reasons and facts. I was happy making the decision, with the information given by the consultant but couldn't help noticing that the registrars did not seem to have any information to add—just their strong preference for an epidural. I also think it would be helpful if monitoring equipment could be made to allow more freedom of movement. Finally, having my own music playing could have made a difference to the experience.

I firmly believe that my decision not to have an epidural meant that I could push and I think this is why I narrowly avoided a caesarean. What I am not sure about is whether by opting for this, I put the health of my second twin at risk. This was something which the consultant had not suggested to me.

For forthcoming mothers I don't have much advice. I'd say find out what you can early and ask for facts and details prior to going into labour. You do have to be flexible according to how things pan out but having a discussion about things you can plan for is much preferable prior to labour than during labour. I did this, but from the above you can see that I wasn't entirely satisfied.

Marion Chatfield

Birthframe 57

Some women only find out the hard way—by having a much better experience for their second birth...

With my first birth, I just felt there were too many people around—I had about five different midwives, one after the other. Also, the approach from the one midwife who started off with me was all wrong. When I arrived at the hospital after my waters had broken, she seemed put out that I'd come in to be checked. She didn't give me a good welcome—just made me feel I was in the way. When another midwife put me on an electronic fetal monitor, she said she wasn't sure how it worked. It was new equipment in a new hospital.

I ended up having lots of pain relief. First I had gas and air, then a couple of shots of diamorphine [heroin] and then—since they didn't think I was dilating enough—an epidural, along with a pitocin drip. After several internal examinations, the midwives and doctor who were in the room decided I needed an emergency episiotomy and forceps as the cord was around my daughter's neck. The forceps damaged her left eye.

When I went into labour with my second daughter I had a relaxed, friendly welcome from the midwife. She stayed with me all the way through my labour, right till the birth (which was only 2½ hours altogether). Everything seemed better and the birth itself was a fantastic experience for both me and my husband.

Birthframe 58

In the second birth in this next account, the contrasting attitudes of the health professionals are quite striking. This woman was clearly under a lot of pressure to give birth 'on time' and she finally managed to thwart other people's attempts to get her into hospital to be induced—as had happened before. As well as showing the potential for conflict between women and professionals, this account does also show how some staff attached to hospitals—obstetricians and midwives—can also tune into a pregnant woman's wishes.

The birth of my first child felt very institutionalised and governed by hospital policy. The midwife was definitely in control of the entire situation with me as her charge. My second birth was a truly wonderful experience that was influenced by an extremely intuitive midwife who encouraged me to do what I felt to be right for me. These experiences have made me highly aware of the dynamics between the birthing mother and the midwife whose main purpose is to provide support for the mother and her partner in labour and who needs to understand both the physical processes and the emotional needs of the mother. I feel that this relationship is one of the most important factors during labour and birth.

In my second pregnancy, when I was fairly overdue, I decided to try acupuncture on Wednesday evening to get my labour started. That night I was woken at about 2.00am with fairly mild contractions and they had completely fizzled out by 6.00am. My husband took Thursday off work as we were hoping that something might happen. I had woken him up at 4.00am to put the TENS machine on me, which I found to be more annoying than helpful.

I had been convinced throughout my pregnancy that my labour would be very short and worried that my husband wouldn't make it home in time for the birth as we live in North Finchley and he works at Bart's hospital in Smithfield. Of course nothing happened that day and we went to bed on Thursday evening thoroughly disappointed.

> The hospital staff phoned me all week, harassing me because I was refusing to go and see an obstetrician

I had had irate hospital staff phoning me all week and harassing me because I was refusing to go and see an obstetrician to talk about induction. We had planned a home birth and had hired a birthing pool and I was really looking forward to it. I had started to feel somewhat despondent and felt that my whole labour and birthing experience was about to be taken over by hospital staff. I reluctantly agreed to go to the Barnet General on Friday morning to be monitored and see an obstetrician, as I didn't think anyone would try and induce me then and there and wouldn't be rushed into any decisions as I would have the weekend to think any choices over.

I was woken up at 2.00am on Friday morning with mild contractions and slept in between them until 4.00am when I felt I had to get up and move around. I spent the early hours of the morning walking around the garden and tidying bits and pieces in the house. I woke my husband at 6.00am and we played Scrabble for an hour and then phoned the midwife at 7.00am to say we wouldn't be going to the hospital that morning as my contractions had started up again. She phoned back half an hour later to say she would come and visit us on her way into work. By the time the midwife arrived (at 9.30am) my contractions had stopped. She stayed with us for about 40 minutes and just before she left I had a fairly mild contraction. She asked me to go to the hospital to be monitored and we agreed and set off at about 10.30 with my first daughter, Milly (aged 2).

We arrived at Barnet General Hospital and I was monitored in the Day Unit. Although my contractions had started up again (at seven-minute intervals) they were relatively mild and not getting closer together. I thought they were probably Braxton Hicks contractions as I was beginning to think this baby was never going to be born.

The obstetrician came to see me at 1.00pm and booked me in for an induction the following Friday because he only does inductions on a Friday. As he was talking he looked at me and asked if I was OK. I replied that I was fine, just having a contraction. He wanted to know why no one had told him I was in labour and I told him I wasn't but I was just having very mild contractions. He wanted to examine me, which he did. I knew something was up by the look on his face and then he said, "If you want a home birth you had better get in the car and hurry because you are 5cm dilated and your waters are bulging." It seemed as though a cheer went up with all the midwives in the Day Unit and everyone, including us, was excited, not to mention surprised. One of the midwives phoned my midwife to get her to meet us at home and I dressed, got our things together and hurried back to the car.

Before you start to think that I have an incredible pain threshold you should be aware that the contractions I had with the birth of my first daughter were started artificially with syntocinon and were so incredibly painful (as any unlucky person who has had it can tell you). These were the only comparison of contractions I had.

We got home at 1.30pm and my husband put Milly to bed (very quickly) and then set about filling the birthing pool we had hired. I got the baby's clothes, etc ready, phoned my mother-in-law to come around and look after Milly and then phoned my Mum in Australia and a couple of friends to let them know my pregnancy was finally coming to an end.

My midwife arrived at 2.15pm and just after that my contractions got serious. The pool was ready at 3.00pm and I got into it. Throughout the whole experience I was amazed with the role the midwife took, as it was so different to my last birthing experience in hospital. She didn't examine me internally and only monitored the baby about three or four times. I kept asking what I should be doing and every time she replied: "What do you feel like doing?"

Rosa was born under the water at 4.11pm weighing in at 9lb 4oz (4.2 kg) and measuring 56cm. I had a small tear along my episiotomy scar that didn't require stitches. By 6.00pm all the family had arrived (truck loads of them) and we were all downstairs singing 'Happy Birthday' to Rosa and eating birthday cake.

Rosa is now 11 weeks old and is the most peaceful, relaxed baby I have ever known. She has always slept well (probably due to her incredible size) but now a bad night's sleep for Rosa is sleeping from 9.00pm to 6.30am.

The midwife who delivered Rosa works out of a Barnet General Hospital and is proof that a terrific midwife makes all the difference. I can't even begin to describe how fantastic she was! We owe our perfect birth experience to her expertise.

Jennifer Jacoby

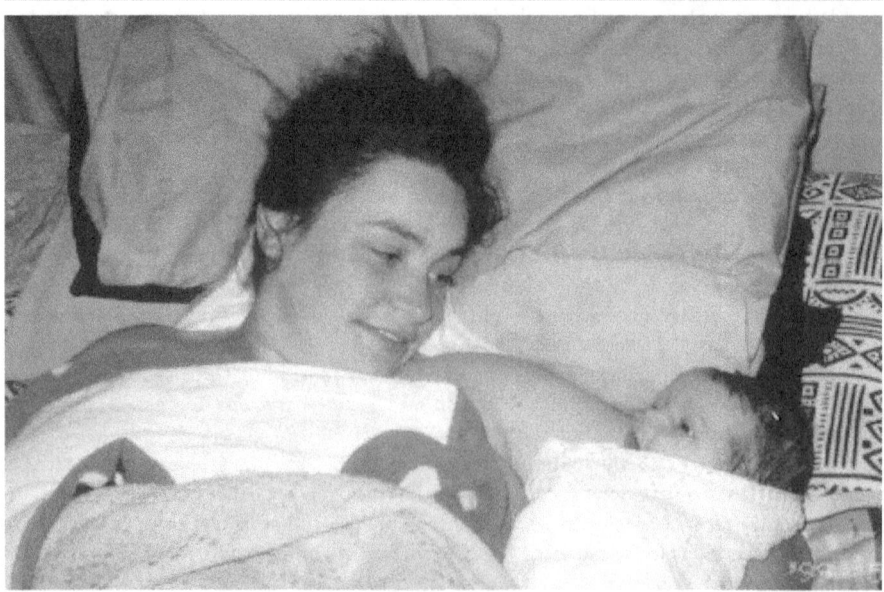

Jennifer Jacoby with baby Rosa, just after the birth

What should a caregiver be like?

Many women planning an optimal birth understand the need to find an appropriate, supportive caregiver. Although many women in Britain today simply go to their GP when they're pregnant, to wait to be 'assigned' someone, increasingly women are realising the advantages of having a midwife they trust.[2] After all, some caregivers are focused on watching out for pathology, while others are more likely to be familiar with the normal, healthy, physiological processes. Jan Tritten, who eventually founded the magazine and website *Midwifery Today* (www.midwiferytoday.com) wrote about this in an article for *The Practising Midwife*:

> I would say the whole experience of birth, the good and the bad, has not only propelled the comeback of midwifery in the US, but also sustains it. We have midwives who are willing to go to jail for their calling of helping women in birth. They are claiming the birthright of women to help other women in the thing that only women can do or truly understand—that is, giving birth. Michel Odent puts forth an interesting theory in his book *The Farmer and the Obstetrician* (Free Association Books 2002). He states that potential midwives should be drawn from women who have had physiological, undisturbed births.

As this comment suggests, ideally, you should find a caregiver who has first-hand experience of physiological birth. If they have this, they will probably realise the importance of not disturbing the pregnant woman's privacy in labour by repeated vaginal examinations, not behaving like an observer and of tolerating a woman's desire to be mobile and noisy—although you will need to check this really is the case! (Michel emphasised all these things in his book *Birth and Breastfeeding* (Clairview Books 2007) and he also stressed that a midwife should be able to monitor a labouring woman just by listening—with no probing fingers.) I would add that it's also vital to have silent birth attendants. The main things I can remember about my labours are the parts where I was spoken to or where I felt forced to speak because I didn't like what was going on. The rest has faded into a dreamy, pleasant memory. Is this perhaps because speech brings us away from our instinctual knowledge of how to give birth, back to the rational, which we can catalogue and recollect more easily? We shouldn't have to discuss our care while we're in labour or giving birth![3]

Why is it sometimes difficult to find support?

It's not actually too difficult to understand why it's sometimes extremely difficult to find someone who is willing to support and facilitate optimal births. Courses in midwifery used to focus mostly on pathology, instead of focusing on what facilitates or disturbs the healthy, physiological processes. (They are now improving.) Even now, while trainees are likely to witness and study many difficult interventionist births, many get no opportunity to witness or study undisturbed, healthy, optimal births. After I had my own first baby I received a letter from my obstetrician, who told me he hadn't seen 'a birth like that' for 14 years! In subsequent appointments with him it was very clear he was delighted to have witnessed an optimal birth.

Here, too, is an extract from an email I received:

> I recently talked with a man who has been an anaesthetist for over 30 years at a medical centre in the USA. He has been at many, many births administering anaesthesia and has never seen a woman give birth without medication. When I briefly described my experience, I could tell he just had no context for it. I think it's so totally different to see a woman birthing in an environment where she feels comfortable, has whatever support she needs, and is not medicated. He probably cannot even imagine the power that moves in the uninterfered-with birthing woman.

Beyond a lack of relevant experience, there are other reasons why some professionals might be reluctant to support women who want an optimal birth. Some don't have the time to research new practices. It must be difficult to constantly evaluate new research (or even old!) when working within an institution whose protocols conflict with it. One GP friend of mine confided that although she reads articles in the *British Medical Journal* with interest, she no longer changes her practice after reading about some new research. She said in the past she'd been discouraged by the spate of 'Letters to the Editor' which often followed articles on new research, making her end up feeling simply confused. Another GP told me she waits until there's a review of literature unless it's something she feels strongly about, or finds especially convincing. Of course, many studies are not repeated or extended because it's difficult for researchers to find funding for some kinds of research, so the 'review' of studies on a particular topic never comes.[4]

In any case, whatever a person's own views, health care professionals are naturally likely to be pressurised by their elders and peers to conform to the protocols of their particular institution. This is not only because of a fear of change but also because of a fear of litigation. Much of the 'monitoring' which takes place would provide clear evidence in a potential court case, even if it had disturbed the birth it was supposed to support.

Finally, it's important to acknowledge the psychological difficulties some professionals might have. Physiological birth inevitably involves professionals giving up control. By contrast, all forms of interventionist 'care' involve the health care professional directly and must give him or her the feeling of being both helpful and in control.[5] Even individuals who can rise above their own insecurities might be unsupportive of new ideas simply because human beings are naturally resistant to change. It's too stressful! In addition, the financial angle might affect the viewpoint of some caregivers or the managers of clinical facilities. After all, electronic fetal monitoring and ultrasound are two of the most expensive components of obstetric care and caesareans are well-known for their expense, largely because of the hours of experts' time they involve, not to mention the need for longer visits to the hospital. Having invested in equipment, some managers may be concerned to make sure it is used, so that the expense can be passed on to the 'client'. Why else would electronic fetal monitoring continue to be used for low-risk mothers when research has clearly shown that its only clear effect is to increase the caesarean rate, as well as the rates of forceps and ventouse use? Why has ultrasound become standard during pregnancy when its effects and usefulness are questionable?

Having said all that, more and more health professionals are reading the research which shows how problematic or unhelpful so many modern obstetric practices are. More and more are also witnessing for themselves the wonder and beauty of physiological birth, which in most cases is free from problems and trauma for both mother and baby, and by extension for their families and friends. Some of them have even experienced it for themselves. Perhaps we are not too far away from a new order of things in which the healthy, physiological model of birth is the standard, with a full technological back-up for emergency situations, in a system free from recriminations. Hey, that's optimal birth!

If you do have trouble finding a caregiver and/or birth attendant who will support your views, do keep exploring possibilities until you find a solution. As demand for 'hands-off' professionals increases, and as physiological birth is witnessed more and more often, so will supply necessarily increase.

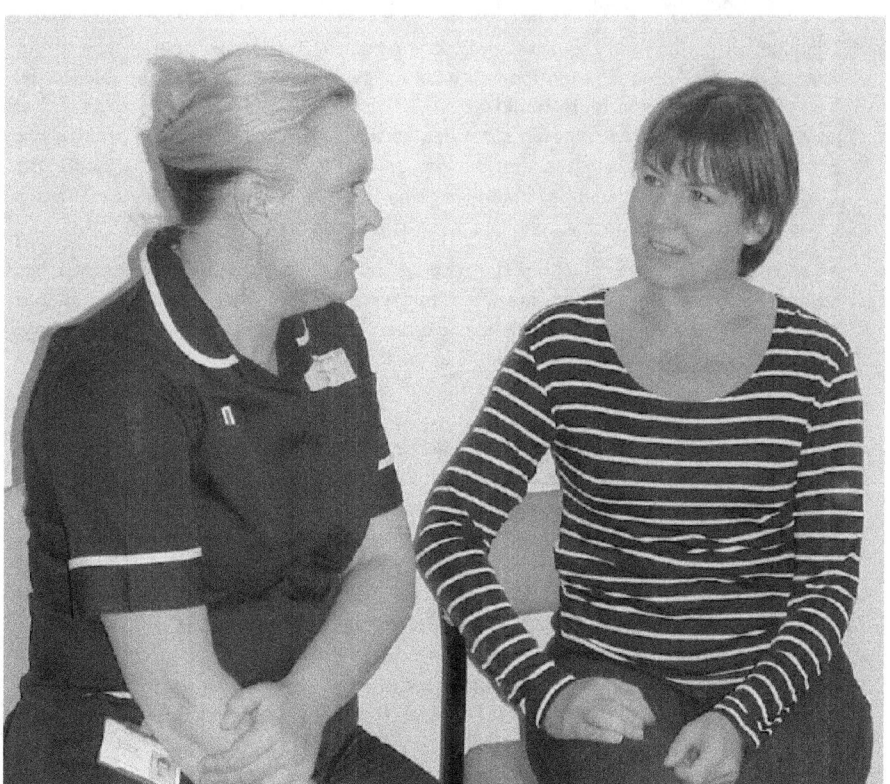

Find someone who is understanding and supportive

Women's experience of searching

A few women describe their experience of searching…

> My GP was aware from the start that I again planned a home birth. The consultant at the hospital told me that I could not have antenatal shared care at the hospital if I was planning to have the baby at home and pressurised me into agreeing to come to the hospital for the birth. The midwife afterwards told me not to worry—that shared antenatal care with delivery at home if all was well, or at the hospital if not, was fine.

> We moved when I was 5 weeks pregnant, and the first thing I did was find a midwife who would deliver my baby at home. At first I approached my GP, who I shan't name, because although he read me the riot act and said officially a home birth would be endangering my life and that of the baby, he, unofficially, was glad I wanted a home birth, and said he would support me. I was relieved. Next, I went to see a midwife who is also pro home birth. But as soon as she heard of my previous caesarean she declined her services. I didn't want to press my case because I wanted to make sure my midwife was 100% on my side. I didn't want to be hauled from home to hospital in labour under any spurious pretext. So I hired an independent midwife.

> I booked with community midwives who are generally supportive of home birth but when my history of a PPH [postpartum hemorrhage] was revealed (by me, voluntarily) I was told that a home birth would be out of the question. I was made to feel that my body was at fault for pouring out a life-threatening amount of blood after giving birth—the truth, however, was that mismanagement had caused the heavy blood loss. I soon booked with independent midwives who had the confidence in my body which I had and I gave birth to a second daughter at home in under three hours.

> At each check-up at the hospital it became apparent that none of the midwives had any experience of delivering twins and after further research and general reading it was clear that a first-time mother having a drug-free normal delivery was quite rare. I was told that my babies were cephalic [head down, i.e. not breech] so a caesarean wasn't absolutely necessary but was told to 'keep my options open'. Even my NCT class teacher (who was wonderful) said a normal delivery was, of course, possible but she wasn't sure whether it was realistic. The only positive response was from the consultant himself who, in an evening talk at the hospital, made it 'loud and clear' that he believes it is every woman's right to have a consultant present in a birth of this kind. However, he also said it is more likely there won't be one, so whoever is there is likely to have had little, if any, experience of delivering twins; therefore he said it would be safer to have a caesarean. He was the most amazing man I have ever met. After the talk, when I told him how important it was to me to at least try for a normal delivery, he wrote on my notes to inform him when I was in labour and he would come in. He gave me his holiday dates which I somehow managed to avoid and he stuck to his word and came in on his 'day off' and delivered my daughters. I know I couldn't have done it without him!

Caregivers who were appreciated...

Those women were not alone in appreciating their caregivers...

❝ Elaine visited my house throughout the pregnancy for tests, and listened to baby's heartbeat through her wooden midwife's trumpet [Pinard]. We got to know her, and she us, and it was a gentle and caring relationship. By the time I was in labour, my trust in Elaine was complete.

❝ Basically, the midwives made themselves invisible. I certainly hardly heard them discussing anything. I do remember hearing them ask Simon to bring clothes and nappies—I couldn't believe I was giving birth already!

❝ Whenever I asked the midwife for guidance about what I was supposed to be doing or how far she thought I was dilated she just told me I was doing really well, coping remarkably well and asked me to feel what my body was telling me to do and to follow that.

❝ Michel was great. He was very calm.

Birthframe 59

My twin daughters, Antonia and Charlotte, are now 13 months old. They are happy and healthy and absolutely wonderful. We decided to try for another baby when my first child, Marcus, was 7. When, at my 12-week scan, we found out it was twins I was absolutely petrified and my partner was delighted—he always had believed he was magic! The pregnancy went remarkably well, despite all the horror stories you hear and the various medical staff telling me to pack my bag at six months and finish work much earlier than I'd intended. The whole family were on tenterhooks for weeks. No one would go on holiday and, by eight months, people were starting to get very impatient. Personally, I was happy to wait as long as possible for the babies to arrive as—having experience of caring for one baby—I was well aware of the amount of work that would be involved.

Finally, six days before the due date, my waters broke at 3.00am. I jumped out of bed and got to the hospital as quickly as possible only to be told that I wasn't in labour and wouldn't be examined due to the risk of infection. I was given a bed on a ward and my partner was sent home.

Later that morning I had a visit from the consultant. She decided that she would give me until the following morning to go into labour naturally but that if I hadn't she felt it best to induce me. She then went on (to my absolute horror) to recommend an epidural. Her reason for this was that, as Twin 2 was breech, if there were any complications and I needed to have an emergency caesarean, I would be ready and wouldn't need to be knocked out. At this point I burst into tears and said that I really didn't want that. I was quite distressed to see how surprised all the staff seemed to be at this and when I later discussed it with a midwife she said that epidurals are now so commonplace that many mothers ask for them!

I'm not sure whether it was the shock of the consultant's visit or just the strength of my desire not to be induced but I very quickly began to experience a lot of pain and, on examination, was told that I was 6cm and really should be in the delivery suite.

I was so relieved that I was given total support in my decision to have no medical intervention when I met the midwife that was to deliver me. The only thing they insisted on was that a drip [a heparin lock] should be inserted into my hand in case I needed glucose. I was also given a gas and air 'contraption', which I didn't use—but I found the mouthpiece great for biting on!

After going into labour at about 12.30pm on 11 June 2001, Charlotte Mary was born at 4.47pm (7lb) and Antonia Grace was born (bottom first and screaming) at 4.59pm (6lb 15oz).

I am so glad that I had the babies normally. I think that it is such an important experience and all part and parcel of becoming a mother. I was very scared of giving birth to twins and I must admit I have never experienced anything so painful but I found that the only way I could get through the pregnancy without being totally freaked out was to have absolute faith in my body. Throughout both the pregnancy and the birth I continued to remind myself that my body had done this before and therefore would be able to cope with it. Thankfully I was right and I do believe that, had I allowed them to give me an epidural, I would have felt I had cheated myself.

Kathryn Clarke

" I feel very privileged to have had such a wonderful birth experience. It must be possible for anybody to have a similar experience but I do feel I had several advantages that made it easier for me: a fantastic midwife who put herself out to give me one-to-one care throughout, a wonderfully supportive consultant, a healthy 'good-at-having-babies' body... and little fear, as I have my midwifery knowledge and experience. *Debbie Brindley*

Taking practical steps to find support

So what can you personally do to find someone supportive?

- ♥ Ask around. Other women and their partners can tell you about their experiences with local birthing attendants.
- ♥ Check out local possibilities by doing a few Internet searches or checking local directories. See the Useful contacts at the back of this book.
- ♥ Talk openly and respectfully with any potential caregivers, with your care guide in hand!
- ♥ Tell any prospective caregivers about the book *Promoting Normal Birth: Research, Reflections & Guidelines* (Fresh Heart, 2011)—see page 494.
- ♥ Consider carefully who else—apart from your main caregiver—you want to have present at the birth itself. Some women have doulas, partners, children and friends at their births... and some prefer not to have so many people around. Only you can decide what is best in your personal case.

Other birth attendants...

DOULAS

Some people feel it's a good idea to have a doula as well as a medically-qualified birth attendant.[6] In case you don't already know, a doula is quite simply a person—usually a woman—who stays with a labouring woman while she labours and gives birth and also perhaps after the birth, sometimes for as long as a few weeks. A doula may also be able to offer you support antenatally or postnatally by helping you to find out information relevant to your particular situation. The amount of training doulas have had can vary tremendously, as can their fees—not to mention their personalities!—so you would need to check out who's right for you. See the Useful contacts for contact details.

You may find it helpful to have a doula if you are feeling very nervous about giving birth, if you want someone to help facilitate conversations or if you want someone to remind you of any issues previously discussed, while you are in labour. A doula may also be useful if you have specific medical needs—her focus will be on viewing you as a person, rather than as a 'case'.

Birthframe 60

I first heard the word doula when about six months pregnant. Like most first-time mothers, I was hungrily searching for clues about childbirth in books and magazines—what would it really be like? Doulas, I was told by the childbirth expert Sheila Kitzinger, are women who help other, less experienced women through birth, mainly by providing emotional and physical support and information. Research has shown, Kitzinger said, that the presence of a knowledgeable doula reduces the need for pain-relieving drugs, shortens labour, makes the birth an easier and happier experience, and results in fewer babies needing intensive care. Wanting as I did a drug-free, non-interventionist birth, it all sounded good to me, but I thought no more of it until a couple of weeks before my baby was due. The baby's head had not yet engaged and this, I was led to believe by the London hospital where I was booked to give birth, might be problematical. A local acquaintance put me in touch with Liliana, a highly experienced doula who lived only five minutes away.

A few days later I was sitting in her kitchen eating homemade soup. At the time, I don't think either of us knew that she would actually be present at the birth but she gave me reassurance. Liliana told me about her own experience of giving birth to four children and, above all, advised me to have faith in my body: simply to let it do what it was programmed to do, leaving the intellect well out of it.

> She advised me to have faith in my body: to let it do what it was programmed to do, leaving the intellect out of it

I had no real concept of the wisdom of these words until about two weeks later when I went into labour. It was then that all the carefully laid plans for my partner Chris's involvement in the birth—offering lower-back massage, quiet encouragement and the sort of 'room service' you'd only ever expect in a five-star hotel—were summarily discarded. Once the contractions started forcefully to take over my body, I had no wish for communication; I wanted to focus unreservedly on the baby.

Liliana had said that she would come over once labour was established, that she'd be able to help us judge the 'right' time to go into hospital—I wanted to leave it until the last possible moment. When she turned up, just before midnight, I was on my hands and knees in the candlelit living room and contractions were coming quite strongly every three minutes. Liliana said hello and then almost immediately left the room. This was how she remained throughout the birth: a dreamlike comforting presence I was vaguely aware of from time to time, but there was never any direct contact or intrusion. About an hour after her arrival, Liliana warned Chris that, if the baby was to be born in the hospital as planned, we should leave at once. She then generously offered to accompany us.

In many ways, Liliana's role—both at home and at the hospital—seemed to be that of a guard; discreetly, firmly she kept people away from me. [Research does in fact show that the sheer presence of a doula will tend to discourage attention from caregivers.][7] She was sympathetic too to the feelings of Chris, who, far from participating in the birth of his child, as laid out in the birth plan, was snarled at every time he came near. Toward the end of the labour, when I had retreated to the total darkness of the bathroom, Liliana stood at the door, reassuring Chris that I was perfectly fine. I knew I was fine, she knew I was fine; for him it must have been perfect agony.

My daughter Bea was born in a birthing pool approximately seven hours after labour had started. She was still encased in the membrane or caul, so her appearance as she slithered out between my legs was awesome and ghostly. I held her and we looked at one another for a long moment, then she rooted immediately for the breast. While I delivered the afterbirth, squatting on a table in the delivery room, Liliana rocked and sang to Bea in the half-light, welcoming her to the world. [Many doulas, including Liliana perhaps, would prefer to involve the father at this and other times.]

I couldn't have wished for a better birth for me and my daughter, except had I known then what I know now I probably would have opted for a home birth. I had wanted no interventions; I had none. I had wanted no drugs; I had none. I had wanted a gentle, natural birth for my child; and this I believe I achieved, though Bea is really the only person who can vouch for this. And all this in a typical hospital setting.

The only other thing I'd do differently now would be to make quite sure that, in the days and weeks after the birth, I had a doula at hand to mother me. A doula's role is often described as 'mothering the mother'. While I certainly didn't want mothering during the birth, I could have done with it after I took my baby home. A doula will come in to see a new mother for a couple of hours a day up to six weeks after the birth, offering support at a time when many women are at their most vulnerable. If I were ever Prime Minister for a day, I'd make this kind of essential care a provision of the state.

Sarah-Jane Forder

Birthframe 61

This account gives even more information about how a doula sometimes supports a woman in labour.

It was an 11th-hour decision to have a doula at the birth of my second child. For eight months, my plan was to go to a local birth centre, as I had for my first. And then as if by magic, a new trust arrived in me. One that told me I could manage at home. It really was a kind of magic. My head didn't convince me, or even my heart. Just as with my first pregnancy, an imaginary hand appeared—deep-down instinct, I suppose—and I took hold of it.

As it turned out, that hand wasn't so imaginary. Two months before my due date, I attended a doula course with Liliana Lammers and Michel Odent. I found their ideas on birth exciting—at times breathtakingly so. I was especially fascinated by their belief in total privacy as being the key to a smooth birth and when Liliana helped me set up a home birth for myself, I knew she was the one I wanted by my side. As it turned out, she offered me more than that. This wonderfully calm and centred doula was more about and behind me, than beside me. Unseen, silent—but absolutely there.

I was over two weeks late and pressure was mounting to get things going. Forget induction. Liliana had convinced me that even gentler nudges, like a sweep or reflexology were to miss the point. It must be the baby that gives the cue, she explained. "If the baby is ready, then the birth will go well." She urged me to feel for myself if everything was OK. Assured me that as the mother, I would know if something was wrong. I'd hang up the phone and feel a fresh energy. Something sure and strong and safe, guiding me. What Liliana was leading me to was my own instinct. [Note here that doulas are generally advised not to provide *advice* to pregnant women. Doulas need to tread a fine line between helping women and standing aside.]

Finally, at 5.00am on a dark November morning, I felt the first twinge. By 9.00am, labour was really established and my husband, Danny, called Liliana. In true style, there was no urgency, no panic. She said she'd see to a couple of things, then cycle over mid-morning. Her ease was contagious. I did some cleaning, made some breakfast—calmly absorbing that most unabsorbable of notions. That at some point that day, I'd have my baby in my arms.

As soon as Liliana arrived, around midday, she made herself scarce—practising absolutely what she and Michel preached. I remember wanting to offer her tea, to make her comfortable, to talk—but she just shushed me and I closed my eyes. As I moved from room to room, from kneeling to standing and back again, I looked like someone alone. But Liliana was there all right. I could feel her unmistakable energy beaming through the walls. Could feel her listening—keeping an eye.

What I wasn't was being watched. I was totally private—and right inside myself as a result. Danny had made himself scarce, the house was silent, the room I'd somehow guided myself to, small and dark, and the world just fell away. I felt absolutely safe, wholly secure in my surroundings and the chemicals just cued themselves up. I could almost feel the hormones firing, ratcheting up the pace—and my labour's progress.

A couple of times I asked Liliana a question: "The contractions pick up when I walk around, so should I keep walking?" She didn't reply. With a shrug, she simply handed the process back to me. Coaxed me back to myself.

After an hour, the pain accelerated and I needed a hand to hold. It was there. A silent squeeze. Liliana gave no encouragement, no commentary. Words would interrupt me, bring me back to thought when what I needed was this flow. My eyes were closed, but her support was surrounding. I could feel her focus on me—saw through half-shut eyes, that her own were shut too. It was as if she was moving through each contraction with me. So much birth assistance seems to tell the woman to turn away from her pain. But Liliana did the opposite. She helped me move to its centre.

It suddenly felt right to get into the pool. As with every stage, she got me to follow instinct—her trust in me made me trust myself, like a circuit. The pain peaked and I practically pulled Liliana in with me. Just then, the doorbell rang—the midwife had finally appeared. Although she was untrained to do water births it was happening anyway—and Liliana's confidence and experience of water births eased the situation.

It was almost a quarter before three and I'd begun to push. There was no cheering me on, no cautioning me to slow down and pant. "Your body knows how to get the baby out," I could remember Liliana saying on the doula course. And so it seemed. Two pushes, and she was there—my beautiful daughter, Pearl, had arrived.

Natalie Meddings

YOUR PARTNER

In this book we're challenging everything!... so let's also reconsider whether or not it's a good idea to have your partner there, when you're in labour and giving birth. On the plus side, you would have an intimate companion who would presumably be 'batting for you' all the way. On the negative side, some people have suggested (including Michel Odent) that relationships might be affected by sharing the birth experience.

Will you feel embarrassed if your partner sees you doing a poo on the floor completely unintentionally? Are you happy for him to see your nether regions fully exposed, stretched and bloody? Is the idea of the sudden revelation of piles an acceptable possibility? Will sex resume its recreational, romantic note, after this interlude of explicit procreative, productive sexuality? These are all questions which are well worth considering.

Your partner might also want to consider these questions. Some men are very happy with the idea of birth, while others are frankly, horrified.

Some men are very happy with the idea of birth, while others are frankly, horrified

Birthframe 62

As we see here, it's not necessarily easy for men to keep their women company at this quintessentially female time.

Please allow to me present my credentials: I am the father of four children, three of which were born without serious medical intervention but the last, being a breech baby, had to make its appearance via caesarean section. I attended all the births (three in hospital, one at home) and therefore you might think I am eminently qualified to write something on the subject of childbirth—but you'd be wrong. I am no more capable of commenting on the pros and cons of the various forms of bringing babies into the world than a professional footballer can offer advice about a good forward defensive stroke in cricket. This is simply because I am male and being male means I will never have the slightest idea of how it feels to give birth. Of course, once the line on the curious spatula thing purchased from Boots turned blue, I read books on the subject, I went to the antenatal classes more or less voluntarily and I did my best to empathise with my wife as she began to slowly swell. But no amount of lectures, films and drinks with midwives could possibly convey the actual experience of labour to those of us with a Y chromosome. This put me in a very tricky situation.

My wife has very strong views about giving birth. She wanted everything to proceed with as little medical intervention as possible and without any painkilling drugs. I could relate to this at least; personally speaking I have always had a peculiar aversion to taking pills (not even an aspirin for a hangover). Covering my face with a mask has induced panic ever since a childhood trip to a drunken dentist and allowing anyone to stick a needle into my spinal column seems like asking for trouble. But it was not me who was going to give birth, it was not me who was going to have muscles and nerves stretched to breaking point and beyond. So when she asked me for opinions on everything from arnica and other homeopathic remedies to using a TENS machine, I felt like a complete fraud offering any advice at all. To compound the problem, there was my own ignorance. I thought a TENS machine was something to do with American bowling alleys and one sip of the foul-tasting raspberry leaf tea made me feel glad I was a man. But if my sense of helpless confusion was bad during the pregnancy, things were about to get a lot worse.

I know everyone is different, but when my male friends say watching the birth of their children was one of the most rewarding experiences of their lives I can't help thinking they are either lying, complete sadists or both. How anyone can describe watching their loved ones suffer extreme pain as 'wonderful' is utterly beyond me— even when the compensation is holding your beautiful baby son or daughter in your arms. I guess the root of my problem was that there was absolutely nothing I could do during labour except to try not to get in the way. Of course, I could hold my wife's hand, offer her words of encouragement and mop her fevered brow as directed, but it all felt so inadequate. I mean how could I help my wife match her breathing with her contractions when I wasn't feeling the contractions?

At the time, it struck me this is why most spectators at sporting events are men. The thousands of males who flock to pitches, tracks and courses every weekend are merely in training for the day when our other halves give birth. Coping with the frustration we feel about not being able to take that crucial penalty kick, take that crucial wicket or ride that crucial winner in the 3.30 at Newmarket is excellent practice for that crucial time in the labour ward, when all we can do is stand, watch and wait. Now don't get me wrong: the midwives and medical staff were absolutely marvellous. They did their best to make me feel included and involved but nothing they said or did could alter my belief that I had contributed nothing positive to the process. I suppose this feeling of helplessness is why some men feel the need to video the births of their children—something which, in my opinion, should be punished by a life sentence of watching endless repeats of *You've Been Framed*. Playing with electronic toys is what we chaps do best and placing a lens between you and reality is an excellent way of coping with stress.

After the birth of No.1, I felt like someone who had got too drunk at a party and made a thorough nuisance of themselves, so imagine my surprise when I was invited back, again, and again, and again! Did it get easier? Yes and no. Every birth is different but the risks remain the same. There is the worry that you are pushing your luck and that something may go horribly wrong. However, the other side of the coin is that the relief gets greater every time it goes right.

So did I do anything right? I suppose I must have done because I am still married to the mother of my four healthy children and she never, not even during our bitterest rows, refers to any mistakes I made during her confinements. If I did contribute anything positive it was, paradoxically, not what I did but what I didn't do. I did not insist she have a natural childbirth but once she had made her decision to do so, I did not insist she stick to it—cf. the medically necessary caesarean required to deliver No.4. I did not allow my natural inclination to 'take charge' get the better of me; instead I let my wife and the midwives take the decisions and get on with it. The 'did not' I am most proud of, though, is that I did not squeal like a stuck pig when she dug her nails into my arm!

I was happy enough to do exactly as I was told but equally my wife knew she had my support whatever her decision. For example, No.2 was three weeks late and the doctors were keen to induce the birth artificially. However, the baby was showing no signs of distress and my wife wanted to wait; if it had been me I would have wanted to be hooked up to every available machine in the hospital… but it wasn't me. I therefore shut up so my wife could listen to what her body was telling her. Our (or should I say her) reward was a bouncing, baby boy weighing an eye-watering 10lb 2oz (!) and delivered without any drugs or intervention.

> Did I do anything right? I suppose I must have done because I am still married to the mother of my four healthy children and she never refers to any mistakes I made.

> Why, you may ask, if I found the births so distressing did I allow myself to be persuaded to attend? Some of you reading this may like to pick up on my earlier football analogy and ask why men spend hours in the wet and cold cheering on a bunch of overpaid, prima donnas, but I would prefer to sum up the whole experience in a single word. I bit the metaphorical bullet, swallowed my pride and allowed myself to be 'persuaded' into taking decisions against my male judgement for one reason and one reason only: it's called love.
>
> *Phil Anderton*

However your partner feels, make sure you discuss your care guide with him in exhaustive detail. It's extremely important that he understands your reasons and feelings on the subject of your baby and your upcoming birth, especially if there is any disagreement about safety issues.

And if you yourself are not keen to have your partner around, for whatever reason, explain this to him too. Even if he very much wants to be at the birth, it would be better if he could be sensitive to your wishes at this important time in your life. If you want your partner to be around but are concerned how he'll behave, do talk to him about birth physiology—perhaps by showing him this book!

> I had initially had a fantasy of my husband being there for me—a time of deep intimacy! But we went to a talk with Michel Odent and someone brought up the question of men attending. Michel questioned the wisdom of it. My husband was relieved—he felt he didn't want to be the main attendant but hadn't felt confident to say so until Michel endorsed this. (My husband had a terrible experience with a birth in a previous relationship where, although he'd been a big support, the birth experience was about as bad as it can get and he was traumatised). When he said he didn't want to be there for me I was initially very disappointed and hurt. Then I came to terms with it, and, of course, it did turn out better for me to focus inwards.

The idea that husbands are supportive and sensitive to pregnant women may be a complete fallacy. I suppose it's not too surprising... with child No.2, 3 or 4, men face increasing worries about finance.

Despite the many chapters in pregnancy books helping men to gain an insight into their pregnant partner's feelings and moods, after travelling as a twosome through a first intriguing pregnancy, I've come to the conclusion from talking to other women that men merely tolerate a pregnant woman's presence a second or subsequent time. Instead of being understanding, supportive and sensitive, men tend to become bad-tempered clods. Pregnancy is then a lonely period for both partners. The children, meanwhile, have to come to terms with this emotional climate and have to somehow work out what on earth's going on in Mummy and Daddy's relationship. They do still have one, don't they?[8]

My husband proved to be a wonderful support

> Although, to be honest, I hadn't really wanted my husband to be with me when I gave birth, I must admit he proved to be a wonderful support throughout my labour. He massaged my back for literally hours on end during my first labour and was always discretely positive and supportive of me. He told me afterwards that he felt offended about being ordered around so much by me during my first labour but he said he was prepared for this the second time round! Again, he proved to be the perfect assistant, perhaps because he really did want to be there.

> When I went into labour, attended only by my husband and a doctor, I had a sudden moment of panic. No one nearby had given birth and I felt a tremendous sense of loneliness—if only a woman could be nearby!

> I felt very strongly that I didn't want my husband to be there, but my husband decided he was going to be and the point was clearly non-negotiable. He took my preference for being alone as an implied rejection and considered it sufficient grounds to end our relationship. I put up with him in the end and I have to admit he was very helpful. I'm not at all sure it helped our relationship, though... It probably had a damaging effect in that respect, as part of me had suspected it might. Some things need to remain private... Strange how the same man will never let me into the bathroom while he's on the toilet!

> My husband was amazing during the entire 36 hours that the birth day lasted, from walking with me during the day to making food in the evening and driving me around in the middle of the night. Neither of us has ever been so physically or emotionally exhausted in our entire lives. The whole thing brought us closer together, I have no doubt. He was an incredible support. I really feel as though we equally gave birth to our baby, especially since I didn't get to experience the delivery, because of the caesarean.

> My husband cooked some sausages (which helped my ongoing nausea no end) and made a few phone calls. I wouldn't be surprised if he didn't switch his computer on and do a bit of work, but he's never told me that. Not because he didn't want to help, but more because I was doing OK on my own and really didn't want any interference.

> I kept sending my husband out of the room, trying desperately to hold on to some of my dignity.

> During second stage Adam had decided that he would put his hands down behind me to catch the baby; unfortunately he caught something entirely different! Apparently, his face was a picture but I was unaware of this until later; I was, however, very amused. A greater love hath no man!

> I insisted on John being at my head-end as opposed to the 'business' end, as I'd heard of men who went off their partners physically after seeing them give birth and I didn't want to risk that.

> When a nurse suggested pushing my haemorrhoids back in, a few hours after I gave birth, my husband immediately said he'd like to come in and watch. Suddenly, I felt as if scales were falling from my eyes. I was not a circus sideshow and I immediately knew—and stated!—that it was not a good idea. It made me wonder about his motivation for watching the whole birth the day before and I remembered I'd read about men dressing up as women in 18th century France so that they could watch women giving birth. If I had a choice another time, I'd want this part of my life to be private. It's not for my man to see.

> I think women should be allowed more privacy at such an instinctual time, when feeling uninhibited and unobserved, and tuning into the natural processes is so important.

A comment from Michel:
> Often the decision as to whether or not the husband should be present is made in an interesting way... One story I remember was typical. I remember it well. The guy said, "I must buy a pint of milk!" And while he was at the shops his wife gave birth. When he came back the baby was born. In another case, the woman was Hepatitis B positive and the man had to go to the pharmacy at the hospital to buy a vaccine for the newborn baby. He had to go before a certain time because it was a Sunday and the pharmacy would be closed after that. As soon as he had gone—poof!—the baby was born.

Birthframe 63

There might be many reasons for wanting to have one's partner present, but the one presented here by a father as being paramount might come as a surprise.

My first child was born when I was 18, my last—fate permitting—when I was 44. I imagine men have been fathering children over that time period and much more for millions of years. Nothing unusual in it, then? Well, not in the time span, certainly, and with many men fathering children in their dotage, it's not even close to an extreme. What is unusual, now I come to think about it, is that my experience spans a revolution in a father's involvement in the birth process, starting as it did at the very time when men were first being tentatively allowed into the sacred labour ward.

Men have been fathering babies for millions of years

Since then, my experience has moved with the times through discouragement of home births, the introduction (re-introduction!) of natural labour, and the latter-day antenatally-trained father oozing calm in the ward, sopping brows and monitoring birth plans (you wish!), while still filming the beautiful scene. Perhaps that's why Sylvie asked me to write a contribution, and I don't know what is about to appear. Much of it I haven't thought about recently.

At 18 (in the late 1960s), my wife was petrified when her waters broke and we took our battered car to the hospital. The nurses spoke to her rather less well than a dog. (Actually a lot worse than a dog. Dogs at least cannot understand uncaring and cruel asides... "Yeah, she's just making a fuss. Look, she's not even one finger yet!") I sat, immature, scared and powerless. Having read all about fathers being welcomed, I was expecting someone might notice I was there, but I was surprised to be told to leave and 25 minutes later was told I had a new son and that I'd be able to go in in an hour or so. I remember throwing everything on my lap in the air. I had never felt ecstasy like it, but then at that stage I hadn't seen what my wife looked like either.

Even with the distance of over 30 years, this is a traumatic memory. My wife and I had never felt so dominated, so insignificant and worthless. I have heard women be critical of male involvement in childbirth but in those days it was the nurses who didn't give a f***. Perhaps fatherly attendance in the labour ward has one positive effect: it may keep medical staff more on their guard about common decency. I vowed to be present for every subsequent birth.

David Newbound

Birthframe 64

This birth story shows just how supportive partners can sometimes be. Indeed, the support this particular partner offered is probably the very best kind of support a pregnant and labouring woman can wish for... This man made sure his wife had caregivers she felt comfortable with by completely supporting her wishes, even under very difficult circumstances.

We had returned late on the Saturday night from a friend's wedding reception and climbed into bed, with me still feeling the effects of an over-indulgence of food and alcohol. Sleep came upon me with ease until I was rudely awakened by a sharp dig in the ribs by Karen, my beloved, who rather nervously announced that she thought it had started. Being a loving, sensitive and supportive partner, my immediate response was to enquire: "Have you had a show yet? No?! Well go back to sleep and don't wake me until you have." Could this really have been Mr Sensitive talking or was it the booze and lack of sleep taking over? (That's my excuse and I'm sticking to it!) A slightly more aggressive dig in the ribs followed and was accompanied by a short, sharp volley of verbal abuse and threatening behaviour. I was stung into action, so crawled out of bed and attempted to look sharp and alert, ready for anything, but in reality of course was a total wreck and looked it—no fooling anyone.

We agreed that we should keep busy, so tidied the house, had a bath, played Scrabble (I won) and before we knew it 3.00am turned into 7.00am. It was now time to call Liz, who had helped and advised us so far and was our 'expert'. She had agreed to help out and had three children of her own, two of which had been born at home. I collected Liz around 9.00am and returned to find that the contractions were regular enough to warrant calling the midwife.

In the months leading up to the birth we had some difficulties (understatement) with 'The Establishment' regarding our desire for a home birth, with a few midwives vehemently opposed. We had expressed our discontent to the Head of Midwifery Services, who had agreed that the attending midwife would not be one of the dissenters. Unfortunately, on that fateful morn, No.1 choice was ill, No.2 had a day off, No.3 was Head Dissenter (didn't even bother calling her, she would have been out on her broomstick anyway) but No.4 answered. Great! Or so we thought. Much to our surprise, Karen was answered with a torrent of abuse for choosing a home birth and for also politely refusing the midwife's offer of having a student in attendance. She said she would be around soon, but was not happy. The effect of this event was to stop the contractions completely, but normal service resumed 20 minutes later.

We discussed and collectively agreed that this lady was not for us. Karen and Liz agreed that I would turn her away at the door while they hid—thanks. Time for my cool, calm approach towards problem-solving to surface. I took control and phoned the hospital to find out the alternatives and demand action. All they could suggest was to make the peace with midwife No.4, as she was all that was available—time for Mr Cool to panic. "We can do it ourselves!" I proudly announced. "Boil some water and fetch towels!" Liz calmed the hysteria by informing us that this was illegal and that she would contact her ex-midwife and now friend, Jo, who was a practising independent midwife. She agreed to come but would have to obtain the appropriate approvals from the State Health Authority first. This was to be a momentous obstacle but she managed to battle through OK and arrived on our doorstep at 1pm—phew! The next stop was to provide her with some assistance and back-up, courtesy of Jan, who we all knew and was an ex-nurse and current antenatal teacher.

The first examination revealed, much to everyone's amazement, that Karen was 8cm dilated. Around 2.00pm the second stage commenced, a time Karen had been dreading, but Jo reassured her by saying that whilst it would probably be painful it shouldn't take too long as she was doing so well. 'Too long' to someone (like me) in intense pain would be 10 seconds.

'Not too long' lasted two hours for Karen, who was by this time starting to tire. Digby (the silly name we had christened the bump once the scan had revealed our baby was to be a boy) started to crown, but a further 25 minutes passed. Jo and Jan constantly reassured Karen that 'one more push will do it' but none of us really believed it until suddenly, without warning, Digby shot out and was fantastically caught one-handed by Jo.

Suddenly, without warning, Digby shot out

On closer examination Digby appeared to be woefully short of a few vital attributes that would make his position as the rightful Captain of the England football team difficult to attain. Digby's attributes were more suited for netball so I found myself wiping the tears of joy away, holding our beautiful daughter, while the third stage commenced. I looked at her and thought, "Just like her mother—late!" It made me want to weep!

Meanwhile, back at the action, Karen had finished the third stage relatively quickly but was haemorrhaging badly, was very pale and was starting to shake uncontrollably as she was going into shock. The scene started to resemble an out-take from *The Exorcist* but, fortunately, Jo and Jan quickly averted any danger and the bleeding subsided.

At the first available moment I dashed downstairs to crack the champagne and returned to find the new mum feeding our daughter, which immediately restored the lump in my throat and dampness to my eyes. By 9.30pm, everyone had left and we were left alone in total amazement looking at the little bundle laid between us. Our first sleepless night was soon to be upon us...

Alan Low

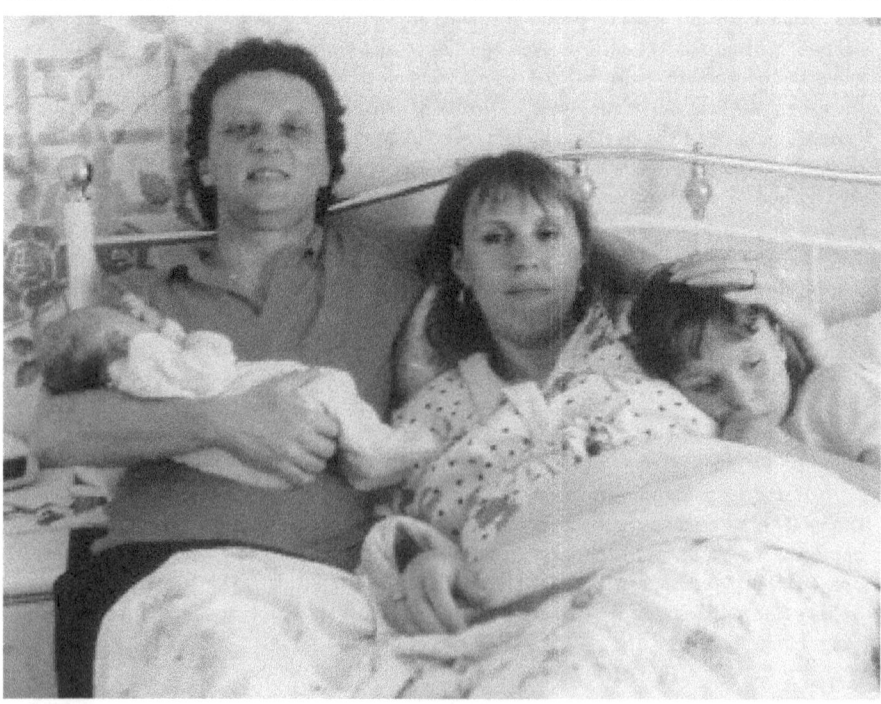

Postnatal family cuddle

CHILDREN

Birthframe 65

The next account was written by the 'baby' whose birth was described in the last birthframe. She witnessed her little sister's birth. Although she had mixed feelings about attending a birth (the birth of her little sister, in fact) this child—who was 7 years old at the time of the birth—was clearly surprised by what happened and it changed her views and expectations of childbirth.

I remember feeling warm all over. I had wanted a sister and now she was finally here. It was truly amazing. I fell asleep momentarily because I was so tired.

Since then, I have learnt a lot more about what happened that day, as at the age of 7 I didn't really take it all in. When I have seen videos at school, I have never seen an account of a home birth. From these videos I had been led to believe that there would be lots and lots of blood and screaming, but it was nothing like that. There had been surprisingly little blood and no screaming or signs of excruciating agony. The overall atmosphere was calm and pleasant and Marie made everyone feel relaxed and excited. We decided to give Christy the middle name of Marie after this wonderful midwife, who made the birth so much easier and relaxed. I am very grateful for the experience and, thanks to Marie, understood and saw all the things I'd seen on videos, in real life. I think it's a shame that so many people are unaware that home births are a possibility. I think that home birth awareness has grown since Christy's birth and it's still becoming more popular. If I have children I think that I will have a home birth and possibly in water too.

Cara Low, 13 years old

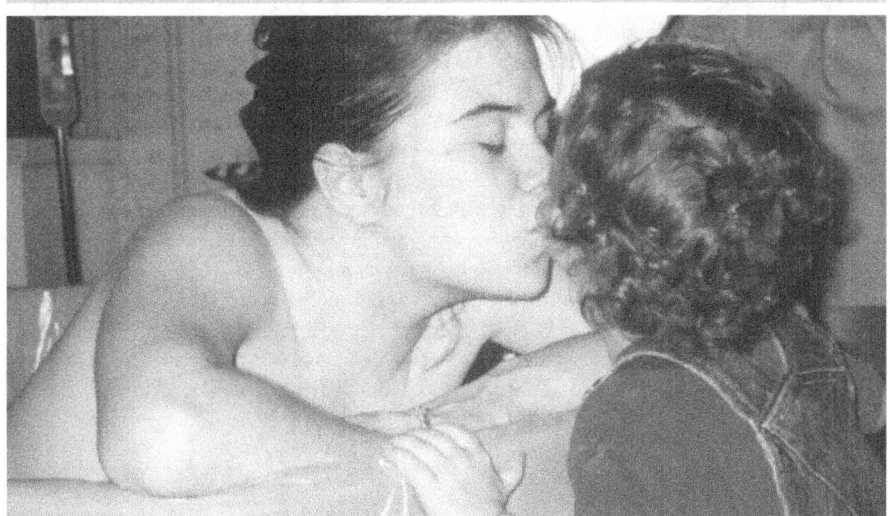

Sometimes it's reassuring for older children if they can be there when the baby's born

Children don't usually get scared unless their parents are scared

In case you were wondering, the photo on the previous page *is* a photo of a labouring woman (in a birthing pool). When I explained my policy of not using photos of women in labour because of the risk of disturbing them and making them feel 'observed', Ashley Marshall, the contributor (see Birthframe 4), made the following comment:

> I'm sorry to say that I was in very active labour when this photo was taken. It was at my request, though, as I wanted the event to be documented. I just love birth!! I think a simple statement about children at birth would justify using the photo.

So, despite my general policy, I am including this photo because it's a beautiful photo of a labouring woman, which shows a positive attitude and good positioning, i.e. leaning forward, which is good for the baby inside. I'm perhaps also using it so as to pander to the rebel in every woman, who might really want to see what a woman looks like when she is labouring normally! Of course, women who are strapped up to monitors on hospital beds, with drips in their arms, and the various other paraphernalia that a 'managed' birth involves look quite different. There are numerous photos of that kind of labouring woman in magazines on pregnancy and birth. So is it OK to have children present when you give birth? Again, there are differing views on this...

> Children don't usually get scared unless their parents are scared. The great thing about home birth is it's so unscary. If anything frightening began to happen, the midwife would see it coming hours before and get you to hospital immediately. I wouldn't wake my kids up to watch, but if I am blessed with another birth at home and the older ones do wake up, I won't worry.

> Very handy that my son woke up at just the right moment. But that's not really the point. What if yours doesn't? Children are very matter-of-fact about things. If you explain to them what you plan to do—have a baby right here in the bedroom—and what might happen—Mummy might make funny noises—then, chances are, if your children wake up at an inopportune moment, they probably won't be fazed in the least. Of course, you want to make sure you have back-up options, such as a neighbour who doesn't mind being woken up in the wee hours. But in the event, chances are it won't be necessary. I rehearsed with my 2-year-old the grunting noises he might hear me making and explained that making a baby come out takes a lot of work. "You can help me practise," I told him, and we made pushing sounds together. *Nina Klose*

Very handy that my son woke up just the right moment. But that's not really the point. What if yours doesn't?

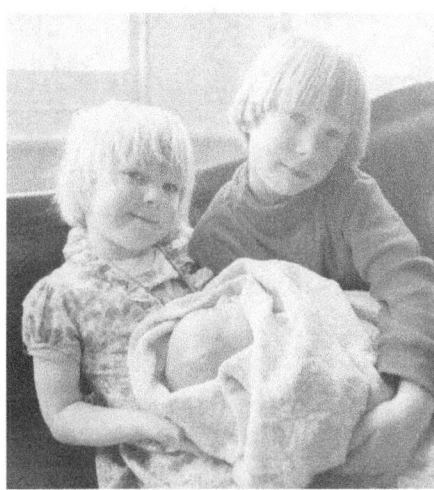

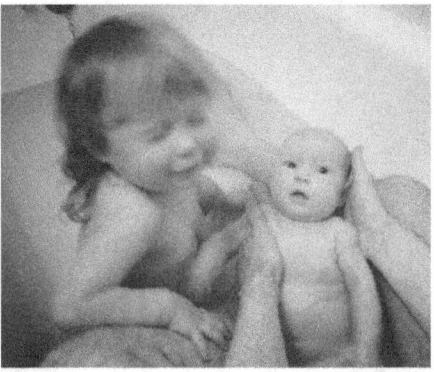

Here a little girl seems delighted to be included in her new sister's bath, with Daddy's help and support, of course

Two big sisters contemplating the new arrival...

Delighted to be included...

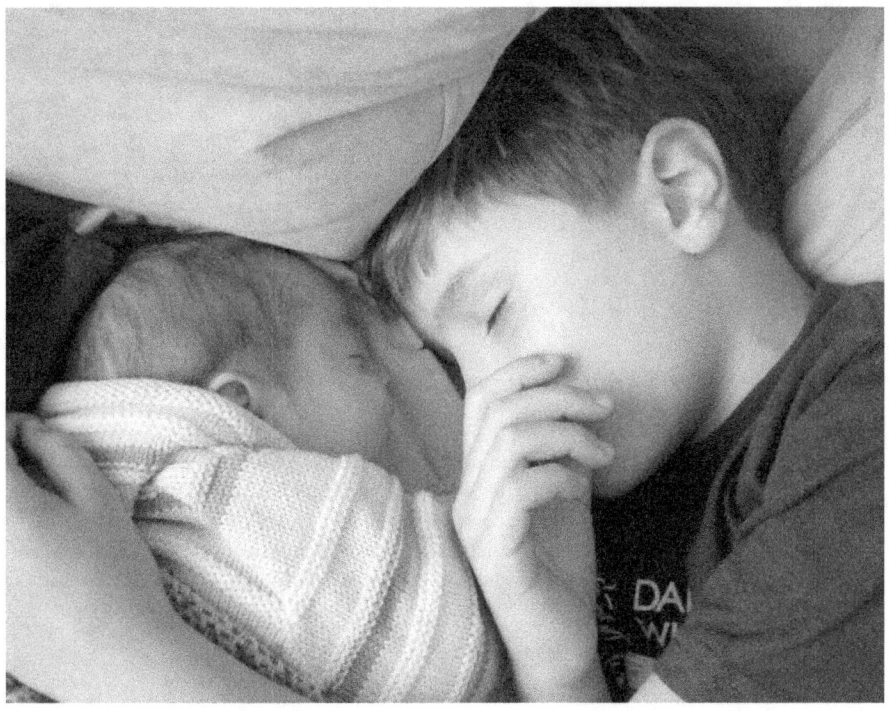

Big brother asleep with his newborn sister

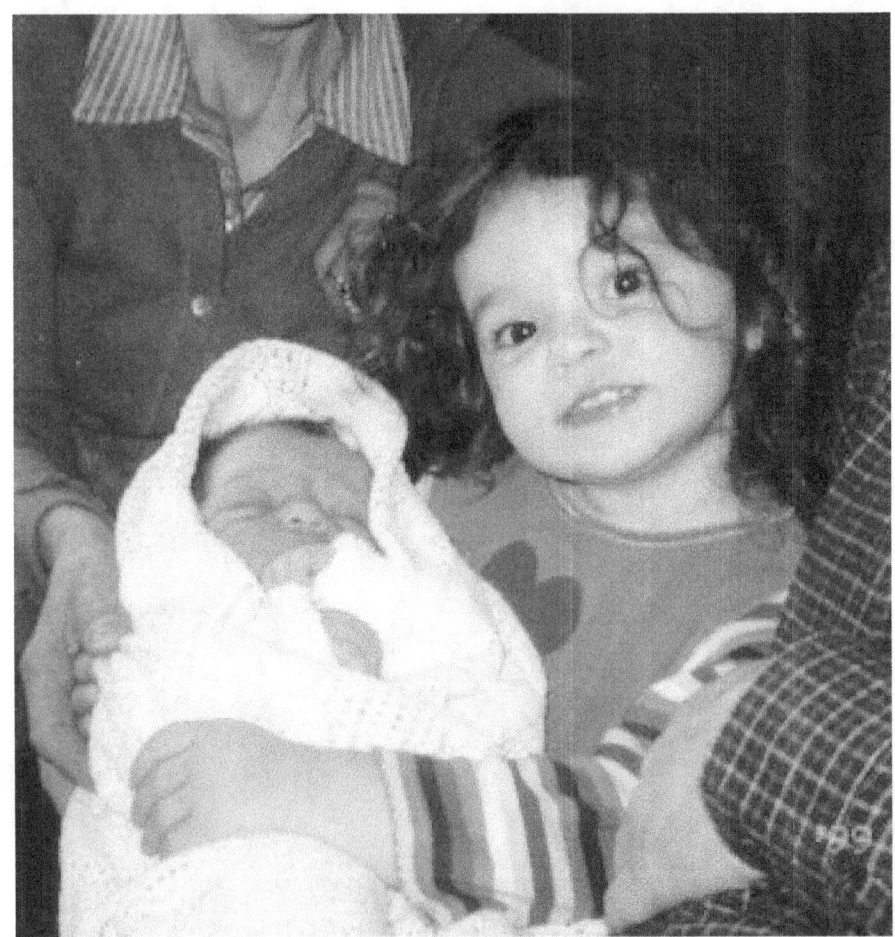

Another little girl who's delighted to be involved, this time with the help of the midwife

❝ It would be nice to be able to give a dreamy, romantic account, but I'm afraid my other children seemed pretty insensitive to my needs as I laboured in front of them. Another time, I'd arrange for someone to be on call, to take them away somewhere to play so that I would be able to labour in peace and seclusion. Yes, I do love my children!—but I need to focus inwards when I'm in labour and I can't do that when my kids are around.

It'd be nice to be able to give a dreamy, romantic account,
but I'm afraid my children seemed pretty insensitive

FRIENDS

Finally, we need to consider these other possible birth attendants... Is it a good idea to have them around?

> Some friends came over for some wine and cheese, and the contractions stopped for 20 minutes or so. If I had it to do over, I wouldn't have anyone besides my husband in the house. I was very self-conscious, and didn't want anyone to see me in pain.

In the end, as with everything else, you need to follow your intuitive sense of what is right for you when making decisions on this issue.

Having said that, it does seem to be the case that having fewer birth attendants will result in a smoother labour and birth. As long as you feel safe, i.e. you have that safety net in place, you don't feel you're being observed and you're not spoken to, you're much more likely to spontaneously tune into your primitive knowledge of how to give birth. This may mean it's necessary to ask everyone, including midwives and friends to be as unobtrusive as possible or to leave the room. You may even want to ask friends to leave the house or the hospital—in the nicest possible way, of course!

Have confidence in yourself and be content to share this very intimate, private time with just yourself and your new baby, and possibly your partner too! Insist that caregivers take a back seat... after all, it's your birth, not theirs!

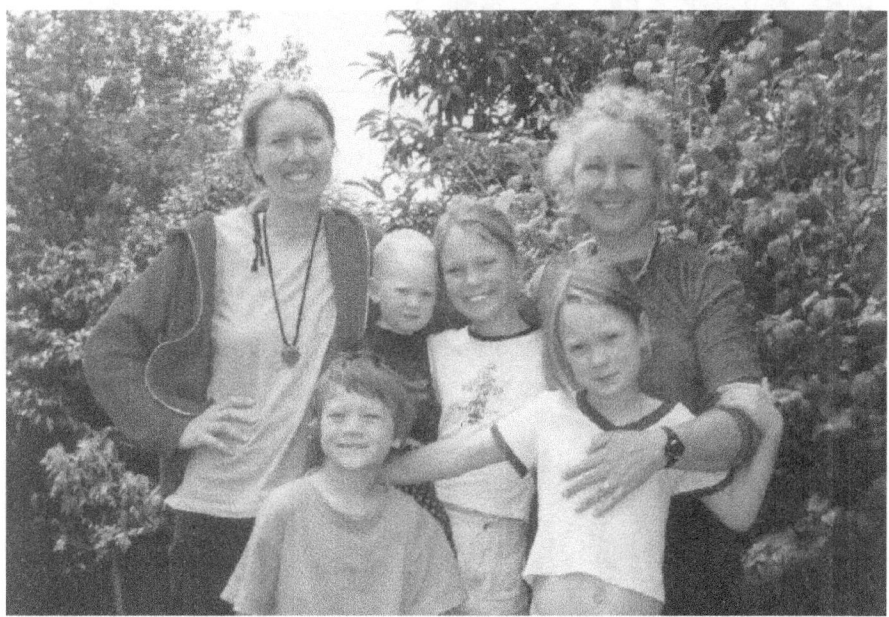

Do you have a friend you're close enough to? This is Sarah Buckley with her four children and a very good friend (see pages 109-111)

The most important people of all…

Above all, remember that this is your one and only chance to bond with your new baby and that you may well need privacy to do this… The first hour of life has been found to be crucial to future relationships, so enjoy!

Remember you need privacy to bond with your baby (or babies)

Photo © Jill Furmanovsky

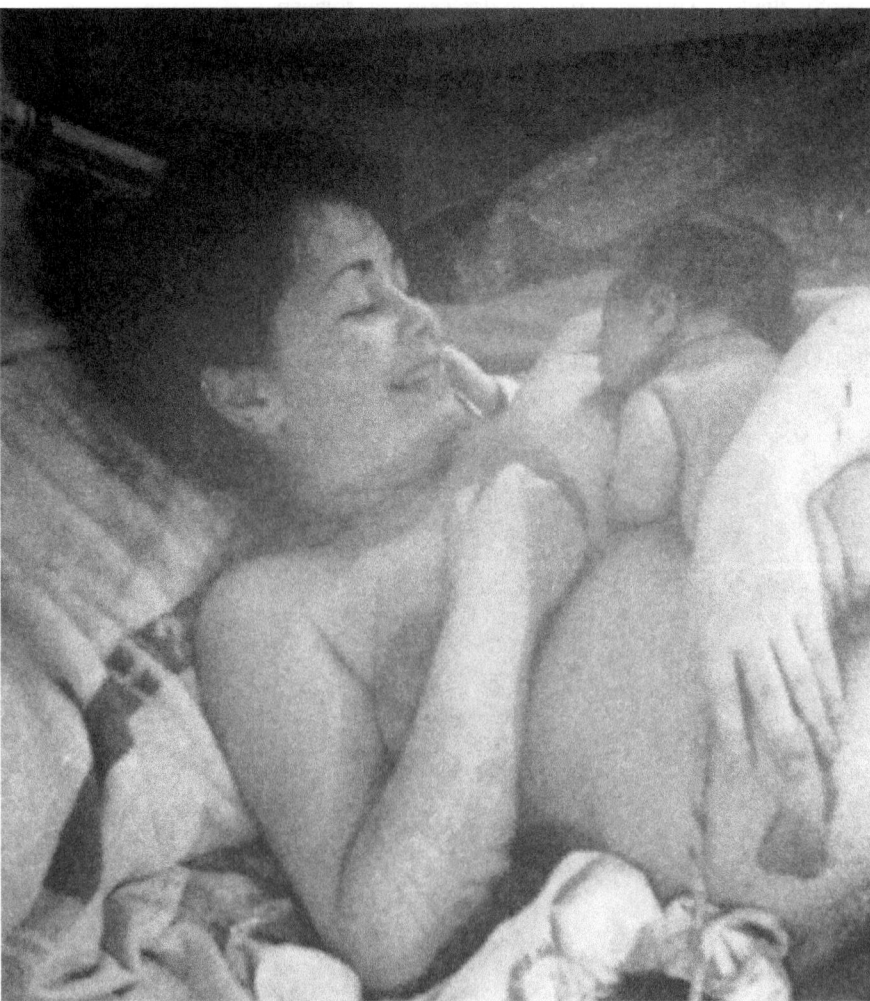

Nuala OSullivan, moments after giving birth, entirely physiologically

3... CHOOSE WHERE

A very practical decision...

This is not necessarily the simple decision you might suppose it to be... And it's a very important one because your birthplace may dramatically affect the type of birth that you and your baby experience. This, in turn, will affect your own mind and body, your early relationship with your baby and your early perceptions of motherhood. So please do take this seriously, again putting aside your assumptions.[1]

> I signed up to have the baby at a birth centre, which offers birthing pools, TENS machines and midwife-only birth. It turned out there were several problems, however. First, it was a 40-minute drive to the birth centre from our house, even without traffic. As a result, I didn't go there very often antenatally—I went to most of my check-ups at the hospital. So the birth centre midwives didn't know me. For them, I was just as anonymous as I was for the doctors at the hospital. Second, because they are a midwife-only NHS birth centre, they are required to follow very strict safety guidelines. They couldn't be flexible the way an independent midwife could. As soon as they saw meconium, they kicked me out. If I had been at home, my midwife might still have transferred me, but only if there had been further cause to suspect fetal distress, such as an abnormal heart rate.[2]

Your own decision about 'where' should involve considering which kind of building you're going to give birth in, which kind of room, whether or not this will involve transfer from one room to another and even whether you're going to be in water or on dry land!

In this chapter we'll focus mainly on the home vs hospital debate because, as we can see from the comment above, a birth centre is like a hospital in the sense that there are inevitably systems and protocols and also because it's someone else's territory. Having said that, some birth centres make an enormous effort to be homely and accommodating and sometimes the people who work in them are aware of the importance of not disturbing women who are labouring and giving birth. So it may be a good alternative to home for women who want to separate their birthing experience from their home life. For others, a birth centre birth may not be anywhere near as good as a home birth—simply because it is not home.

Make your decision in consultation with your partner and caregiver(s), because their support is also incredibly important. Ultimately, though, it is your decision... so be prepared to negotiate and persuade anyone necessary, wherever it is you eventually feel it will be better for you to give birth.

Decide in consultation with your partner and caregiver(s)

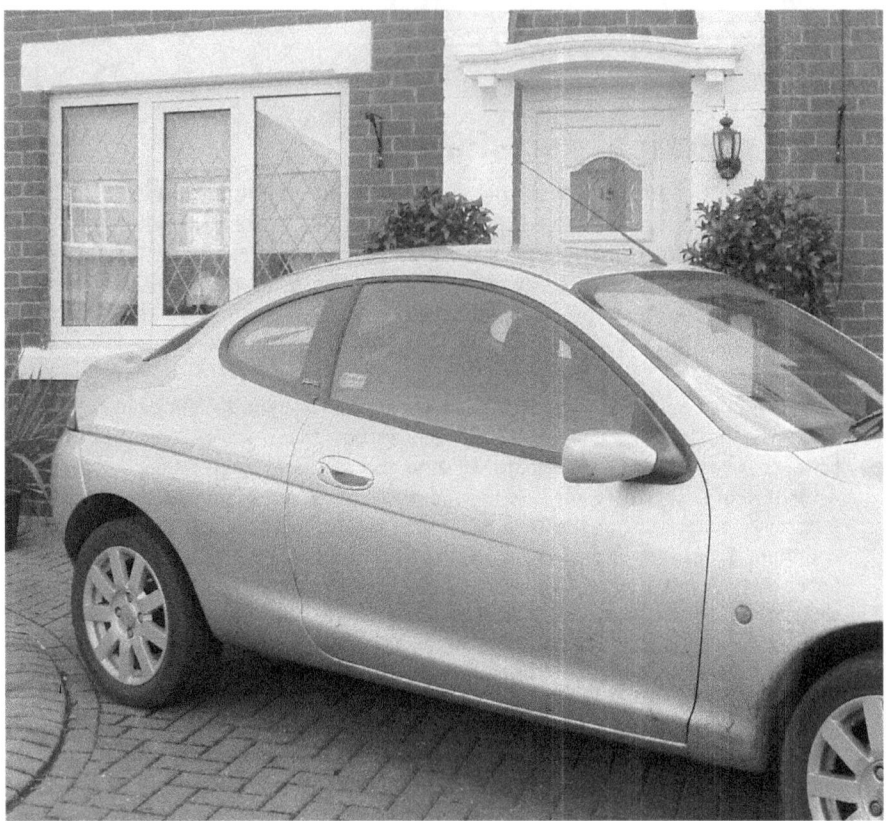
Your decision of 'where' may well depend on where you live and whether you have transport to get to a hospital, if necessary

The historical shift toward the hospital

A few decades ago, most women gave birth at home... Then—in the 1960s in particular—more and more women started going into hospital to give birth. This trend has recently been changing again, due to increased awareness of the disadvantages of hospital birth and the comparative advantages—and even safety—of home births.

However, it is still the case that in many countries around the world the majority of women give birth in a hospital. In some countries (e.g. Sri Lanka, Vietnam, Oman and the UAE), almost the entire female population gives birth in a hospital either because the government has promoted hospital birth effectively or because home births have been made illegal.

Why has there been such a dramatic change in attitudes amongst either health professionals or women? Here are a few possible reasons...

COST

All hospitals are essentially businesses, which need to operate at a profit, and it is in their best financial interests to encourage people to spend time there. At the same time, various companies which manufacture medical equipment promote certain new devices and technologies and once a hospital manager has approved purchase of an expensive piece of equipment it is obviously then necessary to demonstrate that the money hasn't been wasted. A very obvious example is the electronic fetal monitor, which was originally developed for and marketed by Hewlett Packard. Although research studies later showed that these machines have virtually no impact on outcomes—except for unnecessarily increasing rates of caesareans and forceps or vacuum extractor use—they continue to be used widely and in some cases routinely. Their technical appearance and convenience may also be factors in their popularity, as well as the fact that the printouts usefully provide 'evidence' in litigation cases. Both medics and patients *believe* in technology.

Still considering cost as a reason for the shift from home to hospital over the last century, it's probably also significant that hospital really is expensive—because using it then becomes a sign of status. Beyond the general charges which can be made for overnight stays, any technology or treatment used adds to the bill. I became aware of this personally when I received the bill for my first birth, which took place at a private hospital in Sri Lanka. The total was very reasonable, even though tiny items were listed... but I realised it would have been altogether different if I'd had scans, EFM and a caesarean...

CONDITIONS AND CLEANLINESS

In the days when families were larger and modern amenities were not available, homes were not the calm, clean, sanitised places they usually are today. Many women must have been pleased to leave their chaotic homes for the relative calm and cleanliness of the local hospital. Nowadays, because of our increased wealth, improved cleaning products, household appliances and smaller families, many homes are cleaner and calmer than hospitals. What's more, any germs at home are ones you, your partner and new baby are prepared for—they're not 'foreign' hospital ones.

If you feel inclined to disbelieve this, consider that in 2003 the *Reader's Digest* reported that in Britain an estimated 100,000 people were picking up an infection in hospital each year. In the same article they stated that hospital-acquired infections killed more than 5,000 patients and that they contributed to the deaths of some 15,000 more. Has the situation changed so dramatically since then? Is it realistically possible for hospitals to become places which are 'cleaner' than houses, given that their main purpose is to serve people who are sick? Even in maternity wards, bugs can collect on catheters, intravenous lines, computers, watches, curtains and male doctors' ties—not to mention hands which are not washed thoroughly.

Birthframe 66

The reminiscences of the following midwife serve as a reminder of how different people's homes could be only a few decades ago.

Some of the home circumstances were quite appalling and some of the home births I attended were in the most awful places. You just wouldn't want to wash your hands because the facilities were so bad. I remember in one flat, they had done their best to make the bedroom clean and tidy, but you couldn't get into the kitchen for unwashed plates and clothes all over the place. The husband then said to me that he would have made me a cup of tea, but he wasn't expecting me... His wife was nine months pregnant but he wasn't expecting a midwife to call! I was actually quite grateful because I didn't want to drink out of any of their cups, but I wouldn't have wanted to appear rude.

I was shocked by some of the housing areas I had to visit and the very poor circumstances and living conditions people lived in. One evening I once came across a child sitting in the gutter, eating out of the dustbin. Families lived in one room up flights of stone stairs, with one toilet for three flats, halfway down. There was one room with a sink, which did duty for the potatoes, the washing (of course everybody had cotton nappies) and the baby's bath. We would be horrified now at some of the home conditions in which people had home births. A lot of the births I attended were in big families and I assisted many women who already had eight, nine or 10 children. Believe it or not, this was in the UK in the 1960s!

Carol Walton

PAIN RELIEF

Many forms of pain relief can only really be administered in a hospital setting because they necessitate careful monitoring and all kinds of other procedures, for the sake of safety. (There is implicit recognition that disturbing the physiological processes is dangerous.) An epidural, for example, can only be administered in a hospital because when one is used the woman's blood pressure needs to be monitored in case it falls dangerously low; she needs a urinary catheter because she loses all sensation in her lower regions; she also needs a drip in position in case her labour slows down or stops and syntocinon needs to be administered in order to restart or augment contractions. In addition, facilities for performing a caesarean need to be available when epidurals are used as the likelihood of one being needed rises dramatically.

EQUIPMENT

Obstetric equipment (which has been developed over the last few decades) has been marketed aggressively by manufacturers. It is probably attractive to health professionals because it may make them feel they have more 'control' over the natural processes. Marketing campaigns have usually not been supported by research data and sometimes they have even taken place when research data has clearly shown equipment to have a *negative* influence on birth outcomes.

Electronic fetal monitors are a prime example of this: research has clearly shown that their only contribution to birth outcomes is to increase the caesarean rate without improving safety—but they continue to be purchased and used by hospitals around the world. Fetal scalp monitors are shockingly invasive, but since they provide clear data on a baby's condition they are used, even though it is likely they may distress the baby. Any volunteers to try out a metal clip in the scalp? Even if monitors are attached by suction they must be perceived by the baby.

STATISTICS

Outcomes for mother and baby have improved significantly over the last few decades. Health authorities and researchers widely recognise that this is because of general improvements in health and hygiene, not because of any shift toward hospital birth. In places where home births are illegal or discouraged, births at home usually only take place 'by accident', i.e. when a fast birth takes a woman by surprise. This is unfortunate because unplanned home births are not the safest type because the people participating are usually unprepared and frightened. Statistics gleaned from countries where home birth is accepted (such as Holland) show it to be a safe or safer option than a hospital birth.

Statistics show planned home birth to be a safe or a safer option than a hospital birth for the majority of women

Photos by Sylvie Donna, courtesy of the Beamish Living Museum in Co Durham

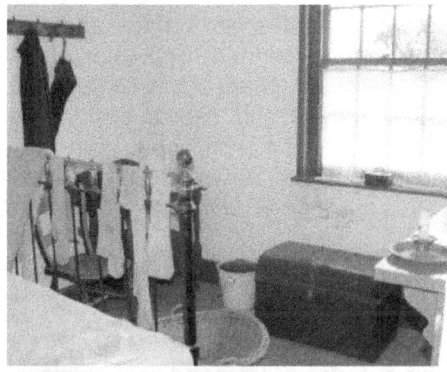

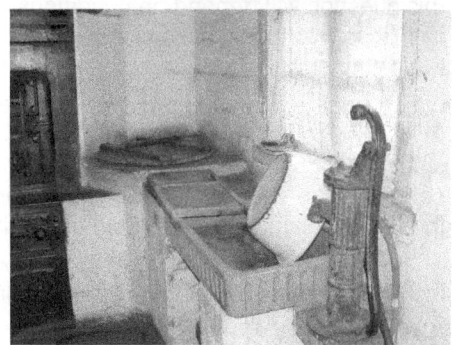

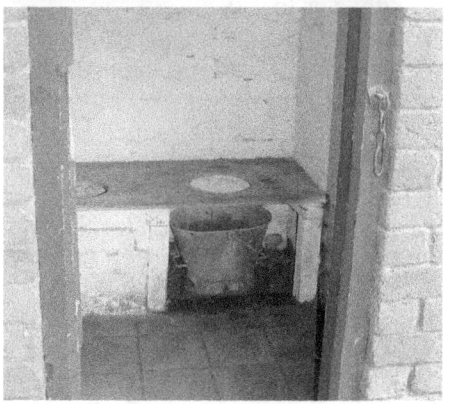

Even recently, home birth would have been a very different prospect for most people. These photographs of a 'living museum' aim to portray life as it was in 1913 in a typical home in Britain.

FASHION

In an age of high-technology, home births are sometimes seen as a primitive 'alternative lifestyle' choice and home birthers are wrongly regarded as unscientific, selfish romantics who are only looking for a good one-off birthing 'high'. Statistics which show low-tech home births as being safe for both mothers and babies are not as readily available to women as birth accounts on TV or in popular pregnancy magazines of highly interventionist hospital births. Because they are well-documented by the media, hospital births are seen as being the only real option.

Is the hospital the best place to give birth?

For a tiny minority of women with specific life-threatening health conditions, the answer is clearly yes. For a woman in relatively good health, the answer to this question will depend on conditions at her local hospital and on the quality, calmness and cleanliness of her home. Of course, the woman's state of mind is also important, as is the accessibility (or otherwise) of the hospital.

The idea that conditions may not be ideal at some hospitals is surprising to many people—even me! One antenatal teacher I consulted told me her students thought she was being extreme when she warned them about the need to take their own cleaning equipment into the hospital. Afterwards, though, she said they'd changed their minds.[3]

If you do decide to have a hospital birth, be reassured that there are many things you can do to help protect yourself from infection...

- ♥ If necessary remind doctors and midwives to wash their hands before attending to you.
- ♥ Wash your own hands carefully after handling any type of body fluids, and especially after going to the bathroom.
- ♥ Take a shower early on in labour, if you're worried about surgery being necessary. This will reduce bacteria on your skin, which may reduce your chances of infection.
- ♥ If you have to have a catheter, or drainage tube, let your midwife know if it becomes loose or dislodged and make sure he or she keeps the skin around the dressing clean and dry. Any intravenous device is a potential entry point for germs, so discuss with your consultant when it can safely be removed.
- ♥ Don't touch any wound or disturb a dressing as this may introduce bacteria. Ask a midwife to replace a dressing that gets loose or wet.
- ♥ Ask well-wishers not to visit if they feel ill.
- ♥ Watch out for early signs of infection: redness, swelling or pain. Early treatment improves recovery.
- ♥ Consider checking out the cleanliness record of any hospital or clinic you plan to attend. Begin by visiting the hospital itself to get an initial impression, then ask around.

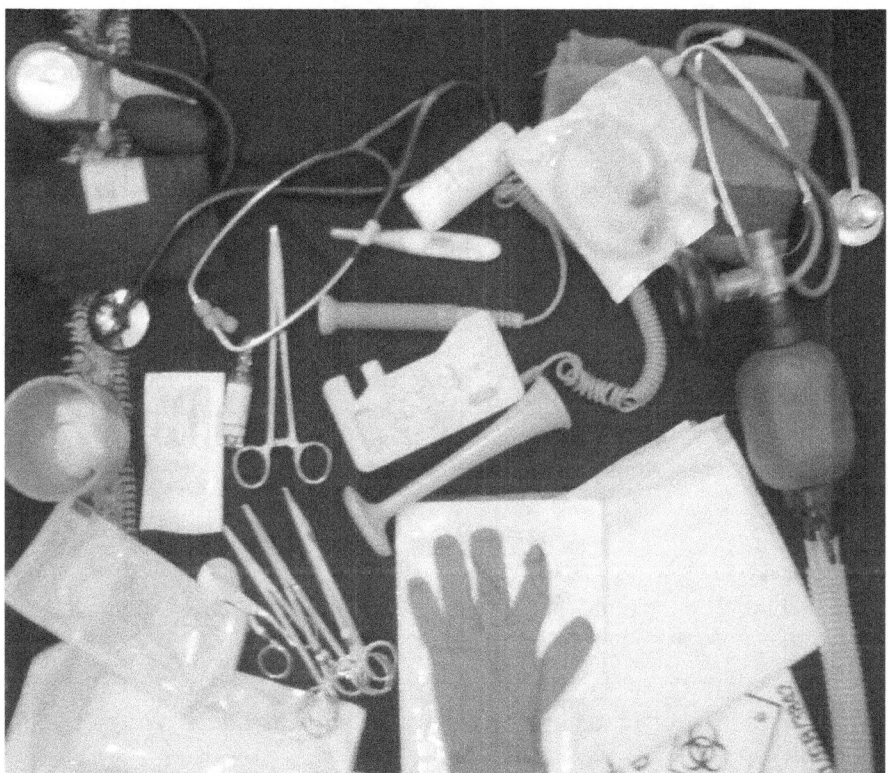

A midwife needs very little equipment in order to attend a woman having an optimal birth at home... Here is a home midwife's kit.

As well as cleanliness and risk of infection, there are other reasons why you might seriously consider not going to hospital, if you have this choice. Firstly, women in a hospital are likely to move into the mindset of a patient rather than an active birther. Signing consent forms, donning hospital gowns and lying on beds may all cause this. Secondly, since most hospitals are relatively unfamiliar women are likely to become tense and fearful. (As we've seen, this usually results in a slower, more painful and less effective labour.) Protocols or even caregivers' habits may mean that procedures are carried out and drugs administered without women being consulted or fully informed. Finally, women in hospitals are less likely to have one-to-one care because more 'efficient' models of care are in place.

Protocols may mean that procedures are carried out and drugs administered without women being consulted

From a purely psychological point of view, you may find that at the hospital the focus is very much more on machines and numbers than on you and your state of mind. You may feel more ready to succumb to any pressure to use equipment simply because it's so readily available—and of course this also applies to so-called pain relief. (It's that chocolate biscuit problem again—if they're there, I'm highly likely to eat them!) You're much more at risk of disturbance in hospital because there's inevitably less privacy and there are usually protocols about moving women to delivery rooms, not to mention postnatal rooms. Protocols after the birth are likely to disturb your baby too.

As we've already recognised, though, there are good reasons to give birth in the hospital in some cases. You might seriously consider it if you have specific medical needs which can't be catered for at home (e.g. kidney failure). It might also be a good idea if you live a long way away from your nearest hospital, if you have several children or if you have a particularly unsanitary home, with poor facilities and inadequate heating.

Birthframe 67

Debbie Brindley, a midwife who we've met before [in Birthframe 45], opted for a home birth when she had her first baby. For her second birth, when she had twins, she chose to go to the hospital. Here she explains why.

I understand your first birth was a water birth at home. Weren't you nervous?

No. I'd worked hard to prepare myself for a good labour—I'd eaten well, I swam daily and practised yoga throughout pregnancy. I had knowledge which reduced fear of the unknown. I was very positive and trusted in my abilities as a woman to give birth. (I also had excellent support from my husband and my midwife.) And I knew home birth is safer than hospital birth in low risk women. All I needed was a bit of luck!

Why did you choose to have a water birth?

I had delivered quite a lot of women in the pool at the hospital I work in and seen for myself its advantages. To me a water birth meant privacy, a quiet environment away from medical intervention, relaxation from the warmth, subdued lighting, music and the ability to change position easily. The water births I attended were straightforward labours, enhanced by gravity, upright positions and reduced pain.

Did you have specially-trained midwives to attend you?

I had my local community midwife who, fortunately, is very experienced in home birth. She hadn't conducted water births but she read as much as she could and spoke to midwives who had done home water births. She was supported by a hospital midwife (a private arrangement) who was confident in water births. They were both fantastic.

When you got pregnant again with twins, you opted to go to hospital. Why didn't you arrange a home birth?

I knew as a midwife that if there were problems they were likely to be acute. I also knew that any problems were likely to affect the second twin, placental separation or malpresentation being the main potential problems. Problems with a singleton can often be anticipated but this was unknown territory for me and I didn't feel it was fair to risk the second baby's well-being. I contacted AIMS [the Association for Improvements in Midwifery Services] at 34 weeks to check if there was any research on twin home births before my final decision and there was none!

If you were ever to go through the same thing again would you consider having them at home or would you make any special arrangements?

Not unless I had a crystal ball that could show me a guaranteed successful outcome for the same reasons as I've already given. The odds of a cephalic second twin malpresenting, or a premature placental separation are likely to be low, but the baby's health is paramount and more important than my choice of birthplace. The hospital was not as bad as I had thought... quite all right, in fact! I was only in for nine hours, overnight. If I had another singleton pregnancy I would definitely stay at home, though.

If you were to get pregnant again, would you change anything about your care or the way you give birth?

No, I don't think so. I would definitely choose a home birth over the hospital, and would always want an active birth, but as long as I had done everything in my power to facilitate a natural active birth, I could accept deviations out of my control, and their consequences.

I wish my mum could have been with me at my second labour, as well as the first. But I needed her to look after my 2-year-old. And I wish someone had changed the Enya tape over instead of leaving it on replay... Not much to grumble about, is it?!

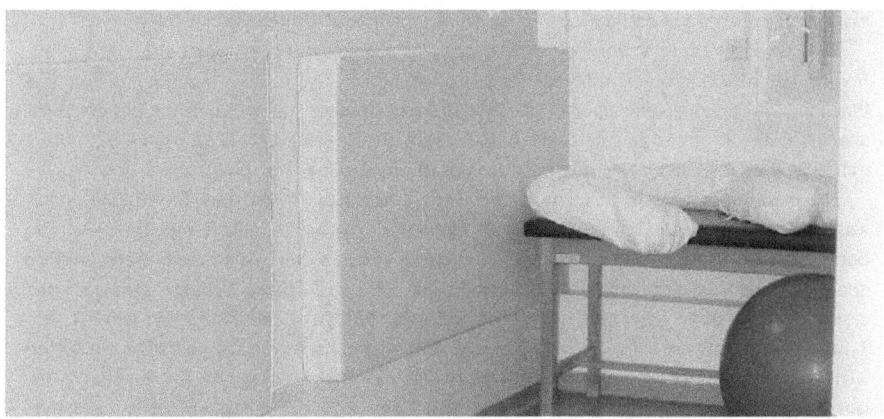

You may feel reassured knowing you're within arm's reach of an operating theatre with staff ready to perform a caesarean. This is a hospital labour room.

Birthframe 68

This account describes another few births which were not much disturbed by hospital protocols. It also raises an interesting question: What is it that makes women give birth quickly and easily? As this account suggests, it's not just down to our choice of birthplace. Attitudes (of the woman and the people around her), genes, past experience, pain relief, disturbance and interventions might all play a part... But then again, some women can clearly override negative factors, when these aren't really ideal.

When I met the woman who contributed this account it was a couple of weeks before she was due to give birth to her fifth child. At the time, I was struck by her carefree attitude towards the upcoming birth, although she later told me she had actually felt far from carefree inside! Anyway, as expected, the birth went fine.

I have always had a lot of contact with babies and children. I have a half sister and brother who are 12 and 18 years younger than I am. I met my children's father when I was 18 and he had a young daughter who we often had to stay with us. I enjoyed looking after children when I was younger and always wanted to have a baby myself. I now have five children: Hannah (7lb 11oz, born in 1986), Faye (7lb 10oz, born in 1990), Liam (7lb 13oz, born in 1993), Ashley (9lb 5oz, born in 1997) and Luke (8lb 9oz, born in 2002).

All my births have been relatively easy. My longest labours were four hours with my first and fourth children. The shortest labour was one hour with my third child. There were no major complications during any of my labours, although I did have to have stitches after each birth. I also bled quite heavily afterwards. My second child became distressed during labour because the cord was wrapped twice around her neck, restricting her breathing. She was given oxygen immediately after delivery. I never used any pain relief during any of my labours, there was never time anyway. I was encouraged to try gas and air during my first labour, but this made me vomit.

I assume my labours were quick and easy compared to other women due to genes. My mother also had quick, easy labours. [Comment from Sylvie: Other women have told me their mothers had long, difficult labours. Could there be another reason?] I never did anything special in any of my pregnancies to help myself give birth easily. I did have a positive attitude towards labour and was not worried at the prospect of giving birth.

I had all my babies in hospital. I did want a home birth with my fourth child, but was told that because I was anaemic it was not advisable in case I bled heavily. The baby's father also preferred the baby to be born in hospital. This labour began with a show, followed almost immediately by mild contractions. These became stronger and close together quite quickly. I stayed at home for the first two hours and when I felt I needed the support of a midwife, was taken to the hospital. The midwife consulted with me throughout labour and allowed me to make the decisions for my care. My waters broke after about an hour and the baby was delivered normally about an hour later, after just three pushes.

With my fifth child, the midwife actually suggested a possible home birth the first time I met her. However, she said I would have to change my doctor temporarily, as the practice I was registered with did not support home births. I decided to have the baby in hospital but was provided with a home birth pack and advice in case I didn't make it to the hospital.

This labour started with quite strong contractions almost immediately. They became very frequent after about an hour. I had to wait for someone to arrive to look after my other children. I arrived at the hospital 10 minutes before I delivered the baby. Shortly after my arrival at the hospital my waters broke and the baby arrived almost immediately after one push. I was allowed home six hours later.

I don't regret having my babies in hospital, although I would like to have experienced a home birth. Since I had my first child, care for pregnant women has improved. The woman has more choice with regard to labour and I found there was much less medical interference.

Even though the choices are there I still think there is room for improvement to encourage women to make these choices. Until my last pregnancy I was never offered a choice of where to have my babies. I had to ask. Even with my last pregnancy when I was offered a choice there was still the problem of the GP practice I was with not being willing to support this choice.

Debbie Shaw

Birthframe 69

This next account presents a rather less positive picture and perhaps explains why many women choose a home birth for their second baby's birth...

My first son's birth was short but traumatic, ending with him being dragged out by forceps and myself being sutured afterwards, surrounded by what seemed like a menagerie of people, watching me in a compromising position. It left me not wanting to ever go through giving birth again. Six and a half years later, after a miscarriage, I got pregnant again.

My second son's birth was a completely natural home birth. After about two hours of manageable contractions, I could feel my baby's head coming down, then sliding back again between contractions. The only real discomfort was in my lower back. I was very quiet and peaceful between contractions, appreciating the lull in between each one until 10.24, when Arion was born. Eventually, I couldn't stop myself from pushing...

I feel the crown of my baby's head and cry out in a very primal way, feeling like I want to almost sing, "My baby's head is born!" Then after what feels like a very long 10 minutes, his body is born... I cradle him in my arms and offer him my breast. We soon get out of the pool and join my other son and my husband on the sofa.

Georgina Taylor

Here are a few comments about hospitals...

> With my second labour my waters broke at home so I went straight to hospital. When I arrived, I was 4cm dilated and having regular contractions, then they all stopped. I do believe it was because I was in a different place and wasn't so relaxed.

> Arrived at the hospital. I remember walking down the long corridor and thinking, "This must have been built by a man, I'll never make it to the end." The staff were really good, although they had a go at me when my contractions were really big— I just did not want to start pushing. I kept telling them off for the pink baby unit when I was having two boys. The original midwife could not stay—it was her shift change—but she did ask after me. The second midwife took over and was having no more of me panting over the contractions—"Come on, now is the time."

> I was afraid of having my first baby at home. Then I experienced birth at a maternity hospital, where no one cared at all. The nurses, midwives and doctors acted as if I and the other patients were unpleasant interruptions in their very important business of drinking tea and watching television. This was at a maternity hospital that was known for being fairly progressive.

> All in all I found it to be a really positive experience as I felt in control the whole time, but I was glad to be at the hospital.

And here's a comment which is ostensibly about home birth...

> A friend recently asked me what it was like giving birth at home. She sounded as though she was afraid of the pain, and sceptical about why she should choose to subject herself to it. I found I was at a loss to explain why I thought it was so worthwhile. I got as far as 'It was important to me to know what birth felt like.' I could pretty safely say it was the best experience of my life. Sure it hurt, but it was more than worth it. But I couldn't think of a reason why *everyone* would want to.
>
> Here's one: quick recovery. After my son's birth by caesarean section, I wasn't allowed to get out of bed—I couldn't even wee for myself, I was hooked up to a catheter. The day my daughter was born, I laughed, cried, slept with her snoring on my chest, and went out for a walk that afternoon. Family and friends came over for a party that evening. The baby and I were up celebrating with everyone else. The next day my diaphragm felt bruised as though I'd run a marathon from the exertion of pushing. A day after that, I felt nearly normal.
>
> Here's another: it's very satisfying. It makes you feel very proud to push a baby into the world all by yourself. It's a deeply carnal satisfaction.

Could these comments actually relate to hospital birth too? The important factors are whether or not women use drug-based pain relief, whether or not they have unnecessary interventions and whether or not they are disturbed while in labour and giving birth. Avoiding interventions and disturbance and getting one-to-one care are the main challenges with hospital birth—but hi-tech interventions are there in the tiny minority of cases when they're really needed.

If, so far, you have decided you want to have a hospital birth, try and lay the groundwork so as to optimise your chances of having a good experience...
- ♥ Make sure that everything you've stated in your care guide has been accepted. (Note this should include details of admissions procedures.)
- ♥ Ask if there are any protocols you need to know about... Do they have any policies about monitoring, 'progress' of labour, episiotomy, caesareans and the third stage of labour?
- ♥ Check whether or not you'll be free to wear your own clothes and eat and drink as and when you wish to.
- ♥ Ask if you'll be free to make any noises you want to make, or play music.
- ♥ Check their view on movement... Will you be able to walk around and use the toilet and bathroom (the shower or bath) whenever you wish?
- ♥ Ask them whether they will require you to adopt any specific positions either during labour or while you are giving birth, and whether they have any rules about being in specific rooms at specific stages.
- ♥ Check what midwives and other staff feel about disturbance and 'coaching' (which is another form of disturbance). Note that you can get advance permission to have either an independent midwife or doula with you. (In many hospitals this is only possible if the person is actually named in your care guide.) She can do a huge amount to ensure that you are not unnecessarily disturbed.
- ♥ Finally, ask what is likely to happen after the birth... Where will you be? What procedures do they consider routine? What policies do they have as regards bottles, dummies and breastfeeding? Remember, you can insist that your baby is not taken from you at any stage, even for a few seconds, for 'hospital procedures'—unless he or she requires emergency treatment.

Yes, there's a lot to get agreed in advance! It may seem tiresome or embarrassing doing this, but it really is very worthwhile and it will save you a lot of possible problems during and after the birth.

Finally, in order to optimise a hospital birthing experience for both yourself and your baby, when you arrive at the hospital and are allocated a labour room, make it as homely and as comfortable as you can. Ask for the hospital bed to be taken out, if necessary, because it's very unlikely you'll need it while you're in labour or giving birth.[4] Also consider putting a sign on the door:

> **DO NOT DISTURB! Optimal birth in progress.**
>
> Please do not offer any drugs and do not suggest any other pain relief. Just let me feel unobserved and undisturbed. Please monitor my progress by simply listening and unobtrusively observing my behaviour.
> Thank you for your support.

By the way, you needn't use the word 'optimal'. How about calling your birth 'new natural', 'healthy' or 'fizzy-logical'? Or...? Think up your own terminology.

Birthframe 70

In case you decide that hospital is the place for you and you want to visualise a positive experience for yourself, here's an example of a well-managed hospital birth, which took place in the hospital for all the right reasons. As with other birth stories in this book, a certain amount of assertiveness was needed at one point but after this hiccup was past, all else went as the woman wanted. Gas and air was used, although it is not clear how much this was really needed by the labouring woman, who seemed to be doing fine without it. The mention of this in this story reminds me of the many cakes I have eaten out of politeness, simply because they were offered and because everyone else was doing the same thing!

I gave birth to non-identical twin boys on 25 December 2001 in the John Radcliffe Hospital, Oxford on Christmas Day. Here is a little background and the birth story for your book.

I already have one daughter, born in 1999 normally without pain relief or intervention until after the birth. I had a retained placenta so having done the 'hard bit' OK, I then had to have surgery to remove the placenta.

In September 2000 I had a missed miscarriage which resulted in surgery to remove 'products of conception'. Unfortunately, during the procedure the surgeon perforated my uterus!

I then conceived twins and was told, without any consideration for what I wanted, that I would have to have a caesarean section at 38 weeks. Once the hospital (not the John Radcliffe) checked my file and saw I had had a retained placenta and perforated uterus they said, well, that basically made it a definite section, no option. I was not happy with this and I asked to be referred to the John Radcliffe (JR) for a second opinion. The consultant at the JR—Lawrence Impey—was actually the consultant who had scanned me at 12 weeks and told me we were having twins; twins also happened to be his specialist area. He understood why I had been told a section at 38 weeks was necessary, due to the possible complications and strain my uterus would be under if I went into natural labour. However, he didn't rule out a normal, vaginal birth and said we would make that decision much nearer the time.

> He didn't rule out a normal, vaginal birth and said
> we would make that decision much nearer the time

Pregnancy went well and I still didn't want a section. At 37 weeks the consultant agreed not to do a section at 38 weeks if the babies had not come naturally by then but he said he would not allow me to go beyond 39 weeks so a section was booked for 39 weeks gestation. When asked if he thought I would get to 39 weeks, he said, "No, we'll see you next week, I reckon—about Christmas time." He was right!

We live about 45 miles from the hospital! Left home at 1.10am, got to the hospital at 1.50am.

On Christmas Eve itself I went into my local hospital to have baby movements monitored as all had gone a bit quiet. Everything was fine. On Christmas Eve whilst being monitored (at 5.00pm) I had the slightest Braxton Hicks, but nothing else. Came home and had supper and watched television. I had lower backache during the evening but no more than usual after a long day. Got into bed at 12.15am and at 12.30am had a show; called the hospital at 12.50am. We live about 45 miles from the JR! The midwife said to come in. Left home at 1.10am, got to the hospital at 1.50am; contractions were now four minutes apart but not severe or too painful. Alexander and Luc were born at 3.00am and 3.20am. They weighed 6lb 7oz and 6lb 5oz. Labour was basically two and a half hours.

The labour and birth... On arrival the midwife started monitoring me and I had one huge contraction. She said she would get the doctor to see if I was in labour properly but there probably was no hurry. I said I really thought this was it. The doctor came, had a look and gasped, saying, "9cm dilated!" and I'm saying, "Yes, and I want to push". The registrar came and said, "OK, we must get you into theatre to give us more room to manoeuvre and in case there's a problem." They wheeled me across to theatre. I had a drip in my arm to keep the contractions going once the first twin was born. I was then offered gas and air, which I used. A few hard pushes and Twin One (Alexander) was born—all healthy and already holding his head up on the table, where the paediatrician was checking him. Twin Two (Luc), who had been breech, turned and the second midwife sort of held my stomach so he could not turn back. I was then asked to do one really good push to push Luc into the birth canal, so he could not turn again. By this time the contractions had subsided and the midwife had to tell me I was having a contraction and to push. A few pushes and Luc was born—all healthy and also trying to hold his head up.

The anaesthetic for the stitching was the worst bit

Alex had come out with his hand along the side of his face, so I had torn and had to be stitched up. The placentas were slow to come but the midwife was fantastic, saying she had never been beaten yet by a placenta and out they plopped, actually fused together, so it looked like one.

And that was it. I had an Anti-D shot as I am Rhesus negative. The anaesthetic for the stitching was absolutely the worst and most painful bit of the whole procedure. By 5.30am or 6.00am I was on a ward.

I hope this helps. I am not sure what more I can tell you. Good luck with the book.

Justine Renwick

What about giving birth at home?
Is this really a realistic option in the 21st century?

Birthframe 71

Here's an email I received while I was writing this book.

> From: Rebecca Wright
> To: Sylvie Donna
> Sent: 16 June 2005, 7.16pm
> Subject: New baby
>
> Hi Sylvie,
>
> Just wanted to say that our new baby was born on 7 June, at home, and all went well. His name is William and he was 7lb 5oz at birth. I used a birthing pool during the labour, but he was born outside it. The birth was a good one, though I do think most are very hard work. I had only a very small tear from which I experienced no pain, and have since been perfectly fit, healthy and relatively energetic. Just to say that I have to agree again that your premise about natural birth is right. It's amazing how many mothers I've spoken with since have looked at me in amazement that I had a home birth with no drugs—like it's utterly inconceivable and I must be incredibly brave or a martyr! To me, it seems a lot more scary—and in most cases risky—to plan for a hospital birth!
>
> Talk to you soon,
>
> Rebecca

Birthframe 72

Here's part of another email I received. I'd just read *Monique and the Mango Rains* by American author Kris Holloway (Waveland Press 2007). As I explained in my email to the author, I'd bought her book to check out my hunch about so-called 'natural' birth in sub-Saharan Africa. However, after reading what she'd written about African women's experiences, I was surprised she chose to have midwife-attended home births herself when she returned to the States— I felt it would be more likely she'd opt for high-intervention/managed births! I asked her if she'd witnessed any positive experiences of birth in Mali, which she hadn't mentioned in the book...

> Mali became my paradigm for what was normal. I didn't want to die in childbirth, but yes, I wanted a midwife!

Yes, I found many positive things about natural childbirth. I hope that came through in *Monique and the Mango Rains*! Mali became my paradigm for what was normal. Just as most women give birth in hospitals here in the US because that's what's considered normal/what most women do, I experienced birth in Mali first, and that became my yardstick. No, I didn't want to die in childbirth, but yes, I wanted a midwife! I think the biggest lesson that I learned from Monique (the midwife I worked with in Mali) was how strong I was as a woman, what power my body had, and what beauty there was in birth as a community event, a women-centred event. I knew that I wouldn't get that in a hospital. Of course, I had the best of both worlds here in the US: home births with midwives and a great hospital only minutes away in case anything went wrong. How I wish all women had such luxury! As I mention in the book, I gave birth to both my sons (one at 8 lb 10oz, and one at 7lb 10 oz) at home with my midwife, sister, husband and friends in attendance.

Kris Holloway

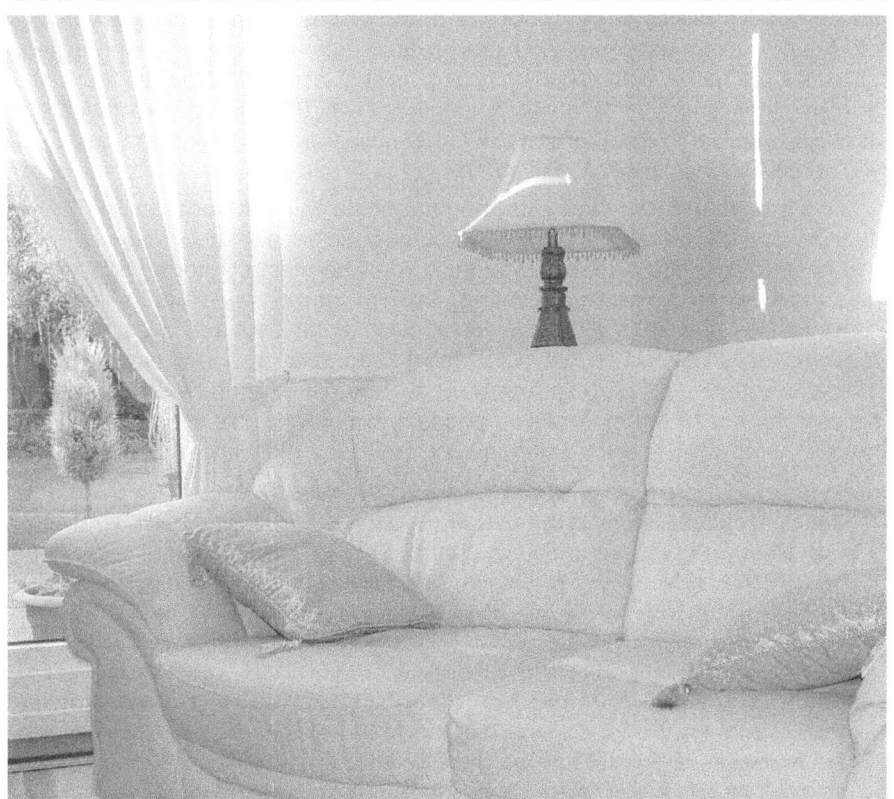

Would you feel better being able to labour and give birth in familiar surroundings? Do you have good hygiene, hot and cold running water and a telephone?

A lot of women do worry about safety. However, if you're basically healthy and have good back-up arrangements in place (i.e. you're registered at your local hospital and you have a phone in good working order), there really is no need to worry. The key to success is to make sure you're undisturbed while you're in labour and giving birth.[5]

Mess is also not something which is a particular problem with births. You will probably need to clear up at least some of your own mess if you choose to give birth at home but this is an advantage in a way, because your privacy and dignity will be safeguarded. After all, do you prefer other people to wipe your bottom after a poo? If you have diarrhoea, do you prefer someone else to come in and help? If the answer is 'No' you'll probably be happier being in control of the mess yourself! There's surprisingly little.

Equipment (or lack of) is also not a problem with a home birth. Your midwives will bring along any medical supplies and equipment which are currently considered necessary for safety. This will allow her to deal with an unexpected haemorrhage or with a baby who is experiencing breathing difficulties—which, incidentally, is a rare occurrence after a gentle, undrugged, physiological home birth. Non-medical supplies, as we've already seen, are also minimal—and people do occasionally give birth without any equipment at all! So you don't need to worry about supplies or equipment particularly, if you're considering giving birth at home.

Finally, some women worry what other people will think of them. As we've already said, the decision as to where you give birth really should be your own. You need to give birth wherever you think you'll be most comfortable. As more and more women return to giving birth at home, with all its modern conveniences and links with emergency care, home birth will once again be regarded as an obvious choice. (Whereas it used to be a case of somebody on a bicycle wobbling off for help, we now have the use of ambulances and even helicopters, not to mention mobile phones.) So don't worry about what other people think... what you yourself think and feel is the most important thing.

> Birth is a delicate process. It's not computer-controlled. Emotions have a lot to do with it. The best place to give birth is where you feel safest and calmest. If, like me, your blood pressure rises the minute you lay eyes on a hospital, you'll probably be better off at home. If you feel more comfortable with lots of professional-looking people in white coats taking care of you, then you probably won't be distressed if the doctors get involved, decide to monitor you and the fetus, and suggest an epidural or other interventions. But if you don't like that idea, best to keep yourself out of harm's way. Doctors have lots of procedures and equipment. They like to use them. That's why they're doctors. They firmly believe that their methods are best for everyone. If you don't share these beliefs, try to make sure your birth is attended by people who feel the way you do, whether you birth at home or in the hospital. At the very least, hire a doula.
>
> *Nina Klose*

Here are a few comments from women who had a home birth only after experiencing a hospital birth for their firstborn...

❝ My first labour in the hospital was very painful and I felt that by having my second baby at home I would be much more relaxed and able to cope with the pain. This was the case.

❝ It was magic, absolutely as life-changing as my first, hospital birth experience, but this was an empowering and enriching experience: strange, seeing as it was such a dangerous, unthinking and life-threatening thing to do, according to the obstetricians.

❝ I was on such a high for ages—I felt empowered and I had regained the confidence in my own body which my first birth had taken away. I do not feel that I did anything either 'brave' or 'dangerous' by giving birth at home. I felt very safe and it was right for me.

❝ My next baby was a planned home birth—I could not imagine going to hospital and going through the same thing [i.e. a forceps delivery, followed by a postpartum haemorrhage because of a mismanaged third stage].

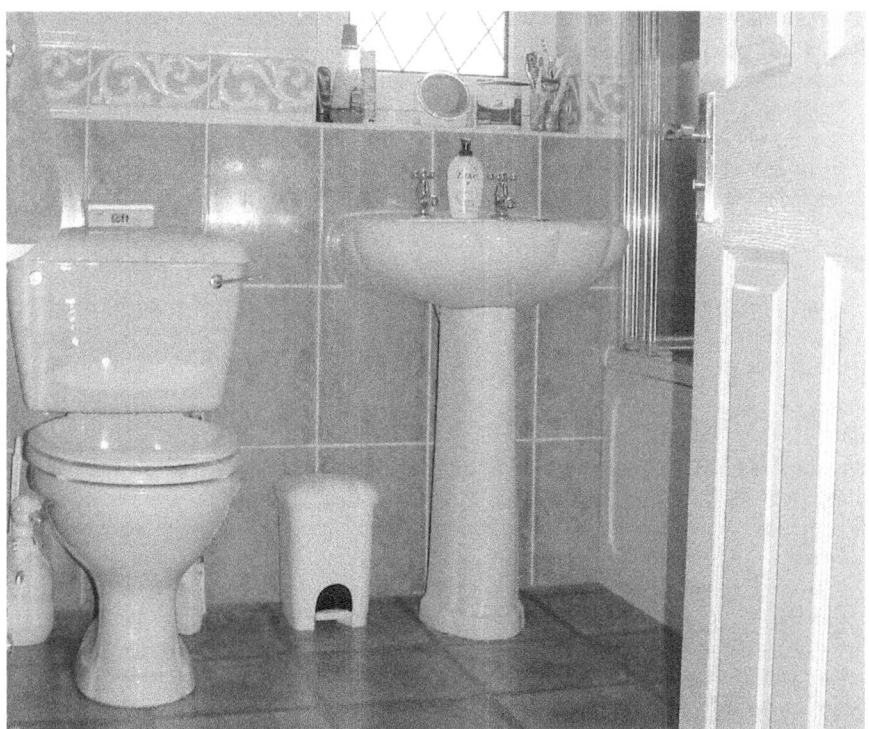

Modern homes are usually clean and comfortable, with good amenities. If they're within easy reach of emergency facilities, they can be the ideal place to give birth.

Birthframe 73

When expecting my first child, I registered in a London hospital, as the most natural thing to do... I was born in the hospital... and my mother too! It was 1983, I arrived smiling and I was told, after an internal, that I was 8cm. One hour later I found myself in a labour ward, surrounded by 10 students, a male doctor and a midwife, and a monstrous fetal monitoring machine was attached to me and sounding very loud. Bright lights, voices everywhere, people coming in and out, my partner at my right... I was soon in a state of shock. Labour almost came to an end. Epidural, episiotomy and a very light and unnecessary forceps followed. "Never again. Never again", I kept repeating to myself, while holding my baby daughter.

Liliana Lammers

❝ I wanted to give birth at home so as to avoid hospital treatment and so as to be as close as possible to what had gone before—after all, I was in my own home when the child was conceived, I was at home while I was pregnant and I wanted to experience the continuity of it all. Birth is just part of the cycle of life.

And when I say 'home' I don't mean just the physical aspect of it, but that confined place where the sacred happens, where the profound experiences of life happen. I didn't want any interruptions. I didn't want this artificial thing of having to leave my home, leave my place of being, where I live, where I sleep, where I dream, where I eat, where I have my friends. It's a normal part of life to give birth and it felt so natural and normal. I would feel it was totally unnatural to go into hospital.

Birthframe 74

It would probably have been impossible for the contributor of this account to relax to the extent she did if she had been anywhere but home. Even though she had MS [multiple sclerosis], she was still scared of the prospect of more pain.

When my first baby Kizzy was born in hospital I felt very empowered by the birth. I had used no drugs of any sort and had no interventions, yet I couldn't imagine wanting to repeat it. "How does anyone ever have more than one baby?" I asked my mum the next day.

However, a year or so later a friend at a La Leche League meeting about birth recommended *Spiritual Midwifery* by Ina May Gaskin. The book is full of stories about peaceful, joyful home births. It was a complete revelation to me that birth could be totally painfree and enjoyable. I thought a lot about changing my view of pain and began to see contractions as 'rushes of energy'. I learned to relax my body and to think of pain as 'an interesting sensation that I needed to concentrate on'.

In the book it is often said that if the mouth is 'soft' (i.e. relaxed), then the pelvic floor area will be too. I practised this by blowing out through my mouth with very relaxed lips when I went to the toilet. I also tried not to tense up when I experienced any sort of pain. For instance, if I stubbed my toe I would relax myself and the pain lessened much more quickly than normally. I was able to combine Ina May Gaskin's theories about pain with Michel Odent's writings about a woman's instinctive understanding of what positions to adopt during labour and birth. (After all, most—if not all?—of the women in *Spiritual Midwifery* had given birth in bed, on their backs or semi-reclined.)

I had a sort of practice run at birth when I had a miscarriage when Kizzy was 20 months old. After two weeks of spotting blood, a mini-labour began when I was 12 weeks' pregnant. I knew the baby had died because I had stopped feeling pregnant around the time the bleeding had started. (I had also had a scan where they 'informed' me there was no heartbeat, as if I didn't know what was going on in my body.) I relaxed through the miscarriage and it was painless. I could sense that the feelings would have been painful, much like strong period cramps, if I had been tense. I felt elated when it was over, as if I had really achieved something by not feeling any pain. I wasn't ready for another baby yet and felt that the miscarriage had been for the best. (I had another scan afterwards where they 'let me know' that my uterus was now empty!)

My next pregnancy was planned and the baby was due when Kizzy was $3\frac{1}{2}$. By this time we had moved from London, where the maternity care was very impersonal, to a small, fairly isolated town. The local hospital has a midwife-run maternity unit and the midwives are friendly, relaxed and have plenty of time to chat. Even so, I knew I would have a home birth this time. I planned a water birth and hired a pool as (even though I was much more confident I could cope with the contractions) I still felt that a pool would provide some pain relief if I needed it and the calm, enveloping warmth of the water was appealing. My team of four midwives seemed keen on the water birth and had special training sessions at another hospital to prepare them. None had delivered a baby in water before and I think they had little experience of home birth. By the end of my pregnancy I felt fully prepared for the birthing to come. Dora was born at home on a beautiful sunny morning in June 2000. The labour was fairly quick. My waters broke at midnight and I tried to sleep, but was too excited. I had a long bath instead and meditated and visualised my womb opening up to let my baby out. I managed some sleep, but by 4 o'clock the contractions were coming regularly. I felt very peaceful and safe as I pottered around the silent, sleeping house, tidying and arranging things for the midwives. When a contraction came, I would lean on a piece of furniture or the kitchen side and sway gently, breathing slowly, out through my mouth. Each contraction was like an exciting journey—enjoyable in itself, but also promising even better to come. I felt the love of friends and family like a warm glow, especially when I was looking at various photos around the house. Even though I was alone physically, I knew there were many people with me in spirit. I often smiled and laughed during contractions and when one was over I waited eagerly for the next.

Jim, my husband, called the midwife at about 7 o'clock, when I felt things were progressing, then began to fill the pool. The midwife arrived and checked me just before 8.00am—I was 3cm dilated. This surprised me as I thought I was further along, but as things turned out maybe I was.

After a few more contractions things began to intensify. I remember moaning 'Woaah' as the feelings suddenly became much stronger. There was still no pain, though I had to work much harder to stay relaxed enough. (I realised after that this was probably transition.) I decided to get into the pool now, thinking I might not be able to cope if things got any stronger. The water felt wonderful, like a big, warm hug. I had two more contractions then, out of the blue, I had an overwhelming urge to push with the next. The midwife, who was waiting for the other midwife to arrive, shouted "No!" when I told her. I understood then that she was scared to be on her own. I didn't let her fear affect me, but when I pushed during that contraction some diarrhoea came out. The midwife insisted I leave the pool as she thought it was too contaminated to give birth in.

Although I had expected to want to squat to give birth, my body knew that it needed to stand and my knees straightened up automatically. I leaned on the side of the pool. During the first push I had felt the baby move down rapidly. With the next, the head crowned and I reached down to touch Dora's soft hair. I had to slow myself down at this stage to be sure I didn't push too hard. I stopped pushing mid-contraction and breathed slowly. I was aware of the beauty of the sunny, blue sky outside and the wonderment of the moment. I felt a strong connection with all of nature. Then the final contraction, and the head was born. I looked down and clearly recall how surreal it seemed to see her head between my legs. I reminded myself to go slowly and within a few seconds her whole body slid gently out.

I held her and she cried with her eyes tight shut for several minutes—it was probably very bright for her. Dora was born at 9.18am, less than an hour and a half since I was examined at 3cm dilated. Kizzy and Jim came into the room, amazed to see a baby. They had been making breakfast in the kitchen when Kizzy said she could hear a baby crying. Jim wasn't sure at first because he thought there was still some way to go!

Dora suckled for the first time and the placenta was delivered a few minutes later. Unfortunately, the midwife pulled on the cord as the placenta was coming out. This was totally unnecessary, felt quite uncomfortable to me and could have created problems.

Dora's birth was serene and peaceful, full of joy and love—something to be cherished. I was on such a high to have achieved my dream of a totally painfree birth and to have my beautiful baby girl in my arms. The only thing to mar the experience was the midwives' interference, however minor. Luckily, I was strong and aware of my body to the extent that I was able to ignore the negative aspects of the midwifery 'care' and still feel I had had the best experience of my life. I was eager to give birth again!

Gemma Shepherd

Birthframe 75

It's easy from many people's experience—and even from the birth stories included in this book!—to get the impression that home births are always better for optimising birth. As the final account in this section shows, how things are done at home is just as important as where a birth takes place. Disturbing the natural processes by disturbing the woman's sense of security, privacy and confidence can have dramatic consequences whether the woman is at home or in hospital.

For the birth of my sixth child, Finn, I had decided on a home delivery for a combination of reasons. The previous five births had been straightforward and progressively quicker and on a practical level it meant not having to worry about where the other children went. The main reason, however, was that by No.6 I had gained the confidence in and awareness of my body and its instincts to want to be left to labour on my own, with as little interference as possible. The birth went beautifully, with the help of some very supportive midwives. Finn is now a very happy and easygoing 4-year-old and I am sure that the peaceful atmosphere into which he was born is responsible.

When I discovered I was expecting No.7 (Joseph) I decided to opt for a home delivery again. The pregnancy proceeded uneventfully and despite the baby lying in a slightly awkward posterior position in the last few weeks, everything signalled another hopefully quick and straightforward birth. 10 days overdue, and after a false alarm (contractions caused by the baby turning into an anterior position), labour began at six in the morning. As before, I kept upright and moving, walking around the house and dealing with the contractions as well as the children's demands for breakfast.

By 8.00am the 'on-call' midwife arrived. On examination, I was almost fully dilated and she prepared for the imminent delivery. At this point the 'day shift' community midwives (plus student) arrived to take over. I was surprised, given the stage of labour, that the on-call team didn't stay to see the birth through to delivery. So at transition I had six people—midwives, students and my husband—in the bedroom, all filling in charts and forms or talking in corners, while I paced around them trying to deal with the contractions and not get in their way. Other visitors into the busy bedroom included two of the older children, who were getting ready for school and needed to know where their PE kits were. By now, I was beginning to feel the first sensation of pressure from the baby's head and was told to push if I wanted by the midwife.

When, half an hour or so later, there was still no sign of the baby's head, an examination revealed that the cervix had swollen, preventing the baby from descending. I was told I would have to allow the swelling to reduce by resisting the pushing urge, possibly for up to two hours. Fighting against my body's overwhelming instinctive urge to push out the baby and the powerful contractions doing exactly that became—after 20 minutes or so of trying—an impossibility.

An epidural was suggested to reduce the pushing urge and help with the pain, but this would mean transferring to hospital to have the epidural administered. By now, the pain of resisting pushing was excruciating even with gas and air, which I had gratefully used for the previous 20 minutes. I agreed, and the midwives called an ambulance, which rushed me into hospital. My husband followed the ambulance in our car and just as he arrived to join me in the delivery room Joseph's head was born with a huge contraction over which I had no control. His shoulder then got slightly stuck but with the midwife pushing me into an almost yoga-like position—bringing my feet up toward my shoulders, while I lay on my back—he slipped out and, despite his shock entry into the world, was fine and didn't need any resuscitation.

Although the birth was not what I had expected, it worked out for the best. Strangely, the noisiest and busiest part of the delivery was at home. It is possible that being distracted by so much activity at a crucial stage in the labour and losing the control that up to then I had had and had always maintained during previous labours, had an adverse effect. Being told to push before my body was ready may have caused the swelling and the resulting battle with my body, and loss of control over what it was doing led to extreme pain and complications. However, being alone with Joseph in the delivery room after his birth was calm and peaceful. We had a few hours alone—uninterrupted, quiet and warm. I lay back and held him and we were both awake but able to recover from the trauma of the birth and rest together, something I'm sure I would not have been able to do at home with Joseph's brothers and sisters desperate to see and hold him.

Sometimes, hospital births can be peaceful and home births quite chaotic! I think this experience taught me that where the birth takes place is less important than how the mother is treated. Too much well-meaning advice, monitoring, admin, instruction and activity can interfere with the mother's control of the labour and result in more pain and unnecessary intervention, whether it occurs at home or in hospital. Being left to follow her natural instincts and urges in a calm atmosphere can only be beneficial for the mother and child.[6]

Clare O'Ryan

In case you are still undecided, here are a few more comments to chew over! First, here's an emailed conversation between me and Michel...

What kind of women would you refuse for a home birth—assuming that you were practising full-time as a home birth midwife?

Today, (1) first baby footling breech and (2) early spontaneous rupture of membranes with tainted liquid, particularly for a first baby. We should not contrast home birth and hospital birth. More often than not it is possible to combine what the privacy of the home can offer and what the hospital facilities can offer. In other words it is possible to decide during the first stage of labour.

3... CHOOSE WHERE

So are you saying that it is ideal if labours begin at home, with a view to transferring to a nearby hospital if there is failure to progress? Would there be any other reasons for immediate transfer to hospital in the case of a woman who began labouring at home?

An unexpected fetal distress during labour.[7]

> I decided that the only way I could be sure of getting the type of birth I wanted and taking charge of the situation was by having a home birth.

> Pregnant women are very sensitive. You need to decide what you want, such as being in hospital or at home, or at a private birth centre. There are a lot of ways to do it, and it's your choice. There's a lot of negative information out there about home birth—people will tell you about babies dying—and you need to be critical about what you hear. There's a very good chance that everything will be OK. But of course there are risk factors you need to be aware of, such as difficult presentation, unusually large baby, the mother's health. If you plan to have a baby at home, you need to be better prepared.

Birthframe 76

I have an identical twin sister who had a very different experience from me. I believe lack of preparation and inexperienced midwives arriving at her home may have contributed to her failed home delivery... she was eventually sent to hospital because of apparent 'fetal distress'. Her labour started with breaking of waters, then slowed down by morning, probably due to her fear and holding back—she was in the bottom-up position. Midwives internally examined her to see cervical dilation, thus risking infection. Later, her temperature went up and she was admitted to hospital... Eventually she had a belt monitor, scalp monitor, etc and finally, a caesarean. Now she's unsure about the whole experience, even though she feels elated that she overcame her fear of childbirth. She wasn't half as committed to home birth as I was and had quite a lot of fear about it—for various reasons. She actually discovered she felt safer in hospital, partly because she found it easier to depend on midwives there, rather than on her partner at home. She is thinking of having another child and wondering what her next choices will be. She wasn't as critical of the hospital as I was, or cynical about the clinical side. She thought the caesarean was necessary. I wasn't convinced.

The goal shouldn't be to have a home birth at all costs. Home is good because it's good for the baby and the mother, if you feel more comfortable there. But if you can't feel comfortable at home, then go to hospital. I feel that some people get too drawn into the whole natural birth thing. Other people just aren't interested in any of it and prefer to go to a doctor. It's not an end in itself.

> There are pluses and minuses to both options.
> For my first birth I chose a hospital birth but
> the whole experience was so harrowing...

There are pluses and minuses to both options. For my first birth I chose a hospital where the baby could be with me. But the whole experience was so harrowing. I lost weight very quickly after the birth. I lost too much, even. My normal weight is 52kg, but after the first birth I dropped to 48kg, and felt nervous and didn't sleep well. On the other hand, staying in hospital you don't have to cook, wash nappies, look after the rest of the family, so that's easier. Supposedly you can rest. But for me, it was worse. I couldn't sleep a wink in hospital. I just didn't like it.

I signed up at a nearby birth centre, and chose to see midwives for my primary care. I did not want to be in the hospital, but both my own fears and the fears of those around me pushed me away from looking into home birth. I know now that there is nothing that can be done in a birth centre that cannot be done at home.

Remember that statistics show that over 95% of all births proceed normally. On the high risk list for home births I would include the following: untreated heart disease, kidney disease, diabetes, gestational diabetes, lung disease, cancer, severe asthma, epilepsy, uncontrolled toxaemia, and emotional illness. If you have any of these, morally you should discuss them fully with a prospective midwife. Also if you take drugs, drink, or smoke, you should not accept the responsibility for a home birth.

One of the things that most frightens women who consider having a midwife-assisted delivery is that a complication may develop suddenly—too fast for the doctor to help. Fortunately, this scene is almost never the case: most problems begin to be evident hours before they become critical. For proof, consider the low mortality rate for home births.

Why hadn't I planned a home birth?

Why hadn't I planned a home birth? My cousin had her first child at home with the NHS and had a good experience—but she told me if she'd had it to do over again, she'd have gone to hospital. A few hours after his birth, her son stopped breathing. By some miracle, one of the midwives was still there, gave him oxygen, suctioned his lungs, and the family rushed to the hospital. The baby was fine. But my cousin says she and her husband couldn't face the prospect of going through such terror a second time. She subsequently had her second child in hospital. She wishes she'd stayed home!

Nina Klose

Land or water?

This is another question to consider. Is it worthwhile taking the trouble to hire a birthing pool? Will a bath do just as well? Here are some different perspectives on water birth, in its various forms.[8] First, an extract from one of Michel's books...

From *Birth and Breastfeeding* (Clairview Books 2007):

We had observed that immersion in a pool full of warm water was an effective way of facilitating the phase of dilation of the cervix. So long as the mother-to-be does not get into the bath until the onset of hard contractions in the middle of this phase, we learnt to expect that once immersed she would be fully dilated quite quickly—after around perhaps an hour, or an hour and a half for a first baby. Although the contractions are apparently less intense and less painful in the water, the mother can feel that they are nevertheless more efficient. But when the baby is not far away, there comes a time when some mothers feel that the contractions are not working effectively any longer. After a series of five or six or seven contractions, there may be no further progress; and then many women feel the need to get out of the pool. As soon as they leave the warm bath and return to the cooler atmosphere of the room, a puzzling phenomenon often occurs. It is as if a kind of reflex were triggered by the difference of temperature and, after a few huge contractions, the baby is born on the floor by the pool. This is a fetus ejection reflex.

In *Birth Reborn* (Souvenir Books 1994) he also mentions that at Pithiviers it was never the practice to insist that the labouring woman remain in the water for the birth itself—or even to encourage her to do so. They also used to prefer it if women got out of the water before the third stage (if the birth had taken place under water) so there was no risk of water entering their bloodstream via the open vessels in the womb, which could cause a life-threatening embolism. Focusing on the needs of newborn babies, Michel emphasises that what they need is warmth and the feeling of their new mums' gentle touch. Here are some more comments and anecdotes from Michel to explain his views...

Personally I don't use the term 'water birth', which implies that the baby is born in water. Birth under water is possible but it should not be the goal. The main objective is to reduce the need for drugs. The best indication for the use of the birthing pool is when the first stage is long, difficult and very painful, in spite of perfect conditions of privacy. When the first stage is straightforward, it may be risky to change the environment. When a woman appears to be having difficulties, a birthing pool can actually be used to check whether or not a caesarean is necessary. It is particularly useful because a decision can be reached before fetal distress has occurred. I call this the 'birthing pool test'. Carrying out this test is very simple: when the woman is in hard labour, she is immersed in water at body temperature for approximately 90 minutes. Usually, within this time period, something spectacular happens. (The period of time is approximate, of course.) By spectacular I mean, for example, if she enters the bath at 5cm she reaches full dilation, or if she enters at 3cm she reaches 7cm. If after an hour and a half in water nothing like that happens, if you can see no difference in dilation, it means something is wrong, that there is some kind of obstacle. So the best course of action is to do a caesarean section—waiting is not at all helpful in this case.

Birthframe 77

Michel told me two interesting stories to illustrate the 'birthing pool test'.

A woman was on a boat and I was with Liliana, the doula. It was obviously a big baby and we first went there early in the morning.

Around 2 or 3 o'clock in the afternoon she was in hard labour but just stayed at 4cm dilation. I suggested she get in the birthing pool. (Amazingly enough, they had hired a birthing pool for the boat!) She then spent two hours in the pool but after these two hours she was still only 4cm dilated. I said, "You know, you need to go to hospital," because I was convinced she should have a caesarean section. I told Liliana to go with her because I could no longer be responsible for the birth. At the hospital, the consultant put the woman on a syntocinon drip and ruptured her membranes. However, in the end she had a caesarean.

Knowing what I knew about her labour I would have done a caesarean immediately, when she arrived at the hospital at around 7.00pm. What happened was that they tried everything and finally she had a caesarean section the day after, in the morning. The baby was OK but it might have been better for both the baby and the woman if the caesarean had been done earlier.

In the second case I was not there myself—it was Liliana who told me the story. It was at a hospital in London. The woman arrived in hard labour, even though she was only a couple of centimetres dilated. Eventually, she got into the birthing pool and no more progress was made so Liliana told them, "I think she needs a caesarean section." She probably mentioned my name but they didn't believe her in any case. Then, a senior obstetrician came along and she said it was a brow presentation—which is completely incompatible with the vaginal route. So without having any other way of diagnosing a problem, apart from through 'the birthing pool test', Liliana said it should be caesarean section. The senior obstetrician gave a reason for the diagnosis... but the result was still a caesarean section.

Birthframe 78

Finally, here's an abridged account of a home water birth. The mother, Angela Horn, founded the Home Birth Reference website www.homebirth.org.uk

Just after the midwife told me my cervix was 4-5cm dilated, I asked Graham to start assembling the birth pool. I found that I needed to devote more effort to dealing with the contractions. I put on some music, turned the lights down and turned on the lava lamp; the Christmas tree was still up, complete with fairy lights, and the whole effect was lovely. I have very fond memories of grooving along to my favourite music, feeling perfectly normal in between contractions and rocking on all fours during them, singing along with the music. Graham needed some help with the pool, so I didn't get to 'groove' for very long. Sorting out the pool was a great distraction, though. Graham and I chatted and worked, and it could have been any normal day—except that every few minutes I had to excuse myself and deal with a contraction.

Our three cats found the pool very interesting and stood on the side watching the water; one of them fell in! I wasn't worried about the hygiene aspect as the pool came complete with a non-chlorine water sterilising kit and filter. The contractions got closer and more intense, and by 11.30am I definitely wanted the pool right away, so I got in while it was still filling. This was a good move, as I could direct the hose on my back and tummy during contractions. Music was playing all the time. Rock and pop songs with rousing choruses which I could sing along to were my main form of pain relief. I didn't need pethidine—Jimi Hendrix and Abba were quite effective and had few side-effects! I am normally very self-conscious about singing when anyone can hear me, because I've been told so often that I have an absolutely dreadful singing voice. However, I was completely uninhibited about singing when in labour, and also about making noises later on.

The pool was a great help. Although it didn't take the pain away, it was warm and soothing and I certainly found it easier to cope with contractions in the pool than out. The support of the water made it very easy for me to switch quickly between positions—I had to be on all fours for contractions, but between them I was floating, squatting, sitting or standing. Squatting positions were far easier to hold than on land. Sometimes I went completely under the water during or between contractions—it was very relaxing to feel surrounded by warm water, and to feel quite alone in this peaceful place. The water helped me to focus on breathing out slowly too. Breathing out under water, or with just my mouth under the water, I could blow bubbles and watch and hear the breath, as opposed to just feeling it. It was a rhythmic process and a good distraction during contractions—duck under the water, breathe out slowly, surface and breathe in, and then duck under again. During some moderate contractions I tried wearing a snorkel and staying underwater for the whole contraction. This was quite fun at first, but having the mask on my face got a bit annoying later. Sometimes I kept my head above the water and sang or made other sounds as I breathed out.

Angela Horn

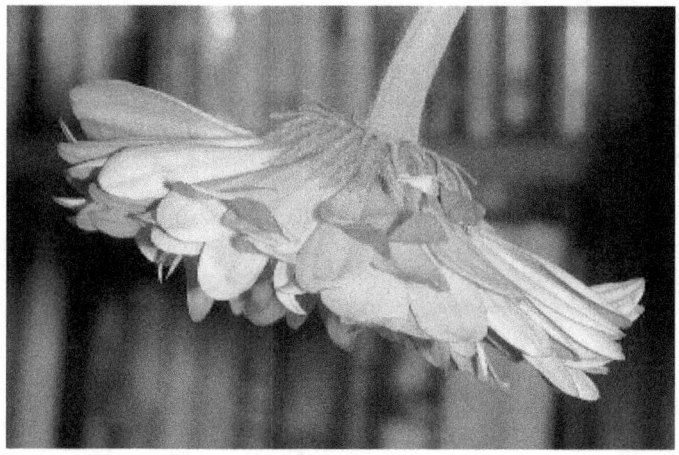

Warm water really can help you open up like a flower so as to release your baby. This is not an outdated, hippy image... it's an age-old truth.

Some other comments on birthing pools...

> I tried the bath but found it too limiting in terms of movement.

> I found the bath perfectly adequate. I leaned forward during contractions then slumped down for a dreamy, sleepy rest between each one. After an hour or so like that, I suddenly wanted to get out and a few minutes later, I gave birth.

> I got into the water and instantly the pain halved. It was beautiful. Mum stroked my head, and Dave my back. The lights were low, the music was on, the water was a giant woman-god warmly holding me together.

> Get a birthing pool if you can. They're wonderful.

> I was a little scared that I would have no official pain relief once in the pool. But I didn't need it—the water was amazing. I could just move around and get into really good positions whenever I had a contraction.

> My partner started to fill the pool, as I'd chosen a water birth. It was so hard for me to get downstairs at this point to the pool in our living room. I just didn't want to move, but with my partner's encouragement I did, and felt so much better for being in water. It just felt the most natural place for me to be.

> Water is fantastic pain relief. Stepping into the birth pool felt like a miracle. Instantly the pain disappeared. No, it was still there, but suddenly it was manageable. I could have stayed in the pool all day.

> Personally I found no need for any analgesic intervention as when I entered the water the pain I was feeling was substantially reduced. I wanted to labour, and possibly give birth, in a birthing pool because I was worried about suffering perineal trauma and, although there is conflicting evidence on the subject, I felt sure that the water would work as an aid in softening my perineum, thereby reducing tearing.

> Before the second stage started there was a complete lull in the contractions. The lull felt like about 20-30 minutes and in this time I just dozed in the pool. When the contractions started up again I wanted to push and my second daughter was born within minutes under the water.

> Baby was born in the water, and I gently brought her to the surface with the midwife's help. She was soft and velvety, purple, wonderful-smelling and crying. I sat there holding and feeling and looking for ages, and then was moved to check she was a girl after all, only to find she had a willie! "It's a boy," I was the one to announce.

When she was checked I found she had a willie!

Water is fantastic pain relief. Stepping into the pool felt like a miracle. The pain was still there but now it was manageable.

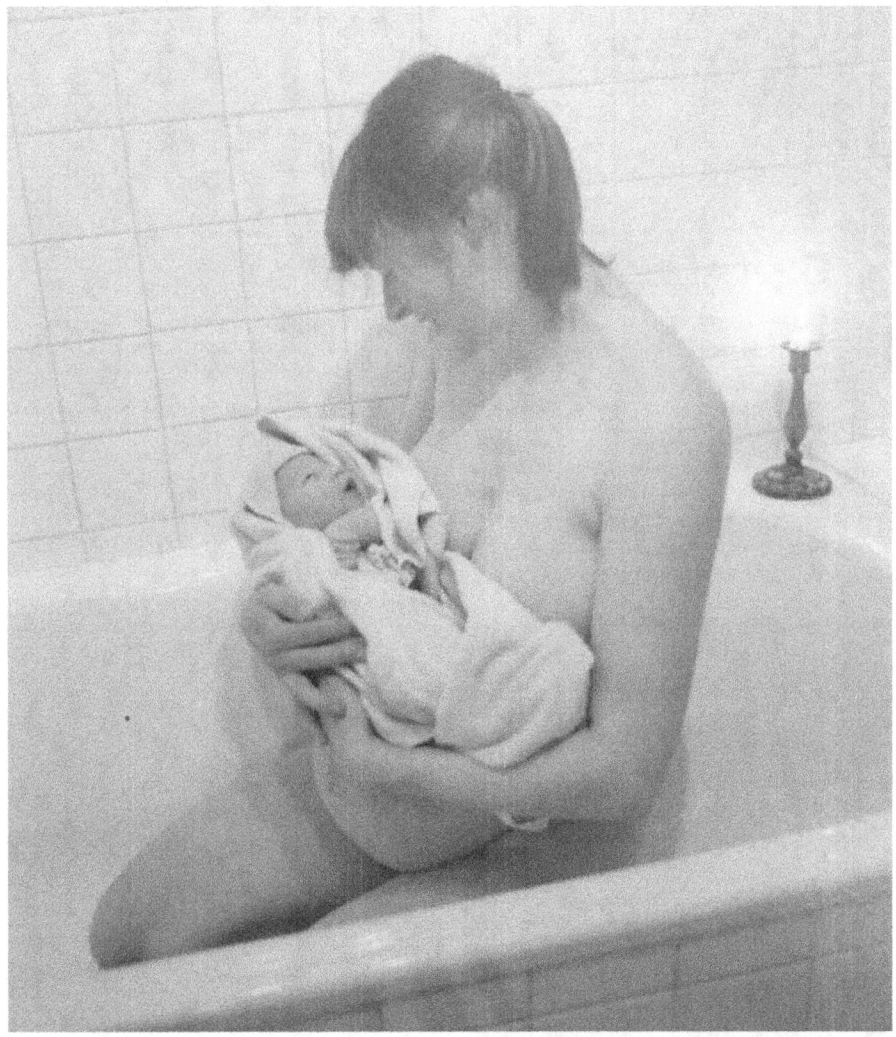

Instead of a pool, you may prefer to just use your bath, as I did. (In case you're wondering... no, this isn't me.) Anyway, with baths the same 'rules' apply—see overleaf.

You may just prefer to use your own bath

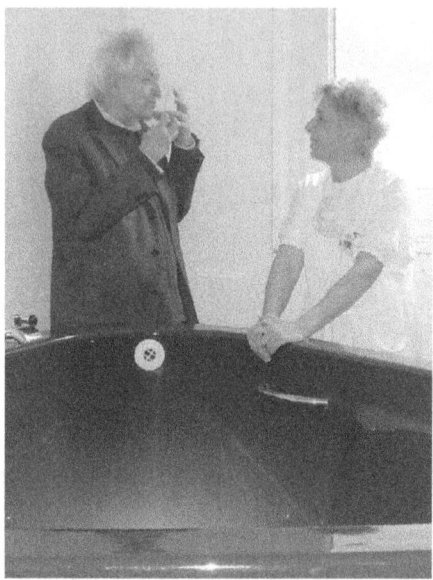

Michel reminiscing with a midwife at the current birthing pool in Pithiviers, where he first introduced the use of paddling pools in the 1970s, followed by specially-designed birthing pools in 1982

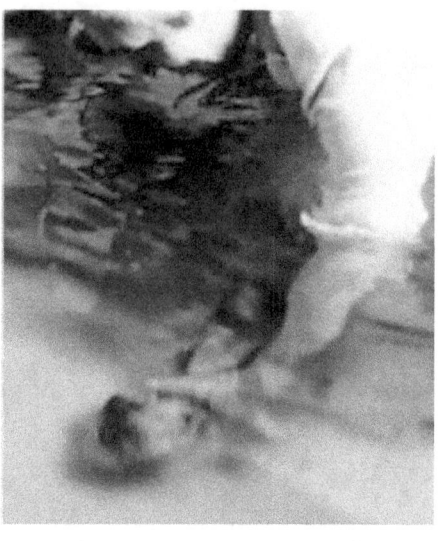

Michel catching a baby as it is born under water

Birth under water is possible, but it should not be the goal

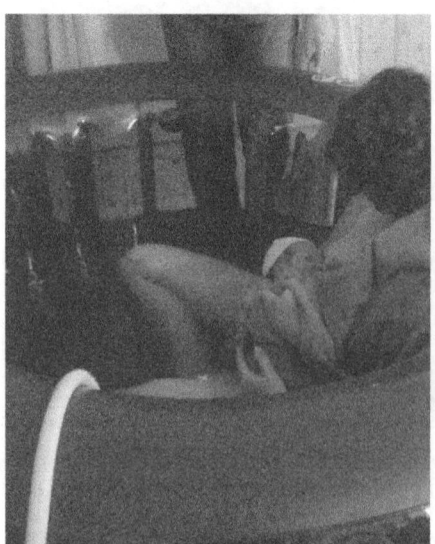

Moments after a home water birth. Here the baby's having her first feed.

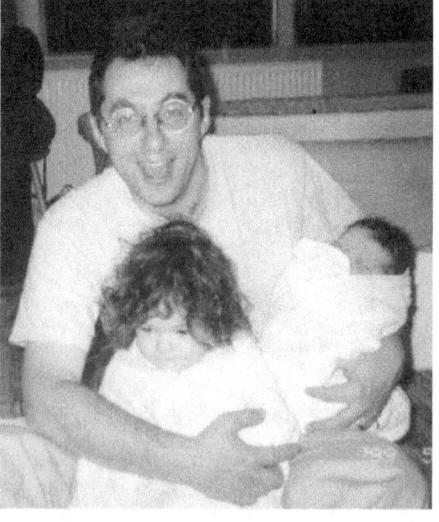

Of course, water births can be fun for the rest of the family too! Here the Jacoby family gets dry after Jennifer Jacoby's home water birth (see Birthframe 58)

Finally, here's a summary of key points to remember when using water... Note the need to plan ahead!

- ♥ Set the pool up in early labour, so nobody's panicking at the last minute.
- ♥ Ensure the immersion heater is switched on, in case extra hot water is needed.
- ♥ Have folded towels available to kneel on underwater.
- ♥ Don't immerse yourself in water until you're at least 5cm dilated. If you're on your own, guess! You need to be having strong contractions thick and fast (perhaps one minute apart) for your labour to have progressed to this stage. (That is, unless you're having one of those low-key painless labours. Your type won't need the water anyway!)
- ♥ Lean forward at all times. This is not a time for lying back in bubbles. The baby needs oxygen and his or her supply might be affected if you recline.
- ♥ It's best to put as little as possible—or preferably nothing—in the water. Hygiene is obviously important.
- ♥ Don't have the water too hot. Heat can be very dangerous for an unborn baby. The water should be at body temperature or very slightly warmer. You can have a nice hot bath after the baby's born—just put up with the cooler temperature for a little while longer!
- ♥ If your contractions become weaker or less frequent after a while, get out. It's likely you've got in too soon. If after an hour and a half or so nothing seems to have happened, remember that might indicate a problem. Seek advice from a professional.
- ♥ If you find the water's not helping you, just get out. Even though some women find water wonderful during labour, others find it annoying. Sometimes it's good to have your feet firmly on dry land. Don't stick to romantic notions about water births if your body and your feelings are telling you to do something else.
- ♥ If you dislike the idea of using water for your labour, consider getting into a warm bath if only for a few moments late on in your labour. This is because the warmth of the water is likely to help soften your perineum, which will then be able to stretch more easily for the birth—and you'll make a tear even less likely.[9]

Wherever you choose to give birth, the key is to make sure you feel as safe and as undisturbed as possible. (As I've explained, this means different things for different people.) Find out the facts, tune into your feelings and make the appropriate practical arrangements. Then be positive about whatever you have organised for yourself. After all, with the appropriate psychological and physical environment, your body and your baby will know exactly how to go about this birthing business... Nevertheless, it's still a good idea to focus on our final two preparatory steps: 'Help your body' and 'Help your mind' because there are still other things you can do to make your pregnancy, labour and birth even easier, safer and more beautiful.

2... HELP YOUR BODY

All I have said about your body's capabilities is true. However, you can actively help your body by taking a few key mini-steps (as it were) while you're pregnant, when you're in labour, while giving birth, and afterwards too.

In case you're not yet pregnant...

If you happen to be reading this book 'ahead of time', it's worth knowing that sperm take 70 days to be produced. This means your partner will need to be in peak condition three months before you hope to conceive. Be aware, in particular, of any chemicals he may be exposing himself to at work or while doing DIY at home.

Be aware of any chemicals you're exposing yourself to

You yourself will need to be healthy for at least a month beforehand, because your ova (eggs) mature each month, so the timescale is slightly shorter. However, since your nutritional status needs to be excellent, it's best to start focusing on being super-healthy three to six months before you hope to conceive so that your body has a chance to readjust to a healthier lifestyle. This mainly means you need to eat a healthy, balanced diet. In other words, make sure you're eating good quality protein (fish is especially good, especially if it's oily fish), lots of fruit and vegetables and as much carbohydrate as you feel you need. Minimise your consumption of 'white', sugary or high-fat foods and cut down on additives and processed food. Also, make sure all the food you eat is very fresh and clean. Improving your overall health may also mean you need to lose weight... Being overweight can sometimes stop women conceiving, believe it or not. Weight Watchers is an excellent re-education program, if you've had trouble losing weight and keeping it off in the past. It's simply based on healthy eating. Useful website: www.weightwatchers.co.uk

Finally, you and your partner might consider signing up for a preconceptual detox program so as to reduce the amount of fat-soluble contaminants accumulated in your adipose tissues... if you can find one taking place locally! If you live near London see if you can register on one of Michel's occasional London-based courses (called 'The Accordion Method of Preconceptual Care'). Perhaps they will eventually become widely available as we come to appreciate the value of preconceptual health more. His programme involves periodic detoxing (through fasting) before conception. For more information on this, see www.wombecology.com/newreasons.html

Consider detoxing by fasting well before conception

What else can you do to help your body?

- ♥ Take daily folic acid supplements. Research is very clear that this kind of supplementation does help to prevent spina bifida. Take 400mg per day from before you want to conceive until approximately Week 14 of your pregnancy, to be on the safe side.
- ♥ Keep a careful record of your periods, including the length of your cycle. One simple way is to mark the day your period is due in your diary with an asterisk, then to use a circled asterisk to indicate when your period actually starts. By looking back, you will quickly be able to find your 'LMP' (first day of your last monthly period) and determine the length of your normal cycle.
- ♥ Just in case it's not totally obvious, stop using any form of contraception! No condoms, no gels, no coils, no pills... What a strange feeling suddenly. You may find you get pregnant the first time you make love 'unprotected', or it may take a year, or longer. Go with the flow, take your time, think open, think love.
- ♥ If you want to be more aware of what might be happening when, note that when your normal creamy vaginal discharge changes to a clear, stretchy jelly you will have just ovulated. (This is usually 14 days before the start of your next period, but can actually be at any time.) Women are usually fertile for two or three days each month. Since sperm survive in your body for about 24 hours, making love every two or three days covers all posts! Lying on your back for half an hour after your partner ejaculates inside you may facilitate the processes necessary for conception to become established.
- ♥ Keep away from anyone with rubella (German measles) or chicken pox. There's a risk of fetal blindness or deafness if these are caught in the first trimester.
- ♥ Because of the risk of listeria and toxoplasmosis, avoid soft ripened cheese, blue-veined cheeses, feta cheese, all unpasteurised cheeses and fresh pâté; pies, pastries, poultry and any other cold buffet/picnic foods sold at deli counters, including ready-made salads and coleslaw. Be careful of any refrigerated or cook-chilled food, again because of the risk of bacterial contamination. (Heating ready-meals very thoroughly is a good way of killing off harmful bacteria.) Because of the risk of toxoplasmosis in particular, avoid all raw meats, such as salami and pastrami, wear gloves for gardening and avoid cats, or at the least wear rubber gloves when you handle cat litter or poo. Be careful, rather than paranoid, washing your hands thoroughly if you think you've touched anything you shouldn't have.
- ♥ Drink as little tea and coffee as possible. We don't know what effect they have on conception, but it's possible they do have some impact on the whole process, so they're best avoided or at least drunk infrequently.

Be careful, rather than paranoid...

- ♥ Stop drinking alcohol completely, if you drink. Even small amounts may be harmful to a newly fertilised egg or to a developing fetus and may result in malformations to the eyes, lips, head and face generally. Alcohol exposure later on in pregnancy is also associated with various problems—so do without it altogether while you're trying to conceive and when you're pregnant.
- ♥ Stop smoking, if you smoke, and keep away from anybody else who smokes.[1]
- ♥ Keep away from any other drugs, unless you have a specific health condition which requires regular monitoring. (Consult your GP for advice, remembering that it's always a good idea to do your own research too.) Recreational drugs are obviously out, but you also need to stop taking over-the-counter drugs or medicines.[2] Even avoid exposing yourself to chemicals through beauty products. That means no aspirin, no throat pastilles, no digestion tablets, no creams, no hair dye... If you have a desperately bad headache and find drinking water and walking in the fresh air does no good, take paracetamol as a last resort. (Certainly do not take aspirin, which can cause problems.) Only use tried and tested cosmetics which you feel really make a difference to you.[3]

Continue with any lifestyle changes for as long as it takes. And try and enjoy the process of conception... After all, it may be rather a long time before you can enjoy undisturbed, unencumbered, romantic sex again.

While you're pregnant...

RELAX AND BREATHE WELL

Relaxation and breathing are intimately connected because our breath usually reflects our state of mind.

How can you relax if you're feeling tense?

- ♥ Developing confidence in the natural processes will help. Re-read any birthframes which are relevant to you, or which you find particularly inspiring. (Also look for intriguing ones in the Birthframes index at the back.)
- ♥ Work out what's causing any tension. Simply doing that will help you understand what you need to do to feel better. Are there any practical issues you need to sort out? Are you feeling unhappy with a particular caregiver? Are there issues you need to resolve in any personal relationships?
- ♥ If you're not sure why you're feeling tense, go for a walk, do some singing or dancing, listen to some music, have a chat with a good friend, ring your mother, cuddle up with your partner, read some more birthframes from this book... try anything at all until you begin to feel better.

- Double-check your diet. Are you having a lot of sugary food and drink? If so, try eating something really healthy—anything containing oats, vegetables, lentils, tofu, salmon, chicken, dried fruit and nuts. (Avoid peanuts if there's any family history of allergy—but eat super-healthy almonds, pistachios, walnuts, Brazil nuts and cashews with gusto! Calming herbs which you can use in moderation to flavour savoury dishes include oregano, dill and rosemary, but others need to be avoided. (Review your use of herbs later, when you're breastfeeding. It's worth remembering that rosemary and sage are particularly unhelpful because they dry up the milk supply.)
- Are you drinking enough water? Being dehydrated can be a problem in pregnancy and can make you feel awful too. If you can't stand the idea of swigging any more water, drink hot water with a squeeze of lemon, very weak tea (black Earl Grey is very refreshing) or some miso soup—a healthy Japanese soup, available in sachets at any major supermarket.[4]
- You'll notice I'm not recommending any breathing exercises. As a result of my personal experience and from my review of hundreds of birth accounts I've come to believe they're not at all helpful. What does help is being aware of your breathing, while observing and accepting any emotions you feel. Amazing as it may seem, simply doing this can calm you down! If you're feeling especially emotional at any time, just stay with those feelings for as long as they last. (This may take as long as a few days or even weeks.) Don't wallow in them—just observe them until they pass away. Try it! (This kind of dispassionate awareness is also useful for labour.)

CONSIDER WHAT MIGHT BE CROSSING THE PLACENTA

Consider how your current lifestyle might be affecting the nutrients and chemicals your baby receives. Then think how you can make positive changes.

- Are your home and workplace both smoke-free environments?
- Do you do a job which exposes you to harmful substances? If so, it's worth informing your employer about your pregnancy very early on, so that changes can be made. Employers have a legal obligation to protect you.[5]
- Can you avoid street pollution any more than you're already doing?
- Can you drink purer water? Is it worth using filtered or bottled water? (If you choose bottled, make sure you go for a low-sodium brand, e.g. Evian.)
- Does your usual beauty care routine involve the use of any products which may contain harmful chemicals?
- Do you buy a lot of vegetables wrapped in plastic which leak oestrogens? Do you store leftovers in clingfilm in the fridge? Are your saucepans made of aluminium? Stainless steel or glass are healthier choices.
- In other words, remember that everything that goes into you will not only contribute toward your own health, it will also affect your baby. Literally everything you expose yourself to may cross the placenta and affect the baby growing inside you.

> Eat healthily, but don't be obsessive. Don't worry about unrealistic statements made in official-looking pamphlets!

As far as your diet is concerned, eat healthily, but don't be obsessive. Don't worry about the unrealistic statements made in official-looking pamphlets and books on health. Just eat as well as you can manage in your personal circumstances. Obviously, what you eat will be affected by your culture, your lifestyle and your budget—but now certainly is the time to spend money on food![6] Look especially for good quality protein—fish is great for the baby—and eat extra-fresh fruit and veg. Obviously, avoid things listed at the beginning of this chapter, which might cause problems. Apart from these items, if you feel like eating something which seems less than ideally healthy—such as chocolate ice cream!—go ahead. (Cravings are common in pregnancy.) Be aware, though, that your baby may well express enthusiasm for the same food when he or she is a toddler! Of course, you'll need to compensate for any treats with extra helpings of super-healthy food later.

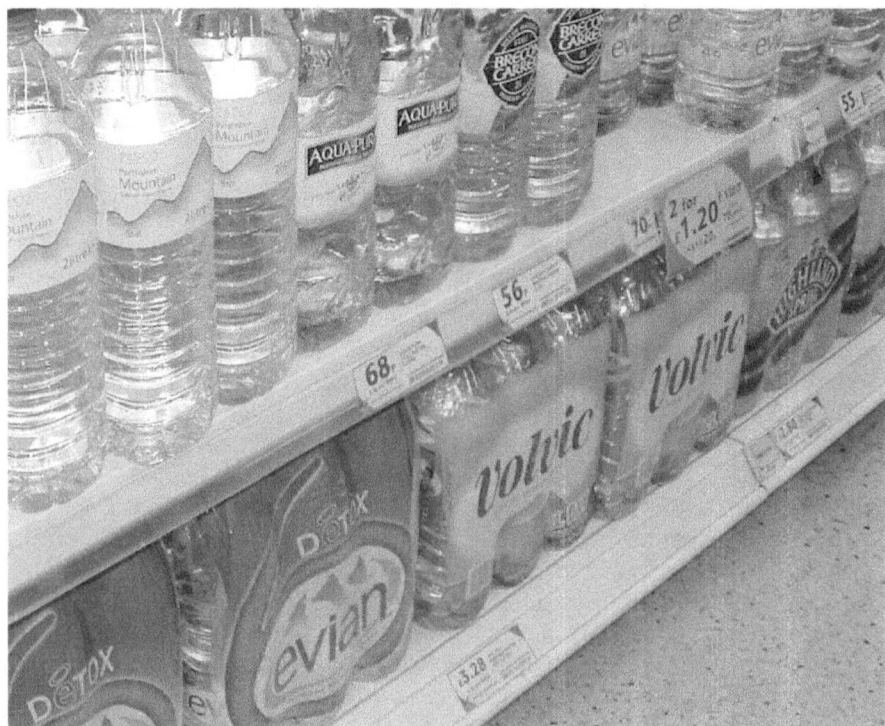

This might be a good time to drink bottled water. However, make sure the type you choose has low levels of sodium. It's time to read those boring labels!

THINK ABOUT USEFUL AND HARMFUL SUPPLEMENTATION

Since your ingestion of nutrients is so important, it's helpful to take certain precautions to make sure your overall intake is adequate. You also need to avoid causing problems...

- ♥ **Folic acid** As we've already mentioned, it's a good idea to take folic acid in the first trimester. This will ensure you have adequate supplies over the period when your baby's spine is developing.
- ♥ **Multivitamins** Unless you have a truly fantastic diet, it might be a good idea to take a multivitamin from the second trimester onwards. Sanatogen *Pronatal* is a specially-designed pregnancy supplement which should not interfere with your bodily balance.[7]
- ♥ **Omega-3 fish oil** Consider taking an Omega-3 fish oil supplement during the last three months of your pregnancy so as to help your little one's brain develop. These supplements are especially useful if you dislike oily fish—salmon, sardine, mackerel, etc.[8]
- ♥ **Iron supplements** It's best to avoid taking any iron supplements, even if you're told you're anaemic (which you're probably not—see the Index for more on this). Iron stops your body absorbing zinc so effectively and this is essential for your baby's growth and brain development.

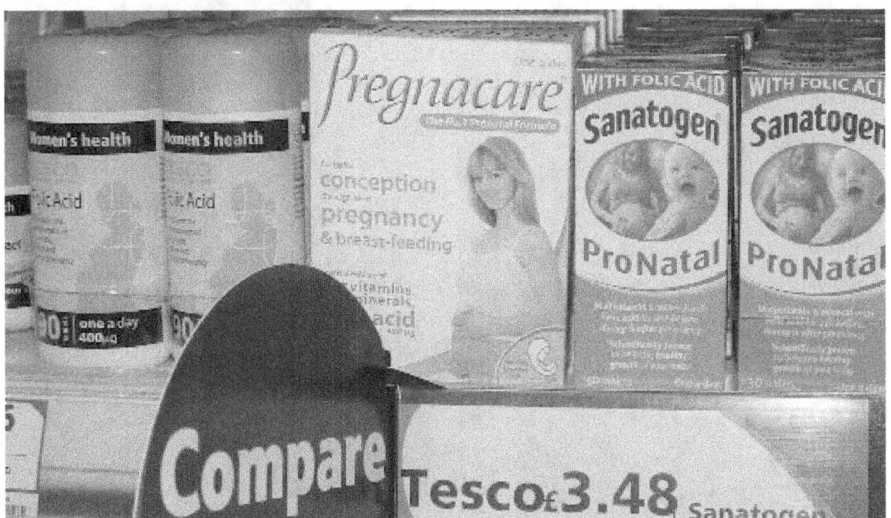

Many supplements are available for pregnant women. Consider what you take carefully.

It's best to avoid taking any additional iron supplements.
Iron stops your body absorbing zinc, which is essential.

372 birth: countdown to optimal

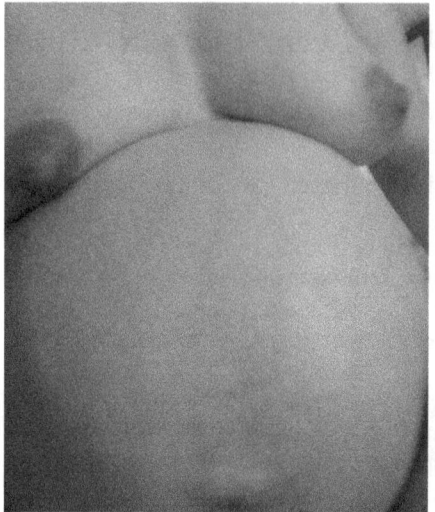

Wow! What a belly... This is what you're going to look like in a few weeks' time. Where else is your baby going to grow?

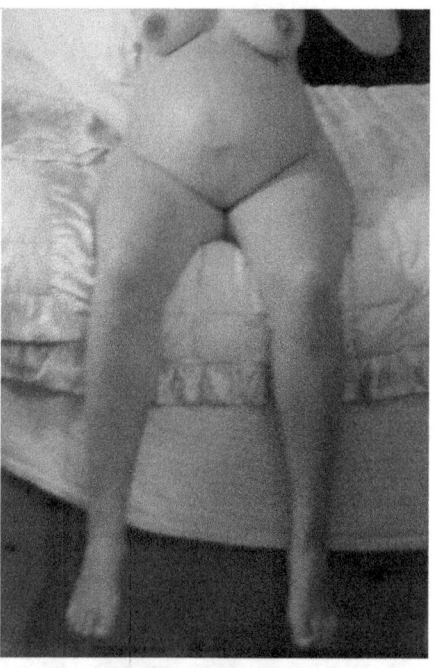

Don't worry, you will eventually regain some elegance

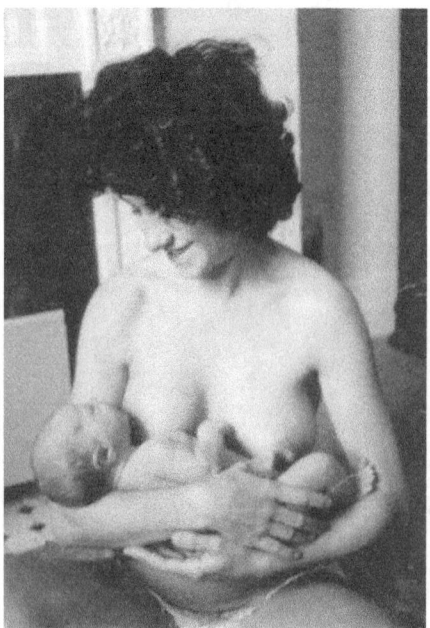

Soon you'll have a new baby in your arms... This is Liliana Lammers (see Birthframe 91)
Photo © Jill Furmanovsky

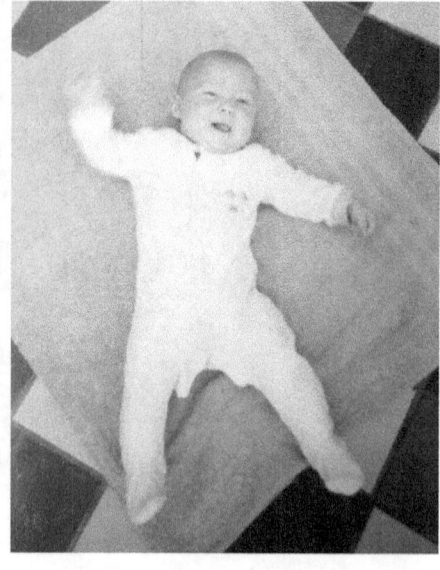

... or kicking on the floor while you do other things in your newly slim body

ENJOY YOUR CHANGING SHAPE

Accepting and even enjoying your changing shape is helpful if you can manage it! Not only will your positive mental attitude affect your posture, it'll also affect your interpretation of ongoing sensations.

To help yourself think positively about your body, revamp and update your wardrobe on an ongoing basis. This needn't cost much... Borrow clothes from friends, explore charity shops and even check out jumble sales or eBay!

Also note that your shape after your pregnancy is likely to be better if you stay (or get) fit during this nine-month period. Consider how much exercise you do and how you might add or adapt physical activities as you become more heavily pregnant. (Many women take up something new, or adapt their current exercise programmes. Avoid anything which might put you at risk of sudden falls or bumps, for obvious reasons.) If you are generally fairly active, i.e. not a total slob, then you needn't worry unduly. I personally feel that walking as much as possible is sufficient, along with a bit of cycling or swimming too, as long as you swim on your front. For reasons of balance cycling becomes a little overly wobbly by about the eighth month of pregnancy! I myself cycled right up until about three weeks before the end of my second pregnancy.

As far as weight gain is concerned, you also don't need to worry too much. Most women find they're left with a little extra flab after they've given birth. If your focus is mainly on healthy eating to satisfy your hunger, you should find that whatever extra you gain can eventually be lost after your baby's birth. This is especially true if you breastfeed, of course.

Consider how much exercise you do and how you might add or adapt physical activities as you become more heavily pregnant

HELP YOUR SKIN

Your skin will be under considerable strain throughout your pregnancy for obvious 'expansion' reasons, but also because of ongoing changes in your hormones.

- ♥ Drink plenty of water so that it remains well hydrated. If you aren't drinking enough, understandably your skin can become dry or itchy. You may be surprised by how much water you need. While I was pregnant in Britain I consumed at least two 1.5-litre bottles of Evian a day... and living in Sri Lanka I consumed at least double this!
- ♥ Avoid taking too many baths because this can dry out your skin. In any case, hot baths can be dangerous for your baby so they may be best avoided altogether until after the birth. (Take warm showers instead.)

- If you find your skin is still too dry, look for a moisturiser which is pregnancy-friendly. Drinking water and using a moisturiser two times daily, you may be able to avoid stretch marks altogether.
- Use a high quality, high-factor UVA and UVB suncream on your face and neck. Your facial skin is particularly prone to unusual sunburn during pregnancy, even in normal weather.
- Obviously, if you use any creams or cosmetics, check the ingredients and avoid any products which contain anything you know or suspect to be harmful. (You might, for example, avoid something such as aloe vera because there are reports that it may have purgative or laxative effects. Some people claim this is only the case when the whole leaf is used—but why take an unnecessary risk when reports are contradictory?) Remember, you can look things up in reference books (in bookshops or libraries), you can do Internet searches, or you can ask professionals, who will use their own reference materials. Consult your intuition too!
- Double-check whatever information you first find. This is important not only because information changes (after new research studies are published), but also because individual experts make mistakes when evaluating products or have different views on potential risks. Remember those thalidomide mothers who trusted their doctors' advice, who in turn trusted the drug companies... If in doubt, do without.

MINIMISE PHYSICAL DISCOMFORTS

Few women get through pregnancy without any niggles. Some even find the physical side of pregnancy extremely unpleasant. Whatever your personal experience, help yourself with a few sure-fire remedies. All of these suggested approaches respect and support the processes going on within you.

Nausea or vomiting

This is a well-known symptom of pregnancy in most cultures, especially in the first trimester. If you experience so-called 'morning sickness'—which can actually occur at any time of the day or night—be reassured that it will probably clear up after about 12-14 weeks, when your placenta takes over 'feeding' your baby. In the meantime, here are a few ways in which you can ease the problem:

- Eat dry biscuits (or something else containing carbohydrate) early in the morning—even before you get up—or whenever you feel nauseous. This will bring your blood sugar levels up.
- In general, eat little and often so as to keep your blood sugar levels stable. This seems to be an important aspect of reducing nausea.
- Eat foods which are nutrient-dense such as nuts, seeds or avocados. This will mean you're more likely to absorb some of the important nutrients you might otherwise miss out on.

- ♥ Drink plenty of water—even more than you would normally expect to be the right amount. If you're vomiting as well as feeling nauseous, the extra water is important so that you don't become dehydrated.
- ♥ Include ginger in your diet because this may help prevent nausea entirely.
- ♥ Eat asparagus. Some research suggests it may also prevent nausea.
- ♥ Consult your midwife or doctor if you are vomiting very often, because you may need salt-replacement therapy in hospital.
- ♥ Take a nap. Nausea may be a sign of low energy levels caused by tiredness.
- ♥ Be aware of your breathing while you're sitting calmly.
- ♥ Explore your feelings—a minority of experts believe that nausea has psychological causes.

Here are some comments from Marina Svechnikova, the Russian author of *Birth Without Trauma* (Astrel; 2001):

> We can fool ourselves, but it is impossible to fool our physical organism. I know a few women who told me during a medical visit that they had planned the pregnancy and were happy about it, but experienced such severe morning sickness that they couldn't stand it, and ended the pregnancy. I am convinced that, in every one of these cases, the woman consciously desired the pregnancy, but at an unconscious level rejected it for one reason or another. Fear of pregnancy and birth, fear of change, of dependence, difficult relations with the child's father are all possible causes of such subconscious rejection of the pregnancy. In any case, if the beginning of your pregnancy is accompanied by nausea, keep in mind that 90% of women experience such symptoms, but some are so absorbed by what is happening inside them that they hardly notice it. Sometimes resolving the psychological problems connected to the pregnancy can completely cure morning sickness.

Most other experts think the problem is caused by pregnancy hormones (which your body is unused to), or by an adaptive mechanism of the placenta. Here are Michel's comments on the subject:

> When a woman is vomiting a lot in pregnancy (hyperemesis), my attitude can be easily summarised ... First, I explain to the mother-to-be that vomiting in pregnancy is almost a guarantee that she will finally have a big and beautiful baby. It is important to start with such considerations, because many women are concerned about the growth of their baby. In fact, morning sickness and vomiting means that the placenta is working hard, asking the mother (on behalf of the fetus) to eat as little as possible. This reduced digestive tolerance is adaptive. In order to compensate for this situation, the placenta is getting bigger, and birth weight correlates with the weight of the placenta. When a woman is first given such explanations, she is less anxious and can more easily accept her condition.
>
> Secondly, I explain in advance that when 'hyperemesis' lasts longer than usual, women often try a great variety of treatments—Vitamin B6, acupuncture or acupressure at the Neiguan point... even antibiotics and corticosteroids in some cases. The final victory is usually attributed to the last treatment that has been tried.
>
> The only role of doctors, in case of real emergency, should be to compensate via drips a possible extreme loss of water and electrolytes.

> I found out I was having non-identical twins at 9 weeks due to very bad morning sickness... it wasn't just morning sickness, it was actually '24-hour sickness'! After 18 weeks the sickness subsided and I had a fantastic pregnancy.

Cravings

These are another symptom typically associated with pregnancy. Perhaps our bodies do have ways of encouraging us to eat certain kinds of things... or could there also be psychological causes here? Whatever the causes of cravings, if you find yourself wanting a particular food or drink, as long as it's basically healthy, go for it! Even good quality ice cream can be justified because of the nutrients it contains. Even if you're worried about weight gain (as in flab), please don't deprive yourself while you're pregnant. Any hunger you feel may well be genuine—after all, you're growing a baby! Just make sure you have a balanced diet with sufficiently high levels of protein and water.

If you find yourself wanting something really weird, get yourself a good, solid, balanced meal, drink some more water or go to sleep. Alternatively, look at what's going on in your mind and encourage yourself to deal with that by writing, painting, dancing, walking, talking... or whatever. Nutritional imbalances, dehydration, tiredness and emotional upsets can all cause unusual behaviour. Whatever you do, make sure you continue to safeguard your baby's health.

Heartburn

This is a symptom often reported in late pregnancy, when the growing baby is putting pressure on the mother's stomach, leaving less room for food! Here are a few ways of dealing with it:

- ♥ Eat smaller, more frequent meals.
- ♥ Try and establish if any specific foods are disagreeing with you and eliminate these, or reduce your intake.
- ♥ Eat foods which are denser in nutrients and higher in calories, such as avocados, halva and nuts.
- ♥ Try eating asparagus. Some research suggests it is as effective as some drugs at reducing heartburn.

Blocked nose

Having a blocked-up nose during pregnancy can be a nuisance. As well as making day-to-day breathing difficult, it can also result in snoring, which isn't exactly romantic or conducive to marital harmony. What can you do?

- ♥ Try eating some ginger because this has a stimulating effect on the circulation and should help the body dislodge phlegm and catarrh. Any type of ginger will do—add half a teaspoon of dried ginger to black tea, or eat a piece of fresh or preserved stem ginger root.

If you have a blocked nose, try eating chillies to clear it!

- Try eating chillies because they also have a stimulating effect. Add fresh, chopped chillies to meals—wear rubber gloves while you chop them!—or go to your local Indian restaurant.

Backache

You may avoid backache entirely by taking the following precautions:

- Buy or make a 'pregnancy pillow', i.e. a wedge-shaped cushion, to put under your bump while you sleep. (The difference to your quality of sleep will probably be substantial.) For your baby's sake (as well as your own), always lie on your *left* side when you use this. Because of the positioning of your internal organs this will mean your baby gets the maximum amount of oxygen (the vena cava won't be compressed) and you yourself will be less at risk of getting high blood pressure.
- Buy or make a belt to support your growing belly and redistribute the weight more evenly around your hips. (A maternity support belt is simply a wide strip of thick cotton which is fixed by Velcro underneath your bump and around your back (rather like a low waistband).
- Hire or buy a pregnancy rocker (e.g. the Stokke 'Variable') or use a high-backed chair to ensure you are tilting slightly forward whenever you are sitting down. As well as easing your back, this kind of chair will also ensure your bump is always tilting forwards and help your baby to get into a good position for the birth.
- Put cushions in your car or on any other chair you use frequently, so as to ensure that you sit comfortably in a leaning forward position at all times.
- Make sure the mattress on your bed is firm enough to be comfortable. If it isn't, place a board underneath your mattress—or sleep on the floor!
- Buy one or more good maternity bras to wear as your breasts expand. Your bust measurements will increase gradually throughout your pregnancy and then again when you begin to breastfeed! It is important to wear a bra that fits properly because incorrectly positioned straps or too tight a band underneath your breasts or underwiring can put strain on your back. See if you can get a bra fitted.
- Wear well-supporting, low-heeled shoes so you can stand and walk well.
- 'Guard' your back by keeping it straight and bending your knees whenever you pick something up or lift something.

Hire or buy a pregnancy rocker or another chair to sit forward. Also, wear good shoes so you can stand and walk well.

Itching

This is both unpleasant, unfeminine and a potential warning sign, to be taken very seriously. If you find yourself scratching, do the following immediately:

- ♥ Drink even more water! You will probably find that the itching subsides after a couple of hours. If it doesn't, seek medical attention immediately because itching can be a sign of a dangerous condition (cholestasis), which can result in premature labour or stillbirth. (See Birthframe 5.)
- ♥ Wear lighter clothing than usual because your temperature naturally increases during pregnancy and your skin is likely to itch if you're too hot.
- ♥ Avoid man-made fibres because it's possible your skin is more sensitive than usual. Wearing cotton close to your skin may well cure the problem.
- ♥ Stop using any creams or lotions you are using for a while or try some different ones.

Other discomforts or symptoms...

If you experience any other discomforts not mentioned here, evaluate your options very carefully. Be wary of complementary therapies precisely because they are powerful. If you can possibly do without treatment, do so. Mention any concerns to your caregivers but do your own research too. This is simply because if you focus too much on worries, this will prompt some caregivers to give you information about all the things that can go wrong! Nevertheless, note:

> **The only serious symptoms of pregnancy are severe, sudden or persistent abdominal pain, persistent itching, vaginal bleeding, severe headaches, dizziness, flashing lights before the eyes and convulsions.**

As long as you have none of these symptoms remember the temporary nature of your situation: whatever it is, it will eventually pass. Extraordinary processes are taking place within you so your body is bound to have some adjusting to do.

HELP YOUR REPRODUCTIVE ORGANS!

Don't forget this all-important area of the body. There are various things you can do...

- ♥ Do exercises to strengthen your perineal muscles—sometimes called 'Kegels', after the man who first recommended them. These muscles support the pelvic organs, rectum, vagina, uterus and bladder, so they're pretty important. (If you ignore them, incontinence may be a problem later in life.) To establish which muscles you need to be exercising, simply stop the flow of urine once when you're going to the toilet. Then, at any time—when you're standing, sitting or lying down—tighten and release those same muscles several times. If you do this, you'll increase your awareness of that part of your body (which might be helpful during labour), you'll be ensuring

that the region has a good supply of blood, you'll be learning how to relax those important muscles and you'll also be learning an exercise which is useful after the birth, for the prevention of incontinence, uterine prolapse and for increasing sexual pleasure. It's certainly worth paying attention to these muscles!
- ♥ Drink raspberry leaf tea in the third trimester of your pregnancy. (This herb has stood the test of time in terms of not appearing to harm women or babies at all. One research study has already confirmed the traditional claim that using this herb in the last couple of months of pregnancy helps the uterine muscles prepare for the second stage of labour.) After comparing the recommendations in various sources, I suggest you drink two cups a day from Week 29 onwards. If you absolutely can't stand the prospect of drinking this rather unpleasant-tasting tea, you can get raspberry leaf in tablet form.
- ♥ Take the homeopathic remedy Arnica 30 once a day for the last month of your pregnancy. Arnica may help you avoid any bruising from the birth, although there's no research evidence to confirm this.
- ♥ Some people also recommend perineal massage with olive oil (or Vitamin E oil) to avoid tearing.[9] I personally don't think this is at all necessary. Your sexual organs (vagina and perineum) are designed to expand and contract according to the situation... just go with the flow and respect the capabilities of your body.

ENJOY YOUR SEXUALITY

Of course, different women have different views of sex and different feelings about enjoying it during pregnancy. Whatever your preconceptions, be aware that pregnancy is a sexual experience for many, if not most, women. After all, the changes taking place within your body are a direct result of having sex! Conception and childbirth, and your sexuality in between the two, are nothing to be ashamed of; they are merely part of the experience of being a woman and, as such, should be celebrated joyfully within your relationship.

Remember, too, as you travel through any new sensations that some women also experience childbirth itself as pleasurably sexual, not painful as many films would have us believe! Physiologically speaking, there is very little difference between an orgasm and a so-called 'contraction', so there's no reason to associate that word with pain. Perhaps our experience of labour is influenced by our attitude toward our sexuality generally... who knows? In any case, be reassured that no research has associated sexual activity during pregnancy with any negative birth outcomes.

Remember that some women experience birth as sexual...

Having said all this, there are two limitations on your sexual activities during pregnancy if you want to optimise outcomes... First, don't use any sex toys! The reason I mention this is because of some surprising statistics produced by a survey conducted by an ultra-respectable women's magazine. The risk of developing an infection is much higher when foreign objects are used near the genitals and unnatural and potentially over-stimulating speeds of vibration could potentially trigger unwanted physical reactions. So, for your baby's sake, stick to natural sex! The second limitation is, of course, to remain loyal to your partner, however aroused you feel. The reasons for fidelity—both physical and psychological—are the same in pregnancy as in relationships generally. Infection and divided loyalties are things you can do without as you're about to embark on motherhood for the first or the fifth time! Again, I mention this not merely to moralise at you, but because of some surprising comments I received while researching this book. There are all kinds of good reasons behind morals!

> Great orgasms—pregnancy's best-kept secret!

> Sex with my lover was gentle and fun when I was pregnant. I loved that he still wanted me, even though my body was so different, and even though it wasn't his baby. I guess he loves me however I am. It did get a little awkward when my bump was really big. I couldn't seem to get a comfortable angle unless I was sitting up on him during intercourse. And then I couldn't kiss him at the same time!

RESPOND INTELLIGENTLY TO SCARES

With the best intentions, caregivers usually scare women several times during each pregnancy. Respond responsibly, but intelligently. Here are some notes on a few common physical problems...[10]

Urinary tract infections

If at any time during your pregnancy you develop a urinary tract infection (the main symptom of which is pain passing urine), you will need to get it treated immediately. This is because of the importance of safeguarding the health of your kidneys, which are working even harder during pregnancy, clearing waste products from your own and your baby's body. To make sure you avoid getting an infection at all, do the following:

- ♥ Always wipe your bottom from front to back to make sure that no faeces (poo) gets on your vagina, or anywhere round the front.
- ♥ Wear cotton knickers and loose-fitting trousers, so as to ensure good circulation of air around your genitals. Avoid wearing nylon tights, or wear the type which have a hole around the gusset area.
- ♥ Never put toilet rolls on the floor or on other potentially unclean surfaces, because any dirt may then get transferred to your bottom when you use the toilet paper.

- Wash your genitals regularly, but don't use much soap.
- Most of the time, you could perhaps avoid using any soap at all, or you could minimise its effect by a) showering, rather than having a bath and b) using a very mild, unscented soap.
- Make sure you do not eat too many sweet things, as this may exacerbate any minor infection you pick up.
- Drink half a cup of cranberry juice each day to prevent or clear an infection.

Strep B

In the UK, NICE [the National Institute for Clinical Excellence] does not recommend routine testing for this infection during pregnancy. (This may be for cost reasons, some think, because a test is available which is non-invasive—involving vaginal and rectal swabs at 35 or 37 weeks of pregnancy.) Anyway, what is Strep B and if a woman gets herself tested and is found to be infected (as one in three women are thought to be), what does it mean? Basically, when a pregnant woman is infected there's a small chance her baby might also become infected and if *that* happens there can be serious consequences (possibly involving septicaemia with pneumonia, or even meningitis). The good news is that babies are much less susceptible to infection if they are born at term (any time from 38 to 42 weeks) at a normal weight, i.e. above 2.5 kg (5lb 8oz). Babies of mothers who are infected are especially low risk if the mother didn't have a fever while she was in labour, if she gave birth within 18 hours of her waters breaking and if she's never had a baby infected with Strep B before.

If you do decide to get tested for Strep B on a just-in-case basis or because NICE guidelines change you have various options if the test comes out positive:

1. You could attempt to get rid of the GBS infection yourself. To do this, insert one whole, peeled, slightly crushed clove of garlic threaded on a string (like a tampon) into your vagina and leave it there for 24 hours. Remove it, then put in another 'garlic tampon' every day for three days. Then get retested. The idea of doing this is based on the fact that garlic contains allicin, a natural antibiotic. One laboratory study already conducted suggested that allicin gel (derived from garlic) might well be an effective treatment.[11]
2. If the test is still positive you might consider refusing a drip while you're in labour (which will probably be the protocol in a hospital) if you consider yourself to be low risk (see above). In this case you could give birth as originally planned—even at home—as long as you can find a midwife who will attend your birth and support you in this. You may wish to arrange for your baby to be given antibiotics immediately after the birth, just in case.
3. Alternatively you could simply stop worrying and take no action at all, except to keep an eye on your newborn baby for any signs of infection particularly in the first six days after the birth and less so for the first three months. Information on signs to look out for, treatments and risks can be found at www.gbss.org.uk. Of course, this is something to discuss with your caregiver if you consider yourself high risk or if the test is positive.

High blood pressure

This is checked routinely at every antenatal appointment because—as we've already noted—high blood pressure in association with protein in the urine is a sign of pre-eclampsia. Even then, in itself, pre-eclampsia is not a problem... it is only taken very seriously because it very occasionally leads to the life-threatening condition of eclampsia.[12]

Another point to be aware of is that pre-eclampsia is very rare indeed in subsequent pregnancies after a first pregnancy with no pre-eclampsia.

Finally, it's important to understand that it's perfectly normal for blood pressure to increase slightly from time to time and also for it to rise slightly towards the end of pregnancy.

If either you or your caregiver are really worried about your blood pressure:

- ♥ Lie on your left side, as I've already suggested, whenever you lie down.
- ♥ Meditate—meditation is scientifically proven to change the patterns of brainwaves and certain patterns of brainwaves are associated with high blood pressure
- ♥ Eat plenty of potassium-rich food (beans, lentils, celery, sweet potato, spinach, apricots, bananas, citrus fruit) and foods which don't inhibit the absorption of potassium (e.g. blackcurrants).
- ♥ Do whatever else you can to ease your stress levels and peace of mind...

Spotting

Even though you should inform your caregiver about any bleeding, however minor, do be reassured that it's quite common. It's only a problem if there's a large amount of blood or you appear to be haemorrhaging. It's quite common to bleed a little for the first month or two at the time when your period would normally have occurred. The bleeding is just a sign that your body is getting your pregnancy hormone levels correctly attuned.

If there is any bleeding late on in your pregnancy, you would need to keep consulting your caregiver. The bleeding could well be a sign of a low-lying placenta, which is only dangerous if the placenta is so low it blocks the exit from the womb or if the placenta actually comes away from the side of the womb. In the first case (where the exit is completely blocked) a caesarean is necessary. In the second case (where the placenta comes away), there would be very sudden, dramatic bleeding, accompanied by abdominal pain, and it would be a complete 999 emergency.

If you notice just a little blood on the toilet paper (or in the toilet bowl) near your due date, this could well be your 'show', i.e. a sign that your mucous plug has come out. This means that you will spontaneously go into labour at any point within the next week—usually within a day or so.

Sometimes a woman is told she has a low-lying placenta. In most cases the placenta moves 'up' as the womb expands.

Low haemoglobin

As we saw before, being told you're anaemic or have a low haemoglobin count can actually be good news, rather than bad. Research has established that the ideal level at the end of pregnancy is between 9.0 and 9.5.

Unfortunately, many caregivers have not read this research and because it is a level which in a non-pregnant woman would indicate anaemia, they recommend iron tablets! Taking iron is problematic from two points of view: a) it usually results in constipation (which can cause varicose veins and haemorrhoids, quite apart from being rather uncomfortable) and b) iron inhibits the absorption of zinc, a mineral associated with growth and brain development. Lower levels of haemoglobin in blood are actually a sign that the blood volume has increased successfully, which is supposed to happen during pregnancy and is necessary for your baby's well-being.

If your haemoglobin level is below the range mentioned above, try and increase your iron levels by increasing your consumption of any of the following foods: lettuce, sweet potato, oranges, cabbage, broccoli, brussels sprouts, kohlrabi, mustard greens, spring greens, swedes, turnips, watercress, beans and lentils, apricots and parsley. In the meantime, don't drink any tea (black or green) because this reduces the absorption of iron from food. Also, don't eat more than 50g of oats per day because oat bran is high in phytic acid, which limits the absorption of iron from other foods.

Low-lying placenta

Many women are told they have a 'low-lying placenta' after a scan at 20 weeks. There is no need to worry because in most cases, the placenta moves up as the woman's womb expands to accommodate the growing baby. In the few cases where it doesn't, a real low-lying placenta would be clearly signalled later on in pregnancy by bleeding. Also see 'spotting' on the previous page.

Prematurity

If you're worried that your baby—or babies—will be born prematurely, you can take a few simple measures to increase your chances of carrying to term:

- ♥ Eat a good, balanced diet.
- ♥ Don't eat any liquorice throughout your pregnancy.[13]
- ♥ Make sure you get plenty of rest.
- ♥ Try to avoid shocks or over-excitement.

Small-for-dates babies/small for gestational age (SGA)

Caregivers are very keen to track growth during pregnancy. Although it is always done routinely, with great care, the main methods used today (measuring the bump with a cloth tape measure, taking measurements from scans) are actually unreliable! (A better way of checking a baby's growth is for a midwife to feel, rather than measure your belly.) There have been numerous reported cases of babies whose growth turned out to have been wrongly assessed in utero. If you are really concerned about your baby's growth, try having a quiet, private chat with your growing baby. Tell him or her that people are concerned that he or she isn't growing fast enough and ask if there's anything he or she can do to help! (I had a surprising experience of this appearing to work for me with my first baby.) Also, eat more protein, especially fish, and make sure your daily calorie-intake is high enough. Eat!

Postmaturity

If your caregiver considers you overdue, again don't worry. Only 1% of babies who are induced because of suspected postmaturity actually display the symptoms of postmaturity when they're born. In other words, 99% of babies who are induced for this reason prove to have been induced unnecessarily and they're deprived of the last few days or weeks in the womb and their right to an optimal birth. If you are considered overdue...

- ♥ Recalculate your dates, taking your normal cycle into account.
- ♥ Deal with any unresolved psychological or practical issues you're aware of.
- ♥ Enjoy the last few days of your pregnancy.

ACCEPT YOUR PHYSICAL SITUATION

Especially toward the end of your pregnancy, there may be many more niggles than before... Here are some examples of things which may be going on in your body, which it is best to simply put up with...

- ♥ **Headaches** Drink more water or get out in the fresh air.
- ♥ **Backache** Check your posture and see the tips earlier in this chapter.
- ♥ **Heavy-feeling legs (especially in the evenings)** Lie down on your left side to rest them, or sit down—leaning forward!—so your weight is on your bottom.
- ♥ **Unusual but mild aches and pains** These are no doubt caused by your baby's changing positions and your body's attempts to attune itself for the birth.
- ♥ **Braxton Hicks contractions** Your body is limbering up for the big day!

Deal with any unresolved psychological or practical issues

- **Cold or the flu (especially near your due date)** In the case of flu, just make sure your temperature doesn't rise too much. Take a couple of paracetamol if it does, to bring it down a bit. (Do not take aspirin in any form, because it's not good for the baby.) You may also get a slight nosebleed if you blow your nose a lot because the membranes are very sensitive. Finally, don't worry if you're a little incontinent if you're coughing a lot.
- **Blocked-up nose or a runny one** Your membranes are more sensitive than usual... Don't worry, this is normal.
- **Feeling hot and sweaty** This just means your body's having a little trouble regulating your temperature. Drink more water!

All kinds of other moods and 'minor' symptoms are typical at the end of your pregnancy. Here are a few, to reassure you you're not alone and that all is well!

- Your baby may be either more or less active... Remember that babies get too big to move around so much just before the birth. On the other hand, movements—when they occur—may be more vigorous.
- You may get a metallic taste in your mouth and feel sick, or feel less hungry... It's also possible you may feel hungrier. Just go with the flow.
- You may get diarrhoea... If this happens consider it a good sign because it may mean labour is not far away.
- If you see a little blood or some clear jelly on the toilet paper after you've wiped your bottom, again that's a sure sign you will go into labour within a couple of weeks, and probably much sooner.
- You may repeatedly feel high levels of sexual arousal... This unusual and unpredictable arousal may be caused by changing levels of hormones, increased blood supply to your vagina and other sexual organs or by the rhythmic practice contractions of your womb. It's nothing to be ashamed about—it's just part of the process! The sensations will eventually pass, even though they may be very difficult to deal with at times. The best approach is to be aware of what is happening within you, while continuing with your daily tasks. Orgasm during pregnancy is fine—it's probably like a cuddle for your baby!—but it's worth noting that some women comment that the pleasure of the rhythmic contractions of an orgasm can sometimes transform themselves into pain and also that the prostoglandins in semen can trigger the onset of labour (which may be a good thing). You will no doubt find ways of coping with the pleasant sensations of pregnancy and birth, in the same way as you will find ways of coping with any pain.

Above all, remember that most seemingly weird symptoms are perfectly normal, so beyond informing yourself and adopting a positive attitude, try to remember that this is a temporary period of your life, which will soon be over. Putting up with a little discomfort here and there might make all the difference to the health of the baby growing within you. A positive, non-interventionist attitude will also help you move towards an optimal birth.

Birthframe 79

In this diary we see how being pregnant does not always give women the 'glow' we sometimes expect to feel. Often a pregnant woman's days are peppered with doubts, irritations and worries. Nowadays, too, as we see here, women mix conventional antenatal care with 'complementary therapies'—which are generally not recommended in this book—and the women might, or might not, mention this to their doctors or midwives! Is this a sign of distrust of the natural processes? Are there other ways of helping our bodies and our babies growing within? Let's step into the private world of one mother's twin pregnancy. At the beginning of this diary, the mum-to-be is 38 weeks + 1 day...

25 Mar — It's Mother's Day. Up really early. Feeling bunged up and snotty. Had a few Braxton Hicks. Feel quite down again. Want to be left alone. Took Sepia (constitutional) before bed.

26 Mar — Feeling really down and have been in tears on and off all morning. Feel really emotional. Have not felt like this in a long, long time. (Mum and Dad are moving next Wednesday.) Had a few Braxton Hicks. Still bunged up and absolutely shattered all day. No motivation to do anything at all.

27 Mar — Feeling much better in myself today. Had a few stronger Braxton Hicks. Tired and still bunged up.

28 Mar — Woke up at 1.00am in a hot sweat! Really tired during the day. A few Braxton Hicks. Feel OK.

29 Mar — Slept well. Have taken Kali bic for sinuses—three a day for four days. Saw midwife. All fine. Head has moved up a bit from 2/5 to 3/5 engaged. Had quite a few niggles. Babies moving well. Slight low backache. Took Caulyphylum at 9.45pm and went straight to bed!

30 Mar — Felt a bit teary in the morning. Fine in the afternoon. No twinges but a few Braxton Hicks. Have had a good day. Sun has shone all day and it's been warm. Babies moving a lot. Still bunged up but feel OK.

31 Mar — Bad night's sleep. Really uncomfortable all night. Woke up early morning with a strong pain across my tummy, with a Braxton Hicks which went away after a bit. Feel all right so far, I suppose!

1 Apr — Babies moving quite a lot. A few Braxton Hicks. Feel really fed up and crabby. Slept for one and a half hours in the afternoon and did feel better afterwards. I now measure 48 inches round my waist!

2 Apr — Babies moving loads. A couple of twinges. Really tired. Feel OK but really fed up. Legs feel really heavy and dragging in the evening by about 7.30pm.

3 Apr — Felt down but OK. Said goodbye to Mum and Dad. Had a few Braxton Hicks.

4 Apr — Had some diarrhoea at 7.30am. Had a few twinges—one light popping sensation about 2.20pm. No water or leakage, though. Felt a bit flat in the morning but better in the afternoon.

5 Apr — Feel OK. Saw consultant. Happy to let me go a bit longer. Babies growing and moving well.

6 Apr	No twinges. No signs. Scott off work. It really helped, him being here. Took Caulyphylum at 2.15pm. Had a bath in the evening and had hot flushes for about an hour afterwards.
7 Apr	40 weeks!!!!!! Holly woke at 5.00am. Been up since then. Metallic taste in mouth. Couple of twinges in the morning. Really tired and a bit teary.
8 Apr	Due date. Feel OK. A bit flat and low. Really tired, but restless too. Couldn't sleep in the daytime. Babies moving well. Can't get comfortable unless lying down.
9 Apr	Feel low and teary. First day of the Easter holidays. Not coping with the girls too well. Want to be left on my own. Don't want to do anything. No energy. Want to just lie down and go to sleep. Legs feel heavy. Right nostril bleeding slightly. Had a few twinges. Felt better later in the afternoon. Took a Sepia at 10.00pm and then went straight to bed.
10 Apr	Feel fine. Took Caulyphylum 200 at 9.00pm. Woke at 12.45am and took another Caulyphylum 200.
11 Apr	Woke up feeling fine. Was sick. Just bile. Metallic taste in my mouth. Had membranes sweeped. 2-3cm dilated and cervix 75% effaced. READY TO GO!!!! Feel OK... apprehensive, excited, nervous, scared... want to be on my own, I think! WATCH THIS SPACE!!!!!!!!!!!!
12 Apr	My birthday! Had a great night's sleep. It has been a lovely sunny day. Felt really good in the morning. Had a bit more of a show. A few niggles, but nothing much. Went out for lunch. Really thought that today would be the day. Really fed up by the end, but had had a nice day. Crushed two Sepia 30 and mixed them with water. Two teaspoons every two hours until bedtime, stirring 20 times each time. Babies moving a fair bit. Took Pulsatilla 30 at 9.00pm then went to bed.
13 Apr	Still having a bit more of a show. Had sex, but it didn't help. Really fed up and teary. Took Caulyphylum 200 at 10.30am. Bit more of a show. Pulsatilla 30 at 12.30pm. Caulyphylum 200 at 2.30pm. Pulsatilla 30 at 5.30pm. Caulyphylum 200 at 6.30pm. Pulsatilla 30 at 8.30pm. Caulyphylum 200 mixture at 9.30pm, then bed. Also went to the hospital and went on the monitor to check that the babies were OK. Both fine. Very similar heartbeats.
14 Apr	Slept really well and dreamt too. Feel much better today. Still having a show. More mucous than anything. Took Caulyphylum 200 mixture every two hours or so. Had a few Braxton Hicks. Not so many as before. Babies moving well, but not so much.
15 Apr	Fine and fed up.
16 Apr	Fine and fed up.
17 Apr	Pulsatilla 200 at 9.30am. Caulyphylum 200 at 12 noon. Pulsatilla 200 at 3.00pm. Caulyphylum 200 at 6.30pm. Pulsatilla 200 at 9.30pm, then bed. Really fed up. Booked into hospital tomorrow to have waters broken to get things going.

Helen Arundell

After being induced on the next day—now 10 days after her due date—Helen finally gave birth (vaginally) to a girl weighing 7lb 4oz and a boy weighing 7lb 10oz. They showed no signs of postmaturity and both had excellent Apgar scores at 1 minute. The mother was delighted to report that she needed no stitches since there was just 'a tiny nick' where the second baby's nose had caught her!

Little Miss Perfect?

As you saw in this last birthframe, and also in many others in this book, outcomes were excellent even when the woman didn't follow all the principles outlined in this book. It's surprising how much we can get away with!

This is reassuring really, given that life is never perfect. Please don't ever let this make you become complacent, though. I have read and heard plenty of accounts where one small intervention or disturbance in a pregnancy, labour or birth resulted in bad outcomes.

In any case, before we continue I would like to say...

1. If ever you meet me face-to-face, rest assured I promise you I will not be a self-righteous advisor! Perhaps I would have been in my 20s, but I've lived too long and made too many mistakes myself for that to be possible now.
2. I wouldn't ever want to judge anybody for whom things didn't work out well. As I've explained, I do think these 10 principles are all crucial if you seriously want to have an optimal birth. However, individuals make decisions and do or don't do things in one way or another for so many reasons: fear, social pressure, difficulty finding supportive caregivers, legal restrictions, lack of money... But maybe we should try to overcome these problems so we can somehow give birth in a way we're really at peace with.

Birthframe 80

Here's an example of a woman who took care of herself in some of the ways I've recommended... Her labour was fast, easy and safe—and, in conventional obstetric terms, non-interventionist. This contributor (who prefers to remain anonymous) took up her midwives' suggestion to use TENS and gas and air even though I feel, having read a longer version of this account, that her body—and mind, for that matter—would have been plenty strong enough to travel through this labour without any pain relief whatsoever. In any case, she mentioned that the TENS pads actually fell off at some point, long before she realised this had happened! What is particularly interesting is the physical preparation that this woman undertook. It no doubt facilitated her easy, fast and safe labour and postpartum recovery, especially since it was clearly underpinned by a very positive mental attitude.

Once I found out I was pregnant I wanted to make sure that I did everything possible to help me with the labour. I was 36 but it was becoming the trend to have babies later in life so I didn't really think about my age. Whilst trying for a baby I took folic acid, as recommended. I did have quite bad sickness for the first three months or so but once that was over I kept as fit as possible. I had always regularly attended a gym and generally used to keep fit and active so couldn't see any reason to change that. I used to enjoy weight training but obviously changed to much lighter weights and started swimming a lot more. A friend of mine had swum regularly throughout her pregnancy and had quite an easy labour so I decided to follow her example. I went to the gym three times a week throughout my pregnancy and swam twice a week. I swam up to 40 lengths at a time, obviously getting slower as my pregnancy advanced! This was the breaststroke, incidentally, which Sylvie tells me would have helped the baby get into a good position for the birth.

I ate as healthily as possible and bought a blender to make fruit smoothies to up my intake of fruit. Constipation is sometimes an unwelcome side effect of pregnancy! I also read an article in a magazine about raspberry leaf tea, which is a herbal remedy and is supposed to help shorten labour. I had nothing to lose so decided to try this too, taking it in tablet form, which I preferred. Each tablet was 400mg and the label said to have one 3 to 6 times a day. It said the tablet could also be broken up and dissolved in hot water—but it tasted awful this way! It seems raspberry leaf is recommended for the last three months of pregnancy but not before. I also read that rubbing Vitamin E oil onto your perineum regularly can help stretch this area and lessen the chance of having to be cut whilst giving birth. Again, I thought, "Why not?" so I used to massage the oil in every night throughout the last 6-8 weeks.

I worked full-time right up to seven days before giving birth and although I was tired toward the end I am glad I did because I believe it is important to keep active for as long as possible. The baby arrived three days before my due date. At 10 o'clock at night my waters broke naturally. I was at home and I had no warning at all—I just got up from my chair to take a glass into the kitchen and that was it! I was relatively calm and was in no pain or discomfort whatsoever. I gathered my bags and got to the hospital for around 11 o'clock. At about 1.00am I started getting contractions—they were quite strong and started coming regularly. It seemed to happen very quickly and I was a bit shocked at how strong they were. At about 3.00am the nurses on the delivery ward examined me and discovered I was around 7cm dilated. I was quite shocked and things started happening very, very quickly by then. The contractions just got stronger and stronger and by about 3.45am I was fully dilated. I had decided beforehand that I wanted to try and squat to give birth and not lie flat on my back but I found that I was not really strong enough because it is very hard on the thighs! The nurses raised the bed up so that I was practically sitting and I had both feet on the bed, which was a huge help. I gave birth at 4.10am, exactly 1 hour 10 minutes after arriving in the delivery suite. I was totally alert and felt absolutely wonderful, apart from being a bit sore. I had no stitches at all, just a graze, which healed itself. The whole experience was amazing.

My body healed very quickly indeed and I had no problems whatsoever. I was back at the gym 10 days later and regained my figure very quickly. I am sure that my easy labour was a direct result of the preparation I did throughout my pregnancy.

While you're in labour and giving birth...

EAT AND DRINK WHENEVER YOU WANT TO

Hospitals used to routinely refuse labouring women all food and drink as soon as they went into labour. Instead, they used to put women on a glucose drip. Professionals were worried there would be a risk of asphyxiation from vomiting if general anaesthesia suddenly had to be given. They have now concluded that withholding food and drink results in even greater risks because stomach contents after fasting are so acidic that chemical irritation and infection can occur. A glucose drip is now also recognised as being unhelpful for other reasons too...[14]

- ♥ The energy provided by the glucose doesn't provide women with enough energy.
- ♥ Putting a drip in a woman's arm exposes her to the risk of infection.
- ♥ Having a drip already in place made many health care workers inclined to encourage women to have other substances 'dripped' in, such as syntocinon to stimulate contractions. Of course, this completely disturbed the normal course of women's labours.
- ♥ Being attached to a drip tended to immobilise women because they were less free to move around, even if this was theoretically possible.
- ♥ Finally, research has shown that having sugar during labour actually lowers a women's tolerance to pain![15]

Once again, taking the natural route turns out to be the best approach. Simply eat and drink whatever you want, whenever you want it throughout your labour—but avoid anything sugary, including fruit juice. Again, water seems to be the best possible thing to drink. (It's especially easy to drink if you use one of those easy-open swig bottles.).

If you find yourself throwing up after you've eaten and drunk various things, don't worry! There's so much internal upheaval going on while your womb is contracting, it's not surprising if your stomach suddenly gets shoved upwards. Having a bucket handy for this eventuality will mean there's less mess to worry about because buckets are very portable! While you're vomiting, incidentally, be reassured that it's a sign your labour is well underway.

If you're vomiting it's a sign your labour is well under way!

MAKE AS MUCH NOISE AS YOU LIKE

Although there are Scientologists and Russian natural birthers who feel that making noises during labour might be distressing for the baby, most people elsewhere recognise the enormous benefits of being noisy. Somehow, the process of letting out deep, sonorous groans—quietly or loudly—seems to help release tension in the woman's body. Most women do it quite spontaneously. There is certainly no need to practice.

If—when you're in labour—you notice that the sounds you're making are tense, constricted and high-pitched, simply open your mouth wider and make an effort to 'let go' of any tension you feel within you. It might be helpful to watch out for tension in your jaw or hips particularly because your moans need to be 'whole body', flowing moans... When you consciously let go of any tension within you, you'll probably notice that the sounds become more sonorous.

The positive side-effect of making deep, sonorous moans is that it seems to have a 'releasing' effect and the vagina usually becomes relaxed too. So moan to your heart's content! Make sure any birth attendants know in advance that you're likely to be noisy, perhaps by making a note of it in your care guide.

Most people recognise the benefits of being noisy during labour

ADOPT HELPFUL POSITIONS

This is the most important thing you can do. Positions will probably come to you intuitively, but so as to give you an idea of the kind of positions you might use, take a look at the photographs on the next few pages.[16]

Don't, incidentally, think I'm recommending anything strange here. The photographs are simply intended to remind you of a womanly tradition, which modern societies forgot for a few years recently. Squatting was normal practice in ancient societies, as is evidenced by the Egyptian hieroglyphic for 'birth', which shows a squatting woman, with a baby's head emerging from below her body. Records have been uncovered of squatting or other upright positions being used in ancient Babylon, Greece, Rome and Central America. In ancient Rome special birthing chairs were even made with cut-away seats and handles for the mother to hang from.

It was only early in the twentieth century that women started being asked to lie down by male physicians who wanted easier access to a woman's sexual organs. It is a great shame that such an unhelpful position, which forces women to push 'uphill' through a smaller opening, while lying on her back and endangering both her own and her baby's oxygen supply should have become the most common one in recent decades. However, knowing that most women who adopted this position were told to, or even *forced* to, does go some way toward explaining why women have become so desperate to use pain relief.

392 **birth:** countdown to optimal

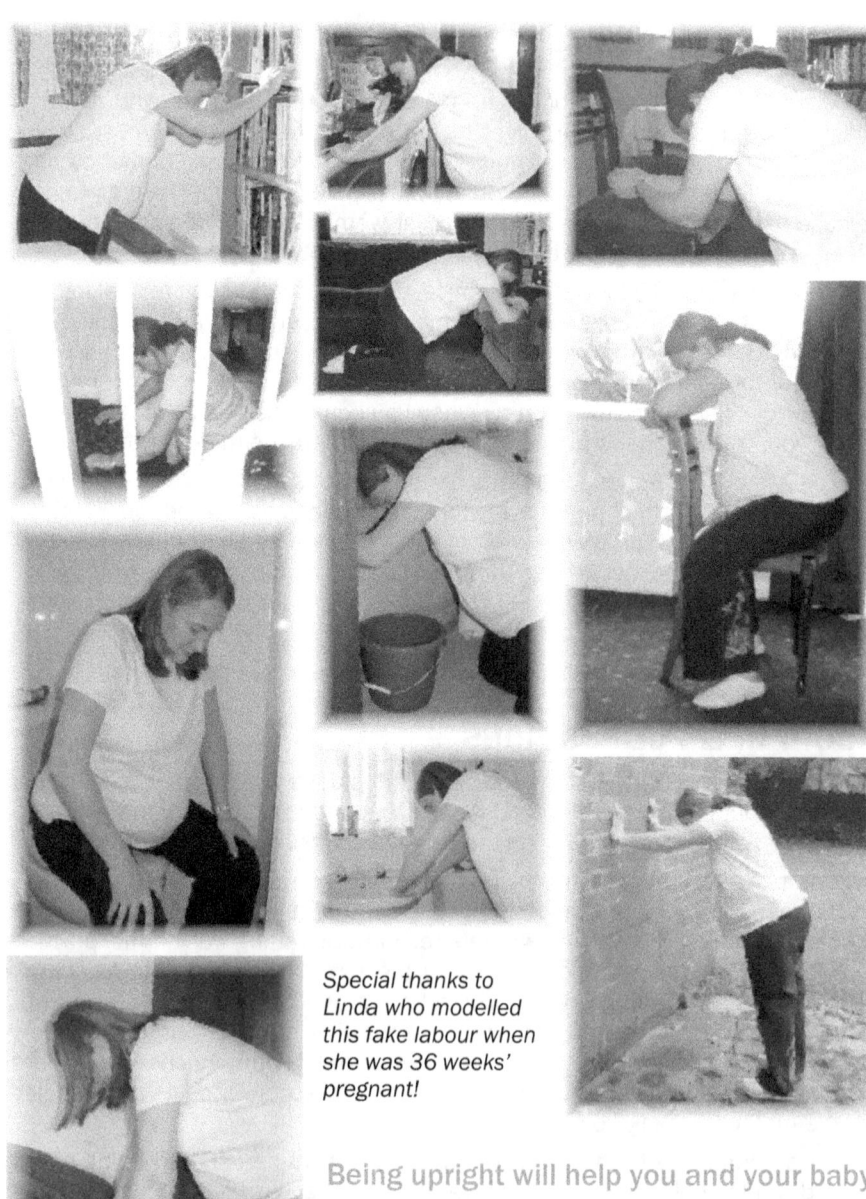

Special thanks to Linda who modelled this fake labour when she was 36 weeks' pregnant!

Being upright will help you and your baby

Do you notice anything special about these positions? Yes! They're all leaning forward positions. Better for the baby—helps him or her get the oxygen necessary to stay alive and intelligent. Being upright will also help you get your baby born more quickly, easily and safely, with no damage to your own body.

Birthframe 81

This next account is interesting in that it clearly shows how one woman's attempts to facilitate her labour—by opting to endure maximum pain!—were misguided. Thanks to our increased knowledge nowadays about what facilitates or impedes labour, this heart-rending mistake seems amazing. Nevertheless, the inappropriateness of the supine position from the fetus' point of view during pregnancy or labour is still sometimes forgotten in maternity units around the world. It is particularly interesting that this particular birth sped up dramatically when the woman made just one small change...

Daniel and his sister Dorothea were born naturally for the main reason, I believe, that we didn't know I would give birth to twins, so neither I nor the doctors would get nervous and I waited and moved about normally until the due date. It was in 1968 and scans were not routinely done yet. As I wasn't aware of any twins in my or Konrad's, my husband's, family—even though I was later reminded that my grandmother had also carried a twin inside her until it was discovered with some surgery after her firstborn baby!—I didn't suspect twins, even though I was enormous. But as my husband was very tall and my first son had weighed close to 9lb we all expected one big baby.

Labor started at 4.00am and when I got to the hospital they told me the baby would be born soon. But then it took hours, during which doctors and nurses and students listened endlessly to the babies' heartbeats, hearing one kind only faintly and never looking for a second kind. The doctor who was attending me at the time (in the USA) was famous for his 'spinals', but women often had problems with them afterwards, headaches etc, and anyway I preferred it all the natural way.

But finally, as by 11.00am nothing seemed to progress any more—I seem to remember that the baby was supposed to turn, which hadn't happened yet—the doctor decided to do a caesarean. When he told me I thought, "Oh well, in that case I'm going to turn over to my side, which would ease the pain somewhat." As I had wanted to move things along I had all the time stayed on my back, the position that gave me the stronger labour pain. Anyway, very soon after I turned over, things began to move inside and I felt the urge to push. They could hardly get me to the birthing room and Dorothea was born with such urgency that I was sure all my lower parts had been ripped out along with her. Then I heard the doctor exclaim, "Oh, there's another one coming!" "Well I have to get on then," I said to myself, matter-of-factly. Nine minutes later Daniel was born quite easily, as his sister had prepared the way for him.

They each weighed close to 7lb, the girl a little over, the boy a little under. After being reassured that they were both all right I was greatly relieved. My husband and I were enormously happy and proud. I still see the other mother in my room receiving her baby for breastfeeding (no rooming-in yet back then) and I remember thinking, "The poor mother, she is only getting one baby." We felt so rich!

Ulrike von Moltke

What if you're told your baby's 'posterior'?

Nowadays—given our comparatively easy lifestyle, compared to our ancestors'—it's not unusual for a woman to be told her baby is 'posterior' when she goes into hospital.[17] If this happens to you, don't despair. Here are a few positive things you can do:

- ♥ Lean forward as much as possible to try to help the baby turn into an anterior position.
- ♥ Use a hands-and-knees position if you can bear to because this may also help your baby turn.
- ♥ While you're on your hands and knees, lift your bottom up slightly. You may find this helps![18]
- ♥ Ask your birthing attendant if he or she will massage your back. You may find it feels best if intensive pressure is applied with both fists during a contraction.[19]
- ♥ Ask your birthing attendant to apply either hot or cold compresses. Experiment and stick with whichever feels better—until you think it might be time to change!
- ♥ Take a hot or cold bath (when you're more than 5cm dilated) or a shower, while still maintaining leaning forward positions.
- ♥ Lie on your left side if you want to rest, or prop yourself into a tummy-down position, using bolsters and large cushions.
- ♥ Continue to try and communicate with your baby by rubbing your bump and simply talking.
- ♥ Be particularly careful that nobody tells you how to push because this can result in the baby getting stuck. Follow your own body's cues and let your baby edge out in his or her own time... Tap into your deepest reserves and make as much noise as you want.
- ♥ Throughout the whole experience remember the pain will disappear completely the moment your baby is born. After that, you'll just have a few afterpains to get through and that'll be it. Incredible, but true.

USE HOT WATER AND *LEAN FORWARD*!

As your labour progresses, you may find it useful to use hot water to help you ease the pain or warm you up—but make sure the water's not too hot. And remember... it's really not a good idea to get into the bath or shower until you're at least 5cm dilated. If you use water too soon there's the risk of slowing down contractions—which really isn't a good idea! (Honestly! You want to get this baby born, remember?!) Just before you give birth, getting into the bath can be wonderful for warming up your nether regions. It will help you to relax and stretch out more easily as your baby emerges.[20] Don't worry about being in an 'ideal' position, by the way, for the moment of birth. Your body will spontaneously find the best possible position for birthing your baby, if you let it!

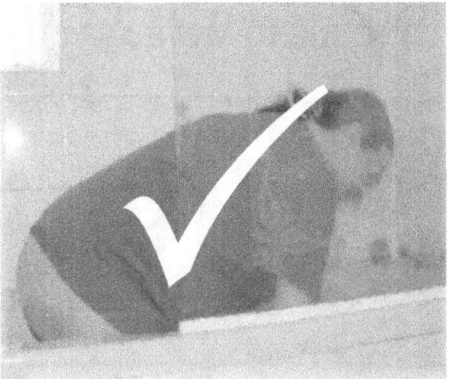

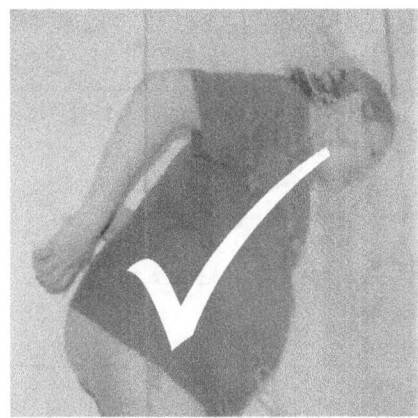

If you need to be sick—which is likely—you may find yourself leaning over a bucket. This is fine, of course, because it's another leaning forward position...

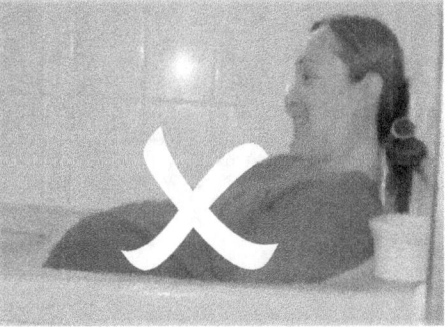

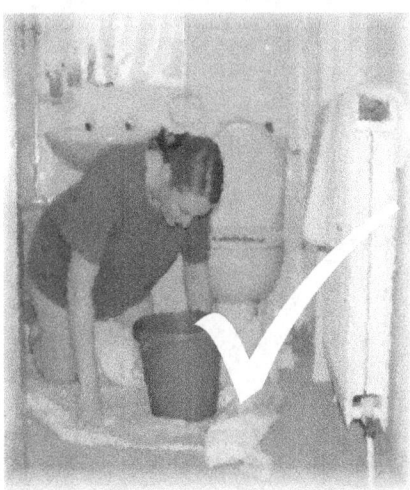

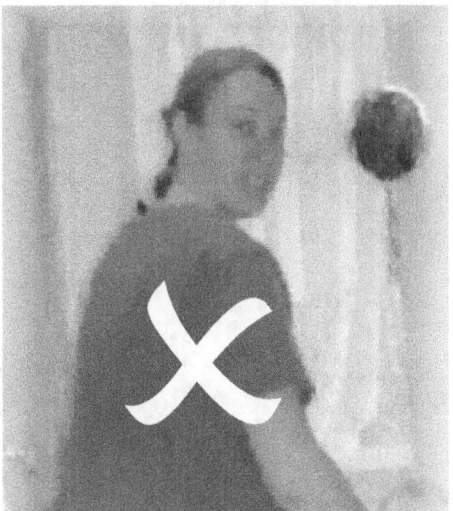

As the birth approaches, try and make sure there's something soft underneath you at all times, just in case the baby does actually choose to come out a little earlier than you expect! He or she really doesn't need to be caught, but a soft landing would make a nicer start to life. In the photo above note the presence of the waterproof tablecloth (which will minimise mess) and the old bathmat to kneel or stand on, which will stop you from sliding around.

By the way, make sure nobody talks to you. You're supposed to be free to 'go to another planet', remember? 'Do not disturb' is the most important rule.

CONTINUE TO MOVE AS YOU WISH

You will spontaneously find a good position in which to give birth. Just so that you realise the possibilities and don't feel inhibited, here are a few positions which optimal birthers often find themselves giving birth in! [21]

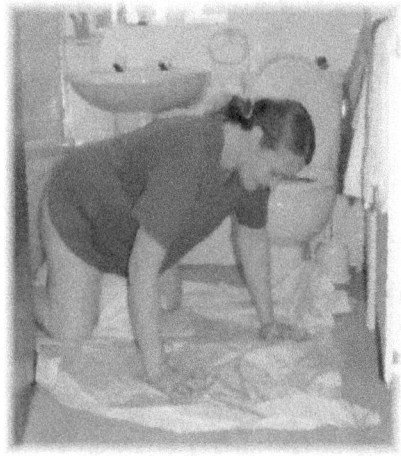
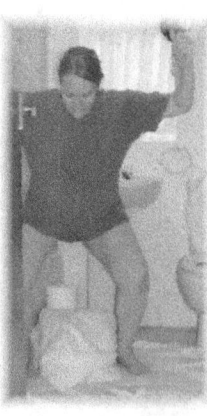

Some typical positions

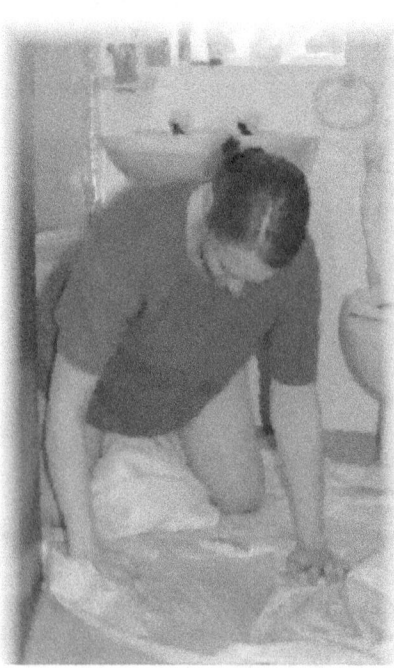
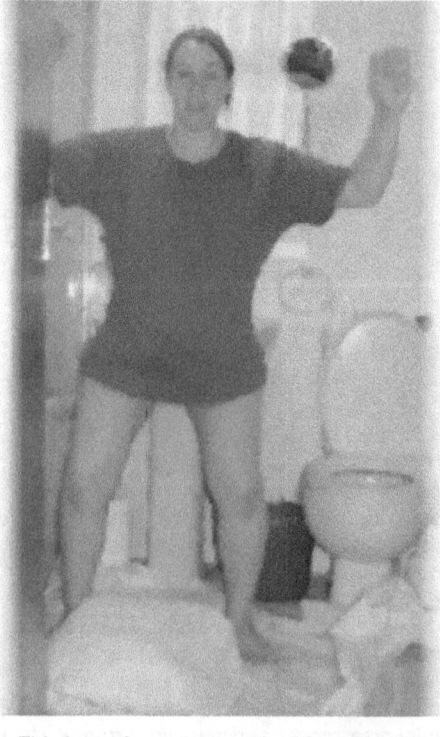

This is my favourite position! Standing like this, I birthed my second and third babies.

DON'T LET ANYONE DISTURB YOU

You will probably find yourself spontaneously breastfeeding your new baby straight after the birth. If you've given birth in the bathroom, sitting on the toilet is a very comfortable place to do this! Notice the extension lead in the corner of the photo on the right—it's there in case the extra, portable heater needs to be brought in to warm up the baby—or the new mummy! After a while, if the placenta hasn't come out yet, you could transfer to a bucket (as in the photo below). This will save your midwife having to fish the placenta out of the toilet! (She needs to check it's all there.) Only sit on a bucket for a few minutes, though, because if you stay too long the vaginal area may get constricted. When it's all over, snuggle up with your baby in bed. Lying on your left side is still best because your baby will be lying on his or her right side—which is the best possible position from the point of view of optimising breathing and blood flow. Keep your new baby's head off the pillow and just keep him or her warm with a baby blanket. And enjoy...

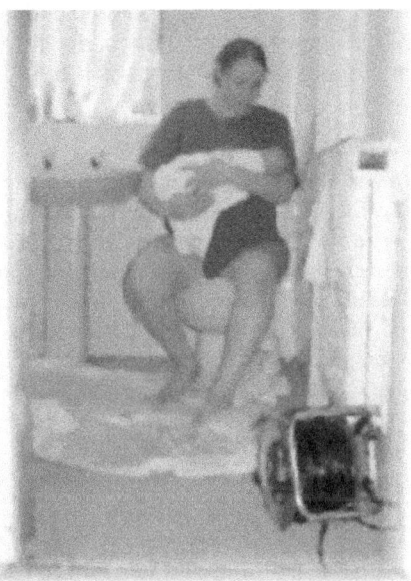

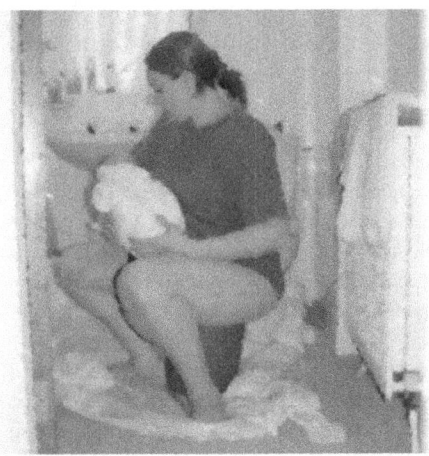

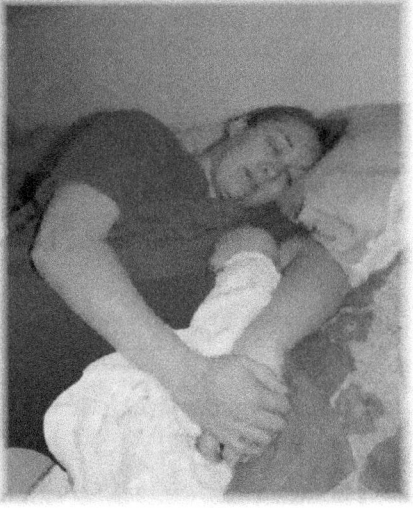

Lie on your left side

By the way, in case you're wondering... this is not Linda's real baby. It's a bald-headed doll borrowed from one of my children. And when she posed for these photos, Linda still had three or four more weeks to wait before her own big day.

Birthframe 82

Nina, who we've met before, had a new experience for her second baby's birth since her first had been born by emergency caesarean. Despite her apprehensions about pushing, she found her body knew exactly what to do when it came to it...

My mother says that newborns look like little angels that haven't fully descended to Earth yet. Newborns do have a faraway look in their eyes. But if you've given birth, you'd hardly say they come from the sky. There is nothing ethereal about pushing a baby into the world. It is just the opposite, a wholly carnal and earthy experience. Pushing out my daughter felt like doing a very large and difficult poo out my vagina.

People keep telling me I had an easy labour. I'm sure it was, relatively speaking. Now that it's over, I'd be ready to do it again next week. But it didn't feel easy. It hurt like anything. The thing is, I was so thrilled that my body was doing what it needed to do, that I hardly minded the pain. With our first child I never went into established labour. During his birth, I had had fairly regular, painful contractions from early in the morning, but labour never became 'well established,' according to the midwives who examined me.

It's hard to pinpoint exactly what went wrong. Was it because I hadn't fully visualised what it meant for the fetus to descend through my pelvis and out into the world? That I couldn't see myself becoming a mother? Was it because I allowed the doctors to 're-date' my pregnancy based on the 12-week scan, even though I *knew* when I had conceived? They pushed the official due date two weeks earlier. This made me more anxious about being induced, so I tried to initiate the labour with nipple stimulation early in the morning of the day my labour started. Maybe trying to induce was the starting point of the problems. Maybe he hadn't got into the right position, and wasn't quite ready to be born yet. My waters broke at 6.00am. I phoned the birth centre, but since nobody asked me, I never mentioned to the midwife that my waters had broken. I figured, since they didn't ask, it couldn't be important. I was in what I thought was labour all day long, but we only went to the birth centre in the evening. I discovered a light green blush of fresh meconium on my sanitary towel. But I had just changed the pad, so when I got there—a long drive all the way across town—the midwives didn't believe me, and sent me home. I phoned again when we got back—I was sure it was meconium. We drove back, this time in the small hours. The birth centre confirmed that it was meconium and sent me straight back across town again to the hospital. Hospital staff were unsympathetic to my desire for a normal, unmedicated birth.

I will never forget the calm before the storm, the two hours' respite they agreed to give us before starting an induction. My contractions had ceased entirely. I stood at the window of the hospital praying for the labour to resume. My womb was still resting as the sun rose. I realised I would soon be forced to acquiesce to the hospital's interventions. I requested an epidural before the induction... but no one told me that the chances of a C-section are over five times higher with an epidural!

(Isn't there a legal requirement to inform patients about the risks they face??) The baby couldn't tolerate the heavy spasms of induced contractions. His heart-rate plummeted. They turned off the drip. His heart rate settled. But there were still no effective contractions, the waters had been broken for over 24 hours and I had not dilated past a few centimetres. If I had been at home, I probably would have gone calmly to sleep, rested up, and then given birth. Or perhaps he was in a funny position. Who knows? The doctor who delivered him couldn't find any clear explanation for the meconium or why he hadn't descended.

For me, agreeing to the caesarean felt like a death sentence. I had so longed to give my son a good birth, and to experience that life-changing moment of pushing him into the world. Why did the caesarean have to happen? I still ask myself. If I had it to do over again, I believe the most important problem was no continuity of care. If I'd been attended by one midwife throughout the pregnancy and birth, I'm sure I wouldn't have felt pressured into trying to induce the birth. And everything might have been different.

Technically, my second labour took only five hours early Thursday morning, from when the first strong contractions began after midnight, until the placenta was born around 5.00am. But I'd call it a 10-hour labour with a day's break in the middle.[22] I was awake most of Tuesday night with contractions every 10 minutes that were strong enough to get me out of bed, but not strong enough to have to shout and holler. I sat up on the couch and breathed hard until about 6.00am when they started to ease off.

"I'm in labour!" I announced proudly to my midwife on Wednesday morning. "I told my husband he could stay home from work. Was that the right thing to do?" "You're not in labour, and he has to go to work," the midwife replied firmly. "You're probably going to have several nights like this before you have a baby." Crestfallen, my husband went off to work, and I went back to bed. I took several long naps during the day, while our nanny took our 2-year-old son to his playgroup and fed him lunch. My back ached, and I had occasional mild contractions during the day, but nothing more.

"It won't be tonight," I thought on Wednesday evening. But just in case, I put the birthing pool together. It was sort of like a blue canvas tent on a 5-foot-wide hexagonal frame, turned upside down. It filled to about 2 feet deep through a garden hose attached to a bathroom tap.

I went to bed at 10.30pm. Around midnight I found myself sitting up in bed in the middle of a contraction. I flopped back to sleep again between a few more contractions. Then I felt a trickle of water as though I'd wet the bed as my waters broke. I went to the bathroom for a pad, and the contractions suddenly became very strong. For a while I sat on the sofa in our bedroom huffing and puffing. My husband kept on snoring. There didn't seem much point in waking him up—what could he do? It was still going to hurt. I went downstairs to try to distract myself.

There didn't seem much point in waking him up...

"It's like running a race!" but that's not quite correct

I guess contractions feel different for different people. I felt a stabbing pain in the small of my back that came in waves. One deep breath in, blow it away, another, another, soon it'll pass. Phew. It's gone. Then a rest before the next one begins. The day after my daughter was born, I told my brother, "It's like running a race," because my diaphragm felt bruised afterwards from breathing hard. But that's not quite correct. During a road race, the pain is psychological as much as physical. You have to force yourself to keep running, because if you don't, you will simply stop running and quit the race. But in labour, there's no quitting.

I could watch TV—would that help? I still hadn't looked at the instructional video that came with the birthing pool, so I put that on. Some stupid woman holding a baby was explaining in great detail how wonderful her water birth was. I switched her off and tried the end of *Singing in the Rain*, which we'd started watching a few days before. Couples in beautiful clothes waltzed to a brass band. Infuriating creatures. No, that wasn't what I needed.

The contractions were coming every few minutes. If I was sitting when one arrived, I stayed sitting and swayed back and forth, taking deep breaths and breathing out with a loud 'Ooooh, ahhhhhh'. Sitting seemed to lessen the pain along the bottom of my bump. If I was standing, I paced to the end of the room and back hollering the words to the *Battle Hymn of the Republic*. After a while, it didn't help to walk away from the pain. "This is no fun," I said to myself. "Remind me I said so next time I have the stupid idea that I want a baby. Nothing can possibly make this worthwhile!"

"Call me if you feel like you don't want to be by yourself any more," the midwife had said. I called her around 1.30am. "I don't like this any more." It was such a relief to do something besides pacing up and down the living room that I didn't even notice the next contraction. "If I can talk through a contraction, does that mean it's not that strong?" I asked.

"Well, usually that's right. But I can come out now if you want me to," she said, polite but unconvinced.

Oh dear. It's going to get much worse than this, I thought. "No, that's OK. Maybe I can survive a while longer."

I survived exactly 15 more minutes before I called her back. This time I was careful to make lots of convincing puffing noises during a contraction.

"I'll come right now," she said.

I can't remember what I did during the next 45 minutes. Knowing that help was on the way made the time fly. When I judged that she was about to arrive, I woke my husband up. His sleepy sense of decorum dictated that he should be fully dressed for her arrival. I went downstairs again to wait. I still remember the elation and relief I felt at the sound of the front gate creaking, then a clunk as she deposited her midwifery equipment on the doorstep.

The midwife kissed me when I opened the door. Another contraction arrived. "Breathe it out. You're doing great," she said, pressing her hands hard against the small of my back. My back felt less like it was going to fall off with her hands pressing against it. My husband came downstairs.

"We haven't filled the pool yet," I said, "Do you think we should?"

"I'll fill it," my husband offered.

"The hose attachment is in the top drawer in the bathroom, along with the spanner," I said. "It attaches to the shower." I had tried attaching the hose a few times myself to make sure it worked, but it hadn't occurred to me that someone else might need to know how to work it.

My husband was up on a stool in the bath when I made it upstairs. "The shower head won't come off," he said. "The spanner doesn't fit." "It fit when I tried it," I snapped, then grabbed for my back again as another contraction arrived.

"Shall I have a go?" The midwife climbed up on the stool, but couldn't make it work, either.

"Who do I have here? Two idiots?" I grumbled. "I don't believe this. I'm going to have to do it myself." I must have been in transition.

But five minutes later, he and the midwife attached the hose. "You can turn it on now," the midwife called from our bedroom. We could hear the water swishing through the hose. A minute later I heard myself exhale hard at the end of a contraction. I was hugging my husband. "That sounds weird," I thought to myself. "Am I pushing? I don't feel like I am. Am I supposed to be doing this?"

"That sounded like a pushing noise!" said the midwife, running in from the other room.

"I think I have to wee." I tried to sit on the toilet. "No, I think I have to poo."

"It sounds like you're pushing," she repeated. "We'd better check how far dilated you are."

After a few more contractions I made it to our bed, where the midwife felt my cervix. "You're fully dilated!" Seeing I didn't look pleased, she added: "That's good news!" I was thinking, "Oh no, now I'm going to have to push the baby out. What if I can't do it?"

"Would you like to get in the pool?" The midwife suggested. It was only half full, but the water was rising quickly. The idea of moving or doing anything different sounded impossible, but I said I'd like to because I figured I was supposed to. I stepped out of my pyjamas and into the pool. The instant I felt the warm water over my ankles I felt better. The warm bath was instantly soothing, just as all the water birth brochures promised. It was even better than the firm pressure of someone's hands against my back. It was like being hugged all over.

The instant I felt the warm water over my ankles I felt better. The warm bath was instantly soothing.

The next contractions were completely different

The next contractions still hurt in the small of my back, but they were completely different. Before pushing begins, it is a matter of passively enduring the pain. But when pushing starts, you feel like you're doing something. It felt sort of like throwing up—or should I say, throwing down, because the involuntary hurling of the stomach muscles went down into my gut, not up into my throat. Pushing was scary, uncontrollable. I didn't know how long I could keep it up before my body ripped apart. "Just go with it," the midwife said. "You're doing great." She was kneeling next to the pool. I held onto the rim and crouched in the water. Before, looking straight into her eyes helped me remember that a contraction would end in another moment. Now I wasn't looking at her any more. I just held onto the rim of the pool and puked my stomach into my pelvis, then closed my eyes and took deep breaths when a break came. I was making heavy, pig-like exhaling noises. Soon after I got into the pool, our son woke up next door. "Mama!" My husband went in to sing him back to sleep. "No…. MAMA!" he protested.

Through the open door I tried to sing him a song between contractions, but quickly realised that he was just as happy listening to his favourite Papa story about the rabbit and the hedgehog.

I started to feel more pressure in my bowels. It sounds strange, but the most pleasurable feeling was the hot sting of the perineum tearing as the baby's head crowned. The feeling of climax. The next push came immediately, and the baby's body squelched out into the water. And then everything stopped. No more pain. Instant peace. The midwife reached down and lifted the baby to the surface. Its face was a purple maroon, with slippery black hair matted down on its head. The baby looked very big to have just come out of my body. It breathed, then cried.

To avoid being disappointed if we ended up with two of the same, we'd convinced ourselves that we were having another son. "Now I get to check that it really is a boy," I thought. "The part I missed last time." I never got to see my first child as he was pulled out of my belly behind the screen on the operating table. The doctors took him away, suctioned his lungs, wrapped him up and presented him like a Christmas present, with nothing but a red, terrified and screaming face sticking out. He might as well have come from a factory. It took months before I was convinced he was my baby.

I lifted the baby's bottom toward the surface. I saw what looked like a scrotum. The rest of the crotch was blocked by the umbilical cord running from the navel, down between the legs and into the water. "Yep, a boy," I decided.

"You have a little girl," the midwife said. I took another look. Indeed, that was no penis I was looking at. Because of all the hormones in the mother's body, the baby's genitals come out all swollen. A daughter! I couldn't believe it. I put her to my breast, and she stopped crying. The midwife tiptoed to the door of our son's room.

"And then Rabbit said to Hedgehog..." my husband was saying.

"You have a little girl," she announced quietly.

My husband said later that he'd heard the baby crying, but couldn't really believe that it had been born already.

"Our client isn't going back to sleep," he reported to me. Our son appeared in the doorway. "Ooh!" he said, taking in the blue pool, the midwife, and his mother in the water. He padded up to the pool. "Baby!" he announced, looking at the slippery beet-red person in my arms.

"That's your sister," my husband said to him, his voice cracking. A few minutes later, sitting in the pool, I was on the phone to my mother and brother in Washington, DC.

My daughter and I sat in the water and breastfed for nearly an hour until the cord stopped pulsing. The midwife clamped the cord next to the baby's navel, then cut through the tough, horny tube. A moment later, the placenta slid out like a big jellyfish.

"Is it true that eating a piece of placenta helps the uterus contract?"

"Yes, though I only know two people who've actually tried it."

"I did last time, but it was probably pointless, because it was after I came back from the hospital. And it must have been filled with epidural drugs and other awful chemicals. I ate a bit raw."

"What did you do with the rest of it? Bury it in the garden?"

"Um, no. I fried it up with onions and ate the whole thing."

"Oh," she said politely. We examined the placenta to make sure no part had been left in the uterus. She pulled off a small, meaty piece. "This is probably enough to help your uterus contract." It was like eating warm, raw liver.

My husband and son came back from cooking up a pot of porridge. I climbed out of the pool carrying my newborn daughter. We all watched as the midwife weighed her in a sling: 8lb 6oz—nearly a pound over her brother's birth weight. Then the midwife sewed me up. My perineum had a fairly long but shallow tear from the bottom of the vagina toward the anus, which the midwife said looked like it wasn't sitting together tidily and might heal in an uncomfortable way if it wasn't sewn up. She injected a surface anaesthetic, the only drug which appears in my birth notes, then put in four stitches. It was nearly 7.00am when we finished our porridge. I can't remember now who was holding the baby. All I can remember is how famished I was. I was watching the clock. I couldn't wait until the nanny arrived, so I could show off my good work. My husband had paged her to come at 8.00am, an hour earlier than usual. When I heard her key in the lock, I wanted to leap down the stairs with the baby in my arms. "But she'll tell me to go right back to bed," I thought. I suddenly realised I was exhausted.

All I can remember is how famished I was.
I suddenly realised I was exhausted.

I was on such a high that day, I even briefly went out. We invited a few friends over in the evening to celebrate with a glass of champagne. Afterwards, I slightly regretted disturbing our baby by inviting other people into her new home. I am ashamed to confess that in the photos of her birthday party, she is screaming her head off as she's passed around. By the time I descended from Cloud 9 enough to feel like resting, the baby had got over her initial post-birth calm and wanted to breastfeed frequently. I should have slept when she slept! (Mental note: Stay in bed next time and keep visitors away.)

During the day my daughter was born, I could still remember exactly what the sickening wave of a contraction felt like. By the next morning I wasn't sure any more. Did it really hurt that much?

Some days I feel weepy and nostalgic. I'd like to be back in the blue plastic pool, pushing my daughter—my daughter!—into the world. She's three weeks old now. Some days I miss being pregnant. How strange from one moment to the next to change from a beautiful, rotund, mum-to-be into a tired, empty-bellied mother. Now that life has gone back to normal, I wish I could be pregnant and special again. I miss the feeling of somebody's feet kicking inside me. But then I reach out my hand to touch our daughter's soft, downy head and I remember how I pushed her out into the world. Life won't ever go back to 'normal'—our daughter is here for keeps.

Post scriptum by Nina:

Our third child was born after a similar five hours of established labour, five and a half years later. The contractions in this labour felt much more painful than in the second one. Boy, did it hurt! (They do say third births are sometimes tougher. Or maybe I noticed the pain more. I was expecting it to be a piece of cake!) This time, I did take it easy and let people wait on me. Like her big sister, the new one was calm and happy after the birth, and so were her older brother and sister.

I would gladly re-live the births of either of my daughters. There is nothing more intensely satisfying than labouring and birthing a baby. I wish I could do it again a dozen times more. It's bringing them up that's hard work!

Nina Klose

Birthframe 83

As we've already noted, moving around during labour and using upright positions during childbirth have not always been encouraged or even permitted by health professionals. For the past three decades, Janet Balaskas has been doing an enormous amount to educate both women and health professionals of their usefulness. As well as founding the Active Birth Centre in London, she has also written several books on the subject. (At www.activebirthcentre.com you can see the original manifesto of her philosophy.)

Here Janet explains how she first came to realise the importance of physical freedom during labour and birth and how it became her mission to help other women understand this.

Surely we can't be the only mammals who can't give birth?

During the late 70s and 80s, when my children were born, the majority of women laboured and gave birth in a highly medicalised hospital environment and almost always in bed and semi-reclining. This was the peak of the hi-tech era when obstetricians launched the concept of 'actively managed birth'—one in which labour was induced at a convenient time, the baby electronically monitored continuously and the mother wired up to an epidural. Large obstetric units were the officially recommended birthplace for all women, whether they needed obstetric care or not. Not surprisingly, outcomes were not good—intervention and caesarean rates soared. No one seemed to know anything about birth physiology. Even 'natural' birth education at the time was geared to teaching coping strategies and breathing techniques for lying-down labours.

This horrified me. Surely, we can't be the only mammals who are incapable of giving birth by ourselves, I thought. I felt sure we must have a similar instinctual capacity to reproduce our species as other mammals do. While I was in labour with my second child I decided to get up from my semi-reclining position and to my astonishment I found that moving around helped my labour to progress more quickly.

I decided to do some research and look into the history of childbirth in different cultures prior to the advent of obstetrics. Availing myself of the amazing libraries in London, I soon discovered that there were many paintings, drawings, carvings and sculptures of birthing women from every continent in the world, some dating back to Neolithic times, some from Europe and as recent as the 17th and 18th centuries. I was struck by the fact that in all of them labouring and birthing women were depicted in upright positions, whether standing, kneeling or squatting. None were lying on their back! I then decided to take a look at existing ethnic cultures not yet influenced by Western obstetrics. Indeed, they too had rich traditions of birthing wisdom going back generations, which involved upright positions, the presence of other women and a generally secluded and private birthing environment.

My next step was to revisit the anatomy books. It was then that it dawned on me that the female pelvis was uniquely shaped for giving birth in upright positions. In a 'Eureka' moment, I realised that women are anatomically designed to be free to move instinctively during labour. This is surely the way, I thought, to make birth easier and safer for the majority of women, reserving the safety net of obstetrics for those who need it. Later, through further research, I confirmed that inevitably, when a woman chooses the positions which are most comfortable, her body aligns with the Earth's gravitational pull.

This makes the contractions of the uterus more efficient and widens the pelvic diameters, making more space for the baby's descent. There is a better blood supply to the uterus and placenta and, not surprisingly, outcomes are much better, with a much greater chance of a vaginal birth and a huge reduction in the risk of complications. By moving, a mother can actually help her baby to be born.

I called this 'active birth'—a deliberate reinvention of the phrase 'active management of labour'. Freedom to move transforms a woman in labour from a passive patient to an active birth giver. No longer disempowered on her back like a stranded beetle, she regains control of her body and recovers her instinctive potential and power to give birth. Again, I experienced the reality of this when I gave birth to my third and fourth babies.

By being upright and free to move, without intervention and disturbance, the woman also reclaims the possibility of generating her own natural hormones. The birth process is governed by the maternal hormones of love and ecstasy, which mother and baby share. An active birth is not only safer and more practical, it also ensures that at the time of birth, babies are bathed in high levels of the hormones which foster love and healthy attachment. Having experienced this myself and witnessed it in thousands of women I have taught, it remains my mission in life to teach this to women and midwives and to continue to challenge the narrow-minded obstetric thinking and practice, which is not grounded in an understanding of birth physiology.

Janet Balaskas

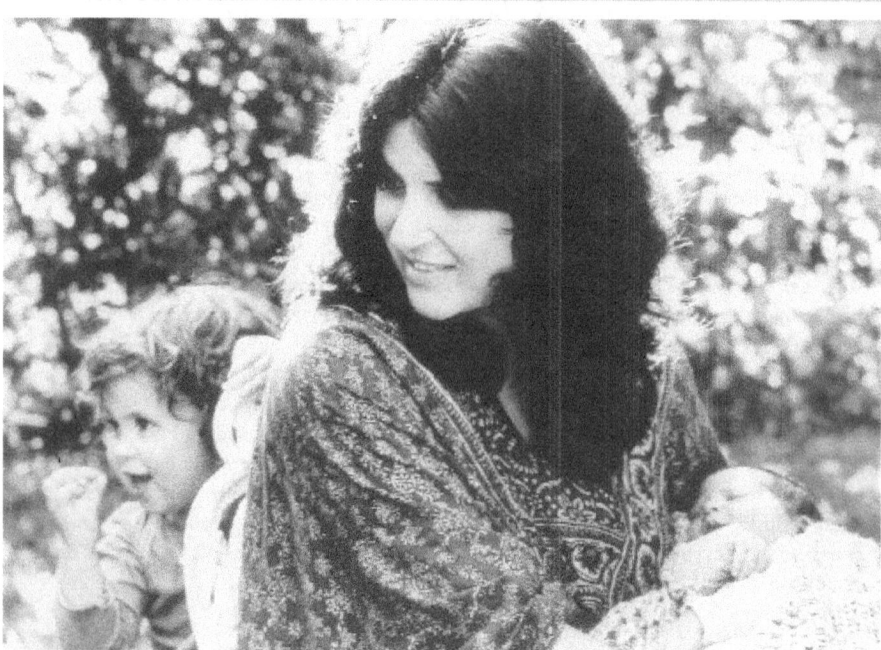

Janet with Kim and Iasona. See another photo of Janet on page 122.

AVOID TEARING

Having read many of the birthframes throughout this book, you will realise that tearing is not inevitable, as many professionals claim, and it also has nothing to do with luck. Full consciousness in an undrugged body, lack of disturbance and an upright position while giving birth seem to be the most important factors. (It may also help to have a warm perineum—warmed up with warm water.) Here is a summary of very specific ways in which you can stop your sexual organs tearing when you give birth...

- ♥ Make sure your caregivers don't put you under any pressure while you're in labour. Unless there's a real medical problem, the baby will be born in his or her own time. Hopefully, you will already have primed your caregivers to expect this and what follows by using a care guide. (See pages 267-275 for more on this.)
- ♥ Labour in a darkened room if at all possible—candlelight is good—so as to help you sink into the right state of consciousness for optimal birthing. If it's broad daylight, at least make sure you're in a completely secluded place.
- ♥ As I've already pointed out, it's vital that you don't let anyone tell you which position to be in when you give birth. If you want to sit on the toilet, fine. If you want to kneel down on all fours, that's also OK. Or squat, or stand. The only position which is unhelpful from the point of view of tearing is lying down on your back—so don't lie down for your caregiver's convenience! Adopt any other position which comes naturally. If you desperately want to lie down—which is unlikely, actually, believe it or not—lie on your left side. Remember, the positions in the photos on page 396 are much more helpful from all points of view, including avoiding a tear.[23]
- ♥ Make sure nobody disturbs you between the first and second stages of labour. If you're alone, you may well not realise when you have moved from the so-called 'first' stage on to the second—which is a good thing! Again, you can ensure no disturbance through the use of a care guide. As I've already explained, if you can manage not to be transferred to a delivery room for the actual birth (again through a pre-agreed care guide), your chances of giving birth easily and safely will be maximised... and of course you'll be least likely to tear. You can give birth anywhere at all—including in the room where you were labouring before—as long as it's warm.
- ♥ When you're sure your labour is well established (and that you're at least 5cm dilated), warm up your bottom! Warming the perineum by immersing yourself in water (in the bath or in a birthing pool) helps the skin to stretch more easily. Even dipping in for a couple of seconds will be helpful.[24]
- ♥ Make sure no local anaesthetic is injected into your perineum on a 'just in case' basis. The liquid swells the tissues, limiting their ability to stretch.
- ♥ Don't let anyone tell you how to push. Instead, tune into what's going on within your body in whatever way you can. (This will probably happen entirely spontaneously.)[25]

- ♥ Don't let anyone speak to you while you're actually giving birth. How will you be able to tune in to what's happening in your body if someone's distracting you? As we've noted before, talking can be a major intervention, especially during labour and birth. Everyone can talk later. Feel free to tell someone to shut up, if necessary, or screen them out by ignoring them or turning away. (Preparation of caregivers through a care guide is obviously helpful in this respect too.)
- ♥ Don't let anyone urge you on with nonverbal cues—e.g. through eye contact or miming. Only you yourself will know exactly when and how to push when your baby is ready to be born. You don't need to commune with anyone except your baby. You're in this 'alone' together!
- ♥ Don't let any caregiver touch your perineum while you're giving birth.[26]
- ♥ Definitely don't allow anyone to perform an episiotomy—you're much more likely to tear if you have one. And *that* would be a tear *and* a cut.
- ♥ Don't let anyone pull the baby's head so as to 'deliver' the shoulders, unless your midwife feels there are clear medical reasons for intervening.
- ♥ Have confidence in your body's ability to release your baby. The more relaxed you are, the better. Sometimes, relaxing your mouth can help you to relax your vagina.
- ♥ Visualise opening images. Flowers, windows, concentric ripples on a pond. All can help you to open up and relax for your baby's passage into the world.
- ♥ Don't strain to get your baby out in an unnatural way. 'Push' is not the right word for what it is that you need to do. Your body and your baby will manage the birth on their own—without any 'help' from you. Just focus inwards, be calm and your baby will just come out. Honestly! And there'll be no tear.
- ♥ Having said all that, if, after following this advice, you find you do sustain a minor tear, remember you have the option of leaving nature to do its own healing. Even without stitches, minor tears tend to heal beautifully, provided you keep your knees together for about two weeks after the birth! That means no vaginal examinations after the initial one (when the tear will have been noticed), no self-examination, no sitting cross-legged on the floor, no squatting. There are two advantages to letting your body heal on its own: firstly, the healing is likely to be more successful (because tears tend to knit together more neatly when left alone) and secondly, you won't have to suffer any pain or discomfort from stitches.[27]
- ♥ If, as is likely, you don't tear at all while you're giving birth, you can simply enjoy the wonderful feeling of having a completely undamaged perineum after childbirth. Many women say that it's worth doing without drug-based pain relief for this advantage alone! Your future sex life will thank you for it...

Many women say it's worth doing without drug-based pain relief because an intact perineum is more likely afterwards

After the birth...

After your optimal birth you'll notice a whole range of changes in your body. The good news is that most of them will sort themselves out spontaneously and the rest can eventually be rectified through entirely natural means. You really only need three pieces of advice...

- ♥ Breastfeed your baby—breastfeeding is best for you and your baby
- ♥ Eat a healthy, balanced diet and drink plenty of water
- ♥ Lose any excess weight and tone up with a little exercise

That's all! You really can regain your body after pregnancy. The only thing is, you need to wait a while to lose the excess weight because your baby's need for good quality milk needs to take priority. (Leave it at least six months.) In any case, you'll probably be too absorbed with the task of looking after your baby in the first couple of years. Breastfeeding may also give you an appetite which is extremely resistant to dieting! Personally, I would suggest you forget about dieting altogether until your baby is at least a year old. Self-acceptance is important, especially when you have an important job like motherhood to be getting on with. After that, as I've said, Weight Watchers is an excellent programme for encouraging healthy eating *and* weight loss, which still allows you to continue breastfeeding, so it's really worth doing.

I personally gained three and a half stone during my three pregnancies (oh dear!) but then lost all the excess weight with Weight Watchers afterwards. Losing weight did make me feel better about my body and it also helped me regain some much-needed energy! Now that my youngest is 7 years old, I feel my body is just as good, if not better than it was when I first got pregnant. I now feel even younger than when I was in my 30s! Strange, but true.

Anyway, in case you still doubt the capabilities of your body, let's take the final step in order to prepare for an optimal birth... *Help your mind.*

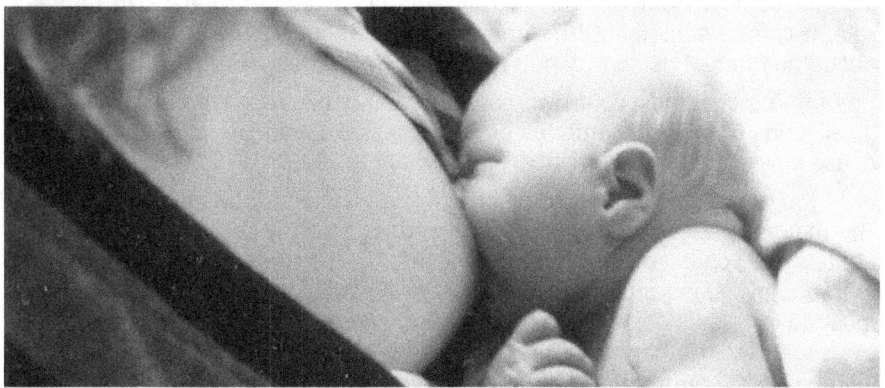

Although it's like being attached to a vacuum cleaner, breastfeeding is a wonderfully tender and intimate experience

1... HELP YOUR MIND

Most of the last few chapters have been about the problem of external disturbance. This chapter's about the kind that might come from within. If you can clear any negativity in your mind before the birth, when you're actually in labour you'll find you instinctively tune in to your primitive knowledge of how to give birth.

Desmond Morris, the famous animal and person watcher, concluded that human beings have difficult births because of the size of our babies' heads and our upright posture.[1] I think he's wrong! My own experience and that of countless other women makes me conclude that many humans have difficult births because they fail to create an environment—both internal and external— in which they are not disturbed.

As we've seen in earlier chapters, things that disturb a woman from the outside include anything that stimulates the new part of our brain, the neocortex. This includes light, speech, noise, movement, unnecessary action and a feeling of being observed. Internal disturbance occurs when there is any kind of psychological problem... If you're preoccupied or upset by something, it makes sense you're going to need to sort that out before giving birth. Only when it's been talked about or accepted in some way will you be in a position to tune into that all-important primitive side of your brain, which knows exactly how to give birth.

So this chapter is about dealing with both the old stuff and the new stuff— including any last-minute anxieties.

Sort through the psychological junk

Most of us have something stored away in our heads that needs to be dealt with. It can be something from the past, something about now, or something about the future. I personally had problems with all three at different stages![2]

Only you can know your own psychological difficulties. We can be affected by all kinds of things—memories of TV births, sexual abuse, partner problems, house-moving, relatives, practical problems...

If you're not sure what's going on in your own mind, how can you find out? The main way is to observe yourself dispassionately whenever you feel tense, unhappy or confused. How are you feeling, talking and behaving? When you feel you have some answers, don't react to anything that you notice. What you must do instead is *act*, i.e. take some calm, carefully considered action to help the situation. In other words, consider how you can respond to what you've learned about yourself, to make things better. On the next few pages there are pointers and birthframes about these steps, which involve identifying your feelings, making some decisions and dealing with major psychological issues.

IDENTIFY FEELINGS AND MAKE DECISIONS

If your feelings are difficult to pin down:

- ♥ Spend more time alone, doing something you love—cooking, gardening, listening to music (or playing it), reading, walking... Or simply sit quietly.
- ♥ Keep an informal diary or write poems. Write things down as and when you feel like it, in note form if necessary so you can keep up with your ever-changing thoughts and emotions.
- ♥ Try drawing, painting or cutting pictures out of magazines to tap into what you're feeling or thinking.
- ♥ Talk to friends and family. Enjoy their company and explore thoughts and feelings together.
- ♥ Try to recall your dreams each morning when you wake up and make notes of anything which seems significant or interesting.
- ♥ Practise bringing your attention to any situation which provokes a strong emotion in you.
- ♥ Finally, think about your beliefs and lifestyle. Are they in tune with your plans for the birth? Is there anything practical which needs sorting out?

Birthframe 84

Here, one woman explains how analytical thinking and soul-searching helped her to make the decisions which were right for her as she approached the birth of her first child.

My first child, Hana, was born at home... I was always planning for a natural birth, and very early on I decided that a natural birth was best achieved at home. Several factors resulted in this strong conviction.

Firstly, personal inclination. I am a believer in a holistic approach to health and the fact that ill health has mental and emotional dimensions which Western medical practices do not always address appropriately or adequately. As part of this philosophy, I see birth as a natural process requiring a sense of security and the ability to relax, requirements not easily met in hospital. A hospital full of sick people and the equipment and training for intervention are not conducive to the normal birth process. Hospital and doctors (rather than midwives) just seem to me a far from ideal set up for childbirth.

Secondly, I was lucky to have the experience of my sister, who having had one section followed by two home births was an excellent natural birth example. She showed me firsthand how seriously traumatising childbirth could be, and also how empowering it could be. Her journey from what she felt was an unnecessary caesarean to home birth, which she shared with me, made me think deeply about all these childbirth issues even before I was pregnant.

As a result, well before I was pregnant, I read widely about childbirth, particularly books about natural birth. I was fascinated with birth stories and was astounded at how clear and easy it was to chart 'things going wrong' in a hospital delivery; the so-called 'cascade of intervention'. The first point of this cascade was often the mother not dilating or 'progressing' because she did not feel sufficiently secure or relaxed, even though she might not even have been fully aware of this or able to articulate it. I just knew I would not be relaxed in a hospital where strangers, however nice, were coming in and out and where I was not in my own comfortable environment.

Thirdly, the risk element seemed just as high, if not higher with a hospital birth. Even if you have enlightened midwives, there is still an element of risk. You don't know these people. Someone possibly giving off nervous vibes, a chance comment about how dilation is slow, etc has panicked many first-time mothers. You are on their territory and I would find it difficult to feel in control enough.

I do believe the instinct of the mother is so important in labour and her lead should be followed. When I was in labour myself I trusted my body implicitly to do what was necessary. It is difficult to have this trust for someone else, and hospital staff just see the need to keep things moving at their pace. In any case, there are risks to the baby with induction, all the pain-relieving drugs, with the supine position of the mother, with forceps and ventouse, with a too speedy labour and removal of the baby, etc, etc. Of course, there are risks with a home birth; there is risk with any birth. However, all the research shows that for a low-risk mother, a home birth is just as safe, if not better in terms of morbidity and mortality levels. This safety factor seems to be what most people have difficulty getting their heads around, but all the research is there. I suspect the real problem that many people have with home birth (and there is a problem—many people act as if you should be committed to an asylum) is the fear of taking responsibility for something we are trained in our society to abrogate control of.

So, based on the research that I had done on the subject, I was absolutely convinced that the best way to give birth for me, and the safest way for mother and baby, was an active birth with no drugs and almost no intervention, unless there were complications, which are less likely with a natural birth anyway. And I was not confident that this kind of birth could be achieved in a hospital, and if it was, I felt it would be lucky. I wasn't prepared to take that risk. I don't think it matters which hospital you go to, as they are all geared to a 'medicalised' birth. So to have a natural birth, you have to fight for it to an extent—a major distraction you don't need during labour. I would want to manage the labour differently from how the medical staff attending me would want. I wouldn't want to be hooked up to a monitor. I wouldn't want any internal examinations. I knew I didn't want to lie down. I didn't want an episiotomy. I didn't want to be in a hospital.

I didn't want to be in a hospital

In my case, I knew birth was going to be hard, and I felt it was only really possible for me at home and with total determination, and secure, away from any temptation of drugs. I am not brave with pain, and needed to keep telling myself that it was only for a certain number of hours and I was just going to have to tough it out for once in my life. I spent a lot of time thinking, planning and visualising the birth, what I would do at each stage, what I could do to help myself. I kept very fit, walking an hour a day and doing yoga and meditation, with affirmations every day. These helped to make me feel confident and strong, rather than actually helping during labour when your body takes over anyway. I was so, so determined that this was how it was best for me personally to give birth—and therefore this was how I would do it—that I didn't allow myself to think of any other option, apart from telling myself that if things were not going well, I would of course accept the need to go to hospital and get help.

Finally, I think it is important to note that my husband was fully involved in my decision-making process. He listened to hours and hours of 'birthtalk' and he agreed with the home birth idea fully and was very supportive. I do think that this is an area where the woman must sort all the issues out for herself and decide what is best for her, and then explain and enlist the support of her partner, if there is one. After all, the fear of the partner often influences decision-making to the detriment of the birth giver!

Justine Rowan

DEAL WITH ANY MAJOR PSYCHOLOGICAL ISSUES

By this stage, I realise it's possible you may be thinking: "Yes, but that's small fry. Those are minor issues. You don't know just how much I've been through." I know what it means to work through heavy stuff. Whatever it is, you can work through it...

If you feel nothing I've suggested so far will work, you may need to consider some other approaches. Here are a few suggestions:

♥ You could follow a course in self-development, such as that provided in the books *Creating a Joyful Birth Experience* (Simon & Schuster 1994) or *Birthing from Within* (Souvenir Press 2007). You may even be able to find a class based on this type of book in your area. In any such course, leave out any activity which you intuitively feel may not be helpful or may disturb your baby. In *Birthing from Within*, for example, I would not recommend any of the exercises involving ice cubes! (They're used to simulate the experience of pain before the birth.) Doing the exercises might have a negative effect on both you and your baby, in my view. Similarly, I would beware of any breathing exercises—they're both unnecessary and unhelpful because the preparation you have done may dominate your instinctive knowledge while you're actually in labour and giving birth.

- ♥ You could try prayer or meditation. The Bible promises remarkable results, so don't pooh-pooh the idea, even if you're a non-believer. Also, the form of meditation called Vipassana, based on the original teachings of the Buddha, is very effective. [Useful websites: www.prayerguide.org.uk and www.dipa.dhamma.org] Again, a couple of words of caution, though... If you decide to pray, remember the Muslim proverb: "Trust in God, but tie your camel first." In other words, there's no point in praying if you're neglecting every other form of preparation—the 10 preparatory steps outlined in this book. And if you meditate, avoid any techniques which involve the use of mantras, visualisation or breath control (although breath observation is fine). The problem with these techniques is that they take you away from reality, rather than bringing you closer to it. You need to observe what is happening within you and become more in tune with what you really feel, not run away from yourself.
- ♥ You could also consult a counsellor, therapist or psychologist. A hypnotherapist may well be able to tap into your deeply-held beliefs or blockages. I remember, years ago, I didn't believe that hypnosis was a real state. Then, while I was attending a lecture on hypnosis, which included demonstrations, I accidentally 'went down'... and I discovered just how wrong I'd been. Oh dear, how embarrassing! In other words, be open to change and try what you feel might be right for you.[3]

Birthframe 85

Dr Nicolette Lawson has a degree in mechanical engineering and used to work as a manufacturing systems engineer. She then moved on to become an environmental manager and gained an engineering doctorate in Environmental Technology. Now she sells baby slings and works as a hypnotherapist and self-hypnosis teacher. I asked Nicolette a few more questions to try and find out why she had so dramatically changed her lifestyle. It seems the services she offers can make a significant difference to women who have worries about childbirth.

What services do you offer your clients?

Using hypnosis I can help women to be healthy and happy during pregnancy, calm and relaxed throughout childbirth and confident in their abilities as a mother, once the baby is born. Occasionally, I also help pregnant women who may have specific phobias related to hospitals, blood or needles.

Can you describe a typical client?

Typically, my pregnant clients come to me with only three or four weeks to go before their baby is due—although it would be even more beneficial if they started earlier. At this stage, they are really starting to worry about the actual birth.

Women are constantly bombarded with all the bad news stories about childbirth and babies—tales of pain and intervention, tales of disrupted sleep and postnatal depression. It's no wonder women approach childbirth with trepidation and anxiety. Women with muscles tense from fear will undoubtedly feel pain, because they will be resisting the natural process that their body is going through. Women who can be calm and relaxed throughout childbirth, who can go with the flow, are naturally more likely to have a problem-free natural birth.

Is there anybody you would refuse, if they came to you wanting hypnotherapy for pregnancy and childbirth?

There are no guarantees with hypnotherapy because everyone has a different belief system and different perceptions. However, anyone can be successfully hypnotised, if they really want to be. So I would be willing to work with anyone that wanted to give it a go—provided they were female!

What first made you interested in hypnotherapy for birth?

I first learnt self-hypnosis to help me finish my doctorate—which of course I did. Then, when I became pregnant with my second child, I decided to use self-hypnosis for both the pregnancy and birth. The birth of my first child was a long and complicated experience that I did not want to repeat.

And did you find it helped with the birth of your next child?

Definitely! During the pregnancy I was much less tired and I had no acne—I had loads with my first pregnancy. Then the birth, which was at home, was calm and relaxed and my $10\frac{1}{2}$lb baby was born with no pain relief—as I couldn't describe any of the process as painful! The midwives were quite impressed! My son was so calm and quiet when he was born—the birth had been so calm—and he was perfectly clean.

Why do you think the birth of your first child was so much more difficult, without self-hypnosis?

I went into hospital 10 days before my due date, because my waters broke. However, it turned out it was only my hindwaters—no one had told me about that possibility—so they didn't start my contractions off. I wanted to go home, but the hospital said I had to stay—because of the danger of infection!—so I did. By the next day, there were still no contractions, so I was induced. This resulted in massive contractions and high blood pressure. The medical staff then insisted that I have an epidural, which was not what I wanted, to bring down my blood pressure and so protect me from the risk of pre-eclampsia. This resulted in me having to lie on my back with monitors strapped on me. The contractions slowed down and I laboured all night, my $7\frac{1}{2}$lb daughter finally being born at 6am with the help of forceps, ventouse and an episiotomy.

The staff insisted I have an epidural

I felt that each intervention by the hospital just led to the next in a long line of problems. The whole situation undermined my dream of having a natural birth, shattered my confidence and left me feeling totally out of control. With my second birth, I was determined to stay in control. Self-hypnosis helped me to have the confidence to do it and to remain calm and relaxed throughout the process, which of course I did!

How many sessions does a pregnant client need?

The majority of pregnant clients—assuming they have not had hypnotherapy before—require two sessions. The first session is to get the client used to going into hypnosis; it is a deep relaxation session that encourages general calmness, relaxation, confidence, competence and better sleep. The second session is specifically for the remainder of the pregnancy—being strong, healthy and sleeping well; the birth—remaining calm, relaxed and in control, going with the flow (with the contractions and the birth process as a whole); and after the birth—recovering easily, feeling confident, happy and competent, getting back to pre-pregnancy size, breastfeeding easily and coping well with everything and everyone. I tape both these sessions and advise that the childbirth session is listened to every day up to the birth. This has the added benefit of ensuring that pregnant women take some well-earned rest and recovery each day. The first session can then be used whenever some calmness and relaxation is required after the birth.

And what kind of results have you achieved?

When I first started, I visited all my clients after they had given birth to see how they got on. Now I simply don't have the time to follow them up, and most new mums don't have the time to let me know how they got on.

However, based on the feedback I collected when I first started and the ongoing calls I get from some of my clients, I can report that all of my clients thought the hypnosis did benefit them. All reported feeling more relaxed and calm. Many had natural births, with minimal pain-relief—even a couple of women who had caesareans for their first baby went on to have natural births for their second babies. Inevitably, some women had to have caesareans, for various reasons, but all that I spoke to reported feeling calm and relaxed, despite the operation, and notably, they healed up and recovered better and quicker than expected. One woman, who hadn't expected to breastfeed because her mother and sister had had difficulties, went on to experience easy and enjoyable breastfeeding. The other common trend was in the babies, who tend to be very calm, happy and easy to look after. I really must collect some more information and write a book!

> Even women who'd had caesareans for their first baby went on to have natural births for their second...
> I really must collect some info for a book!

And do you have any regrets about giving up your life as an engineer?!

Well, occasionally I regret the loss of money... I could have been earning a very handsome salary by now! But I don't regret giving up the long working hours and time away from home.

Being a self-employed hypnotherapist means that I can work from home—hours that suit me and my family—and I have freedom and flexibility that's worth more than any salary. Added to that, I have incredible job satisfaction, knowing that I'm helping so many people to enjoy better lives and experience childbirth as it should be—natural and wonderful. I think being an engineer by background has actually helped me gain credibility with a lot of my clients. They reason that if an engineer—an intelligent, logical, rational, practical person—thinks hypnosis works, then there must be something in it!

Finally, what advice would you give a woman who is not interested in hypnotherapy, but who would nevertheless like to have a positive birth experience, for her own sake and—most importantly—for the sake of her baby?

The most important thing to remember is that childbirth is normal. Women's bodies were designed for it. It's not a medical procedure. Your body knows what it has to do. So, you need to trust your body and trust your instincts. Also...

- ♥ Don't believe all the negative things that other people tell you about pregnancy, childbirth and bringing up babies. Whatever they've experienced was their own experience—it doesn't mean yours will be the same.
- ♥ Learn all you can about the birthing process so that you know what's happening to you and you know what to expect.
- ♥ Stay calm and relaxed. Use whatever methods you want to help you—apart from drugs and alcohol!—and have a birthing partner who is calm and supportive too.
- ♥ Consider using hypnotherapy or learning self-hypnosis after all. It really is a very safe, natural and pleasant experience with so many beneficial side-effects: calmness, confidence, better sleep, more positive thinking and so on. How can you be negative about something unless you've tried it?

For more on Nicolette's work see www.m-power-me.co.uk

Birthframe 86

Here we have an account from an American woman who experienced sexual abuse as a child... Although she did do some exercises which I don't feel are helpful (involving ice cubes!) and the birth did involve some intervention, it's clear that this woman's ongoing focus on being aware of what was happening, on tuning into her instincts and on behaving as she felt was right were key factors in making things as good as possible for both mother and child.

I have been enthralled by stories of empowering births since my college years, when I made the acquaintance of several home birth midwives. However, I was disappointed by the so-called natural childbirth I witnessed during my education as a nurse practitioner, when I was required to attend several hospital births. The nurses were zealously cheering, "Push! Push! I want to see this baby! Push!" No one was encouraging the woman to follow what her body and baby were doing naturally. It seemed the woman was expected to birth her baby for the nurses rather than to be present in her own experience.

When I became pregnant, I knew I wanted something different. I wanted to feel safe and comfortable so that I could open and allow my baby to be born. In addition, I am a survivor of childhood sexual abuse and I knew that the 'wrong' environment could trigger flashbacks and definitely impede the birthing process, possibly even creating further emotional trauma. On the other hand, I hoped that an empowering birth experience could promote healing at a very deep level. In a way my background as a survivor was a gift, as it led me on an intensive inner and outer quest for a healing pregnancy and birth. As I can see now, the process of undergoing the journey, in itself, was healing.

My husband and I spent endless hours reading and discussing aspects of antenatal care and birthing. We interviewed five home birth midwives and two nurse-midwife group practices. We changed caregivers three times, wavered for months when trying to decide between a home birth, birth centre birth, and hospital birth. Finally, we decided we felt most comfortable with a planned home birth, with a nurse-midwife practice as our back-up, should a hospital birth become necessary. We took a great childbirth class based on the book *Birthing from Within* (Souvenir Press 2007), which prepared us for the birth in a very experiential way. In the class, we practised pain-coping techniques (while holding ice cubes to simulate the pain of contractions!), discussed and faced fears, did birth artwork, and watched videos of women labouring and birthing in very non-interventionist settings.

I delighted in the physical closeness I had with my baby during my last few months of pregnancy. I loved to feel him move and to touch and massage his various parts. In fact, even when I was 40 weeks pregnant I felt very comfortable with my baby inside me; I didn't experience the feeling of 'wanting this baby out' or 'wanting to get my body back' that many women describe. And then 41 weeks came and went. As comfortable and wonderful as it was having him so close, I also longed to meet this new person and become a mother. Actually, there was also a sense of urgency because we were due to move to another area a fortnight later! During this period of waiting (and trying many techniques to induce labour) I had plenty of time to worry about various things, mostly related to the birth and the move. At a certain point, my anxieties began to centre on breastfeeding. As a nurse practitioner I was well versed in the benefits of breastfeeding and had a lot of 'book knowledge' on the subject; I was certain that I wanted to breastfeed. I was extremely concerned, however, that I would not be able to comfortably maintain the constant physical closeness and literally the suckling that breastfeeding would require. I was concerned that breastfeeding would trigger memories of my childhood abuse.

My midwives knew about the sexual abuse and we had discussed it in terms of the birth, but I had felt ashamed and afraid to bring up the topic of how my background might affect breastfeeding. As is common with abuse survivors, I carried the shame of the abuse. I felt I was the only one who had ever faced these issues and also, illogically, that admitting their existence might 'jinx' the breastfeeding. I was especially distraught because I believed from the core of my being that I would be failing my child and myself in a very profound way if I were not able to breastfeed.

Eventually, at 41 weeks and still counting, I knew I needed help! I could find no information about survivors of sexual abuse and breastfeeding in any of the literature. I took a courageous step and arranged for a meeting with a lactation consultant who came highly recommended. She listened to my fears and reflections and gave me a lot of reassurance. She said that I had a great chance of successfully breastfeeding. Women who have been sexually abused sometimes have trouble tolerating the physical closeness breastfeeding requires, as was my fear for myself, but different women behave differently when faced with new motherhood as a survivor of abuse. Some lose confidence in their bodies and worry that they will not be capable of producing enough milk. For others, the physical sensations involved with breastfeeding may remind them of the abuse they suffered, which was also something I was concerned about.

After speaking to the lactation consultant, I felt so much freer... my 'secret' was out. I then felt comfortable discussing the issues with my midwives—it turned out they were not at all surprised and had faced these same issues with other women before. I felt so relieved. Both my shame and fear decreased.

Our home birth midwife, Ann, said that many women with abuse backgrounds and/or who do not feel comfortable with nipple stimulation by their partner have no problem when they breastfeed a baby. She said that the hormones released by breastfeeding make women able to tolerate and even enjoy the close contact with their babies. Our nurse-midwife, Valerie, told me that it was the love that mattered in feeding the baby, whether from breast or bottle. She said I should try to breastfeed and see what happened. Of course I still desperately wanted to be able to breastfeed, but I felt less pressure after hearing her words.

At Valerie's suggestion, I took some time to write about my fears and realised that breastfeeding a baby really would be different than the abusive situation I was in as a child. My baby, tiny and in need of food, warmth, and love, would be totally different than the adult who had abused me. And as a breastfeeding mother, I would be in a totally different position than I was as a child suffering the abuse. Instead of being a small child overpowered by someone huge and terrifying, I would be a grown woman responding very naturally to my baby's needs. These insights gave me hope that I would succeed at breastfeeding.

I also prayed that I would be able to breastfeed. To me, being able to successfully breastfeed seemed like a quantum leap. It seemed like it truly would be nothing short of a miracle. I didn't have time to do more therapy, more healing because my baby would be here any day... I needed grace! So I prayed that somehow, just somehow I would be able to successfully breastfeed.

> As the days wore on I continued to be anxious
> that our baby was not yet born

As the days wore on I continued to be anxious that our baby was not yet born. Our move date was rapidly approaching and, to make things worse, I knew that at two weeks after our due date the policy of both our home birth midwife and nurse-midwife practice was for us to have our birth in the hospital. 'Nesting' was difficult, to say the least!

Suddenly at 13 days after our due date, I had a surprising inner shift and felt that the right thing for me to do was go to the hospital and try a very gentle labour induction—prostaglandin gel on my cervix (which is not the same as Cytotec, incidentally). My husband and I spoke to our midwives, who agreed with our plan. It was in fact Valerie who was the nurse-midwife on call. From our earlier conversations, I knew that she was very experienced in working with women with sexual abuse backgrounds. I also knew she recognised and appreciated the inner work I had done and that she welcomed the opportunity to attend our birth. I felt safe with the thought of being in Valerie's care. She said, "We'll make it just like a home birth. Come at 7.30 or 8.00pm and decorate your room. We can start the induction after that." My husband and I spent the day grieving that we weren't having the home birth we had hoped for and packing up everything we wanted to have with us.

We were welcomed warmly by the nursing staff. Valerie had even 'reserved' a specific room for us which had a huge jacuzzi tub. Our home birth midwife, Ann, met us at the hospital which gave me a strong sense of protection. When we saw Valerie and I told her that we didn't want to be there, that we wanted a home birth, she said, "OK. Then go home." But I was clear I did want to try to have my baby right then, so we stayed. However, knowing that no one was insisting on my being at the hospital kept me feeling in control (which was clearly Valerie's intention). We decorated our room a bit. Then Valerie inserted the prostaglandin gel and explained it was a 12-hour slow release. I would need to have fetal monitoring continuously for two hours (to make sure it wasn't releasing too quickly) and then we could go to sleep and see if anything happened in the morning. We never did go to sleep... To my great delight, within two hours I was having strong regular contractions. After the monitor was unhooked, Joel (my husband) and I walked up and down the halls, up and down the stairs, talking and laughing. I was so excited to finally be having regular contractions. I was even happy about the pain.

Wanting to just be alone with Joel, I asked him to ask Ann to leave, that we would call her when labour really got underway (as we were still under the impression that nothing much would happen until the morning). As soon as Ann left, I felt the intensity of the contractions increase. I got in the jacuzzi tub. Lying there in the dark, warm water and listening to the whirring of the jets, I felt like I myself was in the womb. As the contractions got stronger my focus became completely inward.

I remembered a slogan from *Birthing from Within*: 'Relax, breathe, do nothing extra'. I chanted 'Om' during the contractions and then put all my effort into releasing all thoughts and physical sensations in the space between the contractions. Joel chanted along with me and that really kept me going. He was incredible, consistently reading my cues perfectly. One word or one gesture and he knew what to do—rub my back in a certain place with a certain amount of pressure, bring me water... I could really feel that the two of us together were bringing our baby into the world. And quite literally no one else was around. We were in a sleepy hospital on a Friday night and actually Valerie and the nurses were in with another woman who was birthing her baby!

At a certain point the pain was very strong and I had a clear sense the prostaglandin gel should be removed. Joel managed to find a nurse who was doubtful that I could be progressing so fast, but after consulting Valerie, did agree to remove it. My contractions continued to progress. At one point a nurse I'd never seen before strode into the room looking for a piece of equipment. She seemed totally unaware she was entering our space. Later she again strode in, this time probably to listen to our baby's heartbeat. Again, her energy did not feel 'in synch' to me. I felt very 'seated' in my power, like a lioness. I said emphatically to Joel, "Who is that? Tell her to leave." (I later learned that he then took her aside and explained that I was a survivor of childhood sexual abuse and that I needed to feel very safe in my space. And she did improve.)

Eventually I remember making my way to the toilet. During my pregnancy I had the sense I would like to labour on the toilet because my pelvic floor muscles really could relax well there. This proved to be true. Through all the contractions my repetition of 'Om' continued, although the chanting eventually gave way to yelling! I would yell "Om" as soon as the contraction began and continue all the way through it. The sounds that were coming out of me were incredible—they were deep, powerful sounds. I felt myself releasing on a very, very deep level what seemed like lifetimes of accumulated blockages. The process seemed to be freeing me from many of the wounds the abuse had left. I felt so much darkness that had previously taken up residence in my pelvic region being transmuted into light and being released through the sounds.

Unlike the abuse during which I 'left' my body, during the labour and birth, I was fully present. As this moaning and purging was happening, I knew that a miraculous process was occurring. I was simultaneously reaching into the depths of where the abuse memories were stored in my physical body and into a depth of healing power which now seemed to interpenetrate the very same location. Quite literally the site of my childhood abuse was now the canal that my baby was soon to travel through. I tangibly felt that as the darkness was released through the sounds, my pelvis was opening, freeing everything up for my baby to move through. I was also aware even then that the impact of this experience would be far-reaching in my life and that I would be able to offer my child a much healthier mother. I felt grateful for this miraculous process.

At a certain point, I noticed myself very naturally starting to push at the end of each contraction. I had read that grunty pushes at the end of a contraction can help the cervix dilate. I had the sense I was getting close. I told my husband to get Valerie. She arrived and sat on the floor, Indian style, in front of me—and the toilet! She asked me if the sounds I was making were scaring me. I said, "No". In fact, inside I felt very happy about the sounds as I knew what an incredible healing was taking place. I then mentally told the baby that everything was fine and not to be worried about the sounds, but my sense was that he or she was fine with it. From atop the toilet, I yelled and writhed and pushed my feet into Valerie's thighs during each contraction and then when the contraction was over I leaned forward and collapsed into her arms. This was an incredible part of the labour for me because I have never allowed myself to be mothered the way I allowed Valerie to mother me. I had felt engulfed by several women during my childhood and as an adult mostly avoided anything but loose hugs with other women. And here I was collapsing into Valerie's arms! This in itself was a whole other profound healing for me... I felt worthy of being mothered and I realised I wasn't defective in terms of allowing myself to be mothered when I was with a person I truly felt safe with.

Interestingly, at this point, my husband disappeared into the background for me. I specifically needed a woman to travel with me down this leg of the path, someone who had travelled this path before herself and accompanied other women down it. I later learnt Joel had taken a long-needed bathroom break!

I think Valerie noticed those grunty pushes I was doing at the end of the contractions and she asked to check my cervical dilation for the first time since labour had started. She also probably noticed me saying, "I can't do it...," which is apparently a typical sign of being in transition. She checked and I was about 9cm dilated. I said, "Thank God!" Valerie requested I move over to the bed, asking Ann and Joel to 'make it like a seat' since I was so reluctant to leave the toilet.

> It was so clear what my body was doing
> and so easy for me to follow along

I laboured on all-fours for a while continuing to use movement and sound to cope with the pain of the contractions. I distinctly noticed my contractions become half as frequent. I understood I was in 'second stage' (fully dilated and pushing). My urge to push now took up much more of each contraction. It was so clear what my body was doing and so easy for me to follow along. At one point I spontaneously reached my hand into my vagina and I felt this mushiness which I knew to be the baby's head; I was so excited!

At some point I noticed the nurse was concerned that the baby's heartbeat was low. I remembered Ann explaining to us during an antenatal visit that sometimes when the birth is imminent the heartbeat will drop from head compression and that it was not dangerous. I was not concerned and said aloud, "It's just head compression".

Apparently, the baby's heartbeat continued to be low (at times 60 beats per minute). Now Valerie said, "Bring the sound down lower out through your vagina" so I did. Then she said that we needed to have the baby born. By then I had flipped over onto my back. She asked me to pull up on my knees and do some forced pushes. Ann and Joel helped pull my legs up toward my chest. Of course, I didn't want to do this. I wanted to take my time and ease the baby out. I knew that both this position and forced pushing would be more likely to cause a tear and would decrease the oxygenation to the baby. Not wanting to do it and still wanting to do everything 'my way' I said, "I can't". Valerie and Ann said firmly, "Do this for your baby." I pushed about two times and his head was out. One more push and his body swooshed out. The room was dark. Valerie held him up, he let out a cry, she said, "The baby's fine," and immediately placed him on my belly. She said, "It was just head compression."

(It was only two years later, when consulting with another midwife, that I came to believe it to be a sensible practice for a midwife to 'want the baby born' when the heart rate has dropped for quite some time and is not resurging. My husband also told me that Ann said she would have done the same thing had our baby been born at home. I will never know for sure whether pushing him out before I felt ready was medically necessary. However, it was quite a profound moment for me. It was the moment that I did something I didn't want to do because the two midwives, whom I knew wanted to avoid all unnecessary interventions, both made it clear that it was for my baby. I felt Mother Nature was giving me a nudge to step out of the role of the individual 'Beth' and into the role of motherhood. I felt the birth of my motherhood was in that moment.)

Our baby was so full and strong, not like the scrawny newborn I had expected. I rubbed his back and talked and talked and talked to him. It was so amazing to have skin-to-skin contact with him after having him inside me for so long. Since he was face down, I had no idea what he looked like or even if he was a boy or a girl. I just felt his body against mine and held him. Time stood still. After a while my husband suggested we cut the cord and see if we had a son or a daughter. (The placenta had already plopped right out after the baby was born). Then we discovered we had our Theodore and saw his beautiful face and beautiful body.

About 20 minutes after the birth, Ann helped me to breastfeed Theodore. He knew exactly what to do, which thrilled and amazed me and gave me confidence that breastfeeding would work out for us. Ann told us not to be surprised if he didn't feed as well the next few times, that in her experience babies often latch on very well right after the birth and then may need some help. I was so worried it somehow might not work out. I worried about whether Theodore's latch-on was correct. I leaked huge amounts of milk. I struggled with engorgement. I began to feel physically weak and emotionally overwhelmed five days after the birth. All of this while getting ready to move halfway across the country! Luckily, when my friends asked how I was doing I honestly said, "Not well." We asked for help. Friends began coming to our home day and night helping pack, bringing food, feeding me, and giving me emotional support. Their loving assistance touches me to this day.

By the time he was 12 days old, Theodore and I had got into a good rhythm with breastfeeding, my physical strength was gradually returning... and we were living in a new city! I struggled for several months adjusting to the changes in our lives— becoming a mother, leaving my previous employment, caring full-time for a new baby, living in a new city where I didn't know anyone, my husband working at a new job... And as I struggled with these changes, I would remember aspects of my birth experience and feel inspired and proud of my attainment. I also felt very proud and powerful that I was breastfeeding, that my body was nourishing my baby.

For the most part, I was able to tolerate the nearly constant physical closeness that my baby required. Occasionally, I felt overwhelmed at having him attached to my breast so often. During those times I sometimes imagined that the milk was flowing right out of my chest wall into him rather than coming out of my breast. I would concentrate on the sound and feeling of the milk gushing out of me and him gulping it down. This visualisation helped me forget about my breast and the emotional discomfort I was having with his suckling. I imagined myself giving him a person-to-person, life-generating transfusion.

I was amazed and grateful to find that most of the time I relished the physical closeness with Theodore. He wanted either to be held or breastfed day and night. Although it was exhausting to carry and breastfeed him constantly and I did not experience the kind of productivity I was used to in the working world, I was surprised at how often I felt a sense of fulfilment and accomplishment. I attribute this, in large part, to the mothering hormones released as a result of the frequent breastfeeding and nearly constant physical contact. I was surprised to find that my need to be with him was just as intense as his need to be with me.

By the time Theodore was 13 months old, I was able to appreciate how gradually, gently, and naturally the process of him becoming independent and separating occurs. For example, in the early months he breastfed very, very often and was only content if we held him constantly. Then he began to crawl and sometimes preferred exploring to being held and even sometimes to breastfeeding! By 10 months he could walk and eat a little bit of food and could nap without being held, but he still relied very much on breastfeeding, being held and sleeping with us during the night.

Then at 13 months he would breastfeed less frequently because he was really busy doing all his work and explorations. At that age, he would eat some solids but would rely mostly on breastmilk for his main source of nutrition. He slept with us and breastfed about 1-3 times during the night. Although at times he acted very independently such as when he, on his own initiative, went upstairs when I was downstairs or darted off when we were in a shop, I could tell he very much still needed me to be there. I think that his confidence in knowing I was nearby helped him to feel safe to explore.

> I think that my baby's confidence in knowing I was nearby helped him feel safe to explore.

The key for me with breastfeeding a toddler is to make sure that I am comfortable emotionally and physically. As Theodore has grown, I have taken note of any aspects of our breastfeeding relationship that are uncomfortable for me and have sought to make adjustments as necessary. For example, when Theodore was under a year I enjoyed bathing with him and happily breastfed him in the bath. When he was about 18 months I began to breastfeed him in the bath and found that now with his bigger body and both of us undressed I didn't feel comfortable. As soon as I became aware of my discomfort, I stopped breastfeeding, got him involved in something else, and got myself dressed. In general, I noticed that when he breastfed with the intention of drinking milk, usually the milk flowed easily and his suck was comfortable for me. But sometimes when he 'hung out' on the breast I found it irritating. At these times he was usually willing to accept a snack, story, or outing instead of breastfeeding. He often seemed to appreciate a substitution for breast-feeding because it actually better met his current need for attention, food, drink, or interesting activity.

> The key for me with breastfeeding a toddler is to make sure that I am comfortable emotionally and physically.

When I wasn't keen on breastfeeding him but could tell he had a real need, I would breastfeed him then, but with awareness. Rather than sinking into feeling like a victim, I would remember that I'm his mother, a grown woman, choosing to meet my toddler son's needs. Then, as I watched him breastfeed and saw the relaxation and reprieve it brought him, and the relaxation it brought me, my choice was affirmed. Sometimes, when I was breastfeeding a bit reluctantly, it helped if I read while I did it. Reading helped me feel that I was giving something to myself as I breastfed Theodore. At other times I found that focusing fully on Theodore helped me shift into more positive feelings.

Things changed for me when he was about 30 months. One night during that time, he asked to breastfeed. I was sleeping fairly deeply at the time and, and as he breastfed, I had the perception that someone was performing a sexual act on me. It turned out that Theodore's sucking on my breast was triggering a memory of my childhood abuse. Of course, Theodore was still his same little 2-year-old self and doing nothing unusual. But the size of his body (no longer a baby or a young toddler), his larger mouth and the difference in his suck, as well as it being during the night with me half-asleep all resembled the abuse too closely for my subconscious mind to differentiate. After that I gently and firmly discontinued night feeds, making it clear to him that although we wouldn't breastfeed at night, I'd still be there for him, responding to him. Whenever he requested the breast, I offered him a choice of water, a snuggle, or a snack. My husband offered to carry or rock him. We told him he could breastfeed again when it was light outside. Soon he often slept through the night.

As Theodore neared 3 years old, I began to resent his frequent requests for the breast throughout the day. Since, when he was younger, I had offered him the breast readily many, many times a day meeting his needs for food, drink, soothing, etc, he had come to think of breastfeeding as the thing to do whenever a need of almost any kind arose. I think this kind of thing is something many mothers (not only those who are abuse survivors) go through with breastfeeding children of his age. Theodore is quite verbal and I intuitively felt I was short-changing him if I didn't work with him to teach him other ways to meet his needs, verbalising his frustration or need for food or drink, seeking help in completing a project (rather than tossing the project aside in frustration and reflexively yelling, "Milk!"), asking for attention from me (rather than trying to get a 'piece' of me by breastfeeding).

Also, I felt I was short-changing myself since, at this point, I did not enjoy feeding very much. Now, even when I'm fully awake while breastfeeding him, I often feel emotionally uncomfortable feeding such a big boy. My subconscious mind still 'reads' the breastfeeding as abuse and I usually want the feed to end as soon as possible. Two things have helped me during this stage. First, I have explained to him that he can breastfeed three specific times during the day: morning, after lunch, and after dinner. No longer do I have to respond to requests on a case-by-case basis, 20 times a day! I tell him clearly, "It's not time for milk," and offer other options instead. Second, I control the length of the breastfeeding session. Whenever I want it to end, I sing a specific song at a speed I determine. When the song is finished, Theodore stops feeding. He then often proudly says, "I stopped!"

Now, several months after his third birthday, Theodore continues to breastfeed three times a day but has, indeed, found other ways to meet his needs. For comfort he says, "Cuddle me!" When hurt, he calls out woefully, "I am hurt." He readily accepts snacks and drinks. I feel proud to see him growing up, yet continuing to express his needs so clearly and relationally.

What I've learnt...

This process of being attuned to my own experience and making adjustments as needed has been immensely healing for me, a survivor of childhood sexual abuse. When I was abused as a child, my own needs were not considered; I felt incapable and unworthy of asserting my needs.

Now, in relation to Theodore (now that he's 3—this didn't apply when he was a baby), I am able to assert my own needs as being important. Not more important than his needs, but also important. I have found, again and again, that we can find a solution that works to meet both our needs. Through our negotiations, not only am I teaching Theodore about the 'give and take' of healthy relationships, but I am learning about it myself.

Not only am I teaching him about the 'give and take' of healthy relationships—I'm learning about it myself

I now see that not only has breastfeeding been possible for me, a survivor of childhood sexual abuse, it has been immensely healing. My desire to have an empowering birth and fulfilling breastfeeding relationship has forced me to face emotional territory I would probably have otherwise avoided. One wound left by the abuse is an underlying sense of 'I can't do it. It's not even worth trying.' Birthing, breastfeeding, and now the process of weaning Theodore have helped to replace this with a very real sense of capability and trust in myself. I am now confident that I can and will stand up for the well-being of myself and my child whenever necessary. I have also gained a heightened sensitivity to both myself and my son, which continues to serve us in our relationship as we both continue to grow and change.

Beth Dubois

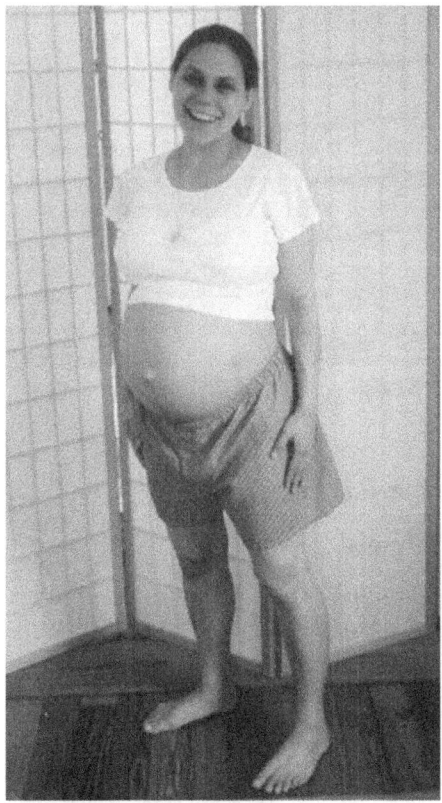
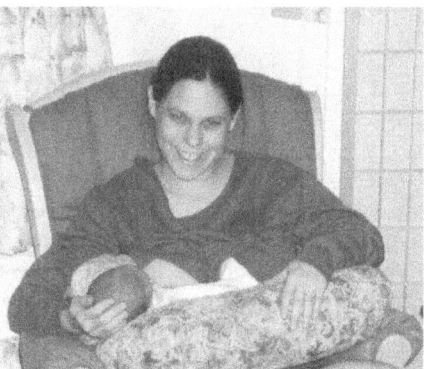
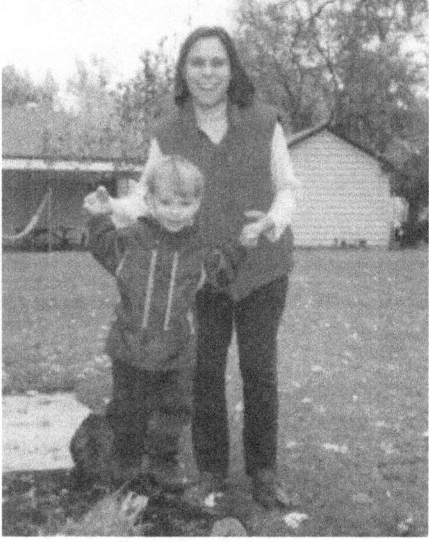

Clockwise from above[4]:
- ♥ *During a non-worrying moment*
- ♥ *Comfortably breastfeeding*
- ♥ *In harmony*

Apart from working through your 'psychological junk', what else can you do? Here's another idea...

Protect your mind

If you're already feeling pretty positive about the prospect of having an optimal birth, or you manage to get to that stage, protect this state of mind. Don't make yourself unnecessarily afraid by watching fictitious or alarmist (highly disturbed) births on TV. Don't overdo your searches on the Internet or at your local library for worst-case scenarios... Know when to stop!

Even be careful generally about watching TV or films, reading newspapers, magazines or novels and playing computer games. None of these are likely to help you get into a good frame of mind for the birth.

Birthframe 87

Why did my waters break? Originally, I thought it was just one of those things. Medical staff had warned me that twins often arrived early and I should be careful but I really thought it wouldn't happen to me. When it did, I couldn't understand it... Again, I thought, "This doesn't happen to me. It's not part of the plan", etc. What physically probably precipitated the event, in hindsight, was that on the Saturday afternoon we went to watch a rugby match—England playing Italy at Twickenham in October 1999. We romped home to a huge victory and there was lots of jumping up and down in great excitement. As I was only 30 weeks, I didn't think about it. The next day was fine, but it was when I was getting out of bed on the Monday morning that my waters actually broke.

Medical staff would not be impressed by my naïveté

I did go into labour naturally six days later. Again, another story... medical staff would not be impressed by my naïveté and lack of appreciation of what was happening... Because I wasn't allowed out of hospital, I had had to forgo my ticket on the following Saturday for another rugby match!—the England game against New Zealand. I was gutted. In the end, my husband heroically gave his up as well and stayed with me in the hospital that afternoon. We watched the game but only because I promised him that I would not get too excited. I was very restrained and everything was fine. He stayed until the late evening and left just as they started to show *Life of Brian* about 11.00pm. I watched it all (again) and laughed too much... A few minutes after it finished I called the nurse to say that I felt a bit 'odd'. The upshot was that we called my husband back an hour or two later when it was confirmed that I was in labour.

Finally, be careful to avoid people who are full of fear or pessimism. Fear produces adrenaline, which inhibits the production of oxytocin, which—as you'll remember—is the hormone which gets contractions going and will get your baby born. Oddly enough, your body will produce adrenaline at the moment of birth, but you don't want it to be doing this too early, when you're supposed to be calmly producing the hormone of love, oxytocin.

Perhaps you're thinking: "Oh no! I don't want to live like some kind of crackpot!" You know, I'm not telling you to avoid everything... I'm just saying that pregnancy is a time for introspection and awareness, rather than distraction, and that you need to protect yourself from negative influences or shocks. Here are a few tips for minimising the risks:

- ♥ Don't set yourself up for a negative reaction. Avoid 'announcing' your intention to give birth naturally to everyone. Many people are only too keen to share their horror stories about the pain of labour and talking may well be their own way of working through their own traumas.
- ♥ Respond constructively to any negativity you do encounter. Remember that health care professionals may have no faith in the physiological processes precisely because they've witnessed so many 'disturbed' births. In the developed world this disturbance has become institutionalised through the environment (bright lights, monitoring, etc) and the use of drugs and interventions. In places like Africa, births are disturbed as a result of local birthing customs, and lack of hygiene does nothing to help mortality statistics. And remember, you don't have to justify yourself. 'Showing' people by actually having an optimal birth is likely to be much more effective than any number of explanations!
- ♥ In cases where it's important to tell people about your plans, help people to travel the same journey you've travelled yourself by providing information. (Suggest they read this book, if necessary!) Be patient and persistent, remembering that you probably asked yourself similar questions.
- ♥ Finally, help your husband and your family understand how important it is not to shock or disturb you while you prepare for labour. In case you think I'm overstating the case, let me tell you about a woman I met at a playgroup. When she told me she'd had her baby five weeks before her due date, I asked her if she had any idea why. Without any hesitation, she said it was because her sister—who lived over the other side of the world, in New Zealand—had suddenly turned up on her doorstep the night before. Apparently, her family had secretly arranged the visit and had picked the sister up from the airport, having said they were going shopping. The shock (albeit pleasant) of opening the door to see her sister on the doorstep was simply too much for this woman, even though she'd been longing to see her! It would have been better if she'd been told about the visit... So, please do tell your family about this kind of problem, if you think there's any chance at all they might do the same kind of thing to you![5]

Birthframe 88

Here's an account from a woman who was consistently positive and proactive in dealing with psychological issues.

It was really important to me to have a natural birth because I'm a rebirther. Perhaps I should explain a bit about rebirthing. It's a breathing technique which opens a person up emotionally and energetically, i.e. physically.

Going through the process of rebirthing allowed me to access deep feelings and old memories, including that of my own birth experience. Rebirthers have actually discovered that the circumstances of a person's birth are mirrored in his or her life patterns. (For example, induced people feel often rushed or pushed into things and people who've had emergency caesareans give things up half way through.) This is why rebirthers feel that the way babies are born is so important, and that a natural birth is a good start to life—it simply results in less emotional baggage. People who are drawn to rebirthing often are aware of birth patterns repeating themselves in their adult life, or they are simply people who feel stuck and want to move on from old patterns and have heard that rebirthing works wonders in unblocking stuff, however old or deep it is (not just birth trauma). It is possible to heal almost anything with breathing and love. Rebirthing also makes you deeply aware of how fully aware a baby is before birth, as during sessions people often revisit antenatal states as well as birth and realise how much they were sensing and feeling and how much they knew about what was happening to their parents and around them.

I believe the positive attitude of my independent midwives also helped me because comments about 'twins always being early' can act like a negative mantra. In fact, our twins were born five days past their due date! I'm sure my midwives' positivity and faith were crucial. People are usually scared of being positive in case things go wrong. But there's really nothing to lose. If things go wrong, people can deal with it and then at least they haven't spent months worrying. It's best to stay positive and open and just have awareness of what's happening.

The only antenatal tests I had were two scans. I had the second one—another ordinary scan (i.e. not a nuchal one)—because I was bleeding, as I was the first time. However, the scan showed us everything was OK. A great deal of pressure was put on me to have more scans but I resisted this because my husband and I had decided we wouldn't have a termination anyway, even if it were recommended. In any case, the early scan had at least made us aware that the babies were non-identical (with two placentas and two sacs), which is useful information for a twin pregnancy.

I had a fantastic pregnancy. I was extremely open, which meant I wasn't always feeling great! However, I was very much in tune with myself—even in terms of what I ate. Although I'd been vegetarian before I got pregnant, when—a couple of months into the pregnancy—I really started fancying meat, I ate it whenever I wanted to. The love of being pregnant can help you be yourself even more strongly than before. I sensed my babies were loving the things they were experiencing through me.

I think babies are living beings the moment they are conceived and what you experience of the world, they also experience. I visualised myself giving birth at 40 weeks because I really wanted them to have plenty of time to grow. I also talked to them a lot, using any positive words I could think of. I also let myself feel excited and curious about the magical process of giving birth. I expected to have a fantastic pregnancy, so I did!

Overall, I'd say the most important thing for me was to stay away from other people's fears. I did not want to be near anybody being negative—which is why I didn't go to the hospital or near some of my friends. We just said, "We know what we're doing. We don't need your opinion." I hardly had any negative feelings myself. As far as comments about my due date went, every time anybody said, "When's your due date?" and I would tell them and they'd reply, "Oh, they're going to be early because they're twins." I'd say, "No! Mine are not!" And they weren't.

My labour lasted about 15 hours, then I had this amazing urge to start pushing. At that point I just wanted to give birth. My heart was set on giving my two babies a beautiful birth, so I made sure I stayed positive—even though I knew one of my babies was breech. (The midwives had been able to tell this just by palpating my bump. Fortunately, they also knew how to deliver breech babies.) Anyway, it went very smoothly—although I was exhausted afterwards! There was no tearing. I started breastfeeding straight away. It really couldn't have gone any better.

Then, when the twins were 8 months old, we bought a big camper van and drove to Italy. The idea was to look for our dream: a property and land where we could start a new life and business. We did find a beautiful house and land, and a year and a half later we moved to Italy permanently.

The twins are now 4 and I'm still breastfeeding them! (They have wanted a lot less milk since they turned 3, so it's only occasionally now.) I became vegan a year after the twins were born, and they were vegan too until they were 3. Then we all started eating other things—I'm far too relaxed to be too restrictive. I just don't eat meat, and neither do my kids, only because by now we are not used to it any more. We now eat cheese, eggs and fish—with pulses every day (which the kids adore)—as well as seeds and a few nuts, soya, quinoa, etc.

If any other mother of twins—or singletons, for that matter—wants to breastfeed, I'd say stick with it, because it really does get easier and easier. The first few months are the hardest because the babies can't hold themselves up at all and with two it is harder, but it becomes second nature quite soon, both for Mum and the babies. One day you won't even remember what was so difficult. I had big problems in the first few days—it was so painful and I was so incredibly tired. Do contact a breastfeeding counsellor if you need to, even in the first week or two. Even if you have to pay it's well worth the money. A breastfeeding counsellor will teach you positions and all the tricks, including breastfeeding lying down—which is a real lifesaver! It is actually easier to breastfeed twins, than prepare bottlefeeds for two. Remember, it does soon become easy.

After the initial problems, I loved it, and so did my kids. Within a week, all the pain was gone for me. I was just tired then! The advice and support I got at the beginning really helped make it a positive experience. And once it became positive and comfortable, there really was no reason to stop.

Before I sign off, I really want to add a bit about John, my husband. He was so, so important in the whole process. He was really positive and supportive and didn't get involved with the fear stuff. If we ever had different opinions, which was rare, he very openly talked about it and we always found solutions that felt right for both of us. He was respectful of my feelings and needs, without forgetting his own, which also needed to be worked through. We actually did the rebirthing sessions together, and a couple of times the sessions ended up with me and the rebirther holding and cuddling and supporting him. Everybody's birth issues come up around birth, not just the mum's! It was so beautiful and free and loving that he could have his process and space around giving birth. It also allowed me to have more support when I needed it, particularly at the birth itself. At that time, he was just so, so amazing. He was there all the way, not just in body, but really with his whole self. We were truly together then just as we are now, as parents. I'm sure our children really feel this. We're in this together, the four of us.

I truly believe that whatever happens to anyone is just the perfect thing for them. Even if I had had a terrible birth, in the end it would have been OK. But, man, am I glad it went the way it did! Life is beautiful. If you're going through all this pregnancy thing now, I'd just say TRUST YOURSELF and allow yourself to feel all you need to feel. Allow yourself to be whatever you are. If you can, surround yourself with people who listen to you and who will support you in what you do. And listen to yourself at least as much as you listen to others, and possibly more. If other people's opinions clash with how you feel, don't dismiss yourself. You're important and special.

Gaia Pollini

Respond effectively

This is also important! How can you respond when you find you are affected by other people's comments, despite all your best efforts to protect yourself?

- ♥ Take note of whether the other person personally had the kind of optimal birth you yourself are preparing yourself for. If their own experience of birth was very different, why take their advice? Why be affected by comments from people who have no first-hand experience?
- ♥ Remember, as you listen to other people's comments and advice, that other people may not have done as much research as you have.
- ♥ Consider why people are taking a certain stand. Professionals may feel the need to prove their own theories so as to maintain their peace of mind. How else can they continue to operate in the way that they do with a clear conscience? Other women, who have not prepared as you have, may feel resentful of your plans. Perhaps it's all simply beyond their imagination.

- When discussing anything with your caregivers, be aware of any differences in emotional reaction when using specific words. I have a theory that what I shall call 'reactivity' is often high in pregnant women while it is low in professionals. For example, while a pregnant woman may react with shock on hearing the word 'episiotomy', a midwife may be unmoved. So before you respond in any interaction consider how your own speech might be affected by these differences in 'reactivity'. Do you feel at a disadvantage because you're having to deal with more emotion? If so, explain that first...
- Whenever you are anticipating or dealing with other people's reactions to what you say (whether over a cup of coffee or at an antenatal appointment), consider the influence you yourself are having on the conversation. Don't you think it's possible that certain ways of speaking might trigger negative reactions? Consider, for example, a woman who has had a caesarean for a previous birth, who is now contemplating a normal, vaginal birth (a VBAC). If she mentions the word 'caesarean' to someone else (whoever that might be) isn't it just possible the word itself might be associated with procedures fit for a queen (or emperor, at the very least)? The word 'vaginal' by contrast, is perhaps hardly an appropriate word for a conversation at work, with people you don't know intimately. Is there perhaps not a bit of sexism involved in the fact that women are almost expected to talk publicly about intimate matters? Imagine a possible equivalent conversation between male colleagues, standing at the photocopier in an open-plan office...

    "No luck with the IVF then..."
    "Oh... right. Well, I've given up on that. I'm going for a PBAV now."
    "P-bav? Sorry, you've lost me..."
    "Penis birth after in-vitro. We're having a trial of penis."

    Extreme? Perhaps... but isn't it odd the way we're so open and isn't it possible that the use of phrases such as 'trial of labour' might provoke a negative response? (The word 'trial' is not always or even often associated with success. Imagine a teenager saying, "But, Dad... Just let me try!")
- Building on the idea that what you say can actually *trigger* responses in other people, consider being creative with your own ways of talking. Even if everybody else calls that flexible passageway between your legs a 'birth canal' (which—as already explained on page 253—sounds solid, instead of expandable and soft) YOU can say the baby will travel 'down through my body'... and that might well change the way other people respond to you. You really can choose what you say to other people and how you say it.
- Finally, work on developing your awareness of any newly-acquired fears and worries. Acknowledge their existence and then take any action necessary to dissipate them. This may mean talking to someone; it may mean lending this or another book to a person who's affecting you; it may mean finding a new midwife (even if that means registering with another GP or consultant); it may mean paying more; it may also mean changing your arrangements for the birth itself. This is important because your own emotional response to the comments other people make to you could actually affect the whole course of your labour—since emotions are so closely linked with hormones.

> I asked my mother to be with me for the birth of our second child, so I had to tell her I planned to have the baby at home. I explained how there are rarely situations when a midwife would let you stay at home if there are any warning signs; that warning signals show up days or hours before there is any real danger to you or the fetus; that we were within a few minutes' ambulance ride of a hospital. I explained why I wanted to be at home. She was comfortable with the idea once she had the facts.

Birthframe 89

Sometimes maybe it really is impossible to avoid other people's negativity. Here's a birth which was not at all straightforward because of a general lack of support... It illustrates very clearly the need to deal with potential psychological issues well before you go into labour.

While I was researching this book I got chatting to an old friend, who said she thought natural birth was all very well as long as it didn't last for five days, as had happened in her case! Five nights actually.

Her story was initially strange and perplexing: when she was 36 weeks' pregnant, for five nights in a row, she experienced strong contractions but each morning, as the sun rose, her contractions came to a complete halt. Eventually, her labour was augmented and her baby pulled out with forceps.

Since I know this woman quite well, I asked her if she'd mind if I asked some questions. Very quickly, I ventured to suggest why she might have had this stop-start labour... My friend immediately agreed with my interpretation. First of all, it was an unplanned pregnancy in a very well-established relationship where it had been agreed there would be no children. Her partner had reacted badly to the news of the pregnancy and had made no secret of his reluctance to go ahead with it. Apparently, even while she was in labour, this woman's partner had complained about her having a baby! Secondly, this woman had conceived just three months after the death of her mother, who she had been very close to; throughout her labour she said she had longed to have her mother's support. With so much emotional baggage, it's hardly surprising this woman couldn't relax into labour. And given the father's strong negative feelings, it was as if she felt she needed to have the baby in secret, in the dead of night, as it were. But on some level of her mind, she was not even allowing herself to have this baby.

This story does have a happy ending. The child is now a healthy and happy 13-year-old. After being looked after by her mother for the first year, her father became her main caregiver because this is what worked out best financially—although her mother continued to breastfeed her until she was 3½ years old. Despite the enormous change this new baby made to her parent's lifestyle, she is now much loved by both parents and they all make a wonderful family. I know this because they all came to visit very recently.

(By the way, the mother did check, edit and approve this account.)

As I've already said, the possibility of being disturbed by professionals also needs to be taken seriously. Often, they tend to disturb women before the placenta is born, which dramatically raises the risk of a life-threatening haemorrhage. (The World Health Organization (WHO) estimates that every year a staggering 14 million women have a postpartum haemorrhage and that around half a million die as a result every year.)[6] It seems this risk arises when women are disturbed precisely because their state of mind is irrevocably changed and this too often causes dramatic physiological consequences.

Birthframe 90

Here, Michel describes how non-disturbance works in practice. You might consider showing this to your midwife and husband before the birth—or at least including a detailed note on avoiding this kind of disturbance in your care guide. (This is an extract from one of Michel's Primal Health Centre's newsletters.)[7]

> Over the years I have come to the conclusion that postpartum haemorrhages are almost always related to inappropriate interference. Postpartum haemorrhage would be extremely rare if a few simple rules were understood and observed. I am so convinced of the importance of these simple rules that twice I have agreed to attend a home birth, even though in each case I knew the woman's previous birth was followed by a manual removal of the placenta and a blood transfusion. These rules result in an approach which is in stark contrast to 'expectant' or so-called 'physiological' management used in randomised studies.
>
> First, it is important to create the conditions for the 'fetus ejection reflex', which is a short series of irresistible contractions which allow no room for voluntary movements. If this is done, the need for privacy and the need to feel secure are met. The fetus ejection reflex typically occurs when there is nobody around but an experienced, motherly, silent and low-profile midwife sitting in a corner and, for example, knitting. Knitting—or a similar repetitive task—helps the midwife to maintain her own level of adrenaline as low as possible.
>
> When conditions are physiological, at the very moment of birth most women tend to be upright, probably because of a momentary peak of adrenaline. They may be on their knees, or standing up and leaning on something. After an unmedicated delivery, it only takes a few seconds to hear and to see that the baby is in good shape. Then, in most cases, my first preoccupation is to warm the room. In the French hospital where I used to work, we just had to pull a string to switch on heating lamps. In the case of a planned home birth, instead of a written list of what to prepare, I focus on the need for a transportable heater that can be plugged in anywhere and at any time (including practical details, such as the need for an extension cord). When the heater is on it is possible, within a few seconds, to warm up blankets or towels and, if necessary, to cover the mother's and the baby's bodies. During the hour following birth women rarely complain that it is too hot. If the mother is shivering, it is not psychological: it means that the place is not warm enough.

It's vital after the birth for both mother and baby to be warm

From that time my main concern is that the mother is not distracted at all and does not feel observed. I want to make sure that she feels free to hold her baby, to look into her or his eyes and to smell her or him. It is easier to avoid disturbances if the light is kept dimmed and the telephone unplugged. I often invite the baby's father (or any other person who might be around) into another room to explain that this first interaction between mother and baby will never happen again and should not be disturbed. Many men have a tendency to break the sacredness of the atmosphere that ideally follows an undisturbed birth.

During the first hour after the birth, I remain as silent as possible and keep a low profile. Either I sit down in a corner behind the mother and baby, or I disappear if there is an experienced doula present with personal experience of this situation. Minutes after giving birth many mothers are no longer comfortable in an upright position. This is most likely the time when their level of adrenaline is decreasing and when women feel the contractions associated with the separation of the placenta. The birth attendant may have to hold the baby for some seconds, in order for the mother to find a comfortable position, almost always lying down on one side. After that there is no excuse for interfering with the interaction between mother and baby.

For an hour I don't go anywhere near either the cord or the placenta. Clamping and cutting the cord before the delivery of the placenta is a dangerous distraction. Suggesting a position to the mother is another unneeded distraction. Her position is the consequence of her level of adrenaline. When her level of adrenaline is low and she feels the need to lie down, it would be unkind and unphysiological to suggest an upright position.

It is only when an hour has passed after the birth—if the placenta has not yet emerged—that I dare to disturb the mother in order to check that the placenta is at least separated from the uterus. With the mother on her back I press the abdominal wall just above the pubic bone with my fingertips: if the cord does not move, it means that the placenta is separated. In practice, the placenta is always either delivered or separated an hour after the birth, and bleeding is minimal, provided the third stage has not been 'managed'. I have never had to inject a uterotonic drug to control bleeding.

Privacy and silence are both essential...

Such an attitude, based first on clinical observation, is based on physiological considerations. An easy delivery of the placenta with moderate blood loss implies that, immediately after the birth of the baby, a surge of oxytocin has been released. It is well-known that oxytocin release is highly dependant on environmental factors. It can be inhibited by adrenaline. This is more than empirical knowledge. A team from Sapporo, Japan (Saito et al 1991)[8] has studied the levels of adrenaline during the different phases of labour extensively by a non-invasive method (recording with a patch and analysing the skin microvibration pattern of the palmar side of the hand) and confirmed the findings of a previous study in which adrenaline levels were measured through indwelling catheters (Lederman et al 1978).[9] The Japanese team clearly demonstrated that postpartum haemorrhages are associated with high levels of adrenaline. The release of oxytocin can also be inhibited by the activity of the neocortex. After a physiological birth, the mother is still in a special state of consciousness, as if 'on another planet'. Her neocortex is still more or less at rest so my advice is: "Don't wake the mother up!" Once again, I must emphasise the need for privacy and silence.

Find friends

You may think I'm being very negative about other people, by suggesting you avoid them in various ways. Actually, they're often wonderful! Let's turn the problem on its head and make it into an opportunity... Whenever you become aware of anybody who might potentially cause you problems, replace him or her with someone supportive! Do this by getting in touch with like-minded pregnant women and professionals. Find them by contacting your local antenatal groups, a local doula, a local independent midwife, a local breastfeeding group, any local home birth organisation—or even by looking through advertisements in magazines. The Useful contacts list at the back of the book should help! Perhaps start by contacting La Leche League, who run monthly meetings for pregnant women and new mothers who are interested in breastfeeding, or contact the National Childbirth Trust (NCT).

> Whenever you become aware of anybody who might cause you problems, replace him or her with someone supportive

Learn from past mistakes

This is another thing you can do to help your mind prepare for the birth. Just as Justine Rowan (in Birthframe 84) thought about her past reactions to hospitals when sorting through her emotions, women who've actually already given birth in hospital need to think about their past experience of that. If you've already had a home birth and it wasn't ideal, you might need to think about what could be done better this time round. After all, the !Kung San tribe think childbirth is just a question of practice! Remember how many people you've read about in this book who learned from previous birthing experiences so as to improve their next experience? (Remember Maria Shanahan and Pauline Farrance?) Liliana Lammers is another person who learned by having a bad experience for the birth of her first baby.

Birthframe 91

In her first labour, Liliana—the doula we met earlier in this book— experienced the effects of having a lot of people watching while she was at the pushing stage. (One doctor, a midwife and 10 students were watching!) This made her decide to avoid hospitals for any future births. With her first birth, the atmosphere of the hospital, the insensitivity of the people, the monitoring—all constituting an atmosphere of feeling very 'observed'—clearly stopped her labour from progressing. The psychological aspect of giving birth is very clear from her three subsequent births. Here, again, we see how positive birth experiences can be when there is no disturbance from outside.

In 1987 I was expecting for the second time. I kept well away from doctors, hospitals and all their machinery. I was feeling wonderful—I knew my baby was well. I wanted to stay at home this time. A friend of mine mentioned Michel Odent... I read a bit about him... "Yes, he will understand me." He did. I had the most beautiful, undisturbed birth one can possibly imagine. Another daughter.

And two years later my son was born. Big boy, 9lb 8oz. Born between lunch and dessert! Literally. I was so lucky to be assisted by Michel Odent again.

I was in labour, but very hungry, to everyone's surprise. I had a big lunch and then, when the cake I had baked that morning was approaching the kitchen table, I stood up suddenly and with an unusually loud voice said, "No pudding. The baby's coming!"—and turning to my partner: "Do the dishes." After this, I rushed into a dark room I had prepared, went on my knees, on the floor, burying my head in pillows.

One and a half hours later I was lying down on the floor, my baby on my chest, both warmly wrapped, the cord not yet cut... and eating the cake! (This child is now 17 and has always had an incredible appetite.)

My fourth child was born at dawn, in a friend's living room, at a time when I could only hear the birds singing... and Michel Odent gently sleeping at the other end of the room. It was so magical, sweet, beautiful. My baby girl found the breast in minutes!

Liliana Lammers

In case this completely non-interventionist, undisturbed approach still shocks you, let's remind ourselves what we're aiming for. We're talking about birth which takes place entirely naturally (as in Liliana's births) unless medical intervention is needed. Remember how intervention proved to be necessary in Birthframe 6, when Liliana's daughter needed a C-section? Some comments by Miranda Castro (in her book on homeopathy for pregnancy and childbirth *Mother and Baby* (Pan Books 1996) may help you to see what I mean here, if you're still doubtful. She was actually writing about illness, but her comments apply just as well to childbirth:

The presence of disease or pain often creates anxiety, which in turn can lead to fear and panic. Most of us have consulted an authoritative figure (a doctor) to allay our anxiety by putting a name to what is happening to our bodies, and to determine how it must be treated. The danger here is that, in looking outside ourselves for the answers and in asking too few questions, we experience a loss of personal control and consequent feelings of helplessness. We give up responsibility for our own health to the people 'in charge' and we become real patients, or, as I see it, victims. We find that we feel unable to confide misgivings, to express our instincts about our own health, or to explore other options. We become passive consumers of medical care.

> Most of us have consulted an authoritative figure (a doctor)... The danger is in looking outside ourselves for the answers and asking too few questions

How can we stop behaving like passive patients, but still stay safe and sensible? We need to become informed by reading and talking to people who are sympathetic to our views (and doubts), and who may have had similar experiences. We must also learn to ask for what we need, to make realistic demands of health care professionals, and to seek the help of doctors and specialists, both orthodox and alternative, who are willing to communicate with us and acknowledge that we too have a part to play. By taking responsibility for what happens to our bodies we can begin to create for ourselves the balance we want in our lives, and tune into our own feelings, or inner sense, of what is wrong. By developing a positive approach, we can also move away from automatically taking a defensive position.

> Believe in nature's ability to get birth right (generally) and try and stay relaxed about it all. Find out as much as you can about your choices and remember who's in charge—YOU are! *Debbie Brindley*

Solve any practical conundrums

This may seem obvious, but it's surprising how often women forget to do this! It's not always deep psychological issues that need resolving. Sometimes worries are about things going on around us.

Birthframe 92

Here's an example of a very straightforward issue that needed to be resolved before labour was able to proceed smoothly.

I was due on 3 July. It came and went with not even a sign of anything happening. As ridiculous as it sounds, I really could not believe that this baby was going to come! My sister, Kate, in South Africa, had long decided that she was coming to visit with her two girls and husband to see the new baby and help me and Matt in the early weeks. I began to get more and more anxious about her visit as she was arriving on 31 July and the later the baby was in coming, the less time Matt and I would have settling in with him. And as I had no idea what it was going to be like to have a newborn baby I was anxious about all of them staying with us.

On Friday, 9 July my midwife, Margaret, visited me. I told her how anxious I was about Kate's visit. She said I should deal with this as my anxiety could be going some way to preventing the baby from coming. What would help lessen my anxiety? I was torn between wanting my sister to stay, on the one hand, because we had this great new house and because I see so little of her and we'd had such a great time when they were out last year for our wedding... and on the other hand, wanting to settle in with the baby, just the three of us.

I got more and more anxious about my sister's visit.
I was anxious about all of them staying with us...

> The other option of having her stay at my Mum's didn't seem any better because I just felt guilty at the thought. We had so much space, whereas my Mum has so little. Matt and I discussed it and decided to ask his parents whether my sister and her family could stay at Bathurst Mews. Matt and I had lived there for a year and had moved out at the end of May. The only problem was that it looked very bare as we'd taken all our stuff and left only a couple of beds, a few chairs and the dining room suite and Alan, Matt's Dad, was planning to move everything out to redecorate the house. Alan agreed that they could stay for the first week and then we would see how I was doing. I felt enormously relieved. Kate was very understanding and happy with the arrangement. At least they could also have their own space as a family.
>
> On Saturday morning, 10 July, I woke early, at about 6.30am with what felt distinctly like period pains. I knew immediately that this was the real thing and not a false alarm.
>
> *Joanne Searle*

Visualise a good birth

Finally, you need to visualise a positive outcome for yourself and your baby.[10] How can you do this?

- ♥ Tell yourself you're going to succeed! If you like the idea, repeat affirmations—for example: "I can give birth easily. My body knows how to do it. I'll be able to cope."
- ♥ Visualise possible scenarios, with positive outcomes. Consider how your labour might start. Consider what kind of disturbance you might encounter and how you might deal with it. It's amazing actually just how much disturbance we can cope with!—especially if we continue to assert our wishes to our caregivers or any birth attendants we have around.
- ♥ Help yourself to overcome the negative imagery of obstetric words by using imaginative alternatives. For example, consider using language like 'baby within', instead of 'fetus' (as I do in this book). Perhaps think in terms of 'expansions', 'waves' or 'zoomings' (instead of 'contractions'), contemplate using the phrase 'vaginal passage' (instead of 'birth canal') and say 'birth' instead of 'delivery'. Have fun creating your new vocabulary... Language is a powerful tool and deserves to be used!
- ♥ Mentally correct people who use 'you' inappropriately to talk about negative possibilities. People merrily say: "If you get [Awful Situation Everyone Dreads], you'll [Awful Experience No. 1] and you'll find that [Awful Experience No. 2]." Aaargh! Have you noticed how I've avoided doing that all through this book? I only want to suggest positive outcomes to you. And don't think, "No, I'm not going to get..." because if I say don't visualise a blue horse, you'll almost certainly 'see' one. Say something positive to yourself, like: "I'm going to have a healthy outcome. My body and my baby are both going to be fine."

♥ Visualise yourself coping well with whatever sensations you experience at each stage. Imagine yourself smiling or in deep concentration. Visualise yourself in a completely new state of mind.

Visualising yourself coping with pain may be helpful. Many women complain after they've given birth for the first time that they were not adequately prepared for the pain. Perhaps, instead of the word 'pain', they've used words like 'pressure', 'contractions' or 'ache' in an effort to visualise things positively (which is fine) but have made this into a form of self-denial. Or maybe they've pushed the possibility of pain right out of their minds because of fear.

As we've already acknowledged, for most women, having a baby really is an extremely painful experience. It's more painful than anything they've ever experienced before. Each time I experienced the pain, in each of my three optimal labours, I was shocked at how extreme it was at times. But it really was possible to edge myself forward from moment to moment, minute to minute, and it was completely over after a few hours, which is not the case when women have so-called 'pain relief'. They experience both physical and emotional pain after the birth, and it seems their babies do too.

If you find yourself unable to imagine yourself coping, remember that you will still have certain things to 'do' to help yourself. You'll be able to move around, listen to music, use hot or cold water (in a shower, batht or birthing pool); you'll be able to make any sounds you feel like making; you can have someone massage you... and you'll have privacy.

Also, remember that when the time comes and you're in labour, if you labour in privacy, without drugs disturbing your system, you will drift into another state of mind which will automatically help you to cope.[11]

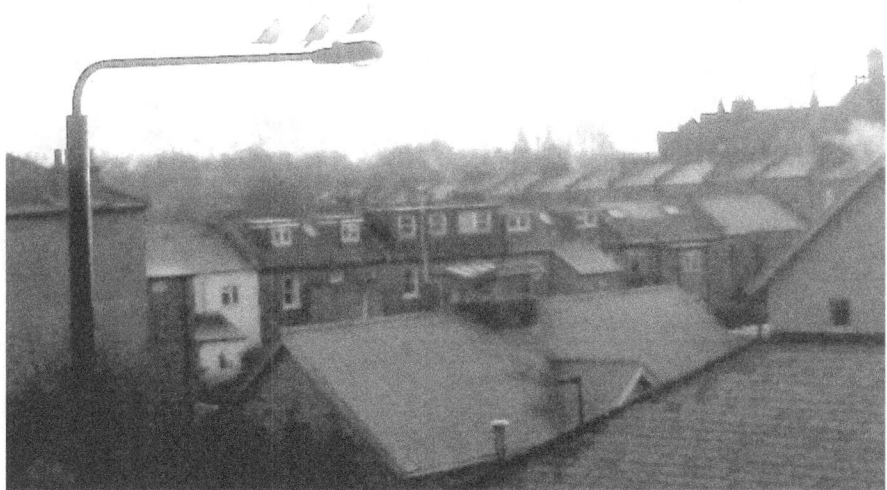

There are other people out there who've done this too, you know

What about the moment of birth itself? Spend a few minutes—perhaps even 30 minutes or an hour—sitting quietly, visualising yourself giving birth. Imagine the sensations developing through labour... Imagine your body gradually opening up. See yourself becoming increasingly active, increasingly powerful, increasingly alive. Then, suddenly—or gradually—your baby will emerge, coming down through your open, supple body, out into the world.

The sensations may be difficult to imagine, particularly if you've never experienced them before, or if you're planning a completely different, optimal birth this time. But you can visualise your future far better than you may think possible. If you find it difficult, or even impossible, the first time you try, do this visualisation exercise again, and again, and again. Allow yourself to experience any emotions which arise. Allow yourself to cry, to feel angry, to experience fear... whatever emotions come bubbling up from deep inside you. Use other ways of releasing these emotions too, so that you can more vividly see yourself really having the optimal birth you're planning: walk, sing, dance, draw pictures, talk for hours to people you trust... Do whatever you feel is going to be helpful.

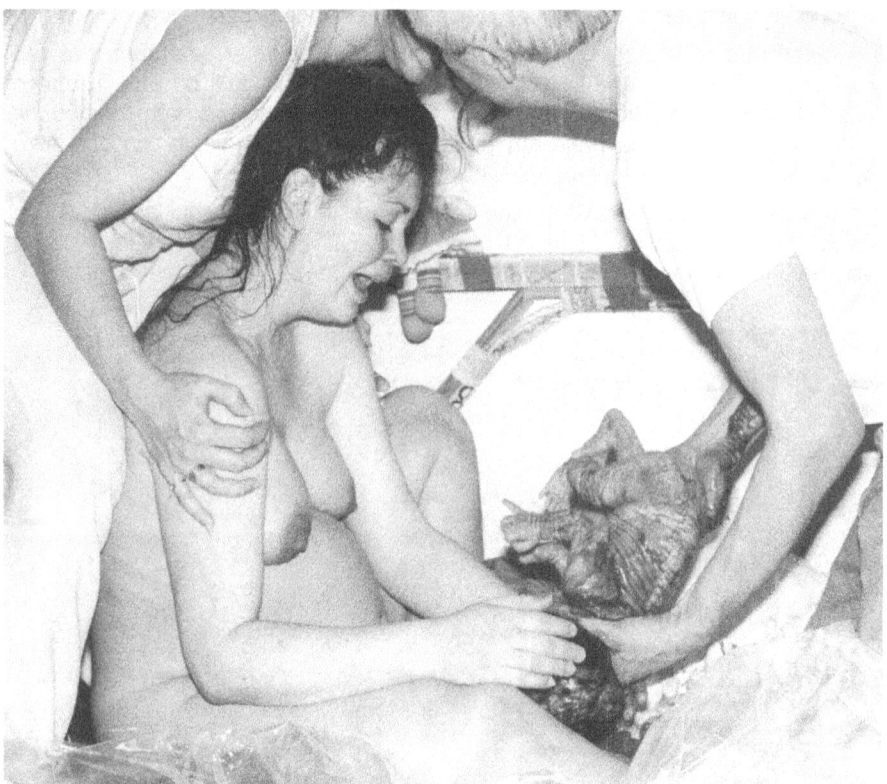

Either you will pick up your baby yourself, or your birth attendant(s) will help you

Photos left and below © Jill Furmanovsky (www.jillfurmanovsky.com)

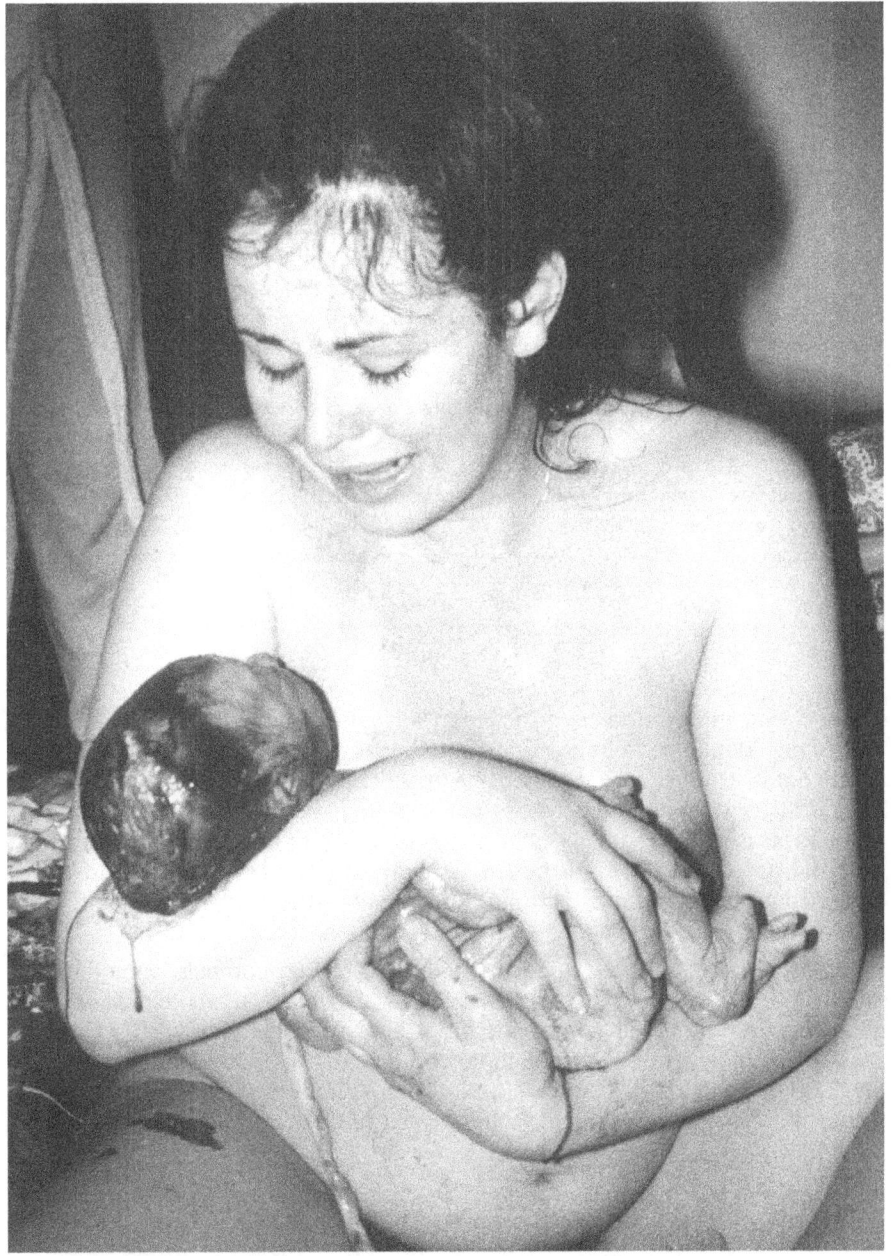

*Don't worry if there's a bit of blood on your baby—it can soon be wiped off...
You will at last be together with your new baby! Your new life will have begun.*

Birthframe 93

Here's an account which beautifully captures the memory of 'going to another planet'… the process which allows women to tune into their instinctual knowledge of how to give birth.

> My waters broke very, very early in the morning and then she wasn't born until after midnight. The labour was all that day—all morning, afternoon and evening—and she was born after midnight. So it was less than 24 hours. It was very slow for a long time. I phoned Michel and he said "Oh it's fine. It'll be all right. I'll come along later." I don't think I was having contractions then—only very slight ones. He came to see me, then he went home again. He was able to go backwards and forwards a little bit, although there was one point when he knew it was getting close and he said he'd stay.
>
> I don't know what I can remember of the labour—it was just very hard work. A lot of resting. Very hard work. Completely closed off from the rest of the world. I remember asking David once to get me a mango and he went out and bought me a mango which I didn't finish. It was actually too much to eat a mango because I had to concentrate. I went really deep, deep within. Quite spontaneously.
>
> And I remember the next morning when I woke up I thought, "Oh, I'm here, back in the world again." I looked out of the window and people were doing normal, everyday things. I felt like saying, "Don't they realise what's just happened here?!"
>
> *Fiona Lucy Stoppard*

Even if you find you don't 'go to another planet' (because of unnecessary and unavoidable disturbance) you will still be able to take things moment by moment. Nature has designed the process such that the sensations get progressively stronger, usually—but not always—becoming most painful at the time of the birth. Having said that, I should add that my second baby's birth, which was the least disturbed, was actually painfree. It was only the contractions leading up to it which were painful—the pushing was fine. And remember it was all completely over after two hours.

In each moment you will need to think only of that particular moment, not of the whole of the rest of your labour. Even the most painful sensations will change and you'll find some way of coping. Imagine yourself doing this. Visualise yourself alone, dressed in an ordinary T-shirt or other loose clothing—or naked!—perhaps in candlelight, with some gentle music playing in the background. (Have you prepared that music compilation as I suggested before? Do it now!)

Each moment think only of that particular moment…
even the most painful sensations will change

Birthframe 94

I got talking to the woman who contributed this account while I was at a playgroup, heavily pregnant with my third child...

I always enjoyed the conversations at playgroups when they invariably came round to the subject of childbirth, a bit like discussing exam results when you know you've done well! It seems that I have been one of the lucky ones and, yes, it does happen.

As the due date of my first child loomed, my mother did admit that she had not had too much trouble giving birth to my three siblings and myself, though you don't know how much gets forgotten over time. In those days it was customary to have the first child in hospital and any further births at home, so in the back of my mind I felt confident that if we had more than one child, I too could enjoy a home delivery. Also, I felt that at long last my wide hips may be coming into their own!

The delivery of your first baby is certainly a surprise. Nothing can prepare you for what is going to happen. I was well planned for the event: I had given up work six weeks before, had rested at home, spent sessions at the local swimming pool building up my stamina, requested a water birth at the hospital and had even spent time taping my favourite music ready for the hours I expected to be in labour.

When the time arrived, not even knowing that I was in labour but wondering why I had been sick and why was I suffering from what I thought to be bad period pains, we drove to the maternity hospital. On arrival at around 6.00am, I was examined by a midwife. To her surprise, she found that I was sufficiently dilated to move to a delivery suite. Once we were there and I had climbed onto the bed, she went in search of pain relief. Within minutes, however, my waters had gone and I was ready to push! As my husband called for someone 'quickly', I couldn't believe that it was all happening so fast. There wasn't sufficient time for any pethidine, so I was offered gas and air. When the moment came to push I pushed as hard as I could and, after a short amount of pain, our son was born at 7.10am weighing in at 8lb 8oz—and I didn't even need any stitches.

So when it came to the due date of our second child, I wondered if I would have a similar easy delivery. Again, things seemed to get going early in the morning (after a good night's sleep) and I awoke again to uncomfortable period pains. I was adamant that I was going to have a shower before the midwife arrived to assess me, and even managed to wash my hair! In the meantime, slightly apprehensively, my husband called the midwife at 6.30am. When she arrived around 7.20am and asked me to lie down on the bed, I knew that as soon as I lay down I wouldn't be going anywhere. Again, after one massive push our daughter was born at 7.42am, weighing in at 9lb 8oz. Throughout the time, I had been totally calm and when I saw how relaxed the midwife was, I felt I too had little to worry about. My body took over.

> When I saw how relaxed the midwife was I felt I had little to worry about. My body took over.

So when it came to the due date of our third child, I felt we ought to be a little more organised at home, and get the midwife to drop off the home delivery pack. My midwife was more than happy with a home delivery, but my doctor certainly did not agree with it. (He believed that babies should be born in hospital.) So I told him that I would endeavour to get to hospital but was fairly sure that I would not make it in time and did not want to be one of those stories in *Woman's Own*—"MOTHER GIVES BIRTH ON HER FRONT DOOR STEP"!

So with everything in place, the due date arrived. My first child had been two days late, the second four days late, so how long did I have to wait for my third? As we got to three days late and me willing things to get going, I went to bed. During the night things started but, as the midwife advised, the baby was lying the wrong way round and I needed him to turn, so off she went. I returned to bed, lay on my side and left it to the baby to get himself into position and after one large contraction, he managed to and was ready to make his entrance. As we called the midwife again at around 8.15am the next day, which was a Tuesday morning, we failed to realise that perhaps the morning traffic would influence her arrival. This time we were on our own, and the thought did cross my mind as to what I was doing. I was worried about being on my own and even began to think that perhaps I should have listened to the doctor and gone to hospital. I felt let down by the midwife because instead of being a perfect delivery I was worried that something might go wrong. However, again, my body (and some say Mother Nature) took over. At 8.55am the midwife arrived just as our son was born. His amniotic sac was still intact, which apparently means that this delivery was slow and controlled.

I had been so lucky. All three of my children's births had been easy and relatively painless. With the second and third I had not had any pain relief. Also, the fact that the deliveries had been quick was a real benefit for my recovery and also my babies', who had not suffered any trauma and were all calm and relaxed babies. It used to cross my mind occasionally whether I ought to offer to be a surrogate mother as really I had enjoyed easy pregnancies and very easy births.

Sue Pakes

As well as visualising fast labours for yourself, like Sue's, also visualise some painfree labours... Why not, after all?! Painfree labours are not myths—some women really do experience them. With the right attitude and awareness, labouring in a supportive but private environment, you may only experience what is happening in your body as unusual or even pleasant. Some women even liken giving birth to having an orgasm. So visualise this as a possibility too! Precisely the same hormone is involved in making contractions happen as the one which causes an orgasm... oxytocin, the hormone of love.[12]

*Life can be even better than we expect,
even if it turns out somewhat different*

Birthframe 95

Rachel, the next contributor, was amazed to find her labour and birth really did happen as Michel had predicted! (He has, after all, witnessed a lot of births.) When we are truly undisturbed in labour and our underlying attitude is right, any pain we might experience goes beyond the 'toothache' type of pain, into something altogether different...

I gave birth at home, at age 38, in water without using any drugs. My [identical] twin sister had had a baby the previous year, with the usual story of failed home delivery due to minor complications followed by the cascade of interventions at hospital ending in a caesarean.

I read Michel Odent's *Birth Reborn* and was inspired at the stories of natural births—the fact that he finally avoided the use of chemical pain relief altogether because it seemed to interfere with the natural pain-relieving processes of the body.

I searched widely for a sympathetic midwife and was so lucky to eventually find one, who visited me at home and helped my confidence. I think state of mind is so important—I also did some hypnosis, or visualisation of the birthing process, which I think helped.

My baby was born after a nine-hour labour. To my amazement, it was like Michel described—I became almost like an animal, or went into another level of consciousness beyond pain. The part I remember as the most difficult was the beginning—moments of fear—then gaining confidence—more moments of fear—reassurance from the midwife—then feeling like a fish in water being thrown about by the contractions and finally roaring as she came out, not with pain (as is so often the stereotype we see of labouring women) but with power.

It left me feeling so proud of my body.

Rachel Urbach

Embrace the unexpected

Sometimes birth is not wildly better or worse than we expect. Sometimes it's just different...

Birthframe 96

This woman's labour rather took her by surprise. Although she briefly and somewhat unnecessarily reached for the TENS machine at one point, her labour was almost entirely normal. Even though it was not ideal that she should have so many interruptions between the birth of the baby and the birth of the placenta from a safety point of view, the third stage also went smoothly. After a highly interventionist first birth, it was obviously a relief for this woman to have a low-tech, completely unsupervised birth, when she was left to follow her own instincts.

The players: Me—Ruth, and Adam—my husband
Ben—the star player
Eddy—our 2-year-old son
Sue—my midwife
Julie—my other midwife
Maggie—supporter for Ruth and Adam
Kerry—supporter for Eddy
Daniel—supporter for Eddy and also my brother

My first birth experience hadn't been as I had hoped. Due to a premature footling breech my plans for a home birth had been well and truly ruined. So this time round I was two times as determined to have my baby at home. I was delighted when I discovered the baby was cephalic (a perfect LOA) and ecstatic once we got past that magical 37 weeks [after which point NHS midwives will cover a home birth]. In fact I was really excited about going into labour, no worries about anything... This was going to be good and everything that my last labour wasn't. My NHS midwives were supportive and we got on really well.

I was woken on 15 January at 5.00am by Eddy, who was crying. As I went in to see him I noticed a slight discomfort in my lower abdomen that was coming and going, I put this down to wind. After dealing with Eddy I went back to bed and listened to him singing and talking to himself until he went back to sleep at 6.15. All this time I was aware of the abdominal discomfort, only slight but enough to keep me awake (I am a light sleeper).

At 6.30 I decided that I needed to open my bowels. I thought I would feel better after this but I didn't, if anything I felt slightly worse. I wondered if, as this was six days before my due date, these were contractions and decided that if they were they must be Braxton Hicks.

At 7.00am I got up and fed the cats (all seven of them). The contractions were now coming about every 10 minutes and were getting stronger and longer but were easily bearable—I just breathed through them. I now also noticed a lower back pain but still did not think that I was in labour.

At 7.15am I needed the toilet again, this time it was much looser and I noticed a show. I wondered if this was the real thing as there were now four signs but I was not convinced.

At 7.30am I thought that maybe I should wake Adam. I told him I thought that I might be in labour; he said OK and did I need him, and then he went back to sleep. I decided I'd better phone the other people who were due to come over. Kerry had just arrived home from working a night shift and she had taken a sleeping tablet and was about to go to bed; she was not going to miss this for the world and set out to walk across town to our house. Daniel was on his way to work so I couldn't get hold of him. Maggie did not answer her phone (it was broken), so I phoned her partner's mobile phone; he was halfway across the country but managed to get a message to Maggie via relatives who live nearby. I got hold of Daniel at 7.55am, I told him there was no rush as he wanted to go elsewhere on the way.

By 8.00am Adam was getting out of bed. I saw him naked at the top of the stairs, and through bleary eyes he told me he needed to go to the toilet. I told him in no uncertain terms: "I need to go first." And once again I opened my bowels. My contractions were now very close together.

At 8.05am, still sitting on the toilet, I had the first really intense contraction. It was very different to the previous ones, which had all been really low down and opening-out type contractions. This one was from the top of my uterus, a really strong pushing contraction. My first thought was that this shouldn't be happening yet, I couldn't possibly be at this part of my labour as I hadn't had the painful bit yet. However my body was pushing and there was nothing I could do that was going to stop it.

I then decided that I needed to do my hair (which is down to my waist), so I unplaited it and asked Adam for my hairbrush. I also decided that I needed my TENS machine on; it was far too late for this but it seemed the right thing to do at the time.

After two or three more contractions I put my hand down between my legs and could feel something sticking out! I lifted myself off the toilet seat and asked Adam what it was... it was the amniotic membranes bulging out and was about the size of a grapefruit. At this point I decided that I needed a midwife rather urgently. She was the one person that I had omitted to phone when I made my calls earlier so she didn't even know I was in labour.

Adam went downstairs and called the labour hotline. He asked to speak to Sue. The person on the other end told him that she was a community midwife and he would have to call their office. He came back up to me moaning about this and how useless they were. "Did you tell them that I am in labour?"... "Oh... no". He went back downstairs and tried again.

At 8.25am Sue phoned back. She heard me shout out at the next contraction and suggested to Adam that he should be upstairs with me. I then shouted down that I could feel the baby's head. Sue said that she would phone back in two minutes once Adam had put the phone on the extension upstairs.

I instinctively kept my hand on the baby's head from when I first felt it. The next contraction came and the head moved out a bit and then back in again. Adam brought the phone upstairs and began to spread a groundsheet on the floor so that I could get off the toilet. As he finished doing this I had another contraction. With this one my waters broke, out came the baby's head followed by his body. As I delivered my baby I lifted myself off the toilet seat, brought him up between my legs and cradled our second son in my arms as I sat back down again. Adam looked round and folded the groundsheet back up again. Then the phone rang, it was Maggie. Adam asked her the time, so we now knew our new son had been born at 8.30am. Almost immediately the phone buzzed again. It was Sue, expecting to talk Adam through the birth. He just said, "Listen!" She heard the cries and asked if we were OK.

She heard the cries and asked if we were OK

She also asked if we wanted to call an ambulance or just wait until she got there. As we were fine we said we would wait and she said that she would get there as soon as possible. I offered baby my breast but he nuzzled at my nipple for a bit and then went to sleep.

At 8.35am Eddy appeared in the bathroom doorway, he looked at me sitting on the toilet and said, "Baby!" and then came to join us. Adam got a big towel to wrap around baby and me to keep us warm and then decided that he'd better get some clothes on before everyone arrived; he'd had no time to dress up to this point and I had been wearing his bathrobe. I then asked Adam to take some photos while the cord was still intact. Kerry arrived first and took some photos of all four of us, she then looked after Eddy.

At 9.00am Julie arrived. She had got dressed in the dark in a hurry and was wearing pink socks with her dark blue uniform and she had also been stopped by the police for speeding on her way to me. (They let her go as soon as she explained the situation.) As the cord had stopped pulsating, I was happy for her to clamp it and Adam cut it. Baby was then wrapped in another towel and Adam had his first cuddle while Julie helped me off the toilet and onto the floor. Adam then put baby on the floor so that I could lean against him while the placenta was born. While I was waiting for the placenta I noticed my window cleaner cleaning the bathroom window! At 9.10 I had a contraction and felt the placenta move down. Two minutes later I had another smaller one with which the placenta was born. Julie examined me and told me that I had sustained a small tear, which I decided not to have stitched. I stayed sitting on the floor while baby was checked and weighed. He was 7lb 12oz.

By this time Daniel, Maggie and Sue had arrived; Sue was later than she had hoped because she had skidded on ice and put her car into a ditch. At some point another midwife arrived but I have no idea who she was and she left once Sue got there. Maggie ran a bath for me and made drinks for everyone. Adam stood on our back doorstep to have a cigarette and shook a bit—poor chap still hadn't been to the toilet. I took baby into the bath with me where he had his first breastfeed for about 20 minutes. Eddy kept coming up to check on us and look at his new brother.

I was then dispatched to my bed even though I felt full of energy and not the least bit tired. I wanted to tell the whole world what a wonderful experience I'd just had; it was a total contrast to Eddy's birth. I was far too energetic and high to sleep, so Adam brought me the phone so that I could call all our friends and family to tell them the news.

It really was the most wonderful and empowering experience of my whole life. I thoroughly enjoyed my labour and birth and I wasn't the least bit worried or frightened about birthing my baby without a midwife in attendance. It was so natural and instinctive. All we needed now was a name for our son. One helpful friend suggested Lou! [Since his birthplace was the 'loo'!] Eddy offered Mr McGregor (he's a big Peter Rabbit fan). Our baby was three days old when we decided to call him Ben.

Ruth Clark

1... HELP YOUR MIND

If things go quickly, it means everything's happening smoothly

In Britain, it's illegal to *intentionally* give birth with a non-expert in attendance, although—interestingly—it's fine to give birth entirely alone. This is called 'unassisted birth'... I'm not recommending it simply because I think it's good if we can take advantage both of what we know about physiological birth and also of all that modern technology and expertise has to offer. If you happen to be outside the UK when you're pregnant, do check out the legal situation there before you go into labour. Actually, wherever you are, in legal terms it has to be OK to give birth *accidentally* before midwives arrive or you get to them, because birth does sometimes happen very quickly. Nevertheless, obtaining a birth certificate after an accidental unassisted birth might be more difficult than it would otherwise be if you're abroad so do make realistic and safe plans.

If you happen to be worried about the idea of birth happening faster than expected, please don't be. See Birthframes 14, 19 and 35 and the notes on pp 178-179 and remember, above all, that if things go very quickly it means that everything's happening very smoothly. It's perfectly safe as long as you have no drugs in your system and as long as you keep yourself and your baby warm after the birth. Oh, and read the next birthframe too...

Birthframe 97

Here is another account of an unexpectedly fast birth which took place before midwives arrived. It is written by the woman I mentioned before (on page 178), Heba Zaphiriou-Zarifi, a movement therapist and Jungian psychotherapist in training. When Heba realised that she might give birth before the midwives arrived for her planned home birth she decided not to panic. Instead, she really did embrace the unexpected. Her comments on this birth serve to remind us of the importance of facing whatever it is we personally have to face as we move through our own individual birthing experience.

My three daughters were born at home and yet every pregnancy was unique and every birth was a new and different experience. Each birth is influenced to some extent by the way the previous one occurred, it contains it as well as goes beyond it. It is also grounded in our maternal lineage with its roots embedded in the timeless, archetypal level of our nature, both personal and universal. Birth and death touch each other, like two sides of the same coin. A letting go, of some sort, is necessary for the birth to occur. Something has to surrender for the new life to emerge. The safety and sacredness of the 'chosen' time and space are a pre-requisite for a fulfilling birth experience. Partners involved, as well as the wider community, will be affected by that powerful experience, be it a hospital or home birth, which will mark and shape patterns of the child's life. The pattern of one's own birth is symbolic of all other transformative life events.

Perhaps one needs to reconnect consciously with the forgotten memory of one's own birth experience or with a major event in the family. Memories are stored in the many different layers of the body and might emerge as the contractions squeeze them out in waves. Like the ebb and flow of the tide, contractions bring to the shore what was trapped at the bottom of the sea, what was held in the tissues of the body. So I believe that whatever knots we can undo will help open a wider path for the birthing process to follow its natural course.

I had thoroughly prepared myself for a home birth the first time, and the second time too, by reading books on home birth, by doing my yoga and singing. Walking in nature was a delight, breathing and listening to birdsong. Harmonisation was a fantastic tool too. (This is a very deep relaxation massage, which puts energies in harmony.) I also had at hand some homeopathic and herbal medicine. Every woman will find in herself all the treasure of knowledge she needs in order to face her pregnancy, birth and mothering experience. Empowering herself and making informed choices is of the essence.

As planned, I contacted my midwife at our nearby hospital while contractions were in progress. No response. The lines were constantly busy. I tried many times until I realised that the hospital's lines must be dysfunctional. There was no time to waste. Nothing can stop life when it is coming forth. So I decided to go with it. I filled my bathtub, breathing, sounding. The flow of the water was magical. I lit a candle and got in the bath. My husband suggested calling the ambulance and asking them to collect our midwife from the hospital. I was very calm... Having had a happy first home birth, there was no reason for me to be disturbed nor alarmed by this one. With total concentration and presence I surrendered to the process. And my baby came rushing out with such power, bursting out with life. I shall never forget her first intake of breath. The transition from water to air is such a significant transition it was a unique and unforgettable moment, something I might have missed had we been in a hospital environment. Hearing her first breath entering her body was a gift beyond words, a most gratifying spiritual experience.

I trusted my instinctive and spiritual ability to give birth— something that all women have in them as an inborn knowledge, waiting to be revealed. In other words, I trusted the wisdom of my body and the circumstances for the birth of my daughter somehow became a manifestation of that basic trust.

I know from my experience as a therapist that the actual birth experience becomes a metaphor for other creative activities involved in one's journey. It is also a metaphor for the deep psychological transformation so necessary in order to find one's wholeness. No wonder women fall into depression and their energy scatters when their initiation from maidenhood to motherhood is tampered with. Other people's need to control them is a substitute for controlling their own fear of this archetypal energy of death and rebirth. Or is it an unconscious jealousy that makes the obstetricians want to take centre stage, when it is truly the woman's realm?

Birth is truly the woman's realm...

Scared men and women who are unable to surrender to the unknown, who are afraid of their own vulnerability tend to medicalise pregnancy, birth and even breastfeeding. Controlling a woman and her baby in their mutual birth experience can leave a scar so deep in the woman's and baby's psychological bodies that it may take many more painful wounds to find the root and meaning of it all. Dis-abling a mother and her baby when entering their heroic journey into the unknown, is a psychological crime committed by many.

Going through a transitional, liminal birthing experience with tremendous vulnerability, a maiden sheds her skin in order to enter her new identity as a young mother. Giving birth is a struggle to be overcome by mother and baby and yet it enables a woman to take on the body of a mother, along with the energy necessary to fill this role. For nine months, her body has been the home of another unique individual and her psyche a land for her baby's development. By giving birth, she is being born unto herself, an experience that will change her for ever.

Heba Zaphiriou-Zarifi

If you're interested in working through problems with Heba using harmonisation, dream work or body therapy, email info@freshheartpublishing.co.uk.

Birthframe 98

My own third birth experience was not actually what I'd expected. All kinds of things 'went wrong'... but there was nothing that couldn't be dealt with.

First of all I went into labour at rather an inconvenient time. Not only was my husband about to go off to work (where he was rather busy), I was also supposed to be taking my other two children along to a morning playgroup. I went ahead as planned, stopping in the street on my way to and from the playgroup, as each new contraction made it impossible to walk for a few seconds. I hadn't felt comfortable with the idea of asking my new friends to help out with the children (since we'd only recently moved to the town). An hour or so after we got home, I eventually decided to phone my husband...

The next 'problem' was that it was broad daylight and we had no curtains in our bathroom. I'd had visions of a candlelit labour and birth because births always take place in the middle of the night, right? Oh well, I'd just have to carry on. Had to stay in the bathroom because I was merrily being sick, and somehow sitting on the toilet seemed the most comfortable position a lot of the time! As I turned on the water to have a shower and run myself a bath I discovered there was no hot water. Aaaargh! What could have gone wrong? A cold bath was hardly likely to have the same effect... I decided to ask my husband if he could prepare me a bath using the kitchen kettle. ("Hot, but not too hot!")

The next minor blip was the NHS midwives. I'd called them as late as possible because I wanted to avoid all possible disturbance. When they turned up, not only did I not know them at all (they had a rota system), I also found them rather overly 'brusque' and business-like. No problem—they'd just need to be locked out of the bathroom! Fortunately, Michel had suggested this idea to me as a possibility by email that very morning.

Perhaps *because* of all these hiccups, I was not as calm and composed as I had hoped. I was even wrestling with some unresolved psychological issues... It's all very well for pregnancy books and magazines to tell us we need to discuss everything with our partner, but what if he's busy or doesn't want to talk? Now hardly seemed the time. I just continued, moment by moment, moving through each contraction as best I could. Somehow the time would pass... I gently talked to my baby to coax her out.

Another thing at the back of my mind was my lack of clarity on what to do with the placenta. Was I going to be really natural and have a lotus birth? [See Birthframe 4.] This question was answered for me very efficiently... The cord snapped as my new baby was born—she shot out with such enthusiasm. And no, I didn't manage to catch her. Landing on our thick-pile carpet covered by a plastic sheet seemed to do her no harm at all. (Giraffes apparently fall about eight feet when they're born!) The broken umbilical cord caused absolutely no problems—she breathed immediately and I myself lost only a small amount of blood. The placenta slipped out then too.

Coming back to glitches in this labour and birth, the post-birth afterpains also took me a bit by surprise. My uterus seemed very intent on getting back to normal as quickly as humanly possible... Vomiting while breast-feeding was not exactly pleasant, but then again the aftermath did only last a few hours in total and I had long breaks between each bout of afterpains. At least the midwives who visited me after the birth were impressed with my involuted uterus, not to mention my intact perineum. (I'd only sustained a few scratches to my vagina this time—no doubt caused by long newborn fingernails!) Beyond the afterpains in the first few hours after the birth, as before I had no postpartum pain and I was full of energy.

All in all, it had gone well, but NOT as expected! Even after the birth there were blips... First, we couldn't agree on a name and the matter was complicated by my wonderful mother-in-law trying to insist on her 'suggestion'. (That ended up being the middle name!) Then—just two days after the birth—I caught a bug off a visitor's baby. As I was throwing up for the umpteenth time that night I did at least console myself with the thought that my new baby, Jumeira, would get my antibodies through my breastmilk. She was fine and I was also back to normal a few hours later. After that I just had the usual problems of early motherhood—sleep deprivation, a messy house and a rather podgy body.

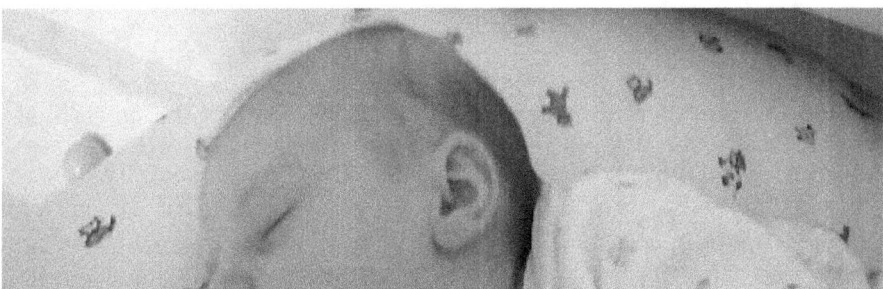
Jumeira (at 6 weeks) asleep on my lap after breastfeeding while I worked at my computer

A few days later, I realised my faith in the natural processes had been reaffirmed. Our bodies and our babies know what to do. We simply need to have the courage not to intervene or disturb the natural processes. We need to observe and move through the sensations as we experience them, even if we perceive these as painful. And we need to hold on to that faith in the natural processes. We can and we must work through these times for the sake of our babies, our children, and the society into which they are born. And we're helping ourselves in doing so because postnatally our lives are likely to be much, much easier than they might otherwise be after a 'managed' birth using so-called 'pain relief'.

18 months later: Since Jumeira's birth I've had no pain, no discomfort—just a little tiredness now and then because of broken nights. The intense but brief pain I experienced during my third labour and birth was just that... strong but short-lived. Jumeira's on my lap, contentedly breastfeeding as I type away at my computer. She's a lovely, lively, happy little girl.

❝ Getting my baby born had all lasted much less than 24 hours overall and, apart from having a strange-looking stomach (my innards needed to rearrange themselves), I was back to my old self. I felt fine. Not only that, I also had loads of energy! Neighbours, friends and acquaintances repeatedly expressed surprise in the days and weeks that followed. How come I was so active? How come I could do so much? Didn't I have any problems? No discomfort? I had no stitches and no soreness – after all, nothing had torn. The midwives who visited me periodically in the days after the birth eventually gave up trying to sniff out problems but they didn't seem to be able to digest what had happened. They'd never before visited a woman after a completely natural birth—it was simply outside their field of experience. They were surprised I had so little lochia (which apparently is associated with having a physiological third stage); surprised that my uterus had shrunk back down so quickly and efficiently; surprised that my baby was so calm and alert, and that she was feeding so beautifully. I had plenty of milk, no soreness or engorgement and loads of energy. Weren't there any problems they could give me drugs for?! Sorry... no, I couldn't think of anything.

Stay focused!

To help you stay focused on what's important, here's a quick revision course, presented in the form of questions and answers. Some of the points were originally presented explicitly, and some were only suggested here and there. Here it's all spelled out for you! Personally, I would have liked to have had something like this to read as I was going into labour.

As you read through each question and answer, remember that you are responsible for each decision you take. Hold this responsibility carefully and intelligently in your heart and mind, remembering that each decision is likely to affect the outcome of your labour for both yourself and your new baby. Trust your intuition too. Deep down you know your own answers to these questions. And your body knows how to give birth…

What if I suddenly start doubting everything?

Perhaps as you read this you're just a few days away from your due date. Perhaps you're 'overdue'. Or perhaps you're actually having your first contractions… It's understandable if you're doubting your ability to give birth. I have every single time!

Women typically experience a range of emotions, as well as some good old-fashioned restlessness and even boredom before they go into labour and give birth… It's normal to feel afraid or very lonely. After all, this really is something you can only do alone—even if other people are there with you. (It's not as if you can say, "Oh, Mum, I don't suppose you could…") And you are entering or re-entering unknown territory, because every birth experience is different in subtle ways—just as every other experience in life is unique.

If you feel fearful or lonely, this is not a sign of weakness—you're only human. You're bound to feel apprehensive if you're in tune with your emotions. You're bound to have a sense of wonder, of questioning. Drug-based pain relief may also suddenly seem extremely appealing. Don't be hard on yourself if you find yourself thinking dramatic thoughts about wanting to be 'cut open' to get the baby out—now, anyhow! Observe these thoughts. Merely be aware of them and continue through each new contraction as best you can.

Why did I opt for no drug-based pain relief or management?!

Here are some of the reasons why you may have decided to trust the natural processes:

- ♥ Unless there is a medical problem, an optimal birth is safer for both you and your baby.
- ♥ You'll feel better both during the birth and afterwards—yes, despite the pain!
- ♥ You'll experience less pain overall.

- ♥ Your baby's experience of birth will be better.
- ♥ There will be no unpleasant short- or long-term side-effects for your baby.
- ♥ It'll be easier to form a relationship with your new baby.
- ♥ You'll experience fewer problems after the birth.
- ♥ If you want to breastfeed, you'll find it's much, much easier.

How am I going to know when I'm in labour?

You can only really know after the birth! The initial signs often continue for some time before the birth. Here's some key information to give you an idea as to how soon the birth might be.

- ♥ Having diarrhoea is a hint that your body may be preparing itself for the big day... but it's no guarantee that things will happen very soon.
- ♥ Seeing a 'show' only means you will go into labour at some point within the next two weeks.
- ♥ If your waters break, there is no cause for alarm. It's possible it is only a hindwaters break, which will soon heal up. If it's a full leak of amniotic fluid from the forewaters in front of your baby's head, the important thing is to prevent an infection. This means staying at home, refusing all internal examinations and not putting anything near your vagina, including your husband's penis or hands—NO SEX! Take your temperature at regular intervals so as to check that all's OK within your body. If it suddenly rises, contact your caregiver immediately. If nothing much changes, you can continue for two or three weeks with no problems before you go into labour. Don't worry about your baby being in a 'dry' environment... amniotic fluid will continue to be produced all the time. Just drink plenty of water.
- ♥ If you only have vague, relatively painfree contractions at irregular, fairly widely spaced intervals it's unlikely the birth will be soon. Just carry on as normal and wait for contractions to speed up. You could easily continue like this for several weeks.
- ♥ If contractions are extremely strong and you find yourself groaning loudly, it's likely you're moving much closer to the birth. However, beware of any disturbances because any kind of disturbance can halt labour, even when it's well-established. Also beware of water—no showers, baths or birthing pools until you're sure you're very near the birth (i.e. more than 5cm dilated). You should know you're at this stage without any vaginal examinations—the contractions will be strong and coming thick and fast.
- ♥ If you are vomiting and/or you're totally involved in contractions, unable or unwilling to speak to other people and have isolated yourself, there's a good chance your baby will be born very soon.

If you're totally involved in contractions that's good news!

When should I tell someone else I'm in labour?

Staying private is important because it's important not to feel observed. When you consider telling someone else you're in labour, think carefully about who you tell and why.

- ♥ Are you looking for sympathy?
- ♥ Will the person you tell respect your need for privacy?
- ♥ Is the person you confide in sympathetic to your intention to have an optimal birth, undisturbed by unnecessary intervention and unsullied by the effects of so-called (very temporary) pain relief?
- ♥ Does this person understand the possible effects of drug-based pain relief on your unborn baby?
- ♥ Will he or she put any pressure on you (indirectly) by asking how you're doing and how much longer you think it'll be?

Keep your labour secret for as long as possible... Simply from a safety point of view, let someone in the house know you think your labour might be beginning, but if you're just experiencing early contractions don't wake your husband up so he can keep you company. You don't need your best friend either. Ringing round other friends would just be asking for trouble—because you'd then be under pressure to 'perform' and produce the baby within a certain timeframe. Not even your other children or your mother need know just yet unless they're actually in your house and noticing you're behaving a little differently. After all, the only way they can really help you is to leave you alone to tune into what's happening within your body. Not even your caregiver can do much for you except check that all is basically OK. (Checks would be made of your baby's position, his or her heartbeat, the amount of amniotic fluid and finally the umbilical cord.) So if you intuitively feel that all is OK, be brave and be strong!

What should I do while I'm in labour?

You could carry on with your normal activities, you could do something different from usual, or you could stop doing anything at all... Which approach is best? Quite simply, do whatever you feel like doing. This is a time when you must sink deep into yourself. If you feel like being busy, that's fine. If you feel like walking, then walk. If you want to do very little, no problem. Just go with your whims and move into each contraction as it waves over you. There are a few provisos...

- ♥ Don't expose yourself to the media in any form—don't watch television, don't turn on the radio, don't leaf through any newspapers or magazines, don't surf the Internet... You're very suggestible while you're in labour and besides, you need to be focusing on yourself at this time, not on the outside world.

Don't expose yourself to the media while you're in labour

- ♥ Don't seek out other people. Birth is something you can and must do alone.
- ♥ Don't go far. This is a time to stay in familiar, safe places where you have everything you need, including privacy.

What positions should I use while I'm in labour?

Remember that leaning forward positions are best for your baby's oxygen supply! (Look at the photos on pp 392 and 395.) Beyond that, experiment and move exactly as you wish to. Your body will tell you what to do.

How am I going to cope with any pain?

There's no special method, but here are a few suggestions...

- ♥ Focus on the sensations you're feeling and try to observe them without judging them as good or bad—they are simply happening.
- ♥ Let your body move in any way that helps you ease the pain.
- ♥ Help yourself to relax by making sure you're in a nice, warm and comfortable environment.
- ♥ Rest or even doze in any breaks between contractions.
- ♥ Put on some music you enjoy.
- ♥ Fill a hot water bottle and hold it against you.
- ♥ Rub yourself or ask someone else to massage you on your back, legs, or anywhere else you feel might help.
- ♥ Make noises if you feel like it, change position—sway, lean and rock—entirely as you feel you want to.
- ♥ Use water—hot or cold—when your contractions are coming thick and fast. (This should mean you're beyond the 5cm mark.)
- ♥ Think about your baby and try to tune into how he or she may be feeling right now.

Don't worry about how you breathe—you've been practising all your life and you'll remember how! Don't try out any complementary therapies—they're only likely to distract you from what you should be concentrating on. Don't use any drugs or artificial forms of so-called 'pain relief'. It'll all be over soon. Somehow, by some miracle, you will find enough strength to move through each contraction. And if things seem really bad, even outrageous, all you need to do is continue for another moment. And then another, then another, then another. Then, before you know it, you will have given birth.

Should I eat and drink something?

It's entirely up to you. If you feel like eating or drinking at any stage, it's likely your body needs the nutrients or the energy. Here are a few things that might help you:

- ♥ Full meals just before you go into labour or in the early stages of labour. Huge platefuls of chicken curry and vegetables! Mounds of potato! Noodles! Pasta! Puddings galore! If you feel hungry, it's a sign you're building yourself up for the very active phase of labour. Starchy foods will give you energy. If there's no time to cook, even oatcakes or toast might help!
- ♥ Water or watered down fruit juice, preferably without sugar or glucose—because this has been shown to lower a woman's pain threshold! The best thing is to simply have a bottle of water at your side while you labour.
- ♥ Fruit, which is easy to digest and very pleasant to eat.

Avoid going purely for carbohydrates because higher glucose levels in the blood have been associated with a lower pain threshold. Give your body a chance to cope and leave the chocolate until after the birth! If you find yourself throwing up, never mind. Keep a bucket or bowl handy, or migrate to the bathroom. If you find you don't want anything to eat or drink, again, don't worry. Just go with the flow. Your body will tell you what to do.

Avoid going purely for carbohydrates because higher glucose levels have been associated with a lower pain threshold

If you have other children:

When shall I get someone to look after them?

When you feel you are drifting away 'somewhere else', this is the time to get help. Don't call people in too early if everything is calm, because as long as you yourself are calm, your children are also likely to take everything in their stride—believe it or not! Also, you may be a long time away from the moment of birth, so just carry on as normal for as long as you feel you can.

When should I call my birth attendant(s)?

Do this when you feel your labour is well advanced. If you call a caregiver too early, you might well feel 'observed' and under pressure to 'perform'. Tuning into your own inner reserves is more important than seeking outside support—after all, nobody else can really help you at this time. You're doing this on your own, however many people are around you, and having other people around while you're in labour is actually likely to have an adverse effect on the progress of your labour. Only call your birth attendant when you intuitively feel it is time to do so... Presumably, you will have thought about logistics—e.g. travelling time—in advance.

If you call someone too early you may feel 'observed'

If you're planning to give birth in hospital:

When should I go in?

Don't go in too early! Unless your contractions are sweeping you along and quickly dilating your cervix, arrival at hospital is likely to slow things down. So only go in when things really seem to be happening—when contractions are coming very regularly and you're fully involved in your labour.

How should I relate to anybody who's around?

Tune other people out. Don't attempt to get strength from other people. All the strength you need is within you. Just tune into each contraction and follow your instincts—and you'll be surprised what you can do. Here are a few other pointers:

- If people around you are distracting you or disturbing you, or if you feel they are watching you, tell them to go away! This is your time and you deserve to have an undisturbed, undistracted, unobserved labour.
- If somebody near you starts asking you questions at this time, explain that you need to be alone now, without any questions, that you want to focus inwards. Again, tell them to go away, if necessary! If the people asking questions are your children, arrange for them to be looked after by someone else—either in your own home or elsewhere.
- If you're giving birth in a hospital, remember that even there you have the right not to be disturbed by staff. Your own internal agenda is a million times more important now than any hospital protocols. Simply say 'No' and assert yourself in whatever way you can, whenever you need to.
- Don't worry about being rude. It's important to get your message across, so speaking directly is probably the best way to do it. If people find you rude, it doesn't matter. What matters is your baby's—or babies'!—birth.

What can I ask of other people?

When you're not ignoring the person or people near you, you may want to get them to do something! Here are some examples of things you can ask them to do:

- Run you a bath, light some candles, put on some music
- Fetch you a hair tie, find you a photo or a picture, pick you a flower... er, find you a bucket
- Get you something to eat or drink, rub your back or thighs
- Telephone your attendant(s) when you want them to
- Persuade unwanted people to go away so you can have more privacy and feel less disturbed...

What must other people not do?
There are quite a few things, actually! For example...

- ♥ They mustn't speak to you, unless spoken to! Even then, their answers must be as short as possible and they mustn't refer to time. When they speak to others, it must be out of earshot.
- ♥ They mustn't encourage you to have pain relief in any way—either by talking about it or by showing it to you, either directly or indirectly (e.g. by mentioning that equipment is working).
- ♥ They mustn't establish eye contact with you unless you seek this out.
- ♥ They mustn't touch you unless you ask to be touched.
- ♥ They mustn't watch you or make you feel you're being observed.
- ♥ They mustn't take photos or film you.
- ♥ They mustn't do anything that bothers or disturbs you.
- ♥ In other words, your birth attendants are there for you and your baby. Use them if you need to. Otherwise, ignore them and just make sure they stay out of your way—both physically and psychologically. You can talk, cuddle and debrief when it's all over. At that time, you may also want to apologise for having been so incredibly bossy and assertive!

How am I going to refuse pain relief?
Here are a few tips...

- ♥ Make sure people know in advance, as far as possible, that you don't want to use any.
- ♥ Have copies of a care guide with you which clearly states that you want no pain relief.
- ♥ If some is offered, simply say, "No, thank you. Please don't offer anything again."
- ♥ If you find yourself wishing for pain relief or a full-blown caesarean, simply be aware of these feelings. Don't mention your thoughts or feelings to anybody around you.
- ♥ Bring your attention to the sensations you are experiencing, while still being aware of your background thoughts and feelings. Observe what is going on in your body with as much equanimity as you can muster. Travel through each contraction—don't fight against it!
- ♥ Remind yourself why each form of pain relief is bad news for either you or your baby. Think about the effects drugs can have on labours, on birth, and on a woman's experience after the birth. Think about the effects drugs might have on your baby, immediately after the birth, in the months after the birth and years later in adolescence. Remind yourself of the positive comments expressed by women who have experienced fully optimal births.

♥ Just keep going. It'll soon be over. Each moment, things are changing. Not one single contraction is like any other... So things are changing, changing, moving forwards toward the birth... And yes, things seem to be getting worse rather than better, but that's good news. You need strong contractions in order to fully dilate your cervix. After all, there's a baby in there who needs to come out! Move deep into yourself, groan as you wish, if you wish, and merely observe your own weakness... Soon it'll turn into strength.

No one single contraction is like any other so things are changing, changing, moving forwards...

How will the birth work in very practical terms?

Your birth attendants will probably be there, keeping an ear out for you, to make sure you're OK. If they don't arrive in time remember that keeping warm is the main thing. If they are there—as they almost certainly will be—remember you can request that they leave you alone in the room while you actually give birth. After all, your body knows what to do without any outside help. Whether you're planning to be alone when you give birth or have people in the background (perhaps over the other side of the room, or in the room next door), just do your best to make sure your baby will have a fairly soft landing. (Nobody needs to catch your baby, unless you particularly want someone to.) A bundled up sheet or towel is fine. You don't need anything special. And a little bump won't hurt your baby. You can then pick him or her up yourself, undisturbed, which will also make things safer because you are more likely—in those completely undisturbed circumstances—to produce the necessary amount of oxytocin to expel the placenta very soon after the birth of your baby.

If you choose to have someone with you while you give birth, make sure that he or she knows that you do not want to be disturbed in any way. Write this on your care guide.

What position am I going to use to give birth?

Any you feel comfortable in. Just remember that an upright position will mean your pelvis can open up more and that gravity will also be able to help you. Just move in and out of positions as you want to, while thinking opening images and relaxing your mouth and jaw. At a certain point you will spontaneously choose a suitable position and give birth.

An upright position will mean your pelvis can open up more and that gravity will also be able to help you

What do I need to have ready for my labour?

Even if you're booked up for a hospital birth, it's a good idea to have quite a few things handy, just in case you have a surprise birth at home! After all, when the physiological processes are truly undisturbed, births are often very fast and smooth. Here's a list of things you might need:

- Bottles of water which you can swig while you're in labour.
- Scrunchies for tying your hair back, if necessary.
- A bucket or bowl in case you need to throw up! Alternatively, a sink or toilet will do fine.
- Something waterproof to put underneath you in the later stages of labour and just before you give birth—a plastic tablecloth, for example.
- An old bathmat or piece of carpet to stand on, which you will not slide around on.
- Some old towels for wiping any blood off you or your baby when he or she is first born.
- A electric fire which can be moved around and an extension lead so it can be moved to a bathroom, or wherever you happen to be when you give birth.
- Some soft clothes and receiving blankets to wrap the baby in when he or she is born, as well as some newborn nappies.
- Some tight-fitting knickers and sanitary towels to use as soon as the placenta has been born.
- Some food to eat afterwards... The easier it is to prepare and eat, the better. Consider stocking up on bottled water, pre-cooked frozen meals, tinned food, nuts, pasta, fruit (fresh, tinned and frozen) and even chocolate!

Just keep on going... different women labour in different ways

What if I keep having contractions but nothing more happens?

As long as you know your baby is in a good position, just keep on going. You don't need to break any records. And different women labour in different ways. Try to accept your own reality and as long as you don't experience any emergency symptoms, don't worry. (See page 378 to check.) If you are worried, then ask your caregiver to check you out. If you feel he or she is putting you under unhelpful pressure to conform to a time schedule, quite simply ask him or her to go away—say you'll call them when you're ready. (Seriously!) Here are a few more suggestions...

- Do something different. If you've been resting, get active—take a walk, do some housework, dance to some of your favourite music!
- Consider your mental state. Are you afraid of something? Is something bothering you? Do you need to talk to somebody? Are you too tired? Then do something about the problem, whatever it is.

- ♥ Think opening images—flowers coming into bloom, ripples on water, windows opening in the sunshine.
- ♥ Get warm. Are you cold? Do you need a shower? Would a bath make you feel more relaxed? (Remember, though, that it mustn't be too hot.) As long as you're at least 5cm dilated, using warm water is likely to help you.
- ♥ Visualise your baby. Talk to him or her! Visualise yourself giving birth successfully.

> Visualise your baby. Talk to him or her!
> Visualise yourself giving birth successfully.

What if I'm told my baby is posterior?

- ♥ Move around however you want to, to try and ease the pain. The baby may turn round to an anterior position before the birth... If this happens, you'll have a rest in between each contraction. If not, never mind. It's still possible to give birth without drugs or interventions. Also...
- ♥ Try kneeling on your hands and knees on the floor, even if this feels especially painful, because this can help the baby turn round. Also try any other position that occurs to you. Any leaning forward position is likely to be helpful.
- ♥ Ask your birth attendants to massage your back—continuously, if necessary—throughout your labour. You will probably find it's good if they exert pressure while they're massaging you.
- ♥ Using a shower nozzle, direct hot water onto your back. If this makes things worse, try cold water.
- ♥ Make deep moaning or groaning noises whenever you want to. Open and relax your jaw as you do so.
- ♥ Remember it's especially important that nobody tells you when or how to push. With a posterior labour there's a very high risk the baby can get stuck if you're told what to do. You're in charge!
- ♥ Use a very upright position for giving birth. A supported semi-squat may be the best position because you will not have to support your own body in any way, so will be able to focus only on the very strong sensations you are feeling. However intense it feels, remember that the second your baby is born, the pain will stop... COMPLETELY! What follows later (afterpains) will be minor compared to this.

> However intense it feels, remember that the second
> your baby is born, the pain will stop... COMPLETELY!

What if something just doesn't feel 'right'?

The following symptoms are all danger signals. If you experience any of these symptoms, take immediate advice from your birth attendant or get yourself to a hospital as soon as you possibly can.

- Waters breaking followed by a dramatic rise in temperature
- Sudden and severe difficulty breathing, possibly accompanied by chest pain and followed by convulsions
- Sudden weakness or collapse, accompanied by severe abdominal pain
- Dizziness and/or spots before the eyes and/or ringing in the ears
- Bleeding which is clearly more than a 'show'
- The sudden appearance of a loop of the umbilical cord
- A strong intuition that something's wrong

What if my caregivers suggest cephalo-pelvic disproportion is the cause of a long second stage?

Remember and remind your caregiver of the following:

- A baby's size is usually proportional to his or her mother—so it's unlikely to be a problem.
- All babies have a head circumference of around 10cm, irrespective of their overall weight.
- Upright positions maximise the space you make available in your pelvis.
- Different women progress at very different rates, so you may just need more time, more silence... or privacy! Ask anyone present to leave you alone for a while. This may be all you need.

What if people put pressure on me to accept drugs, procedures or interventions which I don't want?

Take responsibility for what is happening as it happens and assert your wishes. State what you want and repeat it if necessary, rather than trying to argue. Be assertive and even direct and rude if people are refusing to listen. Remember, you will be fully alert, so this will be easy to do. You are responsible for your own body and your own baby, so take that responsibility and trust whatever faith and intuitions you have. If you have a strong intuition that all is not well, then trust that too and communicate it to a health care professional and insist that action be taken. If you feel uncertain, consider you options using the following framework—use your 'brains' (B-R-A-I-N-S). This is a mnemonic contributed by an antenatal teacher from the NCT (National Childbirth Trust):

If you have an intuition something's wrong, use your B.R.A.I.N.S.

B	is for 'benefits'	Ask what the benefits are of any intervention you're offered.
R	is for 'risks'	Ask about the risks. Do you suspect there might be some as yet undiscovered risks?
A	is for 'alternatives'	Ask what the alternatives are.
I	is for 'intuition'	What do you intuitively feel? Do you suspect the procedure might be harmful or unpleasant for your baby?
N	is for 'nothing'	Ask what would or might happen if your caregivers do nothing.
S	is for 'smile'	If all else fails, smile and accept the intervention, provided you're convinced it's for either your own or your baby's benefit.

What if I feel strange in the days, weeks or even months leading up to the birth?

Just observe whatever you're feeling and accept it all as part of the process. Be aware that...

- You may feel the need to spend more time alone.
- You may feel a little depressed or fed up. You may even feel emotional and tearful.
- You may be grumpy or feel so angry you need to take action on certain issues. This is good because it means you will be sorting out unresolved issues before the birth.
- You may feel apprehensive and have a greater need for reassurance that everything's OK. Remember, even if you suddenly feel nervous or scared, it really is better if you can develop greater confidence in yourself and your own ability to grow and birth this baby. Read or re-read any sections or birthframes from this book which may be relevant to your situation (see the Birthframes index) and try to tune in to the real causes of your feelings. Look up key words in the Index—e.g. 'fear'!
- You may sleep less well. You may dream more or less than usual. You may feel the need to take naps during the daytime. Let yourself rest if you need to.

- ♥ You may feel particularly tired and unmotivated. If this is the case, you will probably experience a rush of energy a day or so before you go into labour. Again, you will have a sudden desire to sort things out. Use this time wisely—it's a good idea to get psychological and physical things sorted before the birth. Just don't waste your energy doing things which really are merely obsessive (e.g. perfectionist cleaning or ironing). Remember, this is your last opportunity (before the birth) to do something you really want to do for your own peace of mind!

Beyond all this, remember... you're a mammal! Your body knows how to give birth and your baby knows how to be born. An optimal birth, involving no drugs or unnecessary interventions, with our modern support networks in place, is entirely safe. All you need to do is let it happen, while intelligently tuning into what you are experiencing. Prepare to let yourself be amazed by your body and its wonderful capabilities.

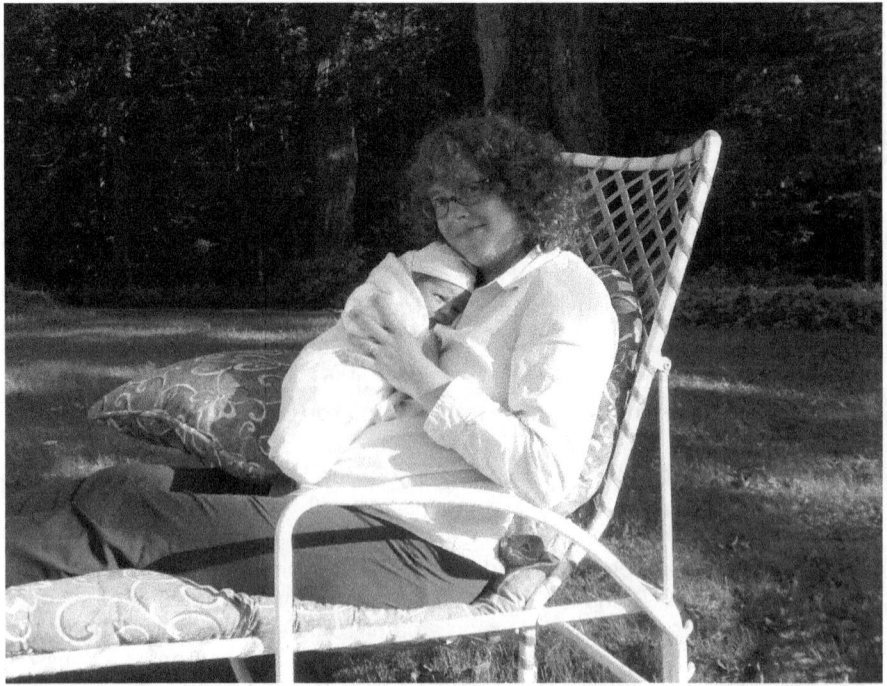

She did it... you can too

Remember... you're a mammal! Your body knows how to give birth and your baby knows how to be born

1... HELP YOUR MIND

You've also read about these women...

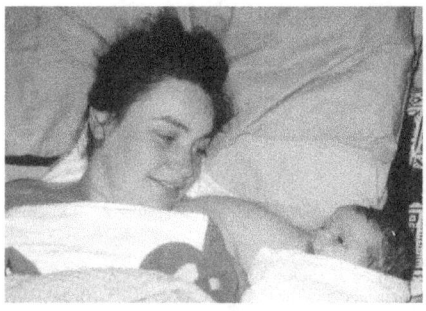

Birthframe 58

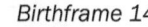

Birthframe 14

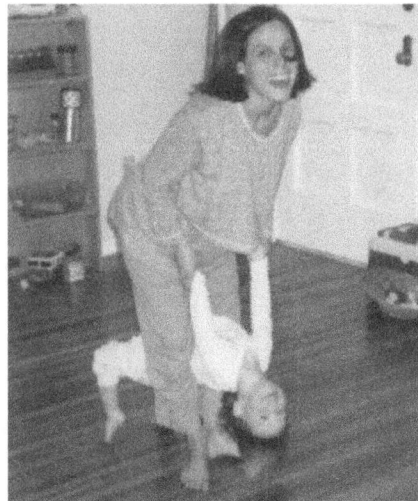

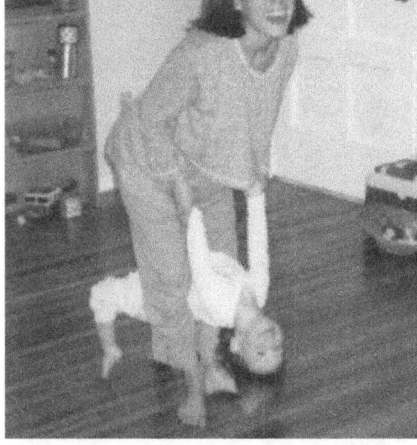

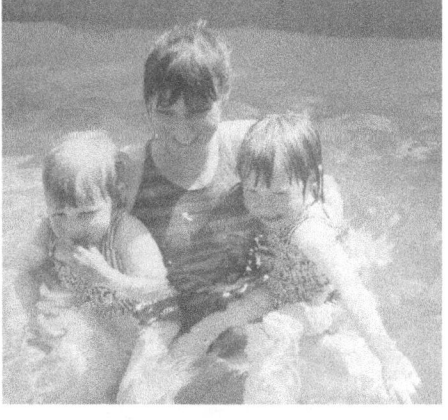

Birthframes 10 and 54

Birthframe 86

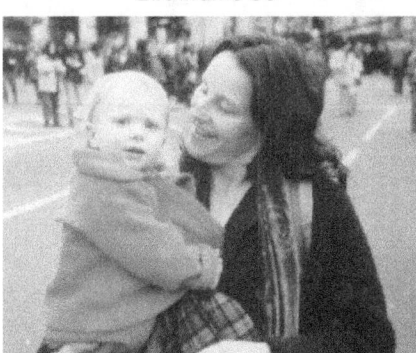

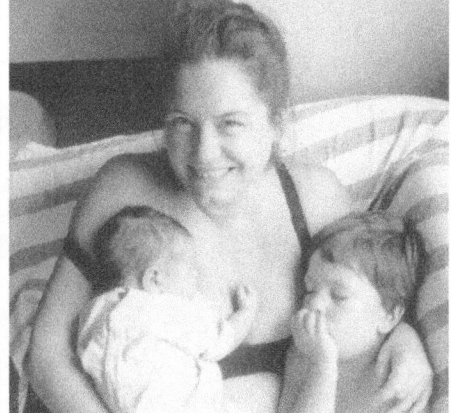

Birthframe 95

Birthframe 12

What about your own birthframe? Here's some space to write up your own account. Also, do please let me know how you get on via the website www.freshheartpublishing.co.uk—simply click on 'Share your experience'.

Above all, remember you're soon going to meet your very own baby!

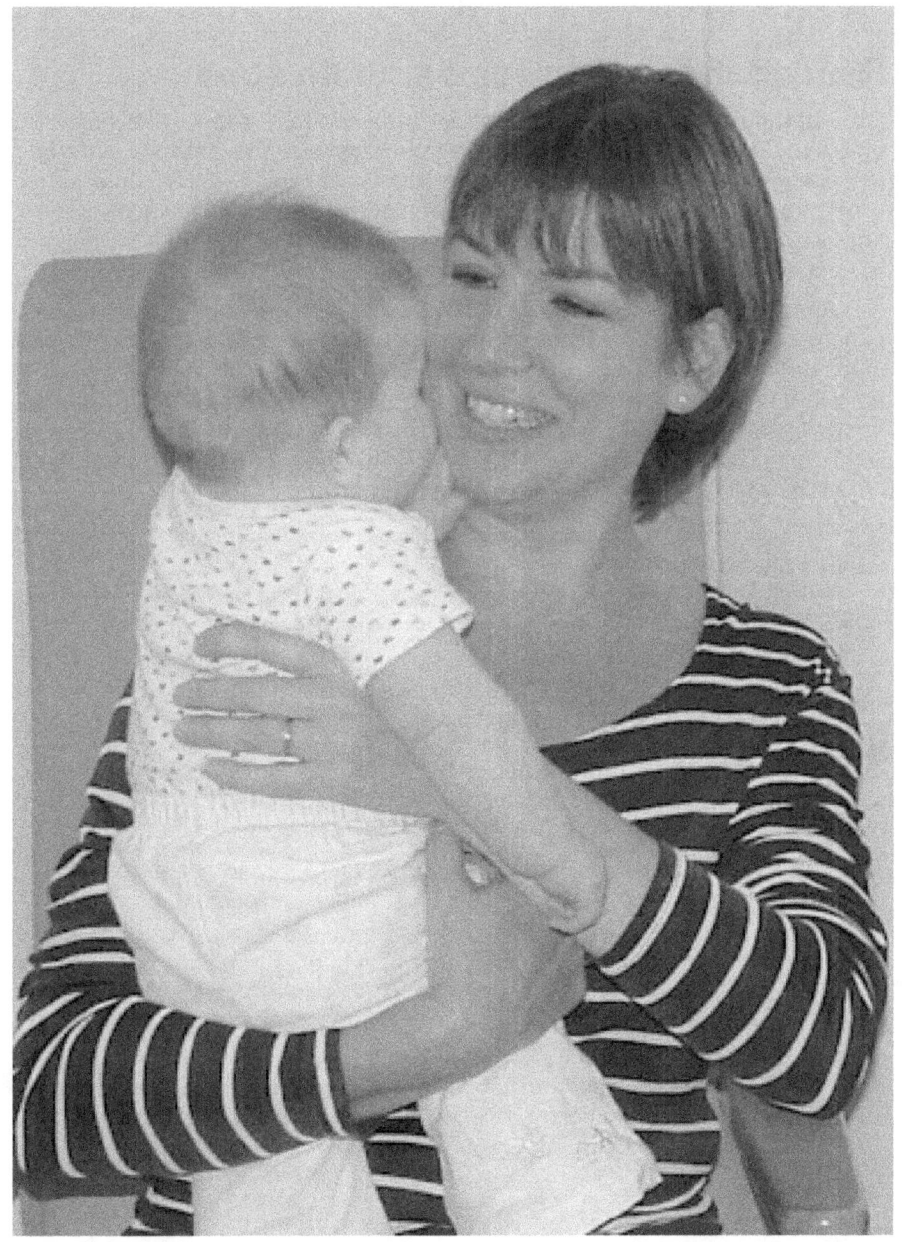

Our cover girl has a chat with her new baby, a few months after her birth

0+1... or 2, or 3

Reminders and tips for a smooth start

Early parenthood can be a real shock to the system, even if it's not your first baby, mainly I suppose because it always involves entering different psychological territory. It's difficult to prepare for, although we must at least try! I remember staring uncomprehendingly at diagrams on nappy-changing before I had my first daughter, but then instantly understanding them with my baby in front of me.

After giving birth, you may well experience elation and joy, as well as quiet periods of contemplation and wonder, and deep feelings of gratitude... Or you may feel strangely flat when you realise that the birth—that big event on the horizon—is now just a memory. There may also be feelings of worry, ineptitude and insecurity when you realise the responsibility involved in looking after a small baby. Both hormones and culture are likely to influence how you feel, as well as your birthing experience, however it turns out.

> Even though the birth was nothing like our plans, I didn't feel let down or disappointed. Eddy was a very healthy and easy baby, he fed well and slept wonderfully. I actually had a very easy time with the labour. I think a lot of women would have been delighted with it but I describe it as a non-experience. It was neither good nor bad.

AVOID EARLY DISRUPTION

It really is vital that you make sure nobody takes your baby away too soon straight after the birth or even in the days and weeks that follow. The first hour or so after birth is especially important for early bonding. In particular...

- ♥ Don't let anybody wash your baby. The smell of a newborn is exquisite and you can enjoy this for a week or more. Just wipe any blood or mucous off.
- ♥ Remember you can refuse any procedures or tests normally carried out on newborn babies. You may well want to refuse heel prick blood tests, Vitamin K (administered in any form), early vaccinations (at 2, 3 and 4 months, for example) and anything else which doesn't seem completely natural. Breastmilk is your baby's biggest protection.
- ♥ Consider carefully whether or not you want your baby to have vaccinations at all. Read, discuss options with other mothers and tune into what you feel is right for you and your baby.

The smell of a newborn is exquisite and you can enjoy this for a week or more. Just wipe any blood or mucous off.

Remember you can refuse any procedures or tests

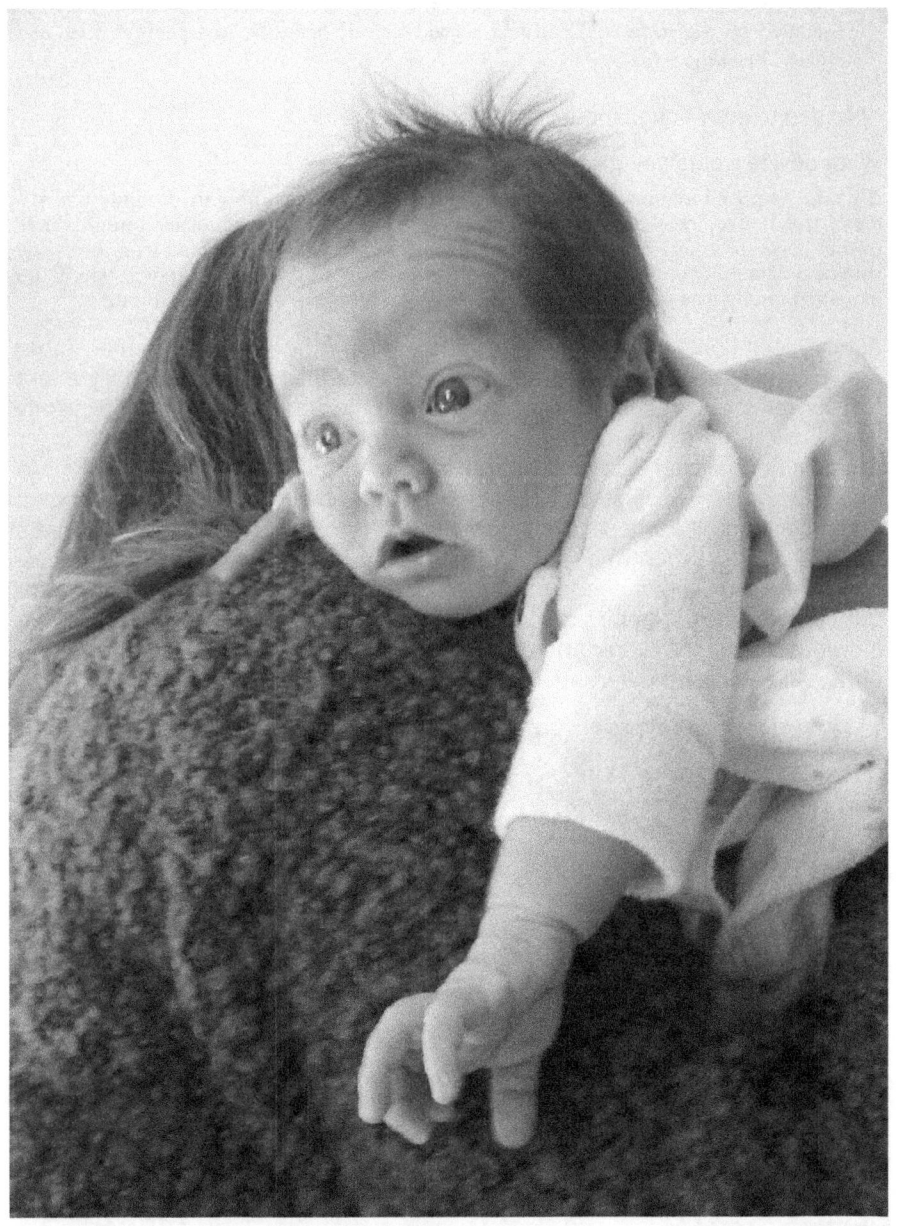

The baby here and on page 483 is another VBAC baby, born entirely naturally

> I spent the whole night looking at Milly and was too scared to pick her up until about 3am. I then put her in bed with me and just watched her until my husband arrived the next morning. When he came we opened her up like a package (she had been swaddled by the midwives) and had a good look at her. She was perfect then and still is 13 months later.

I decided to ask Michel about postnatal care...

What advice would you give a new mother?
If it's at all possible, she should be surrounded by people who can do daily tasks—clean the house, etc—and help her generally. Ideally, a new mother should have nothing else to do but be with her baby. She should try to be liberated from everyday practical tasks. This always used to be the case in traditional societies, when the extended family was around the new mother. Nowadays, it's all more difficult.

Actually, relationships between you and your partner—not to mention other family members!—are likely to be sensitive or strained as you gradually adapt to new roles and responsibilities. Thanks to the relentless daily and nightly reality of having a new baby around, rows and coldness, passion and anger are common. Michel has also noticed that men often seem to suffer from a form of postnatal depression when their women have fully physiological births. Sorry, gentlemen! Perhaps 'penis envy' is not as significant as the envy that's experienced by a man who realises that he can never give birth... We must be sensitive to our man's needs, even if our babies are more at the forefront of our consciousness. As far as your baby goes, he or she will be very much an individual and you will only find out what it's like living with him or her *after* the birth... All babies are different!

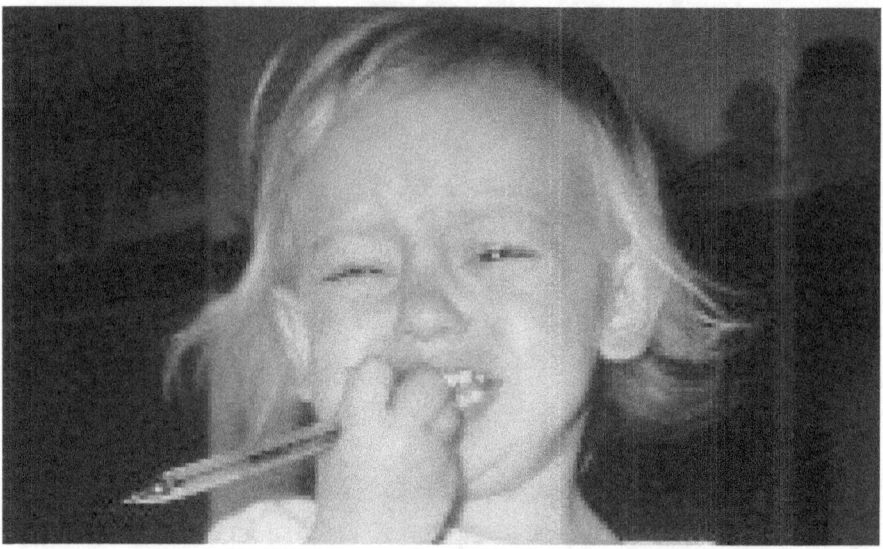

Toddlers can be pretty upset by the arrival of a young sibling...

GET HELP

With all the upheaval, when people ask you how you are you may just find yourself performing a massive cover-up job and saying a breezy, "Fine!"... when in fact things are far from fine. Why not be honest and encourage other people to help you? Here are some things they could do:

- ♥ Phone before visiting
- ♥ Visit with a pre-cooked meal
- ♥ Visit in order to help out with housework!

Don't encourage people to take your baby—because you really do need to have lots of relaxed time with him or her (or them!) so you can get to know each other. Also, make sure you give your partner plenty of opportunities to spend time with your new baby. He's bound to feel left out if you don't, and any feelings of disempowerment he feels may well turn into that anger I mentioned before. Encourage him to do any baby-related tasks you can think of and while he's doing them make sure you don't comment or criticise in any way!

If all these suggestions are rather depressing, because your situation seems particularly difficult, hire a doula! Useful website: www.doula.org.uk

LOVE YOURSELF

Finally, whatever your domestic situation, remember to take your own needs into account. This means you will need to focus on your own feelings from time to time, you'll need to eat well, and you'll also need to get plenty of rest.

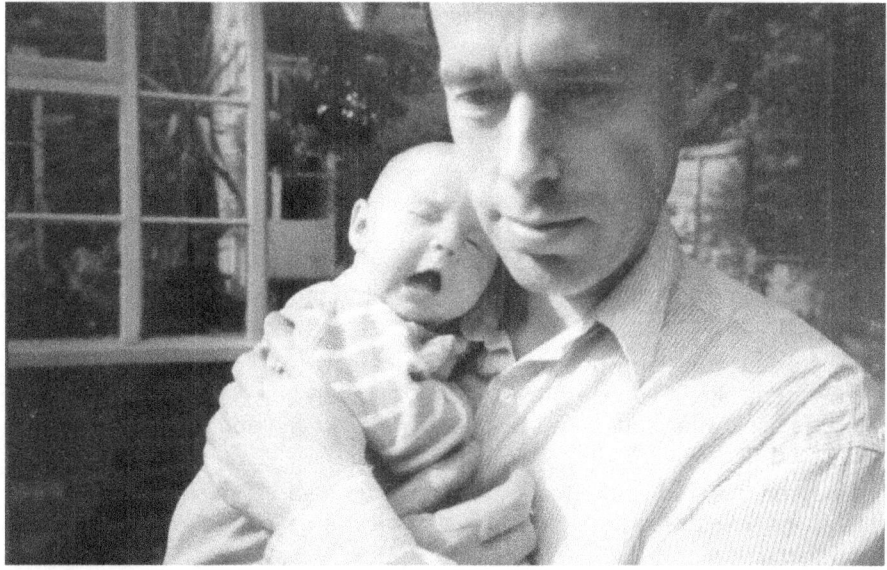

If your partner takes the baby out to get a takeaway, you will get a well-earned break!

Breastfeeding

You probably realise this is the best thing for your baby...

- ♥ Breastfeed immediately. After an optimal birth, you should find you breastfeed instinctively.
- ♥ Use a breastfeeding cushion (or pillow) to raise your baby to a comfortable feeding position, when possible.
- ♥ Offer both breasts every time your baby indicates (letting him or her decide when to switch); start next time with the breast you used last. Don't get paranoid, though, about even use of breasts! It'll all even out eventually.
- ♥ If you experience any soreness or pain at any point, immediately seek help—either from a book, from an experienced breastfeeding mother or from a breastfeeding counsellor (e.g. trained by the NCT or La Leche League). With your baby correctly positioned at your breast breastfeeding should be a painfree experience. Useful website: www.llli.org, www.laleche.org.uk, www.nct.org.uk and www.abm.me.uk
- ♥ Be aware that newborn babies tend to want to suck a lot! As well as having huge needs for milk in the early days, they also need the feeling of safety your breasts offer. Feed on demand and feel confident that your body will cope, whatever the size of your breasts. It will!
- ♥ Note that there are times when your baby will want to feed almost continuously around the clock. These are times of growth spurts or illness. Your body will naturally respond and produce more milk. Never use dummies —doing so would not stimulate your own milk supply enough.
- ♥ Consider allowing your baby to sleep beside you in bed. This will allow you to get enough rest and will help your baby to feel more secure. Note, though, that this is only an option if you don't drink or smoke and use no drugs.

If you ever breastfeed your baby on the sofa, because of the risk of falling asleep simply have your baby lie at the edge of the sofa with your arm cupped round his or her body. This way, there's no risk of smothering. (Put some cushions on the floor too, if you're afraid he or she might fall off. It's actually very unlikely if you're a breastfeeding mother.) Alternatively, or as well, consider using a rocking chair—they're great for soothing babies and helping you to relax too.

Also, note that you don't actually ever need to either express milk or sterilise anything if you are breastfeeding. Life can be very simple if you only start weaning when your baby is 5 or 6 months old and add water, not milk, to baby food...

Beyond this, remember that babies have no idea of your expectations for them. They can't read or tell the time, and they've never studied Dr Spock—so go with the flow!

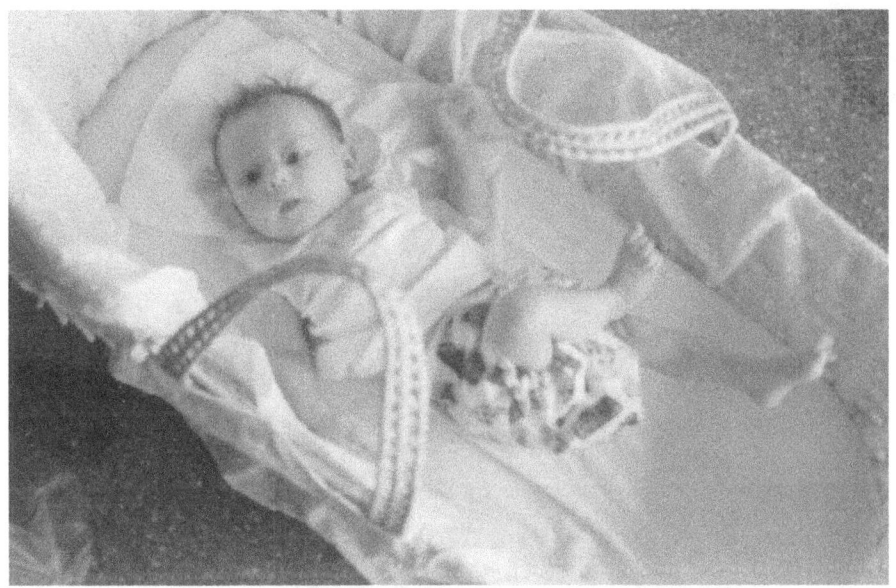

A skinny but spunky newborn fed only breastmilk, having a good kick!

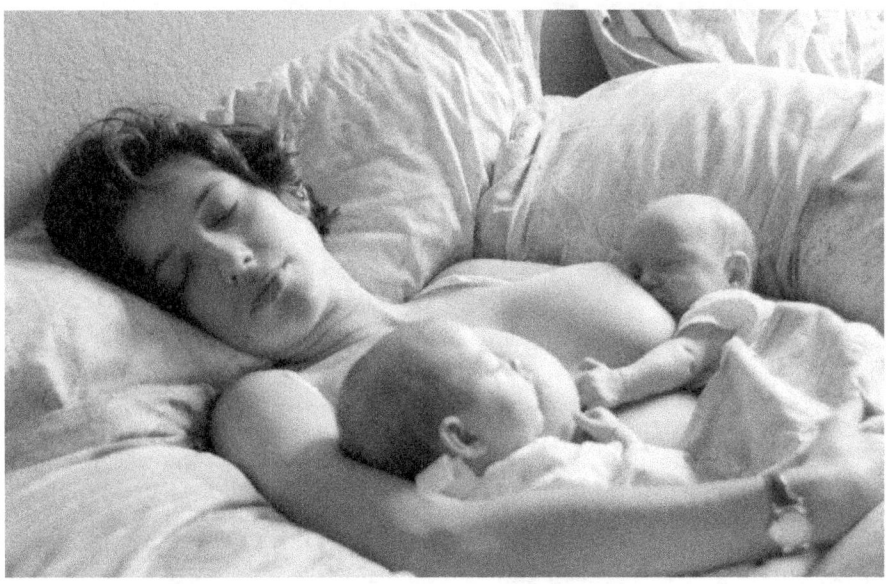

Olga Mellor breastfeeding her twins (see Birthframe 14)

Life can be very simple if you only start weaning at 6 months

Tandem feeding is a great way of keeping a toddler happy too

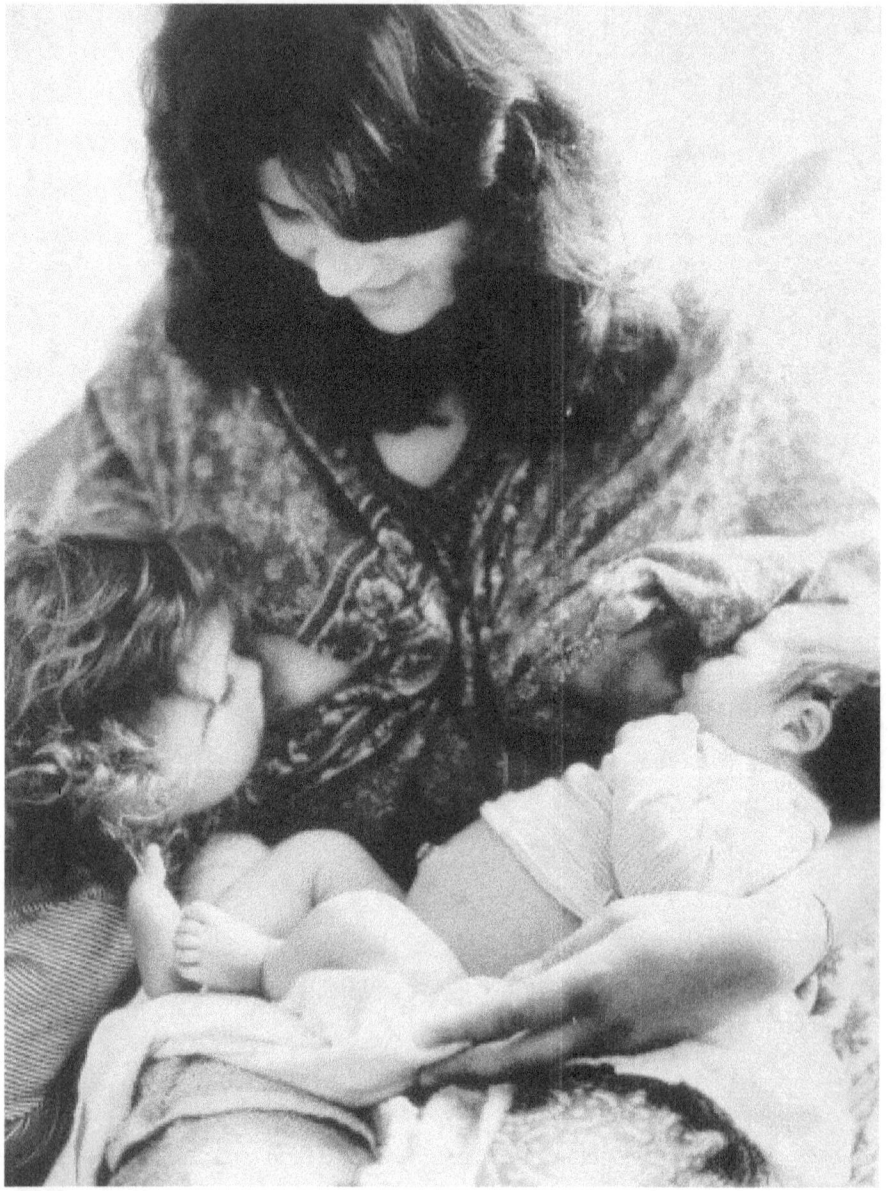

Here Janet Balaskas is tandem feeding. (Remember meeting her in Birthframe 83?) Tandem feeding is a great way of keeping a toddler happy when you have a new baby.

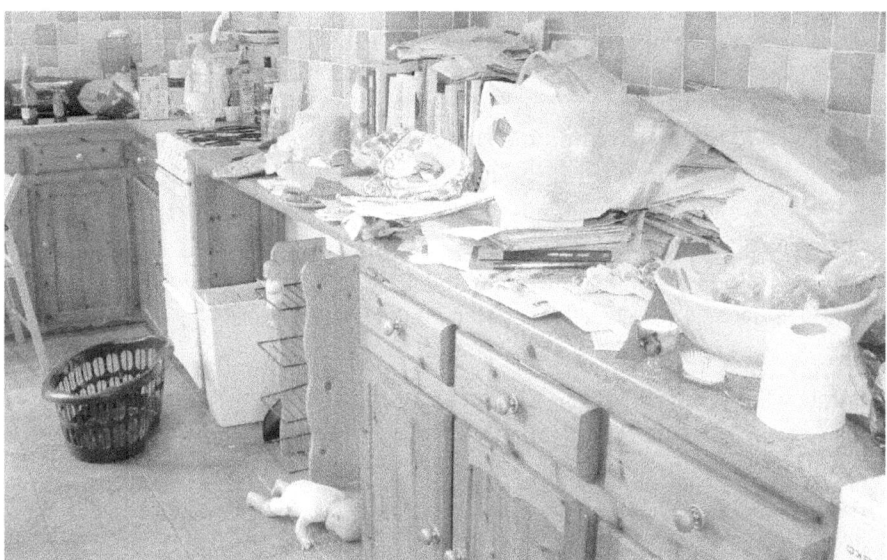
The chaos of the early days. No, that's not a dead baby on the floor...

Mothering

It's constantly both idealised and trivialised... Make it real:

- ♥ Have faith in your own ability to mother your baby. Be kind to yourself. Allow yourself to make mistakes and explore new possibilities all the time.
- ♥ After you've survived the first few days, explore environmentally-friendly nappy options or find out about 'elimination communication', i.e. ways of doing without nappies altogether. (See: Birthframe 99 on the next page.)
- ♥ Remember your baby's a person with feelings and a sense of self, so treat him or her with respect at all times. Whenever possible, give him or her choices—even when he or she is days old! You'll be surprised how well you and your baby will be able to communicate.
- ♥ Try to tune into 'where your baby's at' at all times. Provide him or her with constantly changing stimulation as he or she grows older.
- ♥ As far as is humanly possible, don't sweat the small stuff. Keep the big picture in mind... Only make a fuss about things which are really important.
- ♥ Decide what kind of lifestyle you want for your growing family... Baby groups, play options, childcare, leisure activities and work are all there for you to choose or refuse.
- ♥ Enjoy your time with your child—or children! The years will pass quickly and soon your parenting days will have metamorphosed into something quite different.
- ♥ Finally, here's an important challenge for you... Never lie or conceal the truth from your children. Why not be *real*?

I hope you've enjoyed this book and found it helpful. I'd love to hear about your own experiences of birth and motherhood, especially if you've followed my advice! Email me via the website at www.freshheartpublishing.co.uk

Let's have two more birthframes before we say goodbye...

Birthframe 99

Sarah Buckley, who we've heard from already, tried the environmentally friendly approach, Elimination Communication (EC), when she had her fourth baby [see pages 109-111]. I asked her what it was all about...

Sarah, what is EC exactly?

Elimination communication (EC)—also known as 'infant potty training' (IPT), 'elimination timing' (ET), 'going diaperless' and 'natural infant hygiene' (NIH)—is how most babies are brought up around the world. The 'method', which is so integral and so obvious in most cultures that it needs no name, involves the mother and baby becoming attuned and communicative so that the mother knows when the baby needs to eliminate, i.e. 'wee' or 'poo'.

EC is a new practice for most of us in developed countries, and Westernised mothers and babies have developed their own variations to suit their circumstances. Women may start from birth or with an older baby, make less or more use of nappies, take a long time or a short time to catch on, do EC part-time or full-time and some women even begin work outside the home and train their baby's carers in elimination communication. Although it can be more complex for older babies, some of whom may have already learned to ignore their body's signals, others may welcome the chance to communicate elimination needs.

How did you get into it personally?

I first heard the phrase 'elimination communication' when my fourth baby, Maia Rose, was 3 months old, and a friend pointed me towards the EC website. I was very excited about it and the timing was perfect as I had read in a letter to *Mothering* magazine a few years earlier that African women cue their babies to wee and poo with a 'psss' sound, and I had begun to do this with Maia from birth. EC made sense to me because it felt closer to our genetic imprint and I was drawn to the idea of a deeper physical and psychic connection with my baby. The first time I tried it, I held Maia (aged 3 months) over a tub and made the 'psss' noise. To my delight, she peed straight away and we have been doing it ever since.

From the start, I've had a lot of support from Emma (11), Zoe (8) and Jacob (6), who tell me how much they disliked sitting in wet or soiled nappies as babies. Some believe that we may increase the risk of sexual problems in adulthood by encouraging our babies to disassociate or switch off form their genital areas because of the unpleasant sensation of wearing what some have called a 'walking toilet'. My partner, Nicholas, wondered about the extra effort that I went to in the first year but has been very happy to reap the benefits of a nappy-free toddler.

In the first few months I learnt Maia's signals by carrying her around without nappies or pants and observing her closely. (This was fairly easy as she was very much 'in arms' for her first six months.) I discovered that she would squirm and become unsettled, sometimes with a bit of crying, especially if it took me a while to 'get it'. At other times it was more psychic and I found myself heading for the tub where we usually eliminated, without really thinking. When I was distracted or delayed on acting on my hunch I usually got peed on. (However, she very seldom peed on me when I carried her in a sling.) Learning Maia's daily pattern was also useful. For example, I noticed that she would pee about 10 minutes after breastfeeding or drinking and she almost always pees on awaking. I think it's the need to eliminate that actually wakens her.

At the age of around 6 or 7 months Maia went 'on strike', coinciding with teething and beginning to crawl. She stopped signalling clearly and at times actively resisted being 'weed'. I took it gently, offering opportunities to eliminate when it felt right and not getting upset when, after refusing to go in the tub, she went on the floor. Even on 'bad days', though, we still succeeded most of the time. Then at nearly 10 months we were back on track. I noticed that as she became more independent and engrossed in her activity, she was not keen to be removed to eliminate so I started to bring a receptacle to her. There was a marked shift in things soon after she began walking at 12 months and by 14 months, to my amazement, Maia was out of nappies completely. She now was able to communicate her needs very clearly, both verbally and non-verbally, and her ability to 'hold on' was also enhanced. When she needed to eliminate, she said 'wee' and/or headed for the potty—we had several around the house. Nicholas, her dad, was so delighted when she first did this that he clapped her and so she would stand up and applaud herself afterwards. She began to be very interested in the fate of her body products and joined me as we tipped it onto the garden or into the toilet. She even began to get a cloth and wipe up after herself. Now, at 19 months, she wants to empty the potty herself so she is totally autonomous in her day-time elimination. Compared to other children, she is about the 2½- to 3-year-old stage with her toileting.

Was it all worth it?

It has been more fun and more rewarding for our family than I could have imagined. It has given us more skin-to-skin contact, less washing, no nappy rash and—best of all for me— a deeper respect for Maia's abilities and knowledge of her body and a finer attunement to her rhythms. As well as these advantages, there is obviously less waste and a better time for Mother Earth. And it's fun! Having had three babies in nappies, I have been constantly delighted at Maia's ability to communicate her needs and to keep telling me until I get it. EC also makes a beautiful contribution to my experience of mindfulness in mothering. Like breastfeeding, it keeps me close to my baby, physically and psychologically, and provides very immediate feedback when I am not tuned in. It's been fascinating to learn that mothers and babies are connected very deeply—at a 'gut level'—and that babies (and mothers) are much more capable and smart than our society credits.

Mothers and babies are connected very deeply...

And how does EC fit in with your status as a doctor?

As a GP, the physiology is interesting to me and is totally counter to what I was taught at medical school, where it is asserted that babies do not have sphincter control until close to the second birthday. Obviously, the paediatricians didn't consult the global majority of mothers and babies, for whom knowing their baby's elimination needs is as simple as knowing their own.

Reflecting on my experiences with babies in and out of nappies, I've come to the conclusion that probably ALL babies signal their elimination needs from an early age but, because we're not listening out for it, we misinterpret it as tiredness, needing to feed or just crankiness, especially if our baby is in a nappy and we don't observe the connection with eliminating.

It also interests me that EC babies learn to release before they learn to hold on. This makes EC very convenient because when cooperative, a baby can empty even a small amount of wee from the bladder. (This means, for example, that when I pee Maia before starting a car trip I know that there will then be minimal chance of Maia needing to pee for at least half an hour or so.) In contrast, conventional toilet training is built around the child's ability to 'hold on' to their pee or poo until they can release it in a socially acceptable place. I wonder then about the mind-body implications of this subtle but important difference. Aren't we a society where we tend to 'hold on' to our 'stuff', often needing the help of others (e.g. therapists) to encourage us to 'let it out'?

One of my friends, a bodyworker, commented on Maia's relaxed mouth and this made me wonder if the process might relax the whole digestive tract. I can also feel in my mothering the beauty of supporting her healthy eliminative functions, which many of us feel shameful about and would prefer to deny—hence nappies, which hide the eliminating act itself.

The 'toilet training stage' is, in Erikson's psychological stages, centred on the issue of 'autonomy vs shame and doubt' and it seems to me that Maia has mastered these issues already. She is incredibly autonomous—not to say bossy at times!!!—and I wonder if this might be in part due to being an early mistress of her elimination.

What would you say to other women?

If you feel drawn to EC, I encourage you to have a go. Look on the Internet. It's all I needed to get started and it also gave me invaluable ongoing support. There are also two great books and you can ask other mums and mothers from cultures such as India and China, where this practice is still widespread.

To find out more see:
- www.natural-wisdom.com
- www.White-Boucke.com/ifpt.html
- *Infant Potty Training—A Gentle and Primeval Method Adapted to Modern Living* (White-Boucke Publishing 2000)
- *Diaper Free! The Gentle Wisdom of Natural Infant Hygiene* (Natural Wisdom Press 2001)

Always bear in mind your baby's perspective on things

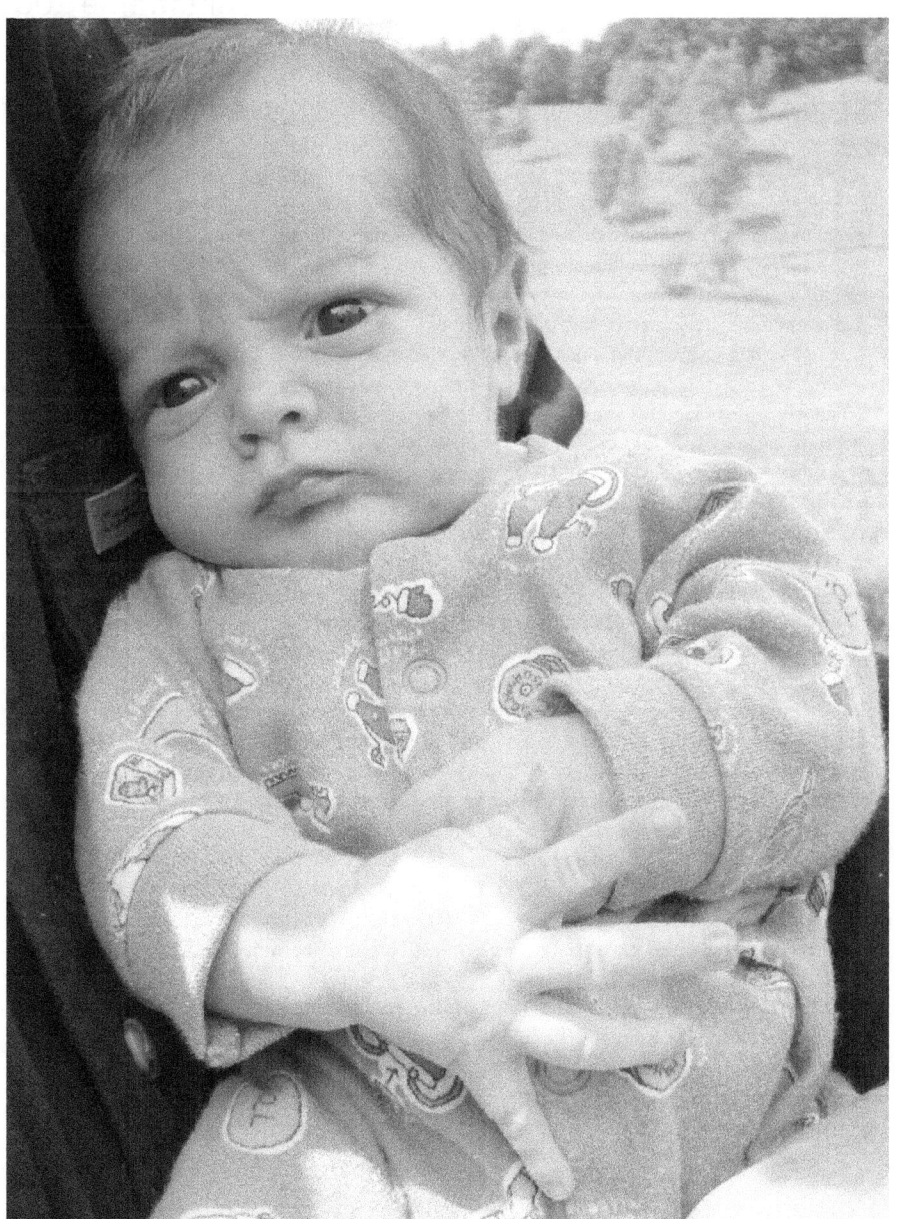

Try out all kinds of possibilities, bearing in mind your baby's perspective on things

Surviving as 'you'

Birthframe 100

Finally, let's think about motherhood in terms of *you*. As we've already hinted, motherhood is not all idyllic blissful bonding... Here one woman recounts how she experienced and coped with a rather unexpected problem.

When I was blessed a few years back with a baby boy, I had a vision. My life would go on much as before, only with a tiny baby keeping me company, smiling and gurgling as I went through the routines of daily living. That vision was almost immediately replaced by a reality where I barely maintained my sanity while struggling to meet the needs of one who, while adorable, was a tyrant. Any time of the day and especially at night I answered his clarion calls for "Milk, milk, milk, and step on it!" In those early weeks I was oblivious to everything but mastering this new role of motherhood.

It was then that I began to notice that not only had my world changed, but also I had changed. Namely, there seemed to be a lot more of me. Twenty-four pounds more, to be exact. I told myself it was all in my breasts, but that myth was dispelled after my husband pointed out that I was wearing maternity jeans. Embarrassed, I packed them away, and was left with a wardrobe of sweatpants and tight T-shirts.

I told my doctor, "I think I have a glandular problem. All the other breast-feeding mothers are losing weight, but I hardly eat anything and I haven't lost an ounce!" She smiled gently and said, "If you burn more calories than you take in, you'll lose weight." She didn't believe me! I left her office in a huff, grumbling about the unfairness of it all. When did I, a new mother, ever have time for a meal? Most nights it was all I could do to grab a spoon and a pint of ice cream while my little one was nestled at my breast. I tried to ignore the growing problem of the larger me by avoiding full-length mirrors and clothes in general, but my new pounds fairly shouted for attention. They stood out in all sorts of awkward bulges, as if they'd been lobbed at me from some distance away and stuck fast. My ankles were thick and my feet were plump, my knees had a double chin and my midsection, well, let's just say I got tired of people asking me when my next baby was due. My upper torso was dominated by 'The Milk Factory', but the novelty of being well endowed quickly wore off. I wanted my old body back and was willing to try anything to get it. "I'll exercise," I declared. The local gym was advertising an aerobics class for new mothers. Babies were welcome. I signed up right away.

On class day, I struggled to get out of the house on time, lugging my son in a car seat that seemed to weigh 100 pounds. I couldn't find parking nearby, so I walked a few blocks with the car seat bashing into my shins. By the time I reached the gym, I was sweating profusely. Class had already started, led by a boyish woman with a body fat percentage of 3.0. She whipped the class through a routine of jumping, step

By the time I reached the gym, I was sweating profusely...

The other women moved smoothly through the programme

The other women moved smoothly through the programme while I focused on not looking like a fool, but I was always a step or three behind. Everyone was kind. I was glad, though, that my son slept through the entire pathetic performance. We went home and I weighed myself. I had lost a pound.

I went to my second class a few days later. This time I managed to keep up somewhat, and even to throw some verve into my moves. As I leapt onto my step and threw my right foot out, I lost my balance and fell, knocking over the woman in front of me. Red-faced, I finished the class and went home to weigh myself. I had gained a pound.

I decided aerobics was not my 'thing'. Instead I bought a fancy jogging buggy, intending to zip around the block a few times a week with my baby riding in style. I had been an enthusiastic runner before my pregnancy, thinking nothing of knocking off two or three miles every other day. It wouldn't take long to fall back into my old habits. Everything went fine with my new programme until I came to my first hill and then I fell apart. It may as well have been Mount Rainier for all the gasping, grunting, and perspiring that went on—and that was just the first 20 yards. [Mount Rainier is a 14,410ft mountain in Washington State, USA.] I felt awkward not having my hands free and altogether discouraged with my outing. "My running days are over," I thought dispiritedly.

Right about then I decided to leave my fat where it was for a while and tackle another problem that had been bothering me—loneliness. My old friends didn't seem to understand my new life very well and sometimes blanched when I whipped out a breast to feed my son. I hadn't really gotten around to making new friends. So, despite my innate shyness, I dragged myself to a La Leche League meeting.

It was astonishing to see so many women brought together by a common interest, cheerfully breastfeeding their babies and discussing the changes motherhood had brought as if they actually relished their new lives. I really enjoyed my first meeting. I met someone there, a woman with a baby girl, who happened to live in my neighbourhood. Before long we had arranged to push our buggies around the lake a couple of times a week. She was such good company and we had so much in common that I really looked forward to these outings.

After a few weeks she suggested that we jog a little way each time we did our three-mile route, and it seemed like a good idea. The pace was never so strenuous that we couldn't keep talking. One day we were so engrossed in our subject (I think it was spit-up) that we jogged the whole three miles. It wasn't long after that that I put my sweatpants and my scales away.

My jogging and mothering buddy lives 600 miles away now... If I had any advice to give to other women in my shoes, it would be this: you are so much more than the sum of your parts. You're somebody's mother, for crying out loud! Life will never be the same, and neither will your body. It will be better. Miraculously, you're nourishing a baby in the best way possible, using only your body, so despite its obvious flaws, strange bulges and odd sagging areas it's amazing.

Focus instead on building and nurturing relationships with your child, your partner and especially other mothers. Have a 'tribe' with which to hang out, share stories, gripe, go to the park, exercise, talk parenting or any other subject... it'll make all the difference. The first year of new motherhood is tough. Establish a support network. You'll be glad you did when you discover how tough the second year is... and the third, fourth, fifth, etc. That would be my advice.

As far as my own weight goes, the less I think about it, the happier I am! I don't look like a model but I feel great: fit, healthy and occasionally like Supermum. I didn't get my old body back... I got a more fun version with bigger boobs! I still exercise regularly and I'm still breastfeeding—my second baby now!

Sarah Hobart

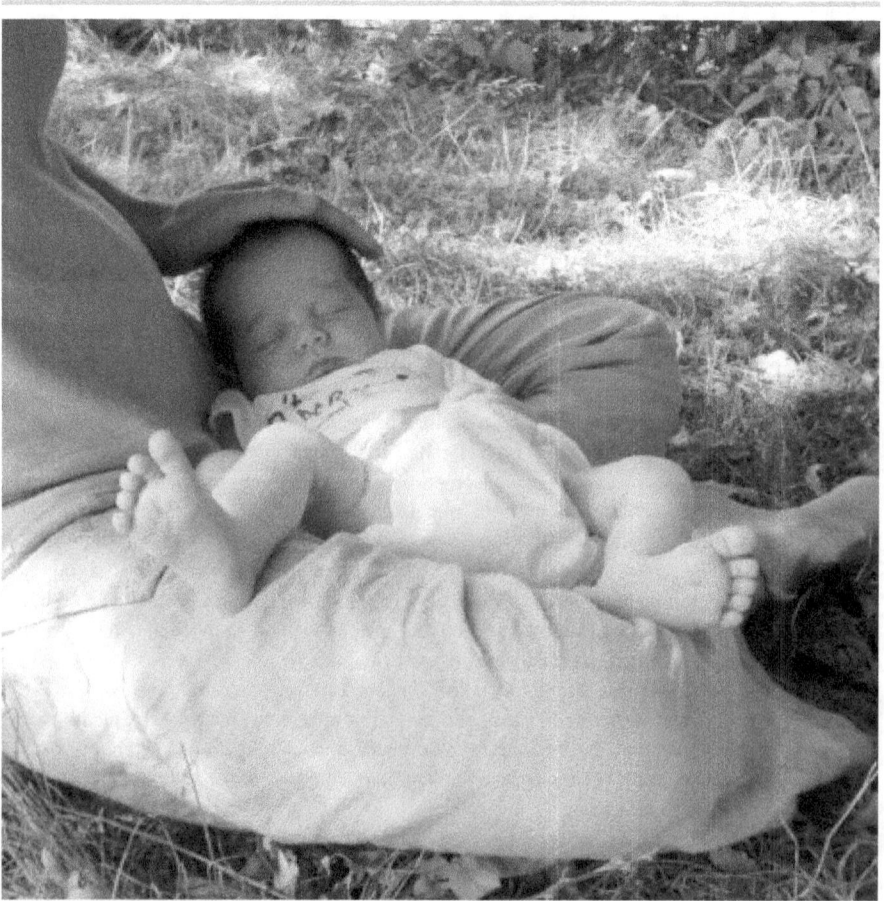

Tune in to a different kind of future...

A summary of the 10 countdown steps...

Keep the countdown steps in mind so you're covering all bases!

10... Understand 'optimal'
Are you clear about this? If you're basically healthy, it means having no unnecessary drugs or interventions during your pregnancy or labour. If you have some kind of medical problem, or experience symptoms during your pregnancy which worry your caregiver, it means judicious use of intervention.

9... Consider your assumptions
If you're in a slightly unusual situation instead of jumping to conclusions, you need to really research your options with a very open mind.

8... Do not disturb
What are you doing or agreeing to which could affect your pregnancy and birth?

7... Help your baby
Are you making decisions with your baby's needs in mind?

6... Care about care
This is all about taking responsibility for your antenatal care. You can choose!

5... Think ahead
What useful preparations can you make? How can you optimise your chances?

4... Choose who
Are you happy with your caregiver? If not, what can you do? Think of all your options—including different ways of communicating with the same person.

3... Choose where
You can choose to go to hospital, stay at home, or give birth in a birth centre...

2... Help your body
Are you taking good care of yourself? Are you doing everything possible?

1... Help your mind
If you feel worried about the actual birth, work through your feelings using all the methods suggested in this last, crucial step. And read the birthframes!

Special circumstances

As you already know, if you've read the whole book, optimal birth is not just for 'perfect women' with 'perfect' circumstances. Consider how you can prepare for the best possible outcomes if you're in any of the following situations:

If everyone around you seems to be pessimistic about optimality...

We live in a world which seems to have forgotten how labour and birth work. What's been particularly forgotten in many places is the way in which an emotion like fear can have such a strong influence on the way a woman's labour goes—because it actually stops her from producing the right hormone, i.e. oxytocin. If people around you are making you fearful, work through the 10th step—Help your mind—and re-read any birthframes which you find inspiring. Also remind yourself about the processes by re-reading step 8.

If you had lots of so-called 'pain relief' last time...

You may wonder how you're going to survive the kind of pain which pushed you to ask for pain relief last time. Actually, a strange thing happens when you optimise conditions for labour (i.e. when you feel safe and you're not disturbed), especially if you have become more confident about the birthing process. The endorphins kick in and you drift towards another state of mind. For more discussion of this problem and very specific suggestions for coping, read *Birth Pain: Power to Transform* by Verena Schmid (Fresh Heart 2011).

If 'everything' went wrong last time...

Remember all the accounts in this book about women who had the same experience. As any midwife will tell you, every labour is different. Ask your caregiver to help you prepare appropriately for your specific circumstances.

If you're preparing for a VBAC (vaginal birth after a caesarean)...

You may still be considering whether or not you're being wise to plan a vaginal birth after having surgery or it's possible you may feel especially lacking in confidence because of what happened last time. The book *Birthing Normally After a Caesarean or Two* by Hélène Vadeboncoeur (Fresh Heart 2011) will give you all the information you need, as well as reassurance and inspiration.

If you're expecting more than one baby...

Research your personal situation and discuss your options with your caregiver.

If you're particularly frightened about birth...

Get to know yourself better... walk, talk, allow yourself to work through you feelings. And read this book all over again with a more open mind this time!

Key decisions to make

Since it's so easy to get swept away by *other* people's decisions, it's particularly useful to remind yourself of the decisions you can and, in fact, *need* to make.

Antenatal care: You can choose when you register and where. You can agree to have antenatal tests, or you can refuse all of them, including ultrasound scans. For every situation you have a right to full information so you can make an informed decision. This means you can also refuse any interventions.

Your caregiver: If you don't like the first person you register with you can go elsewhere. Wherever you live, you probably have far more options than you imagine. Research them and take action, referring to the Useful contacts.

The language you use or refuse to use: How people talk influences outcomes… so use language wisely. If you doubt this, see pages 253 and 432-433.

Antenatal preparation: You can attend classes, or not; you can go to a chiropractor or osteopath, or not; you can do antenatal yoga, or not; you can explore things like the Alexander Technique; you can try out various kinds of new sports; you can do things to help you explore your feelings (or not); and you can read as many books and see as many DVDs as you want… or none!

Your place of birth: You have a lot of freedom of choice. Again, explore your options carefully and choose a place which suits you, even if people around you disagree—but try to get support from key people in your life too. Remember that you probably have a choice of hospitals to register at and that you can also opt to give birth at a birth centre or at home, if that's where you'll feel comfortable and safe. Also consider whether you want to use water for pain relief and if so, what practical arrangements you'll need to make.

Your birth attendants: Don't invite people along to be with you while you're in labour if you're not entirely comfortable with them. Remember that labour and birth are very much like sex: privacy helps. After all, how likely is it that any sensations you initially experience as pain will transform themselves into pleasant sexual feelings… if you have an audience of family and friends?

Your ways of coping with labour: Again, there are various approaches and you need to ensure that you have whatever you want available for your own labour.

The positions you use for labour and birth: Again these are your choice entirely.

Your postnatal care: You can specify what you do or don't want to have happen as long as things are proceeding safely. Would you like some privacy perhaps?

Useful contacts—Starting points for your own research...

AIMS (Assoc. for Improvements in the Maternity Services) - www.aims.org.uk
Support and information about parents' rights and choices. Provides information on complaints procedures.

Active Birth Centre - www.activebirthcentre.com
Tel: 020 7281 6760.
Classes for mothers interested in active, physiological birth. Can put you in touch with local groups and supply birth pools.

Association of Breastfeeding Mothers - www.abm.me.uk
Tel: 08444 122 948. Helpline: 08444 122 949.
Telephone and email advice. Support groups for breastfeeding mothers.

Association of Radical Midwives (ARM) - www.radmid.demon.co.uk
Tel: 01243 671673.
Support for midwives. Helpline for pregnant women.

Back in Action - www.backinaction.co.uk
Tel: 020 7930 8309
Suppliers of chairs and products for good back health. They also supply pregnancy rockers, called 'kneeling chairs'.

BLISS - www.bliss.org.uk
Tel: 020 7378 1122. Helpline: 0500 618140 Mon-Fri 10am-5pm.
Practical and emotional support for parents of premature babies.

Disability, Pregnancy and Parenthood International (DPPI) - www.dppi.org.uk
Tel: 0800 018 4730 or 020 7263 3088.
Information on pregnancy and parenthood for anyone with a disability.

Down's Syndrome Association - www.downs-syndrome.org.uk
Tel: 0845 230 0372.
Information and support for parents of babies/children with Down's syndrome.

Doula UK - www.doula.org.uk
Tel: 0871 433 3103.
Information about birth and postnatal doulas working in your area.

Fatherhood Institute - www.fatherhoodinstitute.org
Tel: 0845 634 1328.
A politically active lobby and information service for fathers.

Foresight – www.foresight-preconception.org.uk
Tel: 01243 868001.
Information on preconceptual care and nutrition during pregnancy.

Independent Midwives Association – www.independentmidwives.org.uk
Tel: 0845 4600 105 (leave message on answering machine).
Association for independent midwives. Can provide list of independent midwives in your area, experienced in homebirth.

Informed Parent – www.informedparent.co.uk
Tel: 01903 212969.
Information about vaccinations to help you reach a decision.

International Cesarean Awareness Netwework (ICAN) – www.ican-online.org
Information and support for women who wish to avoid a repeat caesarean.

La Leche League Great Britain (LLL) – www.laleche.org.uk
Tel: 0845 456 1855 (Mon-Thurs, answering machine at other times).
Support and information for pregnant women and breastfeeding mothers. Network of informal support groups.

Meet-a-Mum Association (MAMA) – www.mama.co.uk
Tel: 0845 120 6162. Helpline: 0845 120 3746 Mon-Fri, 7pm-10pm.
Support for mothers who feel lonely, isolated or depressed. Can put you in touch with other mothers in a similar situation.

Miscarriage Association – www.miscarriageassociation.org.uk
Helpline: 01924 200799 Mon-Fri, 9am-4pm.
Support for mothers who have experienced miscarriage. Also information on cervical stitches and ectopic pregnancies.

NCT (The National Childbirth Trust) – www.nct.org.uk
Tel: 0300 330 0772 (pregnancy and birth); 0300 330 0773 (postnatal line); 0330 330 0771 (breastfeeding line); 0300 330 0770 (general enquiries).
Information and support for all aspects of pregnancy and birth. Antenatal classes and network of informal postnatal groups.

Neal's Yard Remedies – www.nealsyardremedies.com
Tel: 0845 262 3145.
Mail order sales of a wide range of herbs and homeopathic remedies. Will send them anywhere in the world.

The Nursing & Midwifery Council (NMC) – www.nmc-uk.org
Information on the code of conduct by which midwives work and the place to contact if you have a complaint about a midwife or other caregiver.

Parentalk – www.parentalk.co.uk
Tel: 020 7921 4234.
Support for parents in the workplace, as well as for employers and professionals who support parents.

Patients' Association – www.patients-association.org.uk
Tel: 020 8423 9111. Helpline: 0845 608 4455.
Forum for NHS users to raise or share concerns about health care.

Primal Health Research Centre – www.primalhealthresearch.com
Information on research into procedures or drugs used in pregnancy, labour and birth. The quarterly newsletter by Michel Odent is available by subscription.

Rebirthing
- Pat Bennaceur – www.re-birth.uk.com Tel: 01273 727588.
- Binnie A Dansby – www.ecstaticbirth.com Tel: 01 892 890614.
- Gaia Pollini – www.thehillthatbreathes.com Tel: 0870 609 2690.

Courses for pregnant women or new mothers and families.

Society for Teachers of the Alexander Technique (STAT) – www.stat.org.uk
Tel: 020 7482 5135.
Information on classes, teachers or groups in places around the UK.

Stillbirth and Neonatal Death Society (SANDS) – www.uk-sands.org
Tel: 020 7436 7940. Helpline: 020 7436 5881. Email: support@uk-sands.org
Support and information for bereaved parents.

The Carrying Kind – www.thecarryingkind.com
Tel: 020 8509 1660.
Suppliers of a wide range of different baby carriers.

Twins and Multiples Births Association (TAMBA) – www.tamba.org.uk
Tel: 01483 304 442. Helpline: 0800 138 0509.
Encouragement and support for parents of twins or more.

What Doctors Don't Tell You – www.wddty.com
Tel: 0870 444 9886.
Information on medicine and health. Publishes newsletter and booklets.

Wilkinet Baby Carriers – www.wilkinet.co.uk
Tel: 0800 2550 247 (anytime).
Suppliers of Wilkinet baby carriers.

Working Families – www.workingfamilies.org.uk
Tel: 020 7253 7243. Helpline: 0800 013 0313.
Support for parents and families who want to find a better work-life balance.

Further reading

Most of the books below are readily available. If you have trouble finding any, you can do a search on the website www.bookfinder.com. Alternatively, contact the publisher directly or order any book via a bookstore, using its ISBN number.

Books to read while you're pregnant:

- *Birth Pain: Power to Transform* by Verena Schmid. Fresh Heart 2011. ISBN: 9781906619213.
- *Birthing Normally After a Caesarean of Two* by Hélène Vadeboncoeur. Fresh Heart 2011. ISBN: 9781906619152.
- *Birth Your Way: Choosing to Birth at Home or in a Birth Centre.* Fresh Heart 2011. ISBN: 9781906619183.
- *A Guide to Effective Care in Pregnancy and Childbirth* by Murray Enkin (et al). Oxford University Press 2000. ISBN: 9780192631732.
- *Pushed: The Painful Truth about Childbirth and Modern Maternity Care* by Jennifer Block. Da Capo Press 2008. ISBN: 9780738211664.
- *Birth Crisis* by Sheila Kitzinger. Routledge 2006. ISBN: 9780415372664.
- *Born in the USA: How a broken maternity system must be fixed to put women and children first* by Marsden Wagner. University of California Press 2006. ISBN: 9780520245969.
- *A Wise Birth* by Penny Armstrong and Sheryl Feldman. Pinter & Martin 2007. ISBN: 9781905177035.
- *Birth Without Violence* by Frederick Leboyer. Inner Traditions Bear and Company 2002 [first published 1974]. ISBN: 9780892819836.
- *Babies Remember Birth* by David Chamberlain. Ballantine Books 1990. ISBN: 978345364111.
- *Rediscovering Birth* by Sheila Kitzinger. Little Brown 2000. ISBN: 9780316853934.
- *Gentle Birth, Gentle Mothering: A Doctor's Guide to Natural Childbirth and Gentle Early Parenting Choices* by Sarah J Buckley. Celestial Arts 2009. ISBN: 9781587613227.
- *Easy Exercises for Pregnancy* by Janet Balaskas and Anthea Sieveking. Frances Lincoln Publishers 1997. ISBN: 9780711210486.
- *Vegetarian Pregnancy: Definitive Nutritional Guide* by Sharon Yntema. McBooks Press 2004. ISBN: 9780935526219.
- *Love is Not Enough: A Smart Woman's Guide to Money* by Merryn Somerset Webb. Harper Press 2008. ISBN: 9780007235193.
- *Is There Sex After Childbirth?* by Juliet Rix. HarperCollins 1995. ISBN: 9780722529570.

For your partner, relatives and friends:
- *Surprising, Inspiring Birth—accounts to inform, amuse and reassure* by Sylvie Donna (ed). Fresh Heart 2011. ISBN: 9781906619121.

For your caregivers:
- *Promoting Normal Birth: Research, Reflections & Guidelines*—an international collaboration (Sylvie Donna, ed). Fresh Heart 2011. ISBN: 9781906619060.
- *Birth Pain: Explaining Sensations, Exploring Possibilities* by Verena Schmid. Fresh Heart 2011. ISBN: 9781906619145.
- *Welcoming Baby* by Debby Gould. Fresh Heart 2011. ISBN: 9781906619169.

Books by Michel Odent, reflecting on research and his clinical practice:
- *Birth Reborn*. Souvenir Press 1994 [first published in 1984]. ISBN: 9780285631946.
- *Birth Traditions and Modern Pregnancy Care* (by Michel Odent and Jacqueline Vincent-Priya). Element Books 1992. ISBN: 9781852303211.
- *Birth and Breastfeeding*. Clairview Books 2003 [first published in 1992]. ISBN: 9781902636481.
- *Entering the World: The De-medicalization of Childbirth*. Marion Boyars Books 1984. ISBN: 9780714528005.
- *The Caesarean*. Free Association Books 2004. ISBN: 9781853437182.
- *The Farmer and the Obstetrician*. Free Association Books 2002. ISBN: 9781853435652.
- *The Scientification of Love*. Free Association Books 1999. ISBN: 9781853434761.

Books to support you in motherhood—read them in advance to prepare!
- *Breast is Best* by Penny Stanway. Pan Books 2005. ISBN: 9780330436304.
- *The Womanly Art of Breastfeeding* by Judy Torgus (ed.). Plume Books 2004. ISBN: 9780452285804.
- *Diaper Free! The Gentle Wisdom of Natural Infant Hygiene* by Ingrid Bauer. Natural Wisdom Press 2001. ISBN: 9780452287778.
- *Mother and Baby* by Miranda Castro. Pan Books 1996. ISBN: 9780330349253.
- *Sleeping with Your Baby: A Parent's Guide to Cosleeping* by James McKenna. Platypus Media 2007. ISBN: 9781930775343.
- *The Attachment Parenting Book* by William and Martha Sears. Little, Brown 2001. ISBN: 9780316778091.

Bibliography

Babies Remember Birth. Chamberlain, David. Ballantine Books 1990. ISBN: 978345364111.

Babywatching. Morris, Desmond. Jonathan Cape 1991. ISBN: 9780224032599.

Baby Wisdom. Jackson, Deborah. Hodder & Stoughton 2002. ISBN: 9780340793503.

Bill Bryson's African Diary. Bryson, Bill. Doubleday 2002. ISBN: 9780385605144.

Birth and Breastfeeding. Odent, Michel. Clairview Books 2003. ISBN: 9781902636481.

Birthing from Within. England, Pam and Horowitz, Rob. Souvenir Press 2007. ISBN: 9780285637870.

Birth Reborn. Odent, Michel. Souvenir Press 1994. ISBN: 9780285631946.

Birth Traditions and Modern Pregnancy Care. Odent, Michel and Vincent-Priya, Jacqueline. Element Books 1992. ISBN: 9781852303211.

Birth Without Trauma. Svechnikova, Marina. Astrel 2001. (No ISBN available.)

Birth Without Violence. Leboyer, Frederick. Inner Traditions Bear and Company 2002. ISBN: 9780892819836.

Born in the USA: How a broken maternity system must be fixed to put women and children first. Wagner, Marsden. University of California Press 2006. ISBN: 9780520245969.

Breast is Best. Stanway, Penny. Pan Books 2005. ISBN: 9780330436304.

Creating a Joyful Birth Experience. Capacchione, Lucia and Bardsley, Sandra. Simon & Schuster 1994. ISBN: 9780671870270.

Diaper Free! The Gentle Wisdom of Natural Infant Hygiene. Bauer, Ingrid. Natural Wisdom Press 2001. ISBN: 9780452287778.

Diary of a Midwife. Van Olphen-Fehr, Juliana. Bergin & Garvey, 1998. ISBN: 9780897895880.

Face Like a Flower. Anderson, Bill. Dent Dale Publishing 2004. ISBN: 9780954777203.

Gentle Birth, Gentle Mothering: A Doctor's Guide to Natural Childbirth and Gentle Early Parenting Choices. Buckley, Sarah. Celestial Arts 2009. ISBN: 9781587613227.

Immaculate Deception II. Arms, Suzanne. Celestial Arts 1994. ISBN: 9780890876336.

Infant Potty Training—A Gentle and Primeval Method Adapted to Modern Living. Boucke, Laurie and Carlson, Linda. White-Boucke Publishing 2000. ISBN: 9781888580242.

Letting Go as Children Grow. Jackson, Deborah. Bloomsbury 2003. ISBN: 9780747565765.

Mother and Baby. Castro, Miranda. Pan Books 1996. ISBN: 9780330349253.

Mother and Child: The Secret Wisdom of Pregnancy, Birth and Motherhood. Jackson, Deborah. Duncan Baird 2001. ISBN: 9781903296134.

Multiple Sclerosis and Having a Baby. Graham, Judy. Healing Arts Press 1999. ISBN: 9780892817887.

Myles Textbook for Midwives. Myles, Margaret. Churchill Livingstone 2009. ISBN: 9780443069390.

New Active Birth. Balaskas, Janet. Harvard Common Press 1994. ISBN: 9781558320383.

Obstetric Myths Versus Research Realities. Goer, Henci. Bergin & Garvey 1995. ISBN: 9780897894272.

Obstetrics by Ten Teachers. Campbell, Stuart and Lees, Christoph. Hodder Arnold 2000. ISBN: 9780340719862.

Optimal Foetal Positioning. Sutton, Jean and Scott, Pauline. Birth Concepts 1996. Out of print.

Ourselves as Mothers: Universal Experience of Motherhood. Kitzinger, Sheila. Doubleday 1992. ISBN: 9780385403207.

Possessing the Secret of Joy. Walker, Alice. Vintage 1993. ISBN: 9780099224112.

Promoting Normal Birth: Research, Reflections & Guidelines. An international collaboration, Sylvie Donna (ed). Fresh Heart 2011. ISBN: 9781906619060.

Pushed: The Painful Truth about Childbirth and Modern Maternity Care. Block, Jennifer. Da Capo Press 2008. ISBN: 9780738211664.

Sleeping with your baby: a parent's guide to cosleeping. McKenna, James. Platypus Media 2007. ISBN: 9781930775343

Spiritual Midwifery. Gaskin, Ina May. Book Publishing Company 2002. ISBN: 9781570671043.

The Caesarean. Odent, Michel. Free Association Books 2004. ISBN: 9781853437182.

The Complete Book of Pregnancy. Metland, Daphne (ed.) HarperCollins 2000. ISBN: 9780004140995.

The Farmer and the Obstetrician. Odent, Michel. Free Association Books 2002. ISBN: 9781853435652.

The Scientification of Love. Odent, Michel. Free Association Books 1999. ISBN: 9781853434761.

The Trauma of Birth. Rank, Otto. Routledge 1999. ISBN: 9780415211048.

The Womanly Art of Breastfeeding. Torgus, Judy (ed.) Plume Books 2004. ISBN: 9780452285804.

Three in a Bed: The Benefits of Sleeping with Your Baby. Jackson, Deborah. Bloomsbury 2003. ISBN: 9780747565758.

Notes and references

To find abstracts for any studies, go to www.pubmed.com and search using year and key words (e.g. any author's name and main words in the title). If you notice errors of any kind in the Notes & references here, email info@freshheartpublishing.co.uk. Amendments will be made in future editions. Also, please make contact if there's anything in this section which you disagree with, or would like to add to.

If, while you're reading, you encounter words you don't understand, simply go to the Glossary or the Index, for more information. If you're new to the language of birth, you will soon find you feel comfortable with it—although you may feel you want to campaign to change some of the terminology!

Introduction: An interesting challenge

1. There are no references here as I provide plenty—with commentary—later, as topics come up.
2. If you don't believe you really have a choice, read the Darzi report at the following URL: www.healthcareforlondon.nhs.uk/a-framework-for-action-2/

10... Understand 'optimal'

1. In the following article, Michel describes ways of facilitating the natural processes:
   - Odent M. New reasons and new ways to study birth physiology. *International Journal of Gynecology & Obstetrics* 2001, 75:S39-S45

   (He expands further on these ideas in his book *Birth & Breastfeeding*.) In case you feel wary of facilitating the physiological processes of labour and birth *without pain relief* you may be reassured to note that quite a few contributors to this book mention their surprise at the *lack* of pain in their labours or the surprising nature of the sensations. Others—including myself—experienced intense pain but found they were able to travel through it, thanks to the strange hormonal processes which were taking place, which inevitably have an effect on the mind as well as the body. There will be more in later chapters on why and how it's possible to continue through either painful or painfree births. It will soon become clear to you why a drug-free labour is preferable to a medicated, managed one in terms of experience, as well as safety, and why it's so easy to disturb the natural processes if any drugs or interventions are used.

2. For a review and comparison of obstetric approaches (either 'managed' or natural) read any or all of the books listed below. After doing so, it is very difficult to reach the conclusion that intervention enhances the natural processes, unless it's really needed for medical reasons.
   - The book co-authored by seven researchers (Enkin, et al) *Guide to Effective Care in Pregnancy and Childbirth.* Oxford University Press, 2000
   - Enkin's book, written with another eminent researcher Jadad: *Randomised Control Trials: Questions, Answers and Musings.* Blackwell, 2007

- The book written by professor of midwifery and director of a research group, Soo Downe: *Normal Childbirth: Evidence and Debate*. Churchill Livingstone, 2004
- Walsh, D. *Evidence-based Care for Normal Labour and Birth*. Routledge, 2007
- The book written and researched by former WHO director Marsden Wagner: *Born in the USA: How a broken maternity system must be fixed to put women and children first*. University of California Press, 2006
- The book written by Jennifer Block, former journalist and co-editor of the revised classic *Our Bodies Ourselves*: *Pushed*. Da Capo Lifelong, 2008

3   You may think I'm making many assumptions in what I'm saying. The reasons for this should become clear as you read. Breastfeeding is a case in point... if you read any book on the topic, you will find out about its numerous advantages, for both you and your baby. Here's one, which was new to me... The following study found that breastfeeding decreases your baby's chance of getting rheumatoid arthritis later on in life!

- Pikwer M, Bergström U, Nilsson JA, Jacobsson L, Berglund G, Turesson C. Breast feeding, but not use of oral contraceptives, is associated with a reduced risk of rheumatoid arthritis. *Annals of the Rheumatic Diseases*, 2009 Apr;68(4):526-30. Epub 2008 May 13

4   Actually, research into the causative associations between drug use in labour and things such as alertness postnatally and breastfeeding is in its infancy, but results are already suggesting that drugs do have side- or after-effects; these are constantly discussed in the literature on anaesthesiology. Possible (or probable) side- or after-effects are widely accepted as including nausea and vomiting, feelings of confusion, lowering of the blood pressure, sedation, urinary retention, slower emptying of stomach contents and itching (pruritis)—and the pain relief is not always effective. Of course, in all cases, it's not easy to establish what causes what.

In a retrospective study conducted by Jordan, *et al* (Jordan, *et al*, 2009), which looked at 48,366 healthy women birthing singleton babies at term (i.e. women having vaginal births), it was found that at 48 hours after the birth, rates of breast-feeding definitely seemed to be affected by epidurals, opioid analgesia (pethidine, diamorphine, etc) and ergomentrine (used in the third stage of labour). The researchers point out that 'failure to breastfeed increases morbidity and mortality in both mothers and children in developed and developing countries', so the impact of any possible effects of drugs used unnecessarily could be enormous. In this study, beyond sociological factors, which have long been known to affect breastfeeding rates, lower breast-feeding rates were associated with induction with pessaries (prostaglandins), epidurals and opioid analgesia, and ergometrine used for the third stage of labour. (Oddly, they found that first-time mothers who'd had gas and air were more likely to breastfeed. Could this be because these mothers were determined to avoid drugs in labour as much as possible, so as to have as 'natural' a birth as possible, and to breastfeed successfully too? Any determination to avoid everything except gas and air could be a particularly British attitude, which is misguided, in my view, for other reasons, as I shall explain later. The view that it is considered 'nothing' is reflected in the off-hand statement made by many women postnatally: "Oh, I only had gas and air.") Anyway, the study by Jordan, *et al* does provide some evidence that drug use in labour and birth has an impact on breastfeeding rates at 48 hours postpartum, which obviously will affect longer-term rates too, although it must be said that this evidence is not accepted by all anaesthetists as *prospective* randomised studies are seen as more reliable. After all, women usually request epidurals *because* of difficulties, so it is not necessarily epidurals *per se* which cause later problems. Cause-effect are difficult to establish.

Other (prospective) studies reported fairly clear problems with narcotics used in labour (Beilin, *et al*, 2005; Camann, *et al*, 2007; Torvaldsen, *et al*, 2006). In the study by Beilin, *et al* researchers concluded: "Among women who breast-fed previously, those who were randomly assigned to receive high-dose labor epidural fentanyl were more likely to have stopped breast-feeding 6 weeks postpartum than women who were randomly assigned to receive less fentanyl or no fentanyl. (Fentanyl was added to the drug bupivacain, in the epidural cocktail as bupivacain causes paralysis in the lower part of the body; adding fentanyl reduces this effect. Clearly, though, it's a problem if too much is used.) The study by Torvaldsen, *et al* concluded: "Women in this cohort who had epidurals were less likely to fully breastfeed their infant in the few days after birth and more likely to stop breast-feeding in the first 24 weeks"... although the researchers felt they were unable to say whether there was a causal link between epidural anaesthesia and breastfeeding difficulties. This was despite the fact that "Intrapartum analgesia and type of birth were associated with partial breastfeeding and breastfeeding difficulties in the first postpartum week" and the fact that women who had epidurals were more likely to stop breastfeeding than women who used non-pharmacological methods of pain relief. Camann's editorial (below) provides a good overview of this topic. See:

- Jordan S, Emery, S, Watkins A, Evans JD, Storey M, Morgan G. Associations of drugs routinely given in labour with breastfeeding at 48 hours: analysis of the Cardiff Births Survey. *BJOG: International Journal of Obstetrics & Gynaecology*, 2009, online publication on 1 Sept
- Beilin Y, Bodian C, Weiser J, *et al*. Effect of labor epidural analgesia with and without fentanyl on infant breast-feeding: a prospective, randomized, double-blind study. *Anesthesiology*, 2005, Dec;103(6):1211-7
- Camann W. Labor analgesia and breast feeding: avoid parenteral narcotics and provide lactation support. *International Journal of Obstetric Anesthesia*, 2007, Jul; 16(3):199-201
- Torvaldsen S, Roberts CL, Simpson JM, *et al*. Intrapartum epidural analgesia and breastfeeding: a prospective cohort study. *International Breastfeeding Journal*, 2006,Dec11;1:24

Coming back to the issue of alertness, studies do not provide a clear overall picture. Years ago, some practitioners were apparently concerned about the observable depressive effects on newborns of analgesia used in labour. I deduce this because researchers (Bonta, *et al*, 1979) discovered that another drug (naloxone) provided an effective 'antidote' and restored what apparently seemed to be an acceptable level of alertness in newborns. However, is naloxone (or any equivalents) really a solution to reduced alertness or is the mother-baby dyad losing out when natural alertness is not present? (Would you prefer natural sexual arousal when you meet your life partner, or passion produced by sedatives, counteracted by Viagra? Of course, we need to remember that these early interactions can never be repeated, and also that they might have a significant effect on later interactions too.) Mothers, incidentally, are sometimes assessed by anaesthetists for alertness using a four-point scale (1. awake/alert, 2. drowsy, but readily responsive, 3. drowsy and requires shaking to rouse, 4. unconscious). But how awake and alert do people expect women to be just after they've had a baby? Physiological labour usually results in extreme alertness, which is, of course, beneficial for the bonding process.

In a more recent study (Volikas, *et al*, 2005), which looked at potential side-effects of patient-controlled opioid analgesia (remifentanil) postnatally, 22 out of 50 women were reported to have experienced some drowsiness. (44% seems rather a high percentage...) The researchers reported that at the dose used in the study, remifentanil had 'an acceptable level of maternal side-effects and minimal effect on the neonate' (i.e. the newborn baby). Personally, I question whether any level of drowsiness is acceptable during this one-time encounter between new mother and baby. And I wonder how it could be established that there was only a 'minimal' effect on the neonate if there was no control group, i.e. if researchers did not compare these 50 neonates with 50 others, who were born entirely physiologically. What seems a normal level of alertness in a neonate might change if researchers were to document the extreme alertness many people have anecdotally reported when babies have been born without any drugs in their systems. There is an enormous difference, I would suggest, between a dull-eyed look and a vibrant gaze, in terms of bonding and simple joy in new motherhood. And when a newborn looks at his or her mother it's helpful, perhaps, if the mother isn't one of the 22 out of 50 women who were reported in this study 'to have experienced some drowsiness'. Hill (2008) later strongly recommended remifentanil, although Van de Velde disagreed in a follow-up article. Although remifentanil is more effective than pethidine and diamorphine (which perhaps explains why it is popular in Belfast), what price are women paying for their reduced alertness in terms of effective early bonding?

Another study (Wittels, *et al*, 1997) compared the alertness (amongst other things) of newborns exposed to either epidural morphine or intravenous patient-controlled analgesia. Of course, because the focus was on newborns of mothers who'd had a caesarean it was impossible to compare the alertness of babies born with drugs in their systems and that of babies who'd been born with absolutely no drugs in their system, so only 'relative' alertness could be tracked. Yet another study, back in 1981 (Rosenblatt, *et al*) looked at the influence of maternal analgesia (epidural bupivacaine) on the newborn. Significant effects were found: "Immediately after delivery, infants with greater exposure to bupivacaine in utero were more likely to be cyanotic [blue-skinned] and unresponsive to their surroundings. Visual skills and alertness decreased significantly with increases in the cord blood concentration of bupivacaine, particularly on the first day of life but also throughout the next six weeks. Adverse effects of bupivacaine levels on the infant's motor organisation, his ability to control his own state of consciousness and his physiological response to stress were also observed." A recent study by Henrichs, *et al* (2009) considered whether alertness could be affected by a factor such as fetal size in mid- or late pregnancy. (The conclusion was that it could.) In a study such as this, I would imagine there could be numerous confounding factors, the principal one being the use of anaesthesia or analgesia (or not) during labour. Personally, I would only trust the results of this study if all fetuses measured in utero had been born without any drugs in their systems. After all, while the motivation of these researchers appears to have been a desire to investigate behavioural problems in newborns (e.g. infant irritability), they do not appear to have taken into account the fact that one of the primary characteristics of narcotics-addicted neonates is that they are 'substantially more irritable' (Strauss, *et al*, 1975).

Given the vital importance of good bonding in the sensitive one-hour period following birth (from the point of view of later mothering behaviour), I very much hope that other researchers will look further into the issues of alertness and breastfeeding success (or lack thereof), particularly in relation to drug-use in labour. See:

- Bonta BW, Gagliardi JV, Williams V, Warshaw JB. Nalaxone reversal of mild neurobehavioral depression in normal newborn infants after routine obstetric analgesia. *Journal of Pediatrics,* 1979. Jan;94(1):102-5
- Volikas I, Butwick A, Wilkinson C, Pleming A, Nicholson G. Maternal and neonatal side-effects of remifentanil patient-controlled analgesia in labour. *British Journal of Anaesthesia*, 2005, Oct;95(4):504-9. Epub 2005 Aug 19
- Wittels B, Glosten B, Faure EA, Moawad AH, Ismail M, Hibbard J, Senal JA, Cox SM, Blackman SC, Karl L, Thisted RA. Postcesarean analgesia with both epidural morphine and intravenous patient-controlled analgesia: neurobehavioral outcomes among nursing neonates. *Anesthesia & Analgesia,* 1997. Sep;8(3):600-6
- Rosenblatt DB, Belsey EM, Lieberman BA, Redshaw M, Caldwell J, Notarianni L, Smith RL, Beard RW. The influence of maternal analgesia on neonatal behaviour: II. Epidural bupivacaine. *British Journal of Obstetric Gynaecology,* 1981. Apr;88(4): 407-13
- Henrichs J, Schenk JJ, Schmidt HG, Arends LR, Steegers EA, Hofman A, Jaddoe VW, Verhulst FC, Tiemeier H. Fetal size in mid- and late pregnancy is related to infant alertness: the generation R study. *Developmental Psychobiology*, 2009, Mar; 51(2):119-30
- Strauss ME, Lessen-Firestone JK, Starr RH Jr, Ostrea EM Jr. Behavior of narcotics-addicted newborns. *Child Development,* 1975. Dec;46(4):887-93
- Hill D. Remifentanil patient-controlled analgesia should be routinely available for use in labour. *International Journal of Obstetric Anesthesia,* 2008, 17(4),336-339.
- Van de Velde M. Controversy. Remifentanil patient-controlled analgesia should be routinely available for use in labour. *International Journal of Obstetric Anesthesia,* 2008 Oct;17(4):339-42. Epub 2008 Jul 9

5 For more on this subject read *Is there sex after childbirth?* by Juliet Rix. Thorsons, 1995.

6 The term 'cascade of interventions' was first conceptualised and explained by Sally Inch in 1989. See: Inch S. *Birthrights: Parents' Guide to Modern Childbirth.* Green Print, 1989. In Step 8 (Do not disturb) I explain in detail what this cascade of hormones involves.

7 Soo Downe and McCourt (2004) have come up with the concept of 'unique normality'. In other words, they recognise that there is a *range of normality*, which means that women don't have to fit neatly onto charts or into 'mental boxes' so as to be considered normal. See:

- Downe S, McCourt C. From being to becoming: reconstructing childbirth knowledges. In Downe S (ed) *Normal Childbirth: Evidence and Debate.* Churchill Livingstone, 2004

8 This is explained in the following article:

- Steer P, Alam MA, Wadsworth J, Welch A. Relation between maternal haemoglobin concentration and birth weight in different ethnic groups. *British Medical Journal,* 1995;310:489-91

9   Some researchers have pointed out that a midwife's diagnosis of labour in hospital is not a simple, one-sided clinical judgement. Whether or not a diagnosis is made depends on many other institutional constraints. See:
    - Burvill S. Midwifery diagnosis of labour onset. *British Journal of Midwifery*, 2002, 10(10):600-605
    - Cheyne H, Dowding D, Hundley V. Making the diagnosis of labour: midwives' diagnostic judgement and management decisions. *Journal of Advanced Nursing*, 2006, 53(6):625-635

10 As I mentioned, in an earlier note, quite a few contributors to this book mention their surprise at the *lack* of pain in their labours or the surprising nature of the sensations. Others—including myself!—experienced intense pain but found they were able to travel through it, thanks to the strange hormonal processes which were taking place, which inevitably have an effect on the mind as well as the body.

11 Michel S, Rake A, Treiber K. MR obstetric pelvimetry: effects of birthing position on pelvic bony dimensions. *American Journal of Roentgenology*, 2002, 179:1063-1067.

12 Gould (2000) commented on a woman's apparent need to move around during a physiological labour. Many other researchers who have conducted anthropological studies of indigenous peoples have noted that upright positions are generally favoured for birth. See:
    - Gould D. Normal labour: a concept analysis. *Journal of Advanced Nursing*, 2000, 31(2):418-427
    - Gupta J, Hofmeyr G. Position for women during second stage of labour. Cochrane Review in: *The Cochrane Library*, Issue 4. Chichester: John Wiley & Sons Ltd, 2006
    - Jarcho J. *Postures and Practices During Labour Among Primitive Peoples*. Paul Hoeber, 1934
    - Kitzinger S. *Rediscovering Birth*. Little, Brown & Company, 2000
    - Coppen R. *Birthing Positions: Do Midwives Know Best?* Quay Books, 2005
    - Balaskas J. *New Active Birth: A Concise Guide to Natural Childbirth*. Unwin, 1995
    - Lavin J, McGregor J. Native American childbirth on the western plains. *International Journal of Feto-Maternal Medicine*, 1992, 5(3):125-133

13 Control and management at this point often occur because of the mistaken notion (by caregivers) that a time limit needs to be put on the second stage of labour. In fact, large reviews of research has revealed that there is no connection between a long labour and a poor Apgar score, or admissions to a neonatal unit (Saunders, *et al*, 1992; Menticoglou, *et al*, 1995; Janni, *et al*, 2002; Myles and Santolaya, 2003—see below for full references). Some of the women in these studies had had second stages that had lasted more than five hours!—but these long second stages still had no effect on birth outcomes. Only in cases where long stages were linked to special first stage factors or intervention, or when the baby stayed too long on the pelvic floor, was there a link with maternal infection or bleeding, or a deterioration in fetal heart patterns (Nordstrom, *et al*, 2001.) Moreover, research has revealed all kinds of problems with what is known as 'commanded pushing', as follows: 1. It results in the woman holding her breath for prolonged periods, which affects the placenta, and therefore the unborn baby. (Caldeyro-Barcia, 1979). 2. Less oxygen gets to the baby's brain (Aldrich, *et al*, 1995). 3. Babies whose mothers had 'commanded pushing' for more than an hour had a lower pH at birth—which is bad news

(Thompson, 1993). 4. Commanded pushing results in longer second stages (Thompson, 1993; Parnell, et al, 1993). 5. Women tend to become exhausted (Knauth and Haloburdo, 1986; Roberts, 2002). 6. There are more forceps and ventouse births (Fraser, et al, 2000; Hansen, et al, 2002). 7. More episiotomies are performed and more tears occur (Sampselle and Hines, 1999). 8. The pelvic floor is damaged more often, which results in urinary stress incontinence (Handa, et al, 1996). Most surprisingly, perhaps, one hospital audit discovered that although only 8% of midwives attending the births of low-risk women encouraged the women to push as they wished (Walsh, et al, 1999), the practice of commanded pushing only served to shorten the second stage of labour by 14 minutes (Bloom, et al, 2006), which—as I mentioned before—was not helpful in terms of improving outcomes. After reviewing all the research in 2006, Bosomworth and Bettany-Saltikov concluded that pushing while holding one's breath should also be discontinued because of its documented effects on the fetal heartbeat and the perineum. This echoes the guidelines provided by Enkin, et al (2000), which—based on a review of the available evidence—advises against routine directed pushing, pushing by sustained bearing down and breath-holding. See:

- Saunders N, Paterson C, Wadsworth J. Neonatal and maternal morbidity in relation to the length of the second stage of labour. *British Journal of Obstetrics & Gynaecology,* 1992, 99(5):381-385
- Menticoglou S, Manning F, Harman C. Perinatal outcome in relation to second stage duration. *American Journal of Obstetrics & Gynaecology,* 1995, 173(3):906-912
- Janni W, Schiessl B, Peschers U. The prognostic impact of a prolonged second stage of labour on maternal and fetal outcome. *Acta Obstetrica et Gynaecologica Scandinavica,* 2002, 81:214-221
- Myles T, Santolaya J. Maternal and neonatal outcomes in patients with a prolonged second stage of labour. *Obstetrics & Gynaecology,* 2003, 102:52-58
- Nordstrom L, Achanna S, Naka K, Arulkumaran S. Fetal and maternal lactate increase during active second stage of labour. *British Journal of Obstetrics & Gynaecology,* 2001, 108:263-268
- Caldeyro-Barcia R, Giussi G, Storch E. The influence of maternal bearing down efforts and their effects on fetal heart rate, oxygenation and acid base balance. *Journal of Perinatal Medicine,* 1979, 9: 63-67
- Aldrich C, D'Antona D, Spencer J. The effects of maternal pushing on fetal cerebral oxygenation and blood volume during the second stage of labour. *British Journal of Obstetrics & Gynaecology,* 1995, 102(6):448-453
- Thompson A. Pushing techniques in the second stage of labour. *Journal of Advanced Nursing,* 1993, 18:171-177
- Parnell C, Langhoff-Roos J, Iverson R. Pushing method in the expulsive phase of labour. A randomised trial. *Acta Obstetrica et Gynaecologica Scandinavica,* 1993, 72(1):31-35
- Knauth D, Haloburdo E. Effects of pushing techniques in birthing chair on length of second stage of labour. *Nursing Research,* 1986, 35:49-5 1
- Roberts J. The 'push' for evidence: management of the second stage. *Journal of Midwifery & Women's Health,* 2002, 47(1):2-15
- Fraser W, Marcoux S, Krauss I, Douglas J. Multi-centre, randomised controlled trial of

- delayed pushing for nulliparous women in the second stage of labour with continuous epidural analgesia. *American Journal of Obstetrics & Gynaecology,* 2000, 182:1165-1172
- Hansen S, Clark S, Foster J. Active pushing versus passive fetal descent in the second stage of labour: a randomised controlled trial. *Obstetrics & Gynaecology,* 2002, 99:29-34
- Sampselle C, Hines S. Spontaneous pushing during labour: Relationship to perineal outcomes. *Journal of Nurse Midwifery,* 1999, 44(1):36-39
- Handa V, Harris T, Ostergard D. Protecting the pelvic floor: obstetric management to prevent incontinence and pelvic organ collapse. *Obstetrics & Gynaecology,* 1996, 88:470-478
- Walsh D, Harris M, Shuttlewood S. Changing midwifery birthing practice through audit. *British Journal of Midwifery,* 1999, 7(7):432-345
- Bloom S, Casey B, Schaffer J, McIntire D, Leveno K. A randomised trial of coached versus uncoached maternal pushing during the second stage of labour. *American Journal of Obstetrics & Gynaecology,* 2006, 194:10-13
- Bosomworth A, Bettany-Saltikov J. Just take a deep breath. *MIDIRS,* 2006, 16(2):157-165
- Enkin M, Kierse M, Neilson J, Crowther C, Duley L, Hodnett E, Hofmeyr J. *A Guide to Effective Care in Pregnancy and Childbirth.* Oxford University Press, 2000

14 For a discussion on the effects of earlier or later cord cutting, see:
- Gunther M. The transfer of blood between the baby and the placenta in the minutes after birth. *Lancet,* 1957; I:1277-1280
- Kinmond S, *et al.* Umbilical Cord Clamping and Preterm Infants: a randomized trial. *British Medical Journal,* 1993, (6871): 306:172-175
- Pisacane A. Neonatal prevention of iron deficiency, *British Medical Journal,* 1996, 312:136-7
- Wardrop CA, Holland BM. The roles and vital importance of placental blood to the newborn infant. *Journal of Perinatal Medicine,* 1995, 23(1-2):139-43

Basically, suffice to say that delayed cord cutting by up to two minutes was found to be beneficial for premature babies because there was less intraventricular haemorrhage and they then needed less blood transfusion (Rabe, et al, 2006). McDonald and Abbott (2006) found that delaying clamping for full-term newborns meant the babies got 30% more blood and up to 60% more red blood cells—all of which is excellent news! This all means that babies start off life with optimal haematocrit and haemoglobin levels (Prendiville and Elbourne, 1989), better blood circulation to vital organs, better heart-lung adaptation and a better chance of being able to breastfeed for longer (Mercer, 2001). See:

- Rabe H, Reynolds G, Diaz-Rossello J. Early versus delayed umbilical cord clamping in preterm infants. *The Cochrane Database of Systematic Reviews,* 2006, Issue 3
- McDonald S, Abbott J. Effect of timing of umbilical cord clamping of term infants on maternal and neonatal outcomes. (Protocol) *Cochrane Database of Systematic Reviews,* 2006, Issue 3
- Prendiville WJ, Elbourne DR. Care during the third stage of labour. In Chalmers I, Enkin M and Kierse M (eds) *Effective Care in Pregnancy and Childbirth.* Oxford University Press, 1989

- Mercer J. Current best evidence: a review of the literature on umbilical cord clamping. *Journal of Midwifery & Women's Health,* 2001, 46(6):402-414

15 Michel describes this process of transformation in the following article:
- Odent M. New reasons and new ways to study birth physiology. *International Journal of Gynecology & Obstetrics,* 2001, 75:S39-S45

16 Legal requirements for home birth are usually in place to protect both mother and baby. In Britain most NHS trusts stipulate that two midwives need to be in attendance: one midwife should be available to help the mother, and another one should be able to focus on the baby, if necessary. Interestingly enough, it is also legal to give birth at home without *any* professional attendants, providing no unqualified ones are around either. This book does not look at this kind of birth—known as 'unassisted birth'—because it lies outside the concept of 'optimal' which we are defining in this book as being ultra-natural but with support within easy reach. However, guidelines for unplanned, *accidental* unassisted birth (with or without an unqualified person in attendance, both of which are legal) are provided, for the simple reason that physiological birth can sometimes proceed much more smoothly (and quickly!) than people expect, particularly when they've experienced 'managed' births beforehand.

17 After attending approx 16,000 births—in Paris and London—Michel has reported almost never observing breathing difficulties in naturally-born newborns. Getting breathing started effectively and ensuring that any difficulties are overcome is a major preoccupation of caregivers when women have drugs of any kind during labour and/or birth because obviously death or brain damage can quickly follow a lack of breathing after the baby's been born.

18 Bystrova, *et al*,s study (2009) confirmed the earlier, very famous research of Kennel and Klaus (reviewed by the authors themselves in 1988), which indicated that babies and mothers should remain together in the early moments and minutes after birth. Bystrova, *et al* concluded: "Skin-to-skin contact, for 25 to 120 minutes after birth, early suckling, or both, positively influenced mother-infant interaction 1 year later when compared with routines involving separation of mother and infant." One of the original researchers, Marshall Klaus, also offered a commentary on this recently, as you will see from the reference below.
- Bystrova K, Ivanova V, Edhborg M, Matthiesen AS, Ransjö-Arvidson AB, Mukhamedrakhimov R, Uvnäs-Moberg K, Widström AM. Early contact versus separation: effects on mother-infant interaction one year later. *Birth,* 2009, Jun; 36(2):97-109
- Kennell JH, Klaus MH. The perinatal paradigm: is it time for a change? *Clinical Perinatology,* 1988, Dec;15(4):801-13
- Klaus MH. Commentary: An early, short, and useful sensitive period in the human infant. *Birth,* 2009, Jun;36(2):110-2

19 Graham (1997) charts the origins and evolution of the episiotomy; first it was performed as a result of notions about a woman's 'imperfection', then it continued because of a surgical mindset and finally it just became institutionalised in Western birthing practices. Its use was (wrongly) justified because of fears of cerebral palsy (episiotomy, it was thought, would mean the fetal head was 'knocking' against the perineum for a shorter time), because it was felt it shortened the second stage of

labour, and finally—and most persistently—because it was thought to prevent tears into the anal sphincter. Starting with Sleep, et al (1984), research has revealed that its use is inappropriate in most cases, mainly because it results in *more* (not less) tearing and suturing. (This was the conclusion of Carroli and Belizan's Cochrane review in 2006.) Also, it is now considered bad practice for most women because research has also shown that an episiotomy reduces strength in the pelvic floor (Sartore, *et al*,2004), leads to pain in this area (Bick, *et al*, 2002) and even painful sexual intercourse afterwards (Bick, *et al*, 2002). Some studies (Dipiazza, *et al*, 2006; Williams, 2003; Richter, *et al*, 2002) have concluded that episiotomies even *facilitate* bad tears into the anal sphincter. It's also worth noting that some academic papers have condemned the practice of routine episiotomy after a woman has previously had a tear (Peleg and Zlatnik, 1999; Dandolu, *et al*, 2005). According to Dannecker, *et al* (2004), episiotomies should only be performed when the fetus is clearly distressed and needs to be born quickly (e.g. in the case of a breech birth which is not progressing smoothly). See:

- Graham I. *Episiotomy: Challenging Obstetric Interventions.* Blackwell, 1997
- Sleep J, Grant A, Garcia J, Elbourne D, Spencer J, Chalmers L. West Berkshire perineal management trial. *British Medical Journal*, 1984, 289:587-590
- Carroli G, Belizan J. Episiotomy for vaginal birth (Cochrane Review). In: *The Cochrane Library*, Issue 3. John Wiley & Sons Ltd, 2006
- Sartore A, De Seta F, Maso G. The effects of mediolateral episiotomy on pelvic floor function after vaginal delivery. *Obstetrics & Gynaecology,* 2004, 103:669-673
- Bick D, MacArthur C, Knowles H, Winter H. *Postnatal Care: Evidence and Guidelines for Management.* Churchill Livingstone, 2002
- DiPiazza D, Richter H, Chapman V, Cliver S, Neely C, Chen C, Burgio K. Risk factors for anal sphincter tear in multiparas. *Obstetrics & Gynaecology,* 2006, 107 (6):1233-1236
- Williams A. Third-degree perineal tears: risk factors and outcome after primary repair. *Journal of Obstetrics & Gynaecology*, 2003, 23(6):611-614
- Richter H, Brumfield C, Cliver S, Burgio K. Risk factors associated with anal sphincter tear: a comparison of primiparous patients, vaginal births after caesarean deliveries and patients with previous vaginal delivery. *American Journal of Obstetrics & Gynaecology*, 2002, 187:1194-1198
- Peleg D, Zlatnik M. Risk of repetition of a severe perineal laceration. *Obstetrics & Gynaecology*, 1999, 93(6):1021-1024
- Dandolu V, Gaughan J, Chatwani A. Risk of recurrence of anal sphincter lacerations. *Obstetrics & Gynaecology*, 2005, 105:831-835
- Dannecker C, Hillemanns P, Strauss A. Episiotomy and perineal tears presumed to be imminent: randomised controlled trial. *Acta Obstetrica et Gynaecologica Scandinavica*, 2004, 83:364-368

20 Although research into EFM began quite early on, the first *review* of research was carried out in 2005 by Thacker, *et al*, and this prompted a wider re-examination of EFM, which had become routine in so many hospitals up till then. Alfirevic, *et al*'s review of research in 2006 (which covered 37,000 women in total!) concluded that EFM had few benefits and many drawbacks. The rate of caesareans and forceps/ventouse births rose significantly and it brought no improvement in Apgar scores

when 'EFM women' were compared to those who'd just had periodic checks with a fetal monitor (e.g. a Pinard or Sonicaid). (Another study by Madaan and Trivedi in 2006 found that women trying for a vaginal birth after a previous caesarean were more likely to end up with another caesarean if they had EFM, and there was no improvement in outcomes when they had EFM.) In the review by Alfeirevic, et al one benefit was associated with EFM—the number of neonatal seizures dropped—but there was no significant difference in any long-term effects, such as cerebral palsy. (Interestingly, one earlier study—by Luthy, et al in 1987—found *higher* rates of cerebral palsy when EFM was used for pre-term labours.) Overall, given the many documented disadvantages of EFM, the conclusion remains that the procedure is only advisable in certain high risk cases—and even then it is recognised that EFM may not help prevent perinatal deaths or cerebral palsy, so some high risk women opt out too. See:

- Flynn AM, et al. A randomized controlled trial of non-stress antepartum cardiotocography. *British Journal of Obstetrics & Gynaecology*, 1982, 89:427-33
- Kidd LC, et al. Non-stress antenatal cardiotocography—a prospective randomized clinical trial. *British Journal of Obstetrics & Gynaecology*, 1985, 92:1156-59
- Impey L, Reynolds, M, et al. Admission cardiotocography : a randomized controlled trial. *Lancet*, 2003, 361:465-70
- Alfirevic Z, Devane D, Gyte G. Continuous cardiotocography (CTG) as a form of electronic fetal monitoring (EFM) for fetal assessment during labour. *Cochrane Database of Systematic Reviews*, Issue 3, 2006
- Haverkamp AD, et al. A controlled trial of the differential effects of intrapartum monitoring. *American Journal of Obstetrics & Gynecology*, 1976, 126:470-76
- Kelso IM, et al. An assessment of continuous fetal heart rate monitoring in labor. *American Journal of Obstetrics & Gynecology*, 1978, 131:526-32
- McDonald D, Chalmers I, et al. The Dublin randomised controlled trial of intrapartum fetal heart rate monitoring. *American Journal of Obstetrics & Gynecology*, 1985, 152:524-39
- Prentice A, Lind T. Fetal heart rate monitoring during labor—too frequent intervention, too little benefit. *Lancet*, 1987, 2:1375-77
- Wood C. A controlled trial of fetal heart rate monitoring in low-risk obstetric population. *American Journal of Obstetrics & Gynecology*, 1981, 141:527-34
- Thacker S, Stroup D, Peterson H. Continuous electronic fetal heart monitoring during labour. (Cochrane Review) In: *The Cochrane Library*, Issue 1. Oxford: Update Software, 2005

21 It's also useful to consider other forms of common monitoring of labour, such as vaginal examination to track cervical dilation. (This is tracked up to 10cm, when the woman is considered 'ready' to push, although—as we'll see later—some practiners recognise a phase called the 'rest-and-be-thankful phase' when the woman has a spontaneous rest beforehand!) According to Denis Walsh, in 2007 Nottingham City Hospital, which has a large consultant unit, recommended—and, presumably, continues to recommend—a minimum vaginal examination interval of 12 hours for first-time mothers. (Denis Walsh mentions this in his book *Evidence-based Care for Labour and Birth*, Routledge, 2007.) Of course, this recommendation reflects changing attitudes towards monitoring generally, which includes EFM. See Step 5,

Note 1 for other research confirming the limited usefulness of repeated vaginal examinations.

22 Of course, here, Michel was not following protocols typical of a big maternity hospital in the 1980s or 1990s, where constant monitoring was considered essential. Increasingly nowadays, midwives and obstetricians are recognising that 'watchful waiting' is an excellent alternative, which produces better results. This is no doubt because of evidence which is gradually showing that monitoring can be a form of intervention. For example, De Jonge and Lagro-Janssen (2004) linked vaginal examinations in the second stage to the supine position for birth (because it's difficult for women to get up afterwards at this stage)—so they concluded by suggesting no examinations be conducted unless there is cause for concern. Many years before, Carolyn Flint (1986) had recommended that vaginal examinations should be conducted in whatever position the woman happened to be in at the time, and had described how this is possible. See:

- De Jonge A, Teunissen T, Lagro Janssen A. Supine position compared to other positions during the second stage of labour: a meta-analytic review. *Journal of Psychosomatic Obstetrics & Gynaecology*, 2004, 25:35-45
- De Jonge A, Lagro Janssen A. Birthing positions: a qualitative study into the views of women about various birthing positions. *Journal of Psychosomatic Obstetrics & Gynaecology*, 2004, 25:47-55
- Flint C. *Sensitive Midwifery.* Heinemann, 1986

23 If Michel Odent's approach seems negligent to you, you might like to check out the following studies, all of which focus on 'less' being 'more' when it comes to midwifery care:

- Leap N. The less we do, the more we give. In M. Kirkham (ed.) *The Midwife-Mother Relationship.* Macmillan, 2000 (pp 1-18)
- Kennedy H. A model of exemplary midwifery practice: results of a Delphi study, including commentary by Ernst K. *Journal of Midwifery & Women's Health,* 2000, 45(1):4-19
- Fahy K. Being a midwife or doing midwifery. *Australian Midwives College Journal,* 1998, 11(2):11-16

In a presentation at the annual NCT conference in 2004, the late researcher and midwife Trisha Anderson apparently also joked that good midwifery involves 'drinking tea intelligently'. In other words, in order to best facilitate the natural, healthy, physiological processes of birth i.e. optimal birth, a midwife needs to do nothing, while engaging in 'watchful waiting', just to check everything's OK as labour progresses—simply because a good midwife (or obstetrician) knows what to look out for. This contrasts with the obstetric model of care, in which caregivers often have what some researchers (e,g, Grol and Grimshow, 2003) have termed 'a compulsion to act'. See:

- Grol R, Grimshaw J. From best evidence to best practice: effective implementation of change in patient's care. *Lancet,* 2003, 362: 1225-1230

Finally, in the following book, researchers conclude (after conducting an extensive review of midwifery and obstetric practice that 'what really counts, cannot be counted':

- Chalmers I, Kierse M, Neilson J. *A Guide to Effective Care in Pregnancy and Childbirth*. Oxford University Press, 1989

24 After a detailed discussion of the evidence surrounding the use of EFM (and other forms of clinical observation) Denis Walsh has pointed out that 'surveillance' creates an atmosphere of anxiety in the labour room. He reminds us that in 1996 Downs commented that 'gains in technology seem to be resulting in the loss of human essence.' The particular problem with an atmosphere of anxiety is that it prevents the hormones of birth from being produced. (There will be more about this soon.) This explains why Michel wanted to leave me undisturbed. See:

- Walsh D. *Evidence-based Care for Normal Labour and Birth*. Routledge, 2007
- Downs F. Technical innovations: legal implications for nursing. *American Nurses' Association Clinical Sessions*, 1966, 232-237
- Odent M. *Birth and Breastfeeding*. Clairview Books 2003

25 For a discussion of risk on this topic see:

- Berryman J, Windridge K. Motherhood after 35—a report on the Leicester Motherhood Project. Leicester University, 1995

If you are over 35 yourself, you might also want to buy one of several books on the subject, which offer plenty of reassuring statistics too. (Well, I found them reassuring.)

26 As mentioned before, the following recent study did establish links between drug use in labour (either for pain relief or during the third stage) and reduced breastfeeding rates. It's possible there may be other after-effects too, which still need to be researched. See:

- Jordan S, Emery, S, Watkins A, Evans JD, Storey M, Morgan G. Associations of drugs routinely given in labour with breastfeeding at 48 hours: analysis of the Cardiff Births Survey. *BJOG: International Journal of Obstetrics & Gynaecology*, 2009, online publication on 1 Sept

27 See the following articles:

- Kinmond S, *et al*. Umbilical Cord Clamping and Preterm Infants: a Randomized Trial. *British Medical Journal*, 1993, 306:172-175
- Pisacane A. Neonatal prevention of iron deficiency, *British Medical Journal*, 1996, 312:136-7

28 See the following articles:

- Gunther M. The transfer of blood between the baby and the placenta in the minutes after birth. *Lancet* 1957, I:1277-1280
- Wardrop CA, Holland BM. The roles and vital importance of placental blood to the newborn infant. *Journal of Perinatal Medicine*, 1995, 23(1-2):139-43

29 For more about this, see:

- Steinbrook R. The cord-blood-bank controversies. *New England Journal of Medicine*, 2004, 351 (22):2255-7.

30 The following researcher discovered that low-intervention birth brings healing to some women who've previously had a traumatic labour:

- Milan M. Childbirth as healing: three women's experience of independent midwife care. *Complementary Therapies in Nursing & Midwifery*, 2003, 9:140-146

9... Consider your assumptions

1. Michel has written about this phenomenon in the chapter called 'Antenatal scare' in his book *The Caesarean*. Free Association Books, 2004.
2. Again, Michel has written about this in the chapter called 'Breaking a vicious circle' in *The Caesarean*. Free Association Books, 2004.
3. If you are worrying about Judy's risk of infection, see:
   - Ladfors L, Mattsson LA, Eriksson M, Fall O. A randomised trial of two expectant managements of prelabour rupture of the membranes at 34 to 42 weeks. *British Journal of Obstetrics & Gynaecology*, 1996, Aug; 103(8):755-62

   If you believe that electronic fetal monitoring should have been used, see Step 10, Note 19, and to consider the use of EFM in high risk pregnancies specifically, see the references below. Michel's view is that the conditions needed to optimise outcomes for both low and high-risk labours are the same—privacy, non-disturbance, and the feeling of being safe because a competent midwife (or obstetrician) is discretely in attendance. The references:

   - Brown VA, *et al.* The value of antenatal cardiotocography in the management of high-risk pregnancy: a randomised controlled trial. *British Journal of Obstetrics & Gynaecology*, 1982, 89:716-22
   - Haverkamp AD, *et al.* The evaluation of continuous fetal heart rate monitoring in high risk pregnancy. *American Journal of Obstetrics & Gynecology*, 1976, 125: 310-20
   - Leveno KJ, *et al.* A prospective comparison of selective and universal electronic fetal monitoring in 34,995 pregnancies. *New England Journal of Medicine*, 1986, 315:615-19
   - Lumley JC, Wood C, *et al.* A randomized trial of weekly cardiotocography in high-risk obstetric patients. *British Journal of Obstetrics & Gynaecology*, 1983, 90:1018-26
   - Sky K, *et al.* Effects of electronic fetal heart rate monitoring, as compared with periodic auscultation, on the neurological development of premature infants. *New England Journal of Medicine*, 1990, (March 1):588-93
   - Luthy D, Shy K, van Belle G, Larson E, *et al.* A randomised controlled trial of electronic fetal monitoring in preterm labour. *Obstetrics & Gynaecology*, 1987, 69:687-695
   - Madaan M, Trivedi S. Intrapartum electronic fetal monitoring vs. intermittent auscultation in post caesarean pregnancies. *International Journal of Obstetrics & Gynaecology*, 2006, 94:123-125

4. For research on some of the ways in which babies may be affected by drugs in childbirth see the commentary in Step 10 (Note 3).
5. For research on ultrasound see the following, as well as pages 211-215:
   - Ewigman BG, Crane JP, *et al.* Effect of prenatal ultrasound screening on perinatal outcome. *New England Journal of Medicine*, 1993, 329:821-7
   - Bucher HC, Schmidt JG. Does routine ultrasound scanning improve outcome in pregnancy? Meta-analysis of various outcome measures. *British Medical Journal*, 1993, 307:13-7
   - Larsen T, Larson JF, *et al.* Detection of small-for-gestational-age fetuses by

ultrasound screening in a high risk population: a randomized controlled study. *British Journal of Obstetrics & Gynaecology*, 1992, 99:469-74

- Secher NJ, Kern Hansen P, *et al*. A randomized study of fetal abdominal diameter and fetal weight estimation for detection of light-for-gestation infants in low-risk pregnancy. *British Journal of Obstetrics & Gynaecology*, 1987, 94:105-9
- Johnstone FD, Prescott RJ, *et al*. Clinical and ultrasound prediction of macrosomia in diabetic pregnancy. *British Journal of Obstetrics & Gynaecology*, 1996, 103:747-54

6. For research on this policy see:

- Ladfors L, Mattsson LA, Eriksson, M, Fall O. A randomised trial of two expectant managements of prelabour rupture of the membranes at 34 to 42 weeks. *British Journal of Obstetrics & Gynaecology*, 1996, Aug 103(8):755-62

7. A Leboyer birth is a birth inspired by the poetic book *Birth Without Violence* by the French obstetrician Frederick Leboyer. (Originally published in 1974, a 2002 edition is now available from Inner Traditions Bear & Company.) Leboyer births generally involve the use of dim lighting and gentle handling of the baby, who is usually bathed in a small tub of warm water immediately after the birth. This type of birthing approach was very popular in the 1970s. See Step 7, Note 8 for research on Leboyer births.

8. External cephalic version is a procedure where a professional tries to encourage a fetus to turn in the womb (to a head-down position) by manipulating the woman's 'bump' from the outside. Because of the risk that the umbilical cord could get twisted round the fetus' head during this procedure, it is vital for this procedure to be conducted with continuous monitoring, in a place where a caesarean could be carried out immediately, if necessary. Moxabustion is a Chinese procedure which pre-dates acupuncture, which involves burning a herb close to the skin. See:

- Coyle ME, Smith CA, Peat B. Cephalic version by moxibustion for breech presentation. *Cochrane Database of Systematic Reviews*, 2005, Issue 2. Art. No CD003928. DOI: 10.1002/14651858.CD003928.pub2

9. A study by Zanardo, *et al* (2001) found the amount of beta-endorphin in the colstral milk of mothers who'd given birth vaginally was significantly higher than colostrum levels of mothers who had a caesarean section. Having beta-endorphins in milk is thought to be important as these opiate-like substances make the newborn baby 'addicted' to its mother's milk. See:

- Zanardo V, Nicolussi S, Giacomin C, Faggian D, Favaro F, Plebani M. Labor pain effects on colostral milk beta endorphin concentrations of lactating mothers. *Biology of the Neonate* 2001, 79(2):79-86)
- DiMatteo MR, Morton S, *et al*. Cesarean Childbirth and Psychosocial Outcomes— A Meta-Analysis. *Health Psychology*, 1996, 15(4):303-14

10. Although there was a huge breech trial (Hannah, *et al*, 2000), which many caregivers found showed conclusively that a caesarean was the only way forward for breech births, this study has been widely criticised by caregivers who are skilled in vaginal breech deliveries. In the study by Hannah, *et al*—which only looked at hospital births—caregivers had inadequate training and experience and, because of this, most would have been frightened of the possible consequences of a bad outcome. As we shall see in later chapters, fearful caregivers are the last thing a labouring woman needs! Fear inculcates fear and inhibits the production of the hormones a woman needs in order to give birth successfully. For this reason, as well

as because of their long experience of attending successful and safe breech births, many midwives are continuing to agree to attend vaginal breech births. See:

- Hannah M, Hannah J, Hewson S, Hodnett E, Saigal S, Willan AR. Planned caesarean section versus planned vaginal birth for breech presentation at term: a randomised multicentre trial. Term Breech Trial Collaborative Group. *Lancet,* 2000, 356(9239):1375-1383

11 For more on this (including references to research), see the chapters called 'What mothers say' and 'The perineal preoccupation' in Michel's book *The Caesarean* (Free Association Books 2004). Also see Harrison's paper, as follows, which explains why the unborn baby needs to be exposed to the stress of labour if he or she is to be ready for life outside the womb:

- Harrison J. Fetal perspectives on labour. *British Journal of Midwifery,* 1999, 7(10): 643-647

12 To explore the truth of this contention, visit the Primal Health Research Database at www.birthworks.org/primalhealth. Use the keyword 'caesarean' or 'caesarean' to locate the many articles which suggest correlations. One study in 2008 (Cardwell, *et al*) found that children born by caesarean were 20% more likely to get childhood-onset type 1 diabetes. Another study (Thavagnanam, *et al*, 2008) also found that caesarean-born children were 20% more likely to be asthmatic. Another study (Koplin, *et al*, 2008) found that being born by caesarean increased a baby's chances of developing sensitization to food allergens, which might make them more prone to allergies. See:

- Cardwell CR, Stene LC, Joner G, Cinek O, Svensson J, Goldacre MJ, Parslow RC, Pozzilli P, Brigis G, Stoyanov D, Urbonaite B, Sipetić S, Schober E, Ionescu-Tirgoviste C, Devoti G, de Beaufort CE, Buschard K, Patterson CC. Caesarean section is associated with an increased risk of childhood-onset type 1 diabetes mellitus: a meta-analysis of observational studies. *Diabetologia,* 2008, May;51(5): 726-35. Epub 2008 Feb 22
- Thavagnanam S, Fleming J, Bromley A, Shields MD, Cardwell CR. A meta-analysis of the association between Caesarean section and childhood asthma. *Clinical & Experimental Allergy,* 2008, Apr;38(4):629-33
- Koplin J, Allen K, Gurrin L, Osborne N, Tang ML, Dharmage S. Is caesarean delivery associated with sensitization to food allergens and IgE-mediated food allergy: a systematic review. *Pediatric Allergy & Immunology,* 2008 Dec; 19(8):682-7

13 Newton gave the hormone this name in:

- Newton N. The Influence of the Let-Down Reflex in Breast Feeding on the Mother-Child Relationship. *Marriage & Family Living,* 1958, 20:18-20

In 1988 Marchini demonstrated that caesareans involve significantly lower levels of oxytocin. For more details on this see:

- Marchini G, Lagercrantz H, Winberg J, Uvnas-Moberg K. Fetal and maternal plasma levels of gastrin, somatostatin and oxytocin after vaginal delivery and elective cesarean section. *Early Human Development,* 1988, Nov;18(1):73-9

14 It is true that ultrasound examinations have identified micro-damage to the pelvic floor after vaginal births (Dietz and Schierlitz 2005) but—as Denis Walsh points out—there is an enormous difference between mechanical and neural damage, mainly

because neural damage (which is what we're talking about here) involves absolutely no symptoms, so in fact it doesn't affect women. As another research study concluded (Cardozo and Gleeson 1997), the best possible outcome is for a woman to have an intact perineum—i.e. for no tearing *or cutting* to take place—because this is associated with the least pain postnatally, the least amount of incontinence (usually none) and the earliest resumption of normal sexual intercourse after birth. It's also interesting (and perhaps a little perplexing) to note that women who've had an emergency caesarean have virtually the same rates of urinary incontinence postnatally as women who've given birth vaginally—and that even women who've had elective caesareans complain of incontinence postnatally (Chaliha, et al, 2002, Lal, et al, 2003, Rortveit, et al, 2003.) Research conducted by Gordon and Logue 1985, Jolleys 1988, Nygaard 1997 and Viktrup 1992 found no differences in muscle strength or urinary continence between women birthing vaginally and by caesarean. According to these research studies, the women who suffer most after giving birth are those who have forceps deliveries. See:

- Dietz H, Schierlitz L. Pelvic floor trauma in childbirth—myth or *reality? Australian & New Zealand Journal of Obstetrics & Gynaecology*, 2005, 45(1):3-11
- Walsh D. *Evidence-based Care for Normal Labour and Birth.* Routledge, 2007
- Cardozo L, Gleeson C. Pregnancy, childbirth and continence. *British Journal of Midwifery*, 1997, 5(5):277-281
- Chaliha C, Khullar V, Stanton S. Urinary symptoms in pregnancy: are they useful for diagnosis? British Journal of Obstetrics & Gynaecology, 2002, 109:1181-1183
- Lal M, Mann C, Callender R, Radley S. Does caesarean delivery prevent anal incontinence? Obstetrics & Gynaecology, 2003, 101:305-312
- Rortveit A, Kjersti D, Yugvild S, Hannestad S, Hunskaar S. Urinary incontinence after vaginal delivery or caesarean section. *New England Journal of Medicine*, 2003, 348: 900-907
- Gordon H, Logue M. Perineal muscle function after childbirth. *Lancet* 1985;2:123-5
- Jolleys JV. Reported prevalence of urinary incontinence in women in a general practice. *British Medical Journal*, 1988, 296:1300-2
- Nygaard IE, Rao SSC, Dawson JD. Anal incontinence after anal sphincter disruption: a 30-year retrospective cohort study. *Obstetrics & Gynecology*, 1997, 89(6):896-901
- Viktrup L, *et al*. The symptom of stress incontinence caused by pregnancy or delivery in primiparas. *Obstetrics & Gynecology*, 1992, 79(6):945-9

In conclusion, research has shown that the urinary incontinence often results in the following cases: having a forceps birth (Arya, et al, 2001), pushing actively for a long time (Kirkman 2000), having lots of babies, having babies who weigh more than 3,700g, and being over 30 at the time of giving birth (Mason, et al, 1999). (In case you find yourself in any of these categories, it is at least reassuring to note that none of them are associated with increased incidence of tearing.) Research has shown that urinary stress incontinence is best avoided by doing pelvic floor exercises antenatally (Morkved, et al, 2003, Sampselle, 2000) and by insisting on pushing your baby out yourself, according to your own timetable (Kirkman, 2000); postnatal pelvic floor exercises have also been found to be helpful (Glazener, et al, 2001). See:

- Arya L, Jackson N, Myers D, Verma A. Risk of new onset urinary incontinence after forceps and vacuum delivery in primiparous women. *American Journal of Obstetrics & Gynaecology*, 2001, 185:1318-1324
- Kirkman S. The midwife and pelvic floor dysfunction. *The Practising Midwife*, 2000, 3(8):20-22
- Mason L, Glenn S, Walton I, Appleton C. The prevalence of stress incontinence during pregnancy and following birth. *Midwifery*, 1999, 15(2):120-127
- Mason L, Glenn S, Walton I, Appleton C. The experience of stress incontinence after birth. *Birth*, 1999, 26(3):164-171
- Morkved S, Bo K, Schei B, Salvesen K. Pelvic floor muscle training during pregnancy to prevent urinary incontinence: a single-blind randomized controlled trial. *Obstetrics & Gynaecology*, 2003, 101:313-319.
- Sampselle C. Behavioural intervention for urinary incontinence in women: evidence for practice. *Journal of Midwifery & Women's Health*, 2000, 45(2):94-103
- Glazener C, Herbison G, Wilson P. Conservative management of persistent postnatal urinary and faecal incontinence: randomised controlled trial. *British Medical Journal*, 2001, 323:593

Looking at incontinence later on in life, researchers have established the following causes (in order of importance, starting with the most important) (Hannestad, *et al*, 2003, Rortveit, *et al*, 2003): heredity, obesity, smoking, HRT, the number of children a woman's had and how she's had them (noting that forceps is the worst way, from the point of view of incontinence). See:

- Hannestad Y, Rortveit G, Dalveit A, Hunskaar S. Are smoking and other lifestyle factors associated with female urinary incontinence? The Norwegian EPINCONT study. *British Journal of Obstetrics & Gynaecology*, 2003, 110:247-254
- Rortveit G, Daltveit A, Hannestad Y, Hunskaar S. (2003) Vaginal delivery parameters and urinary incontinence: the Norwegian EPINCONT study. *American Journal of Obstetrics & Gynecology*, 2003 Nov; 189(5):1268-74.

Finally, in case all this isn't enough to put you off your dinner, painful sex (dyspareunia) and perineal pain after childbirth have been associated with forceps and ventouse births, episiotomy and anal spincter tears (Buhling, *et al*, 2005). See:

- Buhling K, Schmidt S, Robinson J, Klapp C, Siebert G, Dudenhausen J. Rate of dyspareunia after delivery in primiparae according to mode of delivery. *European Journal of Obstetrics & Gynecology*, 2005, 124:42-46

15 Amu O, Rajendran S and B, Ibrahim I. *British Medical Journal*, 1998, 317:462-465 (15 August)

16 See the following study, as well as Michel's comments on this (with references to research) in the chapter 'Once a caesarean always a caesarean' in *The Caesarean* (Free Association Books 2004):

- Van Ham M, van Dongen P, Mulder J. Maternal consequences of caesarean section. A retrospective study of intra-operative and postoperative maternal complications of caesarean section during a 10 year period. *European Journal of Obstetrics, Gynaecology & Reproductive Biology*, 1997, 74(1):1-6

17 Women who've had a caesarean are also more likely to have a caesarean at the end of their pregnancy, experience post-traumatic stress syndrome and have reduced breastfeeding rates. See:

- Hemminki E, Merilainen J. Long-term Effects of Caesarean Sections: Ectopic Pregnancies and Placental Problems. *American Journal of Obstetrics & Gynecology*, 1996, 174, No 5:1569-1574
- Hemminki E. Impact of caesarean section on future pregnancy—a review of cohort studies. *Paediatric & Perinatal Epidemiology*, 1996, 10(4):366-379
- Ananth C, Smulian J, Vintzeleos A. The association of placenta praevia with history of caesarean delivery and abortion: a meta-analysis. *American Journal Obstetrics & Gynaecology*, 1997, 177(5):1071-1078
- Ryding E, Wijma K, Wijma B. Experiences of emergency caesarean section: a phenomenological study of 53 women. *Birth*, 1998, 25(4): 246-251
- Sackett D. Evidence based medicine: what it is and what it isn't. *British Medical Journal*, 1996, 312:71-72
- Di Matteo M, Morton S, Lepper H, Damush T, Carney M, Pearson M, Kahn K. Caesarean childbirth and psychosocial outcomes: a meta-analysis. *Health Psychology*, 1996, 15(4):303-314

Also see the chapter 'Safer and safer' in *The Caesarean* (Free Association Books 2004).

18 In addition, because of the decreased catecholamine surge, babies born by caesarean are at increased risk of respiratory compromise (Faxelius 1983) as well as low blood sugar (Hagnevik 1984). See:
- Faxelius G, Hagnevik K, *et al*. Catecholamine surge and lung function after delivery. *Archives of Disease in Childhood*, 1983, Apr; 58(4):262-6
- Hagnevik K, Faxelius G, *et al*. Catecholamine surge and metabolic adaptation in the newborn after vaginal delivery and caesarean section. *Acta Paediatrica Scandinavica*, 1984, Sep; 73(5):602-9

19 Enkin 2000 concludes that the risk increases by four times. See:
- Enkin MW, Keirse MJNC, Neilson J, Crowther C, Duley L, Hodnett E, Hofmeyr J. *A Guide to Effective Care in Pregnancy & Childbirth*. 3rd edition. Oxford: Oxford University Press, 2000

20 If you still doubt this, see the following articles:
- Liu S, Liston RM, Joseph KS, *et al*. Maternal mortality and severe morbidity associated with low-risk planned cesarean delivery versus planned vaginal delivery at term. *Canadian Medical Association Journal*, 2007, 176(4):455-60
- Hannah ME, Hannah WJ, *et al*. Planned caesarean section versus planned vaginal birth for breech presentation at term: a randomised multicentre trial. *Lancet*, 2000, 356:1375-83
- Krebs L, Langhoff-Roos J. Elective cesarean delivery for term breech. *Obstetrics & Gynecology*, 2003, 101(4):690-6
- Cheng M, Hannah ME. Breech delivery at term : a critical review of the literature. *Obstetrics & Gynecology*, 1993, 82:605-18
- Lumley J. Any room left for disagreement about assisting breech births at term? *Lancet*, 2000, 356:1368-9

21 Mathai M, Hofmeyr GJ. Abdominal surgical incisions for caesarean section (Protocol for a Cochrane Review). In: *The Cochrane Library*, Issue 2. Oxford: Update Software, 2004.

22 These have also been recommended by Joel-Cohen and Wallin.
23 This is especially important because one study (Nissen, *et al,* 1996) found that after caesareans the first suckling typically took place 240 minutes after the birth, which contrasted dramatically with the 75 minutes in the case of women who hadn't had caesareans. See:

- Nissen E, Uvnas-Moberg K, Svensson K, Stock S, Widstrom AM, Winberg J. Different patterns of oxytocin, prolactin but not cortisol release during breastfeeding in women delivered by caesarean section or by the vaginal route. *Early Human Development,* 1996, 45:103-18

If hormones are inevitably disrupted, it's important that a woman who needs an elective caesarean compensates by making a special request in advance to ensure that herr baby gets put to her breast as soon as possible. Other studies (Salariya 1978, De Chateau 1977) found that early and frequent suckiIng positively influences milk production and the duration of breastfeeding. The full references are as follows:

- Salariya EM, *et al,* Duration of Breastfeeding after Early Initiation and Frequent Feeding, *Lancet,* 2, No 8100, 1978, 1141-1143
- De Chateau P, Wiberg B. Long-term Effect on Mother-Infant Behaviour of Extra Contact during the First Hour Postpartum. *Acta Paediatrica Scandinavica,* 1977, 66:145-151

24 In this chapter there is no focus on possible financial reasons for the rise in statistics, but some writers have suggested this might well be a factor. After all, according to the British Audit Commission in 1997 caesarean sections cost the NHS (at that time) £760 more than a vaginal delivery. Even then, this audit commission estimated that only a 1% increase in the caesarean rate would cost £5 million pounds more. The report noted that hospital stays are on average three times longer after a caesarean. While trends within NHS hospitals for rising caesareans are difficult to understand in financial terms, it is not difficult to see how increasing the rate of caesareans might be financially appealing within the private sector. And of course this is often where fashions and trends are set for the rest of the population because what is 'expensive' is often seen as being desirable, even if it is also 'expensive' in terms of health and a newborn baby's welfare.

25 This issue is also discussed in *The Caesarean,* Free Association Books, 2004.

26 See the discussion of this issue earlier in Step 9, Note 14. Michel has also written about this topic in the chapter called 'The perineal preoccupation' in *The Caesarean* (Free Association Books, 2004). Other differences in the processes have been identified by other researchers. Elective caesareans involve lower levels of endorphins (Facchinetti, 1990), catecholamines (Jones, 1982), and prolactin (Heasman, 1997). The full references are as follows:

- Facchinetti F, Garuti G, Petraglia F, Mercantini F, Genazzani AR. Changes in beta-endorphin in fetal membranes and placenta in normal and pathological pregnancies. *Acta Obstetrica et Gynecologica Scandinavica,* 1990, 69(7-8): 603-7
- Jones CM 3rd, Greiss FC Jr. The effect of labor on maternal and fetal circulating cate-cholamines. *American Journal of Obstetrics & Gynecology,* 1982, Sep 15; 144(2):149-53
- Heasman L, Spencer JA, Symonds ME. Plasma prolactin concentrations after caesarean section or vaginal delivery. *Archives of Disease in Childhood, Fetal & Neonatal Edition,* 1997, Nov;77(3):F237-8

27 One study found that women who had a caesarean were more likely to experience a decline in mood and self-esteem postnatally (Fisher 1997). See:
- Fisher J, et al, Adverse Psychological Impact of Operative Obstetric Interventions: A Prospective Longitudinal Study, *Australia & New Zealand Journal of Psychiatry*, 31, 1997, 728-738

28 The strict protocols based on observations carried out as far back as 1954 (resulting in the 'Friedman curve') are questioned by more modern research. Many studies have concluded that first-time mothers tend to have longer labours than women who've already had at least one baby. The following study concluded that current diagnostic criteria for protracted or arrested labour may be too stringent:
- Zhang J, Troendle J, Yancey M. Reassessing the labour curve. *American Journal of Obstetrics & Gynaecology*, 2002, 187:824-828

This and other papers, such as the following one, suggest that there is more variation in women (labouring naturally) than was thought to be the case in the past:
- Gurewitsch E, Diament P, Fong J, et al. The labour curve of the grand multipara: Does progress of labour continue to improve with additional childbearing? *American Journal of Obstetrics & Gynaecology*, 2002, 186:1331-1338

Also see:
- Gross M, Haunschild T, Stoexen T, Methner V, Guenter H. Women's recognition of the spontaneous onset of labour. *Birth,* 2003, 30(4):2b7-271
- Gross M, Hecker H, Matterne A, Guenter H, Kierse M. Does the way that women experience the onset of labour influence the duration of labour? *British Journal of Obstetrics & Gynaecology*, 2006, 113:289-294

One research study pointed out that the last thing a busy labour ward needs is 'nigglers' (women whose labours aren't progressing 'fast enough') because they are seen to 'clog up the place'. See:
- Hunt S, Symonds A. *The Social Meaning of Midwifery.* Basingstoke: Macmillan,

The following paper reports on latent periods (when nothing happened) during home births, which were (correctly) not interpreted by midwives as pathological:
- Davis B, Johnson K, Gaskin L. The MANA Curve—describing plateaus in labour using the MANA database. Abstract No 30, 26th Triennial Congress, ICM, Vienna, 2002

In the following paper, the conclusion is that midwives and other caregivers need to focus on 'unique normality', which varies from woman to woman:
- Downe S, McCourt C. From being to becoming: reconstructing childbirth knowledges. In Downe S (ed) *Normal Childbirth: Evidence and Debate.* Churchill Livingstone, 2004

Another study demonstrated that women were equally satisfied with longer labours:
- Lavender T, Alfirevic Z, Walkinshaw S. Effects of different partogram action lines on birth outcomes: a randomised controlled trial. *Obstetrics & Gynaecology,* 2006, 108 (2):295-302

One midwife, the late Trisha Anderson, at the NCT conference in 2004, also proposed types of dystocias, which are clearly to be avoided—lack of continuity of care 'dystocia', inexperienced doctors at the start of their rotation 'dystocia', absence of expertise 'dystocia', disagreements between caregivers 'dystocia', inadequate handovers 'dystocia' and intimidation 'dystocia'.

29. For an explanation of this, see the following article:
    - Odent M. The second stage as a disruption of the fetus ejection reflex. *Midwifery Today, International Midwife*, 2000, Autumn; (55): 12
30. See Michel's comments on this in the chapter called 'At the dawn of the post-electronic age' in the book *Birth and Breastfeeding* (Clairview, 2003).
31. If you still doubt this, read Michel's more detailed comments on caesareans at www.wombecology.com/caesareans.html.
32. See Step 9, Note 14.
33. Michel comments on this in the chapter 'Safer and safer' in *The Caesarean* (Free Association Books 2004).
34. See: Odent M Are caesareans the future? *RCM Midwives*, 2004, Jul;7(7):276

8... Do not disturb

1. Sheila Kitzinger has written about the need to 'guard the birth space' and Michel has also written about this topic in detail. See:
    - Kitzinger S. *Rediscovering Birth*. Little, Brown & Company, 2000
    - Odent M. *Birth and Breastfeeding*. Clairview Books, 2003
2. Michel discusses the impact of apparently small interventions, which change a woman's internal chemistry, in the chapter 'The scientification of love' in his book *The Farmer and the Obstetrician* (Free Association Books, 2002). He discusses the problem of stimulating the neocortex (through talking) in the chapter 'Breaking a vicious circle' in *The Caesarean*, Free Association Books, 2004.
3. Michel discusses this further in the chapter called 'Colostrum and civilization' in his book *Birth and Breastfeeding*, Clairview Books, 2003.
4. Relevant issues are explored in the following articles:
    - Rooks J. Low-Intervention Maternity Care. *Journal of Family Practice*, Vol 31,No 2, 125-7
    - Tew M. Do Obstetric Intranatal Interventions Make Births Safer? *British Journal of Obstetrics & Gynaecology*, 1986, Vol 93,659-74
    - Wagner M. *Pursuing the Birth Machine: The Search for Appropriate Birth Technology*. Sydney: ACE Graphics, 1994
    - Wood LAC. Obstetric Retrospect, *Journal of the Royal College of General Practitioners*, 1981, Vol 31,80-90
5. Michel discusses this further in the following article:
    - Odent M. New reasons and new ways to study birth physiology. *International Journal of Gynecology & Obstetrics*, 2001, 75:S39-S45
6. This area will be discussed more fully in the chapter 'Care about care'. If you doubt this idea at all now, explore www.birthworks.org/primalhealth—a website which catalogues academic articles according to topic (autism, anorexia, suicide, etc).

7   It is actually difficult to prove *directly* the improved safety of physiological birth. There is limited research data for this since randomised controlled trials are impossible in the perinatal period because women will not agree to participate in research at this sensitive time. However, it is easy to see the superiority and 'optimality' of physiological birth over other approaches involving unnecessary interventions if a) we realise how complex the natural processes are (and consequently understand their fragility) and b) we understand the consequences of unnecessary interventions (including drugs), which involve upsetting the delicate balance of the natural processes. Research on the former is presented below; research on the latter is presented in the chapter 'Care about care' and also in the books *Pushed* (Da Capo Press 2008) and *Born in the USA* (University of California Press 2006). Even after reading this chapter (Step 8), I hope you be persuaded that disturbance really is something to be taken seriously while you're in labour and giving birth... and even afterwards, while you bond with your new baby.

8   Uvnas-Moberg K, quoted in a report of the Australian Lactation Consultant's Conference, Gold Coast, Australia 1998, published in *Australian Doctor*, 1998, July 8:38.

9   Weiss G. Endocrinology of Parturition. *Journal of Clinical Endocrinology & Metabolism*, 2000, 85(12):4421-5.

10 See the following articles:
    - Jackson M, Dudley D. Endocrine assays to predict preterm delivery. *Clinics in Perinatology*, 1998, 4:837-857
    - Petrocelli T, Lye S. Regulation of transcripts encoding the myometrial gap junction protein, connexin-43, by estrogen and progesterone. *Endocrinology*, 1993, 133: 284-90

11 Russell JA, *et al*, Brain Preparations for Maternity-Adaptive Changes in Behavioral and Neuroendocrine Systems during Pregnancy and Lactation. *Progressive Brain Research*, 2001, 133:1-38.

12 By Michel Odent and Niles Newton.

13 Verbalis JG, *et al*, Oxytocin Secretion in Response to Cholecystokinin and Food: Differentiation of Nausea from Satiety, *Science*, 1986, 232:1417-1419.

14 Fuchs A, Fuchs F. Endocrinology of human parturition: a review. *British Journal of Obstetrics & Gynaecology*, 1984, 91:948-67.

15 Chard T, *et al*, Release of Oxytocin and Vasopressin by the Human Fetus during Labour. *Nature*, 1971, 234:352-354.

16 Fuchs A, Fuchs F. Endocrinology of human parturition: a review. *British Journal of Obstetrics & Gynaecology*, 1984, 91:948-67.

17 Lundeberg T, Uvnas-Moberg K, *et al*. Anti-nociceptive effects of oxytocin in rats and mice. *Neuroscience Letters*, 1994, Mar 28; 170(1):153-7.

18 Dawood MY, *et al*, Oxytocin in Human Pregnancy and Parturition, *Obstetrics & Gynecology*, 1978, 51:138-143.

19 See the following articles:
    - Costa A, De Filippis V, *et al*. Adrenocorticotrophic hormone and catecholamines in maternal, umbilical and neonatal plasma in relation to vaginal delivery. *Journal of*

Endocrinological Investigation, 1988, 11:703-9
- Eliot RJ, Lam R, et al. Plasma catecholamine concentrations in infants at birth and during the first 48 hours of life. *Journal of Pediatrics*, 1980, Feb; 96(2):311-5
- Lagercrantz H, Bistoletti H. Catecholamine Release in the Newborn Infant at Birth. *Pediatric Research,* 1977, 11,No 8: 889-893

20 See the following articles:
- Hagnevik K, Faxelius G, et al. Catecholamine surge and metabolic adaptation in the newborn after vaginal delivery and caesarean section. *Acta Paediatrica Scandinavica*, 1984, Sep;73(5):602-9
- Colson S. Womb to World: a metabolic perspective. *Midwifery Today*, 2002, Spring; 61:12-17
- Irestedt L, Lagercrantz H, et al. Causes and consequences of maternal and fetal sympathoadrenal activation during parturition. *Acta Obstetrica et Gynecologica Scandinavica,* Suppl, 1984, 118:111-5
- Lowe N, Reiss R. Parturition and Fetal Adaptation. *Journal of Obstetric, Gynecologic & Neonatal Nursing*, 1996, 25:339-349

21 Matthiesen AS, Ransjo-Arvidson AB, et al. Postpartum maternal oxytocin release by newborns: effects of infant hand massage and sucking. *Birth*, 2001, Mar;28(1):13-

22 Nissen E, Widstrom AM, et al. Elevation of oxytocin levels early post-partum in women. *Acta Obstetrica et Gynecologica Scandinavica*, 1995, 74(7);530-3.

23 Leake RD, Weitzman RE, Fisher DA. Oxytocin concentrations during the neonatal period. *Biology of the Neonate*, 1981, 39(3-4):127-31.

24 Eliot RJ, Lam R, et al. Plasma catecholamine concentrations in infants at birth and during the first 48 hours of life. *Journal of Pediatrics*, 1980, Feb; 96(2):311-5.

25 Eliot RJ, Lam R, et al. Plasma catecholamine concentrations in infants at birth and during the first 48 hours of life. *Journal of Pediatrics*, 1980, Feb; 96(2):311-5.

26 See the following articles:
- Russell JA, et al, Brain Preparations for Maternity-Adaptive Changes in Behavioral and Neuroendocrine Systems during Pregnancy and Lactation, *Progressive Brain Research*, 2001, 133:1-38
- Axel R. The molecular logic of smell. *Scientific American*, 1995, 130-7

27 Lundblad EG, Hodgen GD. Induction of maternal-infant bonding in rhesus and cynomolgus monkeys after cesarean delivery. *Laboratory Animal Science*, 1980, Oct;30(5):91.

28 Grattan DR. The actions of prolactin in the brain during pregnancy and lactation. *Progress in Brain Research*, 2001, 135:153-171.

29 Brinsmead M, et al, Peripartum Concentrations of Beta Endorphin and Cortisol and Maternal Mood States, *Australian & New Zealand Journal of Obstetrics & Gynaecology*, 1985. 25:194-197.

30 See the following articles:
- Franceschini R, et al, Plasma Beta-endorphin Concentrations during Suckling in Lactating Women, *British Journal of Obstetrics & Gynaecology*, 1989, 96,No 6:

711-713

- Zanardo V, *et al*, Beta Endorphin Concentrations in Human Milk, *Journal of Pediatric Gastroenterology & Nutrition*, 2001, 33,No 2:160-164

31 Bacigalupo's research (1990) suggests that levels subside slowly, reaching normal levels one to three days after the birth. See:

- Bacigalupo G, Riese S, *et al*. Quantitative relationships between pain intensities during labor and beta-endorphin and cortisol concentrations in plasma. Decline of the hormone concentrations in the early postpartum period. *Journal of Perinatal Medicine*, 1990, 18(4):289-96

32 As you may already know, many caregivers and researchers still insist that ultrasound is non-invasive. The situation does not seem clear-cut, though… A review of 16 studies which had all been published since 1990 was conducted in 2008 (Chaimay, *et al*). Surprisingly, I think, the researchers concluded that ultrasound has no adverse effect on child development outcomes (when given during pregnancy) despite noting that "all studies demonstrated that ultrasound examinations during pregnancy increased the risk of undesirable developmental outcomes". It seems the researchers' reasons for dismissing the importance of these possible undesirable outcomes were a) effects were considered "minimal" and b) the studies were criticised on methodological grounds. (The studies which were reviewed by these researchers were 13 randomised controlled trials, one cohort study, and two case-control studies—but they were all deficient in some respect, apparently.) Oddly, perhaps, even though the abstract for this review includes the statement: "Presently, it is not clear whether [ultrasound] has a negative effect on the health and development of children" the conclusion is that ultrasound is safe, after all. Surely more research is needed, particularly since ultrasound has become so common? See:

- Chaimay B, Woradet S. Does prenatal ultrasound exposure influence the development of children? Asia Pacific Journal of Public Health, 2008, Oct; 20 Suppl: 31-8.

33 In case you think that synthetic oxytocin (i.e. a drip of syntocinon during labour) is a solution, please think again. Michel makes some brief comments on this obstetric 'solution' at www.wombecology.com/oxytocin.html. The most important thing to note is that synthetic oxytocin cannot cross from the body back to the brain because of a 'blood-brain barrier'. This means that when it's injected *into the body* it cannot enter the brain and function as the 'hormone of love'. The implication of this is that any synthetic form of oxytocin might impact not only your own ability to feel loving towards your newborn baby, but also your baby's ability to love. (Michel has written about this at length in *The Scientification of Love,* Free Association Books, 1999.) All in all, it's much better if conditions can be created so that your body spontaneously produces oxytocin because loving feelings then also appear as a bonus!

34 Michel explains in detail why it's important that no-one talks to you while you're in labour at www.wombecology.com/physiological.html

35 Michel explains some additional reasons why it's vital that you not be disturbed in the first hour after the birth at www.midwiferytoday.com/articles/firsthour.asp.

36 To read more about these processes see:

- Pearce JC, *Evolution's End: Reclaiming the Potential of Our Intelligence*. Harper, 1995 (pp 178-179)
- Odent M. Orgasmic states, Ecstatic states and Mystical emotions. In: The *Scientification of Love*. Free Association Books, 1999 (pp 75-79)

37 Rosenberg KR, Trevathan WR. The Evolution of Human Birth. *Scientific American*, November 2001 (pp 60-64).

38 Goland RS, *et al*, Biologically Active Corticotrophin-releasing Hormone in Maternal and Fetal Plasma during Pregnancy, *American Journal of Obstetrics & Gynecology*, 1984, 159:884-890.

39 For a discussion of whether or not shoe size and height are related to higher risk see:
- Prasad M, Al-Taher H. Maternal height and labour outcome. *Journal of Obstetrics & Gynaecology*, 2002, 22(5):513-515

40 On this topic, you may be interested to see a DVD called *The Business of Being Born*, which explores possible financial and business motivations for having an extremely interventionist medical set-up for childbirth. You can find out more at www.thebusinessofbeingborn.com.

41 According to Dunn (1991), the instruction to caregivers to have women lying down was first printed in a textbook by Mauriceau in 1678. (Actually, I wonder if it's actually 1668—because copies of a book by him about this with that publication date is still available today!) According to Boyle (2000) the supine position became mandatory with the invention of forceps, which—it was thought, perhaps—might need to be used at any time. Hugh Chamberlain, who translated Mauriceau's book (from the French), belonged to the family who'd invented the forceps... and he tried to sell his secret to Mauriceau, so they obviously communicated. Later on, with the introduction of various forms of drug-based pain relief, women would inevitably end up lying down. The researcher Caldeyro-Barcia (*et al*) revealed the disadvantages of the supine position for labour and birth in 1979, especially for the baby. See:
- Dunn P. Francois Mauriceau (1637-1709) and maternal posture for parturition. *Midirs*, 1991, 66:78-79
- Boyle M. Childbirth in bed: the historical perspective. *The Practising Midwife*, 2000, 3 (11):21-24
- Mauriceau F. *The Diseases of Women with Child and in Child-Bed: as also, the best means of helping them in natural and unnatural labours*. London, 1668—if you want to buy a copy, and can afford the price tag of £380 or £600! By 1727, this book was already in its sixth English edition, so it must have been popular
- Caldeyro-Barcia R. Influence of maternal bearing down efforts during second stage on fetal well-being. *Birth & Family Journal*, 1979, 6(i):7-15
- Caldeyro-Barcia R, Giussi G, Storch E. The influence of maternal bearing down efforts and their effects on fetal heart rate, oxygenation and acid base balance. *Journal of Perinatal Medicine*, 1979, 9:63-67

42 Lieberman R, Davidson K, *et al*. Changes in fetal position during labor and their association with epidural analgesia. *Obstetrics & Gynecology*, 2005, 105(5 Pt 1): 974-82.

43 Many studies, such as the following, conclude that women resort to pain relief less

often when they are outside large hospitals (e.g. at home or in a birth centre) and also when they have continuity of care (i.e. one midwife right the way through their labour and birth):

- Olsen O. Meta-analysis of the safety of home birth. *Birth,* 1997, 24(1):4-13
- Walsh D, Downe S. Outcomes of free-standing, midwifery-led birth centres: a structured review of the evidence. *Birth,* 2004, 31(3):222-229
- Hodnett E, Downe S, Edwards N, Walsh D. Home-like versus conventional birth settings (Cochrane Review). In: *The Cochrane Library,* Issue 2. Chichester: John Wiley & Sons Ltd, 2006
- Waldenstrom U, Turnbull D. A systematic review comparing continuity of midwifery care with standard maternity services. *British Journal of Obstetrics & Gynaecology,* 1998, 105:1160-1170
- Wraight A, Ball J, Seccombe I, Stock J. *Mapping Team Midwifery: A Report to the Department of Health.* Brighton: Institute of Manpower Studies, University of Sussex, 1993
- Harvey S, Jarrell J, Brant R, Stainton C, Rach D. A randomised controlled trial of nurse/midwifery care. *Birth,* 1996, 23:128-135
- Page L, McCourt C, Beake S, Hewison J. Clinical interventions and outcomes of one-to-one midwifery practice. *Journal of Public Health Medicine,* 1999, 21(3): 243-248

44 A Cochrane review conducted in 2006 identified only one study which confirmed that epidurals were more effective than other forms of pain relief. However, the rest of the review discussed the possible complications of epidurals, which makes clear their potential to disturb birth. See:

- Anim-Somuah M, Smyth R, Howell C. Epidural versus non-epidural or no analgesia in labour. *The Cochrane Database of Systematic Reviews,* 2006, Issue 2
- Annandale E. Dimensions of patient control in a free-standing birth centre. *Social Science & Medicine,* 1987, 25(11):1235-1248

45 See Step 10, Note 19 and Step 9, Note 3 for detailed research information on EFM.

46 A new research study has questioned this finding (Viktrup, *et al,* 1993). Liang, *et al* (2007) found that women who had epidurals had a significantly longer first and second stage of labour (which increased the likelihood of forceps or a caesarean), but did not conclude that the epidural *per se* caused the urinary incontinence. See:

- Viktrup L, Lose G. Epidural anesthesia during labor and stress incontinence after delivery. *Obstetrics and Gynecology,* 1993, 82(6):984-6
- Liang CC. Wong SY, Chang YL, Tsay PK, Chang SD, Lo LM. *Chang Gung Medical Journal,* 2007, 30(2):161-167.

47 Denis Walsh also points out the other inevitable effects of having an epidural. These, he says, include the woman becoming a passive patient, restrictions on mobility and tethering to a bed, zero second stage physiology, meaning that 'commanded pushing' becomes necessary, and an increase in the amount of time spent in technical measurement and record-keeping—as well as the disadvantages already listed in the text. This all results in what he calls 'the profound medicalisation of labour and birth'. See:

- Walsh D. *Evidence-based Care for Normal Labour and Birth*. Routledge, 2007

48 In fact, now that the opioid fentanyl has been incorporated into epidurals (alongside bupivacain), I assume the woman is likely to be in an even less alert state because Marucci, *et al* (2003) conclude: "Intrathecal bupivacaine-fentanyl dose produces a larger alertness decrease than single bupivacaine, because the anaesthetic block density increases." See:

- Marucci M, Diele C, Bruno F, Fiore T. Subarachnoid anaesthesia in caesarean delivery: effects on alertness. *Minerva Anestesiologica,* 2003 Nov; 69(11):809-19, 819-24

The reference for Michel's original article is below and he explains the perfect conditions for a fetus ejection reflex at www.wombecology.com/fetusejection.html:

Odent M. The fetus ejection reflex. Birth, 1987, 14:104-5

49 For more on this see:

- Lundell BP, Hagnevik K, Faxelius G, Irestedt L, Lagercrantz K. Neonatal left ventricular performance after vaginal delivery and cesarean section under general or epidural anesthesia. *American Journal of Perinatology*, 1984, 1(2):152-7
- Hagnevik K, Faxelius G, Irestedt L, Lagercrantz K, Lundell BP, Persson B. Catecholamine surge and metabolic adaptation in the newborn after vaginal delivery. *Acta Paediatrica Scandinavica*, 1984, 73(5):602-9
- Christensson K, Siles C, *et al*. Lower body temperatures in infants delivered by caesarean section than in vaginally delivered infants. *Acta Paediatrica Scandinavica*, 1993, 82(2):128-31
- Thilaganathan B, Meher-Homji N, Nicolaides KH. Labor: an immunologically beneficial process for the neonate. *American Journal of Obstetrics & Gynecology*, 1991, 171(5):1271-2
- Molloy EJ, O'Neill AJ, Grantham JJ, Sheridan-Pereira M, Fitzpatrick JM, Webb DW, Watson RW. Labor Promotes Neonatal Neutrophil Survival and Lipopolysaccharide Responsiveness. *Pediatric Research*, 2004, May 5
- Gronlund MM, Nuutila J, Pelto L, Lilius EM, Isolauri E, Salminen S, Kero P, Lehtonen OP. Mode of delivery directs the phagocyte functions of infants for the first 6 months of life. *Clinical & Expermental Immunology*, 1999, 116(3):521-6
- Gasparani A, Maccario R, *et al*. Neonatal B lymphocyte subpopulations and method of delivery. *Biology of the Neonate*, 1992, 61(3):137-41
- Fujimura A, Morimoto S, *et al*. The influence of delivery mode on biological inactive renin level in umbilical cord blood. *American Journal of Hypertension*, 1990, 3(1): 23-6
- Gemelli M, Mami C, *et al*. Effects of the mode of delivery on ANP and renin-aldosterone system in the fetus and the neonate. *European Journal of Obstetrics & Gynecology & Reproductive Biology*, 1992, 43(3):181-4
- Steverson DK, Bucalo LR, *et al*. Increased immunoreactivity erythropoietin in cord plasma and bilirubin production in normal term infants after labor. *Obstetrics & Gynecology*, 1986, 67(1):69-73
- Lubetzky R, Ben-Shachar S, *et al*. Mode of delivery and neonatal hematocrit. *American Journal of Perinatology*, 2000, 17(3):163-5

- Asien AO, Towobola AO, et al. Umbilical cord venous progesterone at term delivery in relation to mode of delivery. *International Journal of Gynaecology & Obstetrics*, 1994, 47(1):27-31
- Lao TT, Panesar NS. Neonatal thyrotropin and mode of delivery. British *Journal of Obstetrics & Gynaecology*, 1989, 96(10):1224-7
- Mongelli M, Kwan Y, et al. Effect of labour and delivery on plasma hepatic enzymes in the newborn. *Journal of Obstetric & Gynecological Research*, 2000, 26(1):61-3
- Miclat NN, Hodgkinson R, Marx GT. Neonatal gastric pH. *Anesthesia & Analgesia*, 1972, 57(1):98-101

50 Even one company which produces bupivacaine (Astra Zenec) acknowledges in its literature that local anaesthetics rapidly cross the placenta and can cause varying degrees of maternal, fetal and neonatal toxicity. See the following articles:

- Fernando R. and Bonello E. Placental and Maternal Plasma Concentrations of Fentanyl and Bupivacaine after Ambulatory Combined Spinal Epidural (CSE) Analgesia during Labour. *International Journal of Obstetric Anesthesia,* 1995, 4:178-179
- Brinsmead M. Fetal and Neonatal Effects of Drugs Administered in Labour, *Medical Journal of Australia*, 1987, 146:481-486

A Cochrane review conducted in 2006 (by Elbourne, et al) into the use of the same opioids administered intra-muscularly (rather than via an epidural) concluded there was insufficient evidence to evaluate the comparative efficacy and safety of different opioids. See:

- Elbourne D, Wiseman R. Types of intra-muscular opioids for maternal pain relief in labour. In: *The Cochrane Library,* Issue 2. Chichester: John Wiley & Sons Ltd, 2006

51 Hale T. The Effects on Breastfeeding Women of Anaesthetic Medications Used during Labour, paper presented at Passage to Motherhood Conference, Brisbane, Australia, 1998.

52 Belfrage P, et al, Lumbar Epidural Analgesia with Bupivacaine in Labor, *American Journal of Obstetrics & Gynecology*, 1975, 123:839-844.

A study conducted back in 1977 (Caldwell, et a) found bupivacaine in babies 18 hours after the birth, compared to just one and a half hours in the case of the mother. See:

- Caldwell J, Moffatt JR, Smith RL, Lieberman BA, Beard RW, Snedden W, Wilson BW. Determination of bupivacaine in human fetal and neonatal blood samples by quantitative single ion monitoring. *Biomedical Mass Spectrometry*, 1977 Oct;4 (5):322-5

53 Mueller MD, Bruhwiler H, et al. Higher rate of fetal acidemia after regional anesthesia for elective cesarean delivery. *Obstetrics & Gynecology*, 1997, Jul; 90(1): 131-4.

54 See the following:

- Bacigalupo G, Riese S, et al. Quantitative relationships between pain intensities during labor and beta-endorphin and cortisol concentrations in plasma. Decline of the hormone concentrations in the early postpartum period. *Journal of Perinatal Medicine*, 1990, 18(4):289-96.

In addition, there is an inhibition of catecholamine release (Jones, 1985) as well as an inhibition of the oxytocin peak, which typically occurs during a physiological labour (Goodfellow, 1983). See:

- Goodfellow CF, *et al*, Oxytocin Deficiency at Delivery with Epidural Analgesia, *British Journal of Obstetrics & Gynaecology*, 1983, 90:214-219
- Jones CR, McCullouch J, *et al*. Plasma catecholamines and modes of delivery: the relation between catecholamine levels and in-vitro platelet aggregation and adrenoreceptor radioligand binding characteristics. *British Journal of Obstetrics & Gynaecology*, 1985, Jun; 92(6):593-9

55 I'm afraid it hasn't yet been possible to track down these specific studies. (Perhaps the one reported at the conference was never published?) However, the following studies also concluded that epidurals provide inadequate pain relief in some cases:

- Agaram R, Douglas MJ, McTaggart RA, Gunka V. Inadequate pain relief with labor epidurals: a multivariate analysis of associated factors. *International Journal of Obstetric Anesthesia*, 2009, Vol 18,10-14,2009.
- Le Coq G, Ducot B, Benhamou D. Risk factors of inadequate pain relief during epidural analgesia for labour and delivery. *Canadian Journal of Anaesthesia*, 1998, Aug;45(8):719-23.

In the first study (Agaram, *et al*) the researchers initially concluded (from women's reports) that 16.9% of women who'd been in the cohort (of 260 subjects) experienced inadequate pain relief. Problems were associated with insertion of the epidural at more than 7cm dilation, women's past experience of opioid tolerance, previous failed epidural and insertion of the epidural by a trainee anaesthesiologist. After adjustments, the researchers concluded that epidurals were ineffective in only 9.3% of cases. The second study (Le Coq, *et al*), which *observed* 456 women (instead of interviewing them), found that epidurals provided inadequate pain relief in labour in 5.3% of cases, and during 'delivery' (birth) in 19.7% of cases. Reasons for inadequacy (in order of importance) included inadequate first doses (so that two top-ups were needed), posterior position, pain when the epidural was sited, epidural being in place for more than six hours, and the epidural being in place for *less* than one hour (meaning it was less effective for 'delivery').

Another related angle is to do with later memories. In one study (which clearly needs to be repeated), even when women reported good pain relief as a result of an epidural, they generally reported lower levels of satisfaction with the birth overall a year after the birth. Another study (by Cooper, *et al*, is due out soon on this too. See:

- Morgan BM, Bulpitt CJ, Clifton P, Lewis PJ. Analgesia and satisfaction in childbirth (the Queen Charlotte's 1000 mother survey) *Lancet*, 1982, 2 (Oct 9) 808-810
- Cooper, *et al* Satisfaction, control and pain relief: short and long term assessments in a randomised controlled trial of low-dose and traditional epidurals and a non-epidural comparison group. *International Journal of Obstetric Anesthesia*, 2009. [Full reference not available at time of going to press.]

56 In any case, Murray, *et al* (1981) reported a higher caesarean rate when epidurals were inserted earlier on in a woman's labour. See:

- Murray AD, *et al*.Effects of epidural anesthesia on newborns and their mothers. *Child Development*, 1981, 52:71-82

57 See McRae-Bergeron 1998 and Behrens 1993. In the study by Behrens, *et al*, average labour times increased from 4.7 to 7.8 hours. The full references are as follows:
- McRae-Bergeron CE, *et al*, The Effect of Epidural Analgesia on the Second Stage of Labour, *Journal of the American Association of Anesthetic Nurses*, 1998, 66, No 2 :177-182
- Behrens O, *et al*, Effects of Lumbar Epidural Analgesia on Prostaglandin F2 Alpha Release and Oxytocin Secretion during Labour. *Prostaglandins*, 1993, 45, No 3: 285-296

58 For confirmation of this claim and a discussion of related issues, see:
- Hughes D, Simmons S, Brown J, Cyna A. Combined spinal-epidural versus epidural analgesia in labour. (Cochrane Review). In: *The Cochrane Library*, Issue 3. John Wiley & Sons, 2006
- Anim-Somuah M, Smyth R, Howell C. Epidural versus non-epidural or no analgesia in labour. *The Cochrane Database of Systematic Reviews*, 2006, Issue 2
- Annandale, E. Dimensions of patient control in a free-standing birth centre. *Social Science & Medicine*, 1987, 25(11):1235-1248

McRae-Bergeron (1998) documented longer second stages of labour and extra need for forceps after epidurals.
- McRae-Bergeron CE, *et al*, The Effect of Epidural Analgesia on the Second Stage of Labour, *Journal of the American Association of Anesthetic Nurses*, 1998, 66, No 2:177-182
- Torvaldsen S, Roberts C, Bell J, Raynes-Greenow C. Discontinuation of epidural analgesia late in labour for reducing the adverse delivery outcomes associated with epidural analgesia. *The Cochrane Database of Systematic Reviews*, 2006, Issue 3

Note too that epidurals are also associated with fecal and so-called 'flatus' incontinence (i.e. having no control over passing wind or poos) because they result in higher rates of forceps births, although—as with other issues around intervention—although problems increase, it's not easy to identify categorically what causes what, i.e. that epidurals specifically are the cause, because they're often requested when many other problems are present, which skews research results.

59 Thorp J, *et al*. The effect of continuous epidural anesthesia on caesarean section for dystocia in nulliparous women. *American Journal of Obstetrics & Gynecologists*, 1989, 161(3), September:670-674.

Also see:
- Lieberman E, Davidson K, *et al*. Changes in fetal position during labor and their association with epidural analgesia. *Obstetrics & Gynecology*, 2005, 105:974-82

60 Lieberman E, Davidson K, *et al*. Changes in fetal position during labor and their association with epidural analgesia. *Obstetrics & Gynecology*, 2005, 105:974-82.

61 Murray AD, *et al*. Effects of epidural anesthesia on newborns and their mothers. *Child Development*, 1981, 52:71-82.

The following researcher has also reported on an increase in the caesarean rate when an epidural is sited in early labour:

- Klein M. In the literature: epidural analgesia: does it or doesn't it? *Birth,* 2006, 33(1):74-76

62 Fusi L, *et al*. Maternal pyrexia associated with the use of epidural anesthesia in labour. *Lancet,* 1989, June 3:1250-1252.

Also see:

- Apantaku O, Mulik V. Maternal intra-partum fever. J Obstet Gynaecol, 2007, Jan; 27(1):12-5

63 Sudlow C, Warlow C. Epidural blood patching for preventing and treating post-dural puncture headache. *Cochrane Database Systematic Review,* 2002, (2):CD001791.

64 See the following articles:

- Rortveit A, Kjersti D, Yugvild S, Hannestad S, Hunskaar S. Urinary incontinence after vaginal delivery or caesarean section. *New England Journal of Medicine,* 2003, 348:900-907
- Ramin SM, *et al*. Randomized trial of epidural versus intravenous analgesia during labor. *Obstetrics & Gynecology,* 1995, 86:783-789

65 Krehbiel DP, *et al*, Peridural Anesthesia Disturbs Maternal Behavior in Primiparous and Multiparous Parturient Ewes, *Physiology & Behavior,* 1987, 40:463-472.

66 Sepkoski CB, Lester G, *et al*. The effects of maternal epidural anesthesia on neonatal behavior during the first month. *Developmental Medicine & Child Neurology,* 1992; 34:1072-80.

67 Murray AD, *et al*. Effects of epidural anesthesia on newborns and their mothers. *Child Development,* 1981, 52:71-82.

68 Walker M. Do labor medications affect breastfeeding? *Journal of Human Lactation,* 1997, Jun; 13(2):131-7.

69 See the following articles:

- Riordan J, *et al*, Effect of Labor Pain Relief Medication on Neonatal Suckling and Breastfeeding Duration, *Journal of Human Lactation,* 2000, 16,No 1:7-12
- Ransjo-Arvidson AB, *et al*. Maternal Analgesia during Labor Disturbs Newborn Behavior: Effects on Breastfeeding, Temperature, and Crying, *Birth,* 2001, 28,No 1:20-21

Michel makes some brief comments about epidurals at www.wombecology.com/epidural.html. For more on epidurals see:

- Beilin Y, Bodian C, Weiser J, *et al*. Effect of labor epidural analgesia with and without fentanyl on infant breast-feeding: a prospective, randomized, double-blind study. *Anesthesiology,* 2005, Dec;103(6):1211-7
- Henderson J, Dickenson J, Evans S. Impact of intrapartum analgesia on breastfeeding duration. *Australian & New Zealand Journal of Obstetrics & Gynaecology,* 2003, 43(5):372
- Ransjo-Arvidson A, Matthiesen A, Lilja G. Maternal analgesia during labour disturbs newborn behaviour: effects on breastfeeding, temperature and crying. *Birth,* 2001, 23(3):136-143
- Torvaldsen S, Roberts CL, Simpson JM, *et al*. Intrapartum epidural analgesia and

breastfeeding: a prospective cohort study. *International Breastfeeding Journal*, 2006, Dec11;1:24

Other studies conclude that tachycardia is more likely, as well as hypoglycaemia. See:

- Lieberman E, O'Donoghue C. Unintended effects of epidural analgesia during labour. *American Journal of Obstetrics & Gynaecology*, 2002, 186:S31-68

70 See: Mander R. *Pain in Childbirth and its Control*. Blackwell Science, 1998.

71 This is because sucking intensity, duration and frequency has been shown to have a dramatic effect on prolactin levels, which are necessary for lactation and breastfeeding. See:

- Grattan DR. The actions of prolactin in the brain during pregnancy and lactation. *Progress in Brain Research*, 2001, 135:153-171
- Ransjo-Arvidson A, Matthiesen A, Lilja G. Maternal analgesia during labour disturbs newborn behaviour: effects on breastfeeding, temperature and crying. *Birth*, 2001, 23(3):136-143
- Jordan S, Emery S, Bradshaw C. The impact of intrapartum analgesia on infant feeding. *British Journal of Obstetrics & Gynaecology*, 2005, 112(7):927-930

72 A Cochrane review conducted in 2006 into the use of opioids administered intra-muscularly concluded there was insufficient evidence to evaluate the comparative efficacy and safety of different opioids. See:

- Elbourne D, Wiseman R. Types of intra-muscular opioids for maternal pain relief in labour (Cochrane Review). In: *The Cochrane Library*, Issue 2. Chichester: John Wiley & Sons Ltd, 2006

73 American College of Obstetricians & Gynecologists, Obstetric Analgesia and Anesthesia, 1996, Technical Bulletin No 225 (July).

74 Thomas TA, et al, Influence of Medication, Pain and Progress in Labour on Plasma Beta-endorphin like Immunoreactivity, *British Journal of Anaesthesia*, 1982, 54: 401-408.

75 Thomson AM. A Re-evaluation of the Effect of Pethidine on the Length of Labour, *Journal of Advanced Nursing*, 1994, 19,No 3:448-456.

76 Lindow SW, Van der Spuy ZM, et al. The effect of morphine and naloxone administration on plasma oxytocin concentrations in the first stage of labour. *Clinical Endocrinology*, 1992, 37(4):349-53.

77 Kimball CD, Do Endorphin Residues of Beta Lipotrophin in Hormones Reinforce Reproductive Functions? *American Journal of Obstetrics & Gynaecology*, 1979, 134, No 2:127-132.

78 Jacobsen B, et al, Opiate Addiction in Adult Offspring through Possible Imprinting after Obstetric Treatment, *British Medical Journal*, 1990, 301:1067-1070.

79 Nyberg K, Buka SL, Lipsitt LP. Perinatal medication as a potential risk factor for adult drug abuse in a North American cohort. *Epidemiology*, 2000, 11(6): 715-16.

80 See the following studies:

- Myerson BJ. Influence of Early B-endorphin Treatment on the Behavior and

- Reaction to B-endorphin in the Adult Male Rat, *Psychoneuroendocrinology*, 1985, 10:135-147
- Kellogg CK, *et al*, Sexually Dimorphic Influence of Prenatal Exposure to Diazepam on Behavioral Responses to Environmental Challenge and on Gamma Aminobutyric Acid (GABA)-Stimulated Chloride Uptake in the Brain, *Journal of Pharmacology and Experimental Therapeutics*, 1991, 256,No 1:259-265
- Liversay GT, *et al*, Prenatal Exposure to Phenobarbital and Quantifiable Alterations in the Electroencephalogram of Adult Rat Offspring, *American Journal of Obstetrics & Gynecology*, 1992, 167,No 6:1611-1615
- Mirmiran M, DF. Swaab, Effects of Perinatal Medication on the Developing Brain. In *Fetal Behaviour*, Nijhuis JG (ed). Oxford University Press, 1992

81 Mirmiran M, Swaab DF. Effects of Perinatal Medication on the Developing Brain. In Fetal *Behaviour*, Nijhuis JG (ed). Oxford University Press, 1992.

82 See the following articles:
- Jacobson B, Nyberg K. Opiate addiction in adult offspring through possible imprinting after obstetric treatment. *British Medical Journal*, 1990, 301:1067-70
- Nyberg K, Buka SL, Lipsitt LP. Perinatal medication as a potential risk factor for adult drug abuse in a North American cohort. *Epidemiology*, 2000, 11(6):715-16

83 Robertson (1997) is one researcher who is concerned that women are inhaling a drug with unknown side-effects. See:
- Robertson A. *The Midwife Companion.* Ace Graphics, 1997

After conducting a systematic review of Entonox, Rosen (2002) concluded with a muted endorsement. However, although women generally speak positively of 'gas and air' when they've used it (usually because they're proud not to have needed anything stronger), they are not commenting from the perspective of a woman who has experienced the alternative— a completely alert, empowered birth, involving only naturally-induced states of mind. Many, who are dismissive of the effectiveness of Entonox as a form of pain relief say its primary role was as a distraction. If this is all it is, it's a shame these women gave up the possibility (for themselves and their babies) of experiencing birth with natural endorphins and—most importantly—the surge of oxytocin (the hormone of love), which is a feature following physiological births, i.e. births without any drugs. See:
- Rosen M. Nitrous oxide for relief of labour pain: a systematic review. *American Journal of Obstetrics & Gynaecology*, 2002, 186:S 110-126

84 We do know that all synthetic morphines—all opiates, in fact—suppress the sucking reflex and since the target of nitrous oxide is the opioid brain receptor there may be cause for concern in this respect. (This was noted in a study by Righard and Alade, for example, who concluded: "It is suggested that contact between mother and infant should be uninterrupted during the first hour after birth or until the first breast-feed has been accomplished, and that use of drugs such as pethidine should be restricted.") A study on other effects of opiates, which may be relevant, is that by Jacobsen, *et al*, as follows:
- Jacobson B, Nyberg K. Opiate addiction in adult offspring through possible imprinting after obstetric treatment, *British Medical Journal*, 1990, 301:1067-70
- Righard L, Alade MO. Effect of delivery room routines on success of first breast-feed. *Lancet*, 1990, Nov 3; 336(8723):1105-7.

85 For clarification, see:
- Emmanouil DE, Quock RM. Advances in understanding the actions of nitrous oxide. *Anesthesia Progress*, 2007, Spring;54(1):9-18, Review

86 This is the advice I'm providing, based on the idea that's it's important not to get distracted and to depend on outside means of support (which might prevent you from getting into the right state of mind to give birth). Nevertheless, it must be said that research has found aromatherapy to be useful. One large study (Burns, *et al*, 2000) found that women used less opioids as a result (pethidine, diamorphine, etc) and another researcher (Mousely, 2005) found similar results and also noted that caregivers were enthusiastic about the use of aromatherapy. See:
- Burns E, Blamey C, Ersser S. The use of aromatherapy in intrapartum midwifery practice: an observational study. *Complementary Therapies in Nursing & Midwifery*, 2000, 6:33-34
- Mousely S. Audit of an aromatherapy service in a maternity unit. *Complementary Therapies in Clinical Practice*, 2005, 11:205-210

87 Research has indeed backed up this assertion. The following review of research concluded that studies of TENS provided no compelling evidence for TENS having any analgesic effect:
- Carroll D, Tramer M, McQuay H, Nye B, Moore A. Transcutaneous electrical nerve stimulation in labour pain: a systematic review. *British Journal of Obstetrics & Gynaecology*, 1997, 104:169-175

88 See the following articles:
- Odent M. La réflexothérapie lombaire. Efficacité dans le traitement de la colique néphrétique et en analgésie obstétricale. *La Nouvelle Presse Médicale*, 1975, 4 (3):188

For more on this, see:
- Bahasadri S, Ahmadi-Abhari S, Dehghani-Nik M, Habibi GR. Subcutaneous sterile water injection for labour pain: A randomised controlled trial. *Australian & New Zealand Journal of Obstetrics & Gynaecology*, 2006, 46:102-6
- Lytzen T, Cederberg L, Moller-Nielsen J. Relief of low back pain in labor by using intracutaneous nerve stimulation (INS) with sterile water papules. *Acta Obstetrica et Gynecologica Scandinavica*, 1989, 68:341-3
- Martensson L, Ader L, Wallin G. Sterile water papules against labor pain. A simple, safe, effective method. *Lakartidningen*, 1995, 92:2395-6
- Matensson L, Wallin G. Labour pain treated with cutaneous injections of sterile water: a randomised controlled trial. *BJOG: International Journal of Obstetrics & Gynaecology*, 1999, 106:633-7

89 This is referred to by Enkin, *et al* on page 252 of their review of research. See:
- Enkin M. Keirse MJNC, Renfrew M, Neilson J. *Guide to Effective Care in Pregnancy and Childbirth*. Oxford University Press 1995

90 This is a difficult topic because, admittedly, research studies into the use of acupuncture during labour have concluded that women receiving acupuncture use less pain relief and have less augmentation. I wonder if this is potentially because

women who arrange acupuncture in advance of their labours set out to have a less medicated birth? As with other topics, it would be very difficult to conduct a randomised controlled trial to test out something like acupuncture because in the UK especially women can exercise choice and they would probably be very unwilling to be 'randomly' assigned to an 'acupuncture' group for pain relief, particularly if they had no expectation of it being effective! For more information, see:

- Ramnero A, Hanson U, Kihlgren M. Acupuncture treatment during labour—a randomised controlled trial. *British Journal of Obstetrics & Gynaecology*, 2002, 109:637-644
- Neisheim B, Kinge R, Berg R. Acupuncture during labour can reduce the use of Merperidine: a controlled study. *Clinical Journal of Pain,* 2003, 19(3):187-191
- Skilnand E, Fossen D, Heiberg E. Acupuncture in the manage-ment of pain in labour. *Acta Obstetrica et Gynaecologica Scandinavica*, 2002, 81(10):943-948
- Ternov N, Buchhave P, Svensson G, Akeson J. Acupuncture during childbirth reduces use of conventional analgesia without major adverse effects: a retrospective study. *American Journal of Acupuncture,* 1998, 26(4):233-239
- Martoudis S, Christofides K. Electro-acupuncture for pain relief in labour. *Acupuncture in Medicine,* 1990, 8(2):51

If you're interested in arranging acupuncture, you could perhaps recommend to your caregiver the following book:

- Yelland S. *Acupuncture in Midwifery.* Blackwell, 2004

Research into the use of acupressure (shiatsu) or reflexology also drew positive conclusions. See:

- Kyeong Lee M, Bok Chang S, Kang D. Effects of SP6 acupressure on labour pain and length of delivery time in women during labour. *Journal of Alternative & Complementary Medicine,* 2004, 10(6):959-965
- Waters B, Raisler J. Ice water for the reduction of labour pain. *Journal of Midwifery & Women's Health,* 2003, 48:317-321
- Yates S. *Shiatsu for Midwives.* Books for Midwives Press, 2003
- Liisberg G. Easier births using reflexology. *Tidsskrift for Jordemodre,* 1989
- Motha G, McGrath G. The effects of reflexology on labour outcomes. *Journal of the Association of Reflexologists,* 1993, June,2-4

91 Tips on massage (for caregivers) are provided at www.midwiferytoday.com/articles/midwifestouch.asp. Also see Step 2, Note 19 for more on massage. This is one complementary therapy (if you would like to call it that), which can be used without disturbing a physiological labour. Of course, it is best if the 'masseur' or 'masseuse' is a person who is sensitive and familiar to the labouring woman and is in the birthing environment *anyway*. (This could be a husband, good friend or midwife.) It also goes without saying, I hope, that anyone doing massage needs to be silent.

7... Help your baby

1   For a justification of this advice, see:
    - Odent M, McMillan L, Kimmel T. Prenatal care and sea fish. European *Journal of Obstetrics & Gynecology & Reproductive Biology*, 1996, 68:49-51
    - Odent M, Colson S, De Reu P. Consumption of seafood and preterm delivery—Encouraging pregnant women to eat sea fish did not show effect. *British Medical Journal*, 2002, 324:1279

2   A study by Kandel, *et al* (1994) showed that mothers who smoke during their pregnancies make their female children much more likely to be smokers when they reach adolescence. See:
    - Kandel DB, Wu P, Davies MK. Maternal smoking during pregnancy and smoking by adolescent daughters. *American Journal of Public Health*, 1994, 84:1407-13

3   The week-by-week guide to fetal development in this chapter was compiled from information in the following publications:
    - *Myles Textbook for Midwives* by Bennett VR and Brown LK (eds). Churchill Livingstone, 1999.
    - *Heart & Hands by* Davis 1997.
    - *The National Childbirth Trust Book of Pregnancy & Birth*
    - *Birth & Parenthood* (Tucker 1996)
    - *The Complete Book of Mother & Baby Care* (Fenwick 1995)
    - *Babies Remember Birth* (Chamberlain 1988)
    - *Babywatching* (Morris 1991)
    - *Birthing from Within* (England and Horowitz 1998)
    - *The Wish, the Wait, the Wonder* (Perry Johnston 1994)
    - *Pregnancy & Birth* magazine, *Practical Parenting* magazine
    - *Pregnancy & Childbirth* (Kitzinger 1989) and the website www.pronatal.co.uk

    I was interested and rather perplexed to note that often information was not consistent between these sources. I obviously had to make decisions as to which source to follow! Measurements (about fetal weight and height) were particularly inconsistent, probably because they're rather difficult to confirm or because of wide variation. In preparation for future editions of this book, I am currently looking at more technical and recent sources, where there should, hopefully, be more consistent information. If you want to check out another, more visual account of fetal development during your pregnancy, you might like to buy:
    - Tallack P. *In The Womb*. National Geographic Society, 2006.

    DVDs are also available. Nevertheless, please be aware—if and when you check out other accounts of fetal development—that subliminal messages (about what 'should' happen at certain stages of your pregnancy) will also, no doubt, be included, many of which may be in conflict with the idea of optimal birth.

4   Actually, false positives are something you need to remember throughout your pregnancy. All kinds of procedures are susceptible to causing a false alarm (or inappropriate delight) In the case of EFM, for example a false positive rate of 99.8% has been observed! See:

- Nelson K, Dambrosia J, Ting T, Grether J. Uncertain value of electronic fetal monitoring in predicting cerebral palsy. *New England Journal of Medicine,* 1996, 334:659-660

In other words, when you definitely know you're pregnant you need to beware of tests which tell you that something 'may be wrong'. The high 'false positive' rate of many tests means that most babies are in fact healthy and well, even though an inadequate test indicates otherwise.

5   A recent review of research has confirmed that skin-to-skin contact at birth has all kinds of benefits (Anderson, *et al,* 2006): longer breastfeeding and less crying from the baby. Finigan and Davies (2005) also concluded that a better emotional connection was established with skin-to-skin contact. See:

- Anderson GC, Moore E, Hepworth J, Bergman N. Early skin-to-skin contact for mothers and their healthy newborn infants. *The Cochrane Database Systematic Reviews,* 2006, Issue 3
- Finigan V, Davies S. "I just wanted to love him forever"—women's lived experience of skin-to-skin contact with their baby immediately after birth. *Evidence Based Midwifery,* 2005, 2(2):59-65

6   For a discussion of the use of kick charts and results considered acceptable, as well as other methods for monitoring (e.g. the use of ultrasound) when women feel their baby is moving around less than usual in late pregnancy, see the following. These studies do suggest that increased monitoring is helpful in late pregnancy in cases where babies are moving around much less. They also conclude that the increased use of ultrasound is helpful (again, only in situations where unborn babies seem to be moving around less in late pregnancy) and that this monitoring results in fewer inductions, and an improvement in stillbirth rates.

- Flenady V, MacPhail J, Gardener G, Chadha Y, Mahomed K, Heazell A, Fretts R, Frøen F. Detection and management of decreased fetal movements in Australia and New Zealand: a survey of obstetric practice. Australia & New Zealand Journal of Obstetrics & Gynaecology, 2009, Aug; 49(4):358-63
- Tveit JV, Saastad E, Stray-Pedersen B, Børdahl PE, Flenady V, Fretts R, Frøen JF. Reduction of late stillbirth with the introduction of fetal movement information and guidelines—a clinical quality improvement. BMC Pregnancy Childbirth, 2009, Jul 22; 9:32

7   There are more comments on postmaturity at www.midwiferytoday.com/articles/timely.asp

8   In 1978 Salter conducted a small study (with only 12 subjects) confirming that newborns who'd had the Leboyer treatment fared better in terms of alertness than those who hadn't; in the same year Oliver and Oliver conducted another small study (with 37 subjects) which also found that Leboyer babies seemed more relaxed (since they less often had tense hands, etc.) and spent more time with their eyes open immediately after their birth. See:

- Salter A. Birth without violence: a medical controversy. *Nursing Research,* 1978. Mar-Apr; 27(2):84-8.

- Oliver CM, Oliver GM. Gentle birth: its safety and its effect on neonatal behaviour. *Journal of Obstetric, Gynecologic and Neonatal Nursing,* 1978. Sep-Oct: 7(5):35-40

9 Xu B, Pekkanen J, Jarvelin MR. Obstretric complications and asthma in childhood. *Journal of Asthma,* 2000, 37(7):589-94.

10 Cnattingius S, Hultman CM, Dahl M, Sparen P. Very preterm birth, birth trauma, and the risk of anorexia nervosa among girls, *Archives of General Psychiatry,* 1999, 56: 634-89.

11 Jacobson B, Eklund G, et al. Perinatal origin of adult self destructive behaviour. *Acta Psychiatriatrica Scandinavica,* 1987, 76:364-371.

12 Jacobson B, Eklund G, et al. Perinatal origin of adult self destructive behaviour. *Acta Psychiatrica Scandinavica,* 1987, 76:364-371

13 Tinbergen N and EA. *Autistic Children: New hope for a cure.* Allen & Unwin, 1983. In correspondence with Michel Odent before his death, Tinbergen wrote that he was considering how to test his hypothesis that there are links between pregnancy and birth practices or situations and autism. He was particularly interested in some children's inability to establish eye contact, which he hypothesised they may not have learnt from their mothers immediately after their birth. It would be nice if someone else could follow up on these ideas.

14 Hattori R, et al. Autistic and developmental disorders after general anaesthetic delivery. *Lancet,* 1991, 337:1357-1358 (letter).

15 Kendell RE, Juszczak E, Cole SK. Obstetric complications and schizophrenia: A case control study based on standardised obstetric records. *British Journal of Psychiatry,* 1996, 168:556-61

16 Kendell RE, Juszczak E, Cole SK. Obstetric complications and schizophrenia: A case control study based on standardised obstetric records. *British Journal of Psychiatry,* 1996, 168:556-61

17 Bakan P, Dibb G, Reed P. Handedness and birth stress. Neuropsychology, 1973, 11: 363-366.

18 Consider the following research studies:
   - Jacobson B, Eklund G, et al . Perinatal origin of adult self destructive behaviour. *Acta Psychiatrica Scandinavica,* 1987, 76:364-371
   - Jacobson B, Nyberg K. Opiate addiction in adult offspring through possible imprinting after obstetric treatment, *British Medical Journal,* 1990, 301:1067-70
   - Nyberg K, Allebeck P, Eklund G, Jacobson B. Socio-economic versus obstetric risk factors for drug addiction in offspring. *British Journal of Addiction,* 1992, 87:1669-1676
   - Nyberg K, Allebeck P, Eklund G, Jacobson B. Obstetric medication versus residential area as perinatal risk factors for subsequent adult drug addiction in offspring. *Paediatric & Perinatal Epidemiology,* 1993, 7:23-32
   - Nyberg K. *Studies of perinatal events as potential risk factors for adult drug abuse.* Thesis: Dept of Clin Alcohol & Drug Addiction Research, Karolinska Institute, Stockholm, Sweden, 1993
   - Nyberg K, Buka SL, Lipsitt LP. Perinatal medication as a potential risk factor for adult drug abuse in a North American cohort. *Epidemiology,* 2000, 11(6):715-16

19 In fact, a review of research conducted in 2005 (by Thacker, *et al*) concluded by recommending the use of fetal blood sampling. However, a new review conducted a year later (by Alfirevic, *et al*) reached the opposite conclusion and did not endorse the practice. These researchers concluded that it does not help to reduce caesearean rates. See:
   - Thacker S, Stroup D, Peterson H. Continuous electronic fetal heart monitoring during labour. (Cochrane Review) In: *The Cochrane Library,* Issue 1. Oxford: Update Software, 2005
   - Alfirevic Z, Devane D, Gyte G. Continuous cardiotocography (CTG) as a form of electronic fetal monitoring (EFM) for fetal assessment during labour. *Cochrane Database of Systematic Reviews,* 2006, Issue 3

6... Care about care

1 For recent studies on independent midwives, compared to NHS care see:
   - Shorten A, Shorten B. Independent midwifery care versus NHS care in the UK. *British Medical Journal,* 2009, Jun11;338:b2210.
   - Symon A, Winter C, Inkster M, Donnan PT. Outcomes for births booked under an independent midwife and births in NHS maternity units: matched comparison study. *British Medical Journal,* 2009, Jun11;338:b2060.

   It's worth noting that the second study's conclusions are mixed. While the researchers state that clinical outcomes are generally much better with independent midwives, they also mention that they found cause for concern. The precise wording of the conclusion in the abstract for this study is: "Healthcare policy tries to direct patient choice towards clinically appropriate and practicable options; nevertheless, pregnant women are free to make decisions about birth preferences, including place of delivery and staff in attendance. While clinical outcomes across a range of variables were significantly better for women accessing an independent midwife, the significantly higher perinatal mortality rates for high risk cases in this group indicate an urgent need for a review of these cases. The significantly higher prematurity and admission rates to intensive care in the NHS cohort also indicate an urgent need for review." It seems likely that since women 'self-select' the independent midwife option, there will be cases where extremely high risk women make this choice, who really shouldn't. The question therefore arises again about risk assessment (which I have discussed to some exent in Step 9: Consider your assumptions). As you will have realised from my own birth accounts, I certainly feel that a woman who is extremely healthy but simply a little older than other women is very different from someone who has serious health problems. In the same way, I think there are enormous differences between a) a woman who honestly feels she had a PPH as a result of a mismanaged third stage in a previous labour, b) a woman who is severely anaemic, and c) a woman who has placenta praevia—because the latter two women really would be seriously at risk if a haemorrhage occurred. In addition, there is an enormous difference between a home birth which takes place (with an independent midwife in attendance) *near* a hospital and one which happens a very long way away from any emergency facilities. Finally, we have to recognise that there must be differences between individual independent midwives... Most are outstanding, but just one with poor judgement can skew the statistics, unfortunately.

2. Thomas P, Golding J, Peters TJ. Delayed antenatal care: does it affect pregnancy outcome? *Social Science & Medicine*, 1991, 32:715-23.
3. Douglas KA, Redman CW. Eclampsia in the United Kingdom. *British Medical Journal*, 1994, 309:1395-400.
4. Michel writes more about his views on antenatal care at www.wombecology.com/newreasons.html.
5. Birlholz J,& Stephens JC. *American Journal of Roentology*. Fetal Movement Patterns: A Possible Means of Defining Neurological Development Milestones In Utero, 1978, Vol 130 (pp 537-540).
6. Meire HB. The safety of diagnostic ultrasound. (Commentary) *British Journal of Obstetrics & Gynaecology*, 1987, Vol 94, (pp 1121-1122).
7. This was Prof. Nicholas Fisk at Queen Charlotte's Hospital in London in 1996.
8. Ewigman BG, Crane JP, Frigoletto FD, et al. Effect of prenatal ultrasound screening on perinatal outcome. RADIUS study group. *New England Journal of Medicine*, 1993, Vol 329, No 12 (pp 821-7).
9. Bucher HC, Schmidt JG. Does routine ultrasound scanning improve outcome in pregnancy? Meta-analysis of various outcome measures. *British Medical Journal*, 1993, 307:13-7.
10. See the following articles:
    - Larson T, Falck Larson J, et al. Detection of small-for-gestational-age fetuses by ultrasound screening in a high risk population: a randomized controlled study. *British Journal of Obstetrics & Gynaecology*, 1992, 99:469-74
    - Secher NJ, Kern Hansen P, et al. A randomized study of fetal abdominal diameter and fetal weight estimation for detection of light-for-gestation infants in low-risk pregnancy. *British Journal of Obstetrics & Gynaecology*, 1987, 94:105-9
11. Johnstone FD, Prescott RJ, et al. Clinical and ultrasound prediction of macrosomia in diabetic pregnancy. *British Journal of Obstetrics & Gynaecology*, 1996, 103:747-54.
12. Wagner M. Ultrasound; More harm than good? *Mothering* magazine, Winter 1995.
13. De Crespigny L, Dredge R. *Which Tests for my Unborn Baby?* Oxford University Press, 1996.
14. Oakley A. The history of ultrasonography in obstetrics. *Birth*, 1986, Vol 13, No 1, 8-13.
15. De Crespigny L, Dredge R. *Which Tests for my Unborn Baby?* Oxford University Press, 1996.
16. Saari-Kemppainen A, Karjalainen O, Ylostalo P, et al. Ultrasound screening and perinatal mortality: controlled trial of systematic one-stage screening in pregnancy. The Helsinki ultrasound trial. *Lancet*, 1990, Vol 336, No 8712 (pp 387-391).
17. See the following for commentaries on this:
    - Olsen O, et al. Routine ultrasound dating has not been shown to be more accurate than the calendar method. *British Journal of Obstetrics & Gynaecology*, 1997, Vol 104, No 11, pp 1221-2
    - Kieler H, Axelsson O, Nilsson S, Waldenstrom U. Comparison of ultrasonic measurement of biparietal diameter and last menstrual period as a predictor of day of delivery in women with regular 28 day cycles. *Acta Obstetrica et Gynecologica Scandinavica*, 1993, Vol 75, No 5, pp 347-9

18 See the following articles:
   - Ewigman BG, Crane JP, Frigoletto FD, et al. Effect of prenatal ultrasound screening on perinatal outcome. RADIUS study group. *New England Journal of Medicine*, 1993, Vol 329, No 12, pp 821-7
   - Luck CA. Value of routine ultrasound scanning at 19 weeks: a four year study of 8849 deliveries. *British Medical Journal*, 1992, Vol 34, No 6840, pp 1474-8
19 Chan FY. Limitations of Ultrasound. Paper presented at Perinatal Society of Australia & New Zealand. 1st Annual Congress, Freemantle, 1997.
20 See the following articles:
   - Ewigman BG, Crane JP, Frigoletto FD, et al. Effect of prenatal ultrasound screening on perinatal outcome. RADIUS study group. *New England Journal of Medicine*. 1993 Vol 329, No 12, pp 821-7
   - Luck CA. Value of routine ultrasound scanning at 19 weeks: a four year study of 8849 deliveries. *British Medical Journal*, 1992, Vol 34, No 6840, pp 1474-8
21 Brand IR, Kaminopetros P, Cave M, et al. Specificity of antenatal ultrasound in the Yorkshire region: a prospective study of 2261 ultrasound detected anomalies. *British Journal of Obstetrics & Gynaecology*, 1994. Vol 101, No 5, pp 392-397.
22 Sparling JW, Seeds JW, Farran, D. C. The relationship of obstetric ultrasound to parent and infant behavior. *Obstetrics & Gynecology* 1988, Vol 72, No 6, pp 902-7.
23 In 1975 a study of scans on unborn babies using Doppler ultrasound was published in the *British Medical Journal*. The researchers didn't tell the mothers whether the ultrasound machine was switched on, but when it was the fetuses were found to move about much more. See:
   - David H, Weaver JB, Pearson JF. Doppler Ultrasound and Fetal Activity. *British Medical Journal*, 1975, Apr 12; 2(5962):62-4
24 Jumping Babies, *Aims Quarterly Journal*, 1993, Vol 5/7, pp 15-17.
25 American Institute of Ultrasound Medicine Bioeffects Report 1988. *Journal of Ultrasound Medicine*, 1988, Sept 7S1-S38.
26 American Institute of Ultrasound Medicine Bioeffects Report. *Journal of Ultrasound Medicine*, 1988, 7S1-S38, Sept.
27 Liebeskind D, Bases R, Elequin F, et al. Diagnostic ultrasound: effects on the DNA and growth patterns of animal cells. *Radiology*, 1979, Vol 131, No 1, pp 177-184.
28 Ellisman MH, Palmer DE, Andre MP. Diagnostic levels of ultrasound may disrupt myelination. *Experimental Neurology*, 1987, Vol 98, No 1, pp 78-92.
29 Brennan P, et al. Shadow of doubt. *New Scientist*, 1999, 12 June, p 23.
30 Testart J, Thebalt A, Souderis E, Frydman R. Premature ovulation after ovarian ultrasonography. *British Journal of Obstetrics & Gynaecology*, 1982, Vol 89, No 9, pp 694-700.
31 See the following articles:
   - Lorenz RP, Comstock CH, Bottoms SF, Marx SR. Randomised prospective trial comparing ultrasonography and pelvic examination for preterm labor surveillance. *American Journal of Obstetrics & Gynecology*, 1990, Vol 162, No 6, pp 1603-1610

- Saari-Kemppainen A, Karjalainen O, Ylostalo P, *et al*. Ultrasound screening and perinatal mortality: controlled trial of systematic one-stage screening in pregnancy. The Helsinki ultrasound trial. *Lancet*, 1990, Vol 336, No 8712, pp 387-391

32 See the following articles:
- Newnham J, Evans SF, Michael CA, *et al*. Effects of frequent ultrasound during pregnancy: a randomised controlled trial. *Lancet*, 1993, Vol 342, No 8876, 887-91
- Geerts JGM, Brand E, Theron B. Routine obstetric ultrasound in South Africa: cost and effect on perinatal outcome—a prospective randomised controlled trial. *British Journal of Obstetrics & Gynaecology*, 1996, Vol 103, pp 501-507

33 See the following articles:
- Thacker SB. Quality of controlled clinical trials. The case of imaging ultrasound in obstetrics: a review. British Journal of Obstetrics & Gynaecology, 1985, Vol 92, No 5, pp 437-444
- Newnham JP, *et al*. Doppler flow velocity wave form analysis in high risk pregnancies: a randomised controlled trial. *British Journal of Obstetrics & Gynaecology*, 1991, Vol 98, No 10, pp 956-963

34 Davies J, *et al*. Randomised controlled trial of doppler ultrasound screening of placental perfusion in pregnancy. *Lancet*, 1992, 340:1299-1303.

35 Stark CR, Orleans M, Havercamp AD, *et al*. Short and long term risks after exposure to diagnostic ultrasound in utero. *Obstetrics & Gynecology*, 1984, Vol 63, pp 194-200.

36 Campbell JD, *et al*. Case-control study of prenatal ultrasonography in children with delayed speech. *Canadian Medical Association Journal*, 1993, Vol 149, No 10, pp 1435-1440.

37 See the following articles:
- Salvesen KA, Vatten LJ, Eik-nes SH, *et al*. Routine ultrasonography in utero and subsequent handedness and neurological development. *British Medical Journal*, 1993, Vol 307, No 6897, pp 159-64
- Kieler H, Ahlsten G, Haguland B, *et al*. Routine ultrasound screening in pregnancy and the children's subsequent neorological development. *Obstetrics & Gynecology*, 1998, Vol 915 (pt 1), pp 750-6
- Salvesen KA, Ein-nes SH, *et al*. Ultrasound during pregnancy and subsequent childhood non-right handedness- a meta-analysis. *Ultrasound Obstetrics & Gynecology*, 1999, 13(4)241-6
- Kieler H, Cnattingius S, Haglund B, *et al*. Sinistrality—a side-effect of prenatal sonography: A comparative study of young men. *Epidemiology*, 2001, 12(6):618-23

38 See the following articles:
- Odent M. Where does handedness come from? *Primal Health Research Quarterly*, 1998, Vol 6, No 1
- Kieler H, Cnattingius S, Haglund B, *et al*. Sinistrality—a side-effect of prenatal sonography: A comparative study of young men. *Epidemiology*, 2001, 12 (6):618-23

39 Newnham J, Evans SF, Michael CA, *et al*. Effects of frequent ultrasound during pregnancy: a randomised controlled trial. *Lancet*, 1993, Vol 342, No 8876, pp 887-91.

40 If you would like to read some other expert comments, find former World Health Organization Director Marsden Wagner's comments at www.midwiferytoday.com/articles/ultrasoundwagner.asp or comments from Beverley Beech (honourary chair of the Association for Improvements in the Maternity Services (AIMS)) at www.midwiferytoday.com/articles/ultrasound.asp.

41 See the following articles:
- Symonds EM. Aetiology of pre-eclampsia: a review. *J R Soc Med*, 1980, 73:871-5
- Naeye EM. Maternal blood pressure and fetal growth. *American Journal of Obstetrics & Gynecology*, 1981, 141:780-7
- Kilpatrick S. Unlike pre-eclampsia, gestational hypertension is not associated with increased neonatal and maternal morbidity except abruption. SPO abstracts, *American Journal of Obstetrics & Gynecology*, 1995, 419:376
- Curtis S, *et al*. Pregnancy effects of non-proteinuric gestational hypertension. SPO Abstracts, *American Journal of Obstetrics & Gynecology*, 1995, 418:376

42 See the following articles:
- Brown VA, *et al*. The value of antenatal cardiotocography in the management of high-risk pregnancy : a randomised controlled trial. *British Journal of Obstetrics & Gynaecology*, 1982, 89:716-22
- Flynn AM, *et al*. A randomized controlled trial of non-stress antepartum cardiotocography. *British Journal of Obstetrics & Gynaecology*, 1982, 89:427-33
- Haverkamp AD, *et al*. A controlled trial of the differential effects of intrapartum monitoring. *American Journal of Obstetrics & Gynecology*, 1976, 126:470-76
- Haverkamp AD, *et al*. The evaluation of continuous fetal heart rate monitoring in high risk pregnancy. *American Journal of Obstetrics & Gynecology*, 1976, 125: 310-20
- Kelso IM, *et al*. An assessment of continuous fetal heart rate monitoring in labor. *American Journal of Obstetrics & Gynecology*, 1978, 131:526-32
- Kidd LC, *et al*. Non-stress antenatal cardiotocography—a prospective randomized clinical trial. *British Journal of Obstetrics & Gynaecology*, 1985, 92:1156-59
- Leveno KJ, *et al*. A prospective comparison of selective and universal electronic fetal monitoring in 34,995 pregnancies. *New England Journal of Medicine*, 1986, 315:615-19
- Lumley JC, Wood C, *et al*. A randomized trial of weekly cardiotocography in high-risk obstetric patients. *British Journal of Obstetrics & Gynaecology*, 1983, 90: 1018-26
- McDonald D, Chalmers I, *et al*. The Dublin randomised controlled trial of intrapartum fetal heart rate monitoring. *American Journal of Obstetrics & Gynecology*, 1985, 152:524-39
- Prentice A, Lind T. Fetal heart rate monitoring during labor—too frequent intervention, too little benefit. *Lancet*, 1987, 2:1375-77
- Sky K, *et al*. Effects of electronic fetal heart rate monitoring, as compared with periodic auscultation, on the neurological development of premature infants. *New England Journal of Medicine*, 1990, (March 1):588-93
- Wood C. A controlled trial of fetal heart rate monitoring in low-risk obstetric population. *American Journal of Obstetrics & Gynecology*, 1981, 141:527-34

- Impey L, Reynolds M, *et al*. Admission cardiotocography: a randomized controlled trial. *Lancet*, 2003, 361:465-70
43 Steer P, Alam MA, Wadsworth J, Welch A. Relation between maternal haemoglobin concentration and birth weight in different ethnic groups. *British Medical Journal*, 1995, 310:489-91.
44 Valberg LS. Effects of iron, tin, and copper on zinc absorption in humans. *American Journal of Clinical Nutrition*, 1984, 40:536-41.
45 Rayman MP, Barlis J, *et al*. Abnormal iron parameters in the pregnancy syndrome preeclampsia. *American Journal of Obstetrics & Gynecology*, 2002, 187(2):412-8.
46 Wen SW, Liu S, Kramer MS, *et al*. Impact of prenatal glucose screening on the diagnosis of gestational diabetes and on pregnancy outcomes. *American Journal of Epidemiology*, 2000, 152(11):1009-14.
47 Kenyon SL, Taylor DJ, Tarnow-Mordi W. Broad spectrum antibiotics for spontaneous preterm labour: the ORACLE II randomized trial. *Lancet*, 2001, 357:989-94.
48 Guise JM, Mahon SM, *et al*. Screening for bacterial vaginosis in pregnancy. *American Journal of Preventive Medicine*, 2001, 20 (suppl 3):62-72.
49 MRC/RCOG Working party on cervical cerclage. Final report of the Medical Research Council/Royal College of Obstetricians & Gynaecologists multicentre randomized trial of cervical cerclage. *British Journal of Obstetrics & Gynaecology*, 1993, 100: 516-23.
50 Enkin MW, Keirse MJNC, Neilson J, Crowther C, Duley L, Hodnett E, Hofmeyr J. *A Guide to Effective Care in Pregnancy & Childbirth*. 3rd edition. Oxford University Press, 2000.
51 See the following articles:
- Odent M. The Nocebo effect in prenatal care. *Primal Heath Research Newsletter*, 1994, 2(2)
- Odent M. Back to the Nocebo effect. *Primal Heath Research Newsletter*, 1995, 5(4)
- Odent M. Antenatal scare. *Primal Heath Research Newsletter*, 2000, 7(4)
52 This view is confirmed by Nolan (2005), who concluded that antenatal education packages do not consistently reduce intervention rates, which in turn suggests that they do not help. However, carefully designed (somewhat non-typical) antenatal classes did result in an increase in the use of upright positions and/or a decrease in the number of epidurals. See:
- Nolan M. Childbirth and parenting education: what the research says and why we may ignore it. In Nolan M and Foster J (eds) *Birth and Parenting Skills: New Directions in Antenatal Education*. Churchill Livingstone, 2005
- Nolan M and Foster J (eds) *Birth and Parenting Skills: New Directions in Antenatal Education*. Churchill Livingstone, 2005
- Foster J. Innovative practice in birth education. In M. Nolan and J. Foster (eds) *Birth and Parenting Skills: New Directions in Antenatal Education*. Elsevier Science, 2005
- Walsh D, Harris M, Shuttlewood S. Changing midwifery birthing practice through audit. *British Journal of Midwifery*, 1999, 7(7):432-345

53 The study by Haverkamp, *et al* (1976) found that caesarean rates increased by 160%. The use of forceps or ventouse also increased by up to 30% (MacDonald, *et al,* 1985), which in turn increases the rate of urinary stress incontinence (Arya, *et al,* 2001), anal sphincter tears (MacArthur, *et al,* 2005) and increased difficulty—or pain—when having sex (Bick, *et al,* 2002). See:

- Haverkamp A, Thompson H, McFee J. The evaluation of continuous fetal heart rate monitoring in high-risk pregnancy. *American Journal of Obstetrics & Gynaecology,* 1976, 125(3):310-320
- MacDonald D, Grant A, Sheridan-Pereira M. The Dublin randomised control trial of intrapartum fetal heart rate monitoring. *American Journal of Obstetrics & Gynaecology,* 1985, 152(5):524-539
- Arya L, Jackson N, Myers D, Verma A. Risk of new onset urinary incontinence after forceps and vacuum delivery in primiparous women. *American Journal of Obstetrics & Gynaecology,* 2001, 185:1318-1324
- MacArthur C, Glazener C, Lancashire R. Faecal incontinence and mode of first and subsequent delivery: a six year longitudinal study. *BYOG: An International Journal of Obstetrics & Gynaecology,* 2005, 112:1075-1082
- Bick D, MacArthur C, Knowles H, Winter H. *Postnatal Care: Evidence and Guidelines for Management.* Churchill Livingstone, 2002

54 Inductions do not always—or often—mean that labour suddenly starts efficiently and continues without interruption. This perhaps explains why some studies have revealed that as many as 57% of low-risk first-time mothers have syntocinon (artificial oxytocin through a drip) to speed up their labours. Walsh (2007) says this suggests 'a collapse in physiological ability to labour spontaneously'. See:

- Mead M. Midwives' perspectives in 11 UK maternity units. In S. Downe (ed.) *Normal Childbirth: Evidence and Debate.* Churchill Livingstone, 2004
- Walsh D. *Evidence-based Care for Normal Labour and Birth: A guide for midwives.* Routledge, 2007

55 This was an informal study by Perez P and Snedeker C, who are the authors of *Special Women: The Role of the Professional Labor Assistant.* Cutting Edge Press, 2000.

56 Maternity Center Association, 2002.

57 Maternity Center Association. *Listening to mothers: report of first national US survey of women's childbearing experiences.* New York: MCA, 2002 (www.maternitywise.org/listeningtomothers/index.html).

58 Many people have written about the dangers of administering pitocin. To provide just two reasons, Freidman 1978 found that artificial oxytocin (synotcinon) causes the resting tone of the uterus to increase and this can result in abnormal fetal heart rate patterns, fetal distress and even uterine rupture (Stubbs 2000). What's more, research has found that artificial oxytocin has minimal effects on cervical dilation, compared to labour without drugs (Bidgood 1987) and other research showed that women who'd had artificial oxytocin did not experience an increase in beta endorphin levels in labour (Genazzani 1985).

- Freidman EA, Sachtleben MR. Effect of oxytocin and oral prostaglandin E2 on uterine contractility and fetal heart rate patterns. *American Journal of Obstetrics & Gynecology,* 1978, Feb 15; 130(4):403-7

- Stubbs TM. Oxytocin for labor induction. *Clinical Obstetrics & Gynecology*, 2000, Sept; 43(3):489-94
- Bidgood KA, Steer PJ. A randomized control study of oxytocin augmentation of labour. 2. Uterine activity. *British Journal of Obstetrics & Gynaecology*, 1987, Jun; 94(6):518-22
- Genazzani AR, Petraglia F, *et al*. Lack of beta-endorphin plasma level rise in oxytocin-induced labor. *Gynecologic & Obstetric Investigation*, 1985, 19(3):130-4

59 The only effect of EFM identified by research is to increase the caesarean rate; it does nothing to improve either fetal or maternal morbidity or mortality. The following studies have all show the same results—forcing us to conclude that EFM is never actually a useful practice, beyond providing caregivers with 'data' in case of litigation. McKay's study in 1991 revealed how an electronic fetal monitor took midwives' focus off women and Munro, *et al* (2002) confirmed this, while also noting that EFM was often the starting point for a cascade of interventions. For a full list of references relating to EFM and more commentary, see Step 10, Note 19 and Step 9, Note 3.

As noted elsewhere, attitudes towards monitoring really are changing amongst caregivers... For example, one large British consultant unit has recommended a minimum vaginal examination interval of 12 hours for first-time mothers. See:

- Thorton J. Natural labour guidelines. Nottingham City Hospital. Personal Communication with Denis Walsh, 2006. Reported in *Evidence-based Care for Labour and Birth,* Routledge, 2007

60 In case this information is useful to you, a study reported in the *Journal of Pain & Symptom Management* (October 2000, 20(4):273-279) reported as follows: Between 1 and 2% of pregnant women experience hyperemesis gravidarium, or severe morning sickness. A randomized, placebo-controlled crossover study found that stimulating acupuncture point PC6 helps ease nausea and vomiting. Information to consider if this is a serious problem...

61 A review of the scientific basis of obstetric interventions is provided in the following book:

- *Obstetric Myths Versus Research Realities: A Guide to the Medical Literature.* Bergin & Garvey, 1995.

5... Think ahead

1 The following systematic literature review failed to identify any research basis for vaginal examinations to assess the progress of labour:

- Devane D. Sexuality and midwifery. *British Journal of Midwifery*, 1996, 4(8):413-20

The following researchers also concluded that vaginal examinations were not necessary for facilitating physiological birth:

- Chalmers I, Kierse M, Neilson J. *A Guide to Effective Care in Pregnancy and Childbirth.* Oxford University Press, 1989

The practice of routinely conducting vaginal examinations was shown, in the following study, to be a ritual which legitimized intrusion into the very private birth place during the second stage of labour:

- Bergstrom L, Roberts J, Skillman L, Seidel J. "You'll feel me touching you, sweetie": Vaginal examinations during the second stage of labour. *Birth,* 1992, 19(1):10-18

Also see:
- Stewart M. "I'm just going to wash you down." Sanitizing the vaginal examination. *Journal of Advanced Nursing,* 2005, 51(6):587-594
- Warren C. Invaders of privacy. *Midwifery Matters,* 1999, 81:8-9

2   Michel explains the importance of a woman's labouring environment at www.wombecology.com/physiological.html

3   Nevertheless, as I've already pointed out, research has generally shown the use of aromatherapy to be helpful, although I consider it inadvisable in certain respects. As with other controversial practices (which haven't been—or could never be—confirmed as useful by research), the important thing is probably to consider the usefulness of a particular practice for you personally, while also considering it within the context of principles generally for facilitating optimal birth. See Step 8, Note 86 for my earlier comments and references on aromatherapy.

4   Some research has demonstrated that music helps to reduce anxiety and/or helps women cope with labour and stress, or give them a greater feeling of being in control. See:

- Spintge R. Some neuro-endocrinological effects of so-called anxiolytic music. *International Journal of Neurology,* 1989, 19/20:186-196
- Browning C. Using music during childbirth. *Birth,* 2000, 27(4):272-276.
- Browning C. Music therapy in childbirth: research in practice. *Music Therapy Perceptions,* 2001, 19(2):74-81

5   *Midwifery Today,* 1996, Issue37, Spring.

6   In a typical study (Feldman, *et al,* 2002), which compared preemies which had had kangaroo care with preemies who hadn't, results of kangaroo care were seen to be quite dramatic. "After KC, interactions were more positive at 37 weeks' GA [gestational age]: mothers showed more positive affect, touch, and adaptation to infant cues, and infants showed more alertness and less gaze aversion. Mothers reported less depression and perceived infants as less abnormal. At 3 months, mothers and fathers of KC [kangaroo care] infants were more sensitive and provided a better home environment. At 6 months, KC mothers were more sensitive and infants scored higher on the Bayley Mental Developmental Index..." The researchers concluded by saying: "KC had a significant positive impact on the infant's perceptual-cognitive and motor development and on the parenting process." For this and other studies on kangaroo care, see:

- Feldman R, Eidelman AI, Sirota L, Weller A. Comparison of skin-to-skin (kangaroo) and traditional care: parenting outcomes and preterm infant development. *Pediatrics,* 2002. Jul;110(1 Pt 1):16-26.
- Rey, ES, Martinez, HG (1983). Manejo racional del nino prematuro. In *Curso de Medicina Fetal.* Universidad Nacional, Bogota
- Charpak, N, Ruiz-Pelaez, JG, Figueroa de Calume Z (1996) Current knowledge of kangaroo mother intervention. *Curr Opin Pediatr.* (8:108-112)
- Doyle, LW (1997). Kangaroo mother care. Lancet 350:1721-1722.

7   Rey Sanabria E. A l'autre bout du monde accueillir le prématuré. In *Les cahiers du nouveau-né, No 6. Un enfant prématurément.* Stock, 1983.

8   If you personally have a history of going into labour prematurely, you may benefit from reading an article at www.midwiferytoday.com/articles/timely.asp

9   Some researchers feel that a managed third stage is 'safer' than a physiological third stage. However, like Esther—who is a very experienced and well-qualified midwife, incidentally—in this book I am wholeheartedly advocating you have a natural third stage for all kinds of reasons. Firstly, it's part of the natural process. As we've seen countless times before, intevening in a healthy process can actually *cause* pathology. If a birth has gone well up till this point, I see no reason why we can't assume the natural hormonal cascade will continue right through to the birth of the placenta. Secondly, it needs to be noted that the use of a synthetic hormone (usually a cocktail in the UK) in order to speed up birth of the placenta comes with a price: side effects. In the case of syntometrine (the drug which is injected into a woman's thigh when there is a managed third stage), side effects include nausea and vomiting, abdominal pain, headaches, dizziness and skin rashes. Personally, I do not want to be feeling nauseous when I first meet my newborn babies. As I know from experience, the alternative is so much better. Thirdly, active management of the third stage of labour involves an enormous amount of disturbance from a caregiver… This is very unfortunate because this is precisely the time (never to be repeated) when a mother first meets her baby, when they first interact and, crucially, when the baby has his or her first feed of breastmilk. It is a magical time if there is no disturbance and the natural processes are allowed to proceed smoothly, without unnecessary disturbance. Having said all that, syntometrine needs to be available with a caregiver in case there is a postpartum haemorrhage (PPH), for any reason, because syntometrine can stop the haemorrhage extremely quickly and effectively. Because the very slight risk of haemorrhage exists, the caregiver also needs to be discretely present until after the placenta has been born.

   In case you're wondering about the *safety* of a physiological third stage, after examining the research I personally am convinced it is safe, provided syntometrine is available, in case it's needed, and provided—of course—you have an expert caregiver (i.e. a midwife or obstetrician) in attendance while you're waiting for the placenta. The research is difficult to present, mainly because so many points in studies are contentious. For example, when 500ml is taken as being the ceiling for PPH, results 'show' that more women having a physiological third stage have a 'haemorrhage'. However, what is a haemorrhage? If a woman loses up to 1,000 ml of blood, but blood loss does not continue, why should that be called a postpartum haemorrhage? And since it doesn't have a bad effect on a new mother, why do we need to worry about it? (It's only really a cause for concern in cases where new mothers are very anaemic, which is often the case—because of inadequate diet—in developing countries. Women who are severely anaemic are much more seriously affected by even small levels of blood loss.) Going back to talking about healthy women, researchers have hypothesised that perhaps a greater level of blood loss during the third stage (i.e. 1,000 ml, rather than 500 ml) may be a feature of an undrugged physiological stage and they see possible reasons for this (Harris, 2001; Wickham, 1999; Buckley, 2009). Perhaps because of these considerations, some researchers (e.g. Burchell 1980) have advocated that the ceiling should be increased to 1,000 ml (i.e. the point at which blood loss is considered 'haemorrhage'). If the level is increased to 1,000 ml, two studies have shown (Rogers, et al, 1998 and Herschderfer, 1999) that the difference in outcomes between 'managed' and 'physiological' third stages is not significant. In any case, when considering all this, we need to bear in mind that blood loss is estimated *visually* and the accuracy of estimates is very variable (as confirmed by Glover, 2003; Read and Anderton, 1997; and Bose, et al, 2006). (Consider how easy—or difficult!—it is to judge how much blood is soaked into a bedsheet or blanket and how an estimate of this might differ from an estimate of blood pooled on a waterproof sheet.) In addition, we need to remember that in almost all the studies conducted most women who had a 'physiological' third stage had had all kinds of interventions (and drugs) in the first and second stages of labour—so the natural processes had no doubt been severely disturbed already. (We could only really draw accurate conclusions if only fully physiological births were included in the 'physiological third stage' cohorts of studies.)

Finally, the whole issue is compounded by the possibility that *disturbance* to the mother of any kind between the second and third stages might well actually *cause* a haemorrhage, because the hormonal cascade would be disturbed. Since disturbances could include even one word comments to the new mother, there must be numerous cases of disturbance in the studies.

In conclusion, then, although some studies conclude that active management is safer (e.g. Prendiville, et al, 1988 and 2006), I question many of the issues surrounding set-up of studies and am concerned mostly with their conclusion that active management was *worse* than a physiological third stage in terms of nausea, vomiting and hypertension (even though this was apparently only in the case of the use of ergomentrine)... Another study, which compared the effectiveness of different mixtures (McDonald, et al, 2006) found that syntometrine (not ergometrine) caused more nausea, vomiting and raised blood pressure—even though it was found to be most effective in terms of reducing PPH. Of course, my reason is that I think it's rather a tragedy if a new mother is experiencing these symptoms when she first meets her newborn baby and I wouldn't like to guess what the babies think about it. Given how desperately young children look forward to special events, I can well imagine that a fetus also anticipates his or her first meeting with his or her new mother with great interest. See:

- Harris T. Changing the focus for the third stage of labour. *British Journal of Midwifery*, 2001, 9(1):7-12
- Wickham S. Further thoughts on the third stage. *The Practising Midwife*, 1999, 2 (10):14-15
- Buckley SJ. *Gentle Birth, Gentle Mothering: A Doctor's Guide to Natural Childbirth and Gentle Early Parenting Choices*. Celestial Arts, 2009
- Burchell R. Postpartum haemorrhage. In E. Quilligan (ed.) *Current Therapy in Obstetrics & Gynaecology*. Philadelphia: W.B. Saunders, 1980
- Rogers J, Wood J, McCandlish R, Ayers S, Truesdale A, Elbourne D. Active versus expectant management of third stage of labour: the Hinchingbrooke randomised controlled trial. *Lancet*, 1998, 351:693-699
- Herschderfer K. Results of RCT expectant versus active management within setting of Dutch midwives' independent practices (home births). Presented at National Study Day on Third Stage Issues, Manchester, 1999

- Glover P. Blood loss at delivery: how accurate is your estimation. *Australian Journal of Midwifery*, 2003, 16:21-24
- Read M, Anderton J. Radioisotope dilution technique for measurement of blood loss associated with lower segment caesarean section. *British Journal of Obstetrics & Gynaecology*, 1997, 84:859-861
- Bose P, Regan F, Paterson-Brown S. Improving the accuracy of estimated blood loss at obstetric haemorrhage using clinical reconstructions. *BJOG: An International Journal of Obstetrics & Gynaecology*, 2006, 113:919-924
- Prendiville W, Harding J, Elbourne D, Stirrat G. The Bristol third stage trial: active vs physio-logical management of third stage of labour. *British Medical Journal*, 1988, 297:1295-1300
- Prendiville W, Elbourne D, McDonald S. Active versus expectant management in the third stage of labour (Cochrane Review). In: *The Cochrane Library*, Issue 3. Chichester: John Wiley & Sons Ltd, 2006
- McDonald S, Abbott J, Higgins S. Prophylactic ergometrine-oxytocin versus oxytocin for the third stage of labour (Cochrane Review). In: *The Cochrane Library*, Issue 3. Chichester: John Wiley & Sons Ltd, 2006

10 Hannah ME, Hannah WJ, *et al*. Planned caesarean section versus planned vaginal birth for breech presentation at term: a randomised multicentre trial. *Lancet*, 2000, 356:1375-83.

11 We can at least be reassured that birth outcomes are good overall in Britain. For more information on the situation in Britain see:
   - Health Committee of the House of Commons, Report on Maternity Services, March, 1992
   - www.dh.gov.uk/en/Publicationsandstatistics/Publications/PublicationsPolicyAndGuidance/DH_065053
   - The latest national statistics for the UK at www.statistics.gov.uk/STATBASE/Product.asp?vlnk=5768

4... Choose who

1 The importance of a midwife's attitudes and behaviour is emphasised in the following paper:
   - Downe S, McCourt C. From being to becoming: reconstructing childbirth knowledges. In Downe S (ed) *Normal Childbirth: Evidence and Debate*. Churchill Livingstone, 2004

The potential impact of antenatal care on birth outcome was confirmed in the following study:
   - Foster J. Innovative practice in birth education. In M. Nolan and J. Foster (eds) *Birth and Parenting Skills: New Directions in Antenatal Education*. Elsevier Science, 2005

The helpfulness of a 'working with pain' attitude, rather than a 'pain relief' orientation was emphasised in the following paper:

- Leap N, Anderson T. The role of pain in normal birth and the empowerment of women. In Downe S, McCourt C (eds) *Normal Childbirth: Evidence and Debate.* Churchill Livingstone, 2004 (pp 25-40)

2   See the following articles:
- Boyer EL. Midwifery in America: A Profession Reaffirmed, Journal of Nurse-Midwifery, 1990, Vol 35,No 4,214-19
- Declercq E. The Trials of Hanna Porn: The Campaign to Abolish Midwifery in Massachusetts, American Journal of Public Health, 1994, Vol 84,No 6,1022-8
- Myers S, *et al.* Unlicensed Midwifery Practice in Washington state, *American Journal of Public Health*, 1990, Vol 80,726-8
- Schrader C. The Memoirs (1693-1740) of the Frisian Midwife Catharina Schrader. 1987. Translated and annotated by Hilary Marland, with introductory essays by M.J. van Lieburg and G. J. Kloosterman. Rodopi, Amsterdam (available from Mrs. L. J. Brooke, 4595 Club Dr, NE, Atlanta, GA 30319
- Tyson H, Outcomes of 1001 Midwife-Attended Home Births in Toronto, 1983-1988, *Birth*, 1991, Vol 18, No 1,14-9
- Van Alten DM, Treffers PE, E. Midwifery in the Netherlands. The Wormerveer Study; Selection Mode of Delivery, Perinatal Mortality and Infant Morbidity, *British Journal of Obstetrics & Gynaecology*, 1989, Vol 96,656-62

3   Continuity of care is clearly a way to avoid this problem. A study by Haggerty, *et al* (2005) emphasised the importance of different types of continuity—informational, management and relational—so it's good to aim to achieve this, if at all possible, although admittedly, in some cases it's difficult to have control over this, because it depends on where you live. Nevertheless, making advance arrangements for care that seems likely to maximise continuity can increase the chances that you will actually have continuity of care yourself. In Britain, the easiest way of achieving this is to find an independent midwife, although unfortunately you have to pay for this service. See:
- Haggerty J, Reid R, Freeman G, Starfield B, Adair C, McKendry R. Continuity of care: a multidisciplinary review. *British Medical Journal*, 2005, 327:1219-1221

The first of the following studies emphasised the importance of registering with a small team of midwives (numbering at the most six), while the other studies concluded that continuity was most important during labour, birth and postnatally (and perhaps not such a concern antenatally):
- Flint C. *Midwifery Teams and Caseloads.* Butterworth-Heinemann, 1993
- Flynn A, Hollins K, Lynch P. Ambulation in labour. *British Medical Journal*, 1978, 2(6137):591-593
- Green J, Curtis P, Price H, Renfrew M. *Continuing to Care: The Organization of Midwifery Services in the UK A Structured Review of the Evidence.* Books for Midwives Press, 1998
- Walsh D. An ethnographic study of women's experience of partnership caseload midwifery practice: the professional as friend. *Midwifery,* 1999, 15(3):165-176
- Page L, McCourt C, Beake S, Hewison J. Clinical interventions and outcomes of one-to-one midwifery practice. *Journal of Public Health Medicine,* 1999, 21(3): 243-248

- North Staffordshire Changing Childbirth Research Team. A randomised study of midwifery caseload care and traditional 'shared-care'. *Midwifery,* 2000, 16(4):295-302

4   Research has actually confirmed the inability of caregivers to appraise research (Veeramah 2004) and—perhaps needlessly!—research has also revealed that lack of time is a factor (Hundley 2000). Another research study (Richens 2002) mentioned the problem that an individual caregiver may feel he or she does not have the necessary authority or autonomy to change his or her practice, and another mentioned more generalised institutional constraints (Scott, *et al,* 2003). Nevertheless, as Denis Walsh has exemplified (in the case of one patient who insisted on having a lotus birth, despite extreme pressure not to), when women assert themselves they can actually succeed in demonstrating to caregivers that fears are ungrounded and that there are possible improvements to current practice. See:

- Veeramah V. Utilisation of research findings by graduate nurses and midwives. *Journal of Advanced Nursing,* 2004, 47(2):183-191
- Hundley V. Raising research awareness among midwives and nurses: does it work? *Journal of Advanced Nursing,* 2000, 31(1):78-86
- Richens Y. Are midwives using research evidence in practice? *British Journal of Midwifery,* 2002, 10(1):11-16
- Scott T, Mannion R, Marshall M, Davies H. Does organisational culture influence health care performance? A review of the evidence. *Journal of Health Service Research and Policy,* 2003, 8(2):105-117
- Walsh D. *Evidence-based Care for Normal Labour and Birth.* Routledge, 2007

5   Grol and Grimshaw (2003) have written about doctors' impulse to act. Other writers have written about the way in which midwives tend to be dominated by obstetricians, when they work closely with them (Donnison 1998, Coombs and Ersser 2004). See:

- Grol R, Grimshaw J. From best evidence to best practice: effective implementation of change in patient's care. *Lancet,* 2003, 362:1225-1230
- Donnison J. *Midwives and Medical Men: A History of the Struggle for the Control of Childbirth.* Historical Publications, 1988
- Coombs M, Ersser S. Medoca; hegemony in decision-making—a barrier to interdisciplinary working in intensive care. *Journal of Advanced Nursing,* 2004, 46(3):245-252

6   The following systematic review of nine randomised controlled trials concluded that continuous support during labour reduced the rates of caesarean sections, pharmacological analgesia, assisted vaginal birth, low Apgar scores and labour length and also helped women achieve more enjoyable births:

- Hodnett ED. Continuity of caregivers for care during pregnancy and childbirth (Cochrane Review). In: *The Cochrane Library,* Issue 2. John Wiley & Sons Ltd, 2006

The following study also supported the idea of woman having a 'known' support person during labour, although the conclusion was that a known *untrained* layperson provided the most effective care (so maybe you don't need to worry about how well-trained a doula is!):

- Rosen P. Supporting women in labour: analysis of different types of caregivers. *Journal of Midwifery & Women's Health*, 2004, 49(1):24-31

This strange conclusion was explained in the following study, which analysed women's stress response:

- Taylor S, Klein L, Lewis B, Gruenewald T, Gurung R, Updegraff J. Biobehavioural responses to stress in females: tend-and-befriend, not fight-*or-flight*. *Psychological Review*, 2000, 107(3):411-429

7 Bertsch TD, Nagashima-Whalen L, Dykeman S, Kennell JH, McGrath S. Labor support by first-time fathers: direct observations with a comparison to experienced doulas. *Journal of Psychosomatics in Obstetrics & Gynaecology*, 1990, 11:251-260.

8 Michel is of the opinion that childbirth has been 'masculinised' over the last few centuries and that having a partner at the birth is part of this. Read his full comments on this issue at www.wombecology.com/masculinisation.html

3... Choose where

1 In her book about birth in different cultures, Sheila Kitzinger provides evidence for the notion that place of birth has usually been highly significant. See:

- Kitzinger S. *Rediscovering Birth*. Little, Brown & Company, 2000

2 Despite this one negative comment, several papers have concluded that giving birth in a birth centre (rather than a hospital) can help women avoid unnecessary interventions. At recent conferences I have also met or heard about many midwives who are setting up birth centres which sound amazingly well designed. A birth centre might, therefore be a good option for a woman who is not confident about arranging a home birth. See the following papers:

- Tracy S, Sullivan E, Dahlen H, Black D. Does size matter? A population-based study of birth in lower volume maternity hospitals for low risk women. *BJOG: An International Journal of Obstetrics & Gynaecology*, 2005, 113:86-96
- Jackson D, Lang J, Swartz W, Ganiats T, Fullerton J. Outcomes, safety and resource utilization in a collaborative care birth centre program compared with traditional physician-based perinatal care. *American Journal of Public Health*, 2003, 93:999-1006
- Walsh D. Subverting assembly-line birth: childbirth in a free-standing birth centre. *Social Science & Medicine*, 2006, 62(6):1330-1340
- Stewart M, McCandlish R, Henderson J. *Report of a Structured Review of Birth Centre Outcomes*. Oxford: NPEU, 2004
- Walsh D, Downe S. Outcomes of free-standing, midwifery-led birth centres: a structured review of the evidence. *Birth*, 2004, 31(3):222-229
- Reddy K, Reginald P, Spring J, Nunn L, Mishra N. A free-standing low-risk maternity unit in the United Kingdom: does it have a role? *Journal of Obstetrics & Gynaecology*, 2004, 24(4):360-366
- Green J, Coupland B, Kitzinger J. *Great Expectations: A Prospective Study of Women's Expectations and Experiences of Childbirth*. Cambridge: Child Care & Development Group, 1998

- Hodnett E, Downe S, Edwards N, Walsh D. Home-like versus conventional birth settings (Cochrane Review). In: *The Cochrane Library,* Issue 2. John Wiley & Sons Ltd, 2006

The following studies also mention that less pharmacological analgesia is used in settings which are *not* large hospitals (i.e. in people's homes, in free-standing birth centres or in integrated birth centres):

- Olsen O. Meta-analysis of the safety of home birth. *Birth,* 1997, 24(1): 4-13
- Walsh D, Downe S. Outcomes of free-standing, midwifery-led birth centres: a structured review of the evidence. *Birth,* 2004, 31(3):222-229
- Hodnett E, Downe S, Edwards N, Walsh D. Home-like versus conventional birth settings (Cochrane Review). In: *The Cochrane Library,* Issue 2. John Wiley & Sons Ltd, 2006

3   In addition, some studies have found that the ethos of hospitals tends to be hierarchical, institutional and medically-led, which has the effect of making women feel like 'patients' and of making birth seem abnormal and unhealthy. The studies are as follows:

- Hunt S, Symonds A. *The Social Meaning of Midwifery.* Macmillan, 1995
- Machin D, Scamell M. The experience of labour: using ethnography to explore the irresistible nature of the bio-medical metaphor during labour. *Midwifery,* 1997, 13: 78-84
- Kirkham M. The culture of midwifery in the National Health Service in England. *Journal of Advanced Nursing,* 1999, 30:732-739
- Ball L, Curtis P, Kirkham M. *Why Do Midwives Leave?* Royal College of Midwives, 2002
- Stapleton H, Kirkham M, Thomas G, Curtis P. Midwives in the middle: balance and vulnerability. *British Journal of Midwifery,* 2002, 10(10):607-611

4   During my very first labour in 1997, when my consultant asked me what I thought of my hospital room and I said, 'Er... it looks a bit like a bed with walls around it'—he immediately arranged for the bed to be taken out! (This was one of many reasons he was a wonderful obstetrician.) The researchers Spiby, et al (2003) recommend that hospital beds be removed from birth spaces, or at the very least pushed against a wall so that women have more space. See:

- Spiby H, Slade P, Escott D, Henderson B, Fraser R. Selected coping strategies in labour: an investigation of women's experiences. *Birth,* 2003, 30:189-194

5   If you would like to consider whether it would be possible to arrange a home birth in your personal case, see the articles at www.aims.org.uk. To consider the relative safety of home birth over hospital birth, in general, around the world, see the following, noting that studies generally draw very favourable conclusions, based on data collected and analysed:

- Gyte G, Dodwell M, Newburn M, Sandall J, Macfarlane A, Bewley S. No rising trend in home birth mortality. *BJOG: International Journal of Obstetrics & Gynaecology,* 2009, Nov; 116(12):1686-7
- Groenendaal F. Homebirth: as safe as hospital? *BJOG: International Journal of Obstetrics & Gynaecology,* 2009, Nov; 116(12): 1686-5; author reply 1685-6
- Hutton EK, Reitsma AH, Kaufman K. Oucomes associated with planned home and planned hospital births in low-risk women attended by midwives in Ontario,

Canada, 2003-2006: a retrospective cohort study. *Birth*, 2009 Sep;36(3):180-9
- Janssen PA, Saxell L, Page LA, Klein MC, Liston RM, Lee SK. Outcomes of planned home birth with registered midwife versus planned hospital birth with midwife or physician. *Canadian Medical Association Journal*, 2009 Sep 15;181(6-7):377-83. Epub 2009 Aug 31
- Olsen O, Jewell M. Home versus hospital birth. *The Cochrane Database of Systematic Reviews*, Issue 3, 2006
- Johnson K, Daviss BA. Outcomes of planned home births with certified professional midwives: large prospective study in North America. *British Medical Journal*, 2005, 330(7505):1416-1418
- Chamberlain G, Wraight A, Crowley P. Home births. Report of the 1994 confidential enquiry by the National Birthday Trust Fund, 1997, Parthenon (pp 107-113).
- Wiegers TA, Keirse MJNC, van der Zee J, Berghs GAH. Outcome of planned home and planned hospital births in low risk pregnancies: prospective study in midwifery practices in the Netherlands. *British Medical Journal*, 1996, 313:1309-1313 (23 November).
- Tew M. *Safer Childbirth? A Critical History of Maternity Care*. Chapman & Hail, 1998
- Campbell R. Place of birth reconsidered. In Alexander J, Levy V and Roth C (eds) *Midwifery Practice: Core Topics 2*. Macmillan, 1997
- Abel S, Kearns RA. Birth Places: A Geographical Perspective on Planned Home Birth in New Zealand, *Social Science & Medicine*, 1997, Vol 33,No 7,825-34

In the study by Hutton, *et al* (2009) the conclusion was: "Midwives who were integrated into the health care system with good access to emergency services, consultation, and transfer of care provided care resulting in favorable outcomes for women planning both home or hospital births." In the study by Janssen, *et al* (2009), the conclusion was: "Planned home birth attended by a registered midwife was associated with very low and comparable rates of perinatal death and reduced rates of obstetric interventions and other adverse perinatal outcomes compared with planned hospital birth attended by a midwife or physician."

In the American study by Johnson and Daviss (2005), the conclusion was: "Planned home birth for low risk women in North America using certified professional midwives was associated with lower rates of medical intervention but similar intrapartum and neonatal mortality to that of low risk hospital births in the United States. Despite all these positive research conclusions, home birth is very seriously under threat in some countries where it is legal now and many caregivers in all countries still tend to try and undermine it. Perhaps their motivation is to do with convenience, rather than safety or client satisfaction. Sorry, but I refuse to call a pregnant woman a 'patient'... but is the use of this word to describe a woman in labour also a clue to why some caregivers prefer births to take place in hospital? Could it be to do with control? Or is it just that so many caregivers and pregnant women cannot imagine birth without 'pain relief', which clearly needs to be managed in hospital settings, simply because it increases risk... See:

- Starr L. Legislation may drive homebirths underground. *Australian Nursing Journal*, 2009, Aug;17(2):31

6   If you're worried about pushing (at the wrong or right time), you might find it helpful to also read an article at www.midwiferytoday.com/articles/ruleof10.asp

7   Some more reasons and rationales for homebirth are presented at www.midwiferytoday.com/articles/homebirthuk.asp and www.midwiferytoday.com/articles/homebirthissues.asp, along with some research statistics.

8   The following research study established that hydrotherapy (i.e. the use of water) was far superior to augmentation with syntocinon when first-time mothers in labour experienced a 'prolonged' labour:

- Cluett E, Pickering R, Getliffe K. Randomised controlled trial of labouring in water compared with standard of augmentation for management of dystocia in first stage of labour. *British Medical Journal*, 2004, 328:314

Another study, as follows, concluded that more women who immersed themselves in warm water used no analgesia during labour than women who laboured on a bed:

- Eberhard J, Stein S, Geissbuelher R. Experiences of pain and analgesia with water and land births. *Journal of Psychosomatic Obstetrics & Gynaecology*, 2005, 26(2): 127-133

The following researchers found that women who laboured in water had a high sense of control:

- Hall S, Holloway M. Staying in control: women's experiences of labour in water. *Midwifery*, 1998, 14(1):30-36

Finally, the following study concluded that after waterbirths more women had an intact perineum:

- Geissbuehler V, Stein S, Eberhard J. Waterbirth compared with landbirths: an observational study of nine years. *Journal of Perinatal Medicine*, 2004, 32(4):308-314

9   Michel makes his own comments and recommendations about using water during labour and birth at www.midwiferytoday.com/articles/landmark.asp, basing his comments on research and clinical observations.

2... Help your body

1   In one study (Zammit, *et al*, 2009), pregnant women who smoked during pregnancy and drank more than 21 units of alcohol a week more often had babies who were at increased risk of suspected or definite psychotic symptoms. (Fathers smoking while their partners were pregnant was also found to be associated with increased risk.) Even if you generally drink less than this, please don't relax too much because another study (which draws tentative initial conclusions) (Sayal, *et al*, 2007) found that having more than one alcoholic drink per week during the first trimester of pregnancy was associated with childhood mental health problems in girls (behavioural and emotional) at 47 months (approx. 4 years old) and these problems apparently persisted—according to teacher reports—when checked when the child was almost 7 years old (81 months). So maybe it really is best to abstain from alcohol altogether. See:

- Zammit S, Thomas K, Thompson A, Horwood J, Menezes P, Gunnell D, Hollis C, Wolke D, Lewis G, Harrison G. Maternal tobacco, cannabis and alcohol use during pregnancy and risk of adolescent psychotic symptoms in offspring. *British Journal of Psychiatry*, 2009, Oct; 195(4):294-300

- Sayal K, Heron J, Golding J, Emond A. Prenatal alcohol exposure and gender differences in childhood mental health problems: a longtitudinal population-based study. *Pediatrics,* 2007, Feb;119(2):e426-34

2 In the following study, babies who'd been exposed to opiates while in the womb were more at risk of neurodevelopmental problems throughout early childhood. Good reason to keep off the heroine. (But could it also perhaps be a reason to keep off the diamorphine in labour too? After all, as I've mentioned elsewhere, diamorphine is simply another name for heroin.) See:

- Hunt RW, Tzioumi D, Collins E, Jeffery HE. Adverse neurodevelopmental outcome of infants exposed to opiate in-utero. *Early Human Development,* 2008 Jan;8(1): 29-35. Epub 2007 Aug 28

3 It is really important to be careful about drugs you take during pregnancy, whether these are prescribed or over-the-counter medicines. (And even if your doctor says the drugs are OK, you might want to do some research and reflection yourself because, after all, both thalidomide and DER were prescribed by doctors until they were found to result in deformities (in the case of thalidomide) or later infertility in girls (in the case of DER).

Since antidepressants are now taken by so many women, unfortunately, I shall mention them particularly here. One study looked not at whether or not babies were affected, at how to categorise the various effects! The researchers (Boucher, *et al,* 2008) considered 73 newborns who'd been exposed to antidepressant late on in their mum's pregnancy, and 73 who hadn't. Three statistically significant clusters of symptoms were identified and these related to a) increased risk of alertness alteration, b) altered muscle tone, feeding and gastro-intestinal problems, and c) neurological problems. This reminds me of when I lived in Singapore. Shortly after arriving, I remember reading that there were eight varieties of poisonous snake. I thought, "Aaaargh!" —or words to that effect— "I don't just have to worry about stepping on *eight* snakes while I'm here. I have to worry about stepping on (and being killed by) eight *varieties* of snake—in a place the size of Birmingham!" What I'm trying to point out here is that there really is something to be taken seriously here. So please do consider the possible after-effects (on your baby) of any drugs or medications. See:

- Boucher N, Bairam A, Beaulac-Baillargeon L. A new look at the neonate's clinical presentation after in utero exposure to antidepressants in late pregnancy. *Journal of Clinical Psychopharmacology,* 2008, Jun;28(3):334-9

4 My main justification for this advice is the following study, which established that when pregnant women consumed large quantities of water, the volume of amniotic fluid increased, but only for a limited time period:

- Malhotra B, Deka D. Duration of the increase in amniotic fluid index (AFI) after actue maternal hydration. *Archives of Gynecology & Obstetrics,* 2004, Mar;269(3): 173-5. Epub 2003 Oct 24

You might also be interested to see the following study, which mentions that amniotic fluid is 98-99% water:

- Modena AB, Fieni S. Amniotic fluid dynamics. *Acta Bio Medica.* 2004, 75 Suppl 1: 11-3

The researchers admit that, even though different hypotheses have been advanced on the mechanisms regulating the turnover of amniotic fluid, the inflow and outflow mechanism that keeps amniotic fluid volume within the normal range is not entirely clear. They explain that regulatory mechanisms act at three levels: placental control of water and solute transfer; regulation of inflows and outflows from the fetus; and, maternal effect on fetal fluid balance. We might guess that consumption of water by the mother could well be extremely helpful in the whole process. The following text (written by Tomasz N from the Polish Gynaecological Society, published in *Ginekologia Polska*, 2009, Jul; 80(7): 538-47. Polish) articulates why it might be a good idea to make sure you drink plenty of water: "Water is a substance essential for life. It creates the environment of our body, keeps it's homeostasis, enables every biochemical reaction and metabolic processes in human organism. Maternal hydratation is essential for homeostasis of two organisms and drinking water influences the amniotic fluid volume, fetal well-being and removes toxic metabolic products. The chemical contaminants of drinking water and products of it's chlorination and ozonization could be responsible for spontaneous abortion, birth defects and perinatal complications. Therefore it is recommended to drink natural mineral water for women in reproductive age."

5   A study by Opler, *et al* (2008) confirmed the previous finding that exposure to lead prenatally increased the likelihood that a baby would later suffer from schizophrenia. See:
    - Opler MG, Buka SL, Groeger J, McKeague I, Wei C, Factor-Litvak P, Bresnahan M, Graziano J, Goldstein JM, Seidman LJ, Brown AS, Susser ES. Prenatal exposure to lead, delta-aminolevulinic acid, and schizophrenia: further evidence. *Environmental Health Perspectives*, 2008, Nov;116(11):1586-90. Epub 2008 Jul30

6   If you're worried about your own weight—or your baby's future slimness—read Michel's research-based comments on this subject at www.wombecology.com/obesity.html. It really isn't a good idea to eat too little while you're pregnant. (Worry about your weight only when your baby is about six months old or older! And see Birthframe 100 if you don't believe me!) One recent study found there was an association in grown female babies of women who'd lived through a famine while pregnant with higher cholesterol levels, which obviously aren't helpful.
    - Lumey LH, Kahn HS, Stein AD, Romijn JA. Lipid profiles in middle-aged men and women after famine exposure during gestation: the Dutch Hunger Winter Families Study. *American Journal of Clinical Nutrition*, 2009 Jun;89(6):1737-43

7   Taking a multivitamin designed for pregnancy does not seem to be dangerous, as long as normal dosages are followed, of course. In the following study, which looked at the use of vitamin supplementation in the *first* trimester, researchers concluded "In the final adjusted model, any use of vitamins during pregnancy was associated with decreased odds of miscarriage ... in comparison with no exposure." I am not recommending vitamin-use until the second trimester simply because there is so much very delicate fetal development going on in the early weeks, which it could be very easy to disturb. Focus on eating healthily instead!
    - Hasan R, Olshan AF, Herring AH, Savitz DA, Siega-Riz AM, Hartmann KE. Self-reported vitamin supplementation in early pregnancy and risk of miscarriage. *American Journal of Epidemiology*, 2009, Jun 1;169(11):1312-8. Epub 2009 Apr16

8   Michel explains briefly why fats are so important during pregnancy at www.wombecology.com/nutritionpregnancy.html

9   It has actually been confirmed as being useful for protecting the perineum from damage by three randomised controlled trials:

- Shipman M, Boniface D, Tefft M, McCloghry F. Antenatal perineal massage and subsequent perineal outcomes: a randomised controlled trial. *British Journal of Obstetrics & Gynaecology*, 1997, 104:787-791
- Labrecque M, Eason E, Marcoux S. Randomised controlled trial of prevention of perineal trauma by perineal massage during pregnancy. *American Journal of Obstetrics & Gynaecology*, 1999, 180:593-600
- Davidson K, Jacoby S, Scott Brown M. Prenatal perineal massage: preventing lacerations during delivery. *Journal of Obstetric, Gynaecological & Neonatal Nursing*, 2000, 29(5):474-479

10 Michel wrote an article discussing this issue of pregnancy 'scares'. He also explains what he means by 'cul-de-sac epidemiology'—an off-shoot problem—at www.birthpsychology.com/primalhealth/primalone.html

11 Cutler RR, Odent M, Hajj-Ahmad H, Maharjan S, Bennett NJ, Josling PD, Ball V, Hatton P, Dall'Antonia M. *In vitro* activity of an aqueous allicin extract and a novel allicin topical gel formulation against Lancefield group B streptococci. *Journal of Antimicrobial Chemotherapy*, 2009, Jan;63(1):151-4. Epub 2008 Nov 11.

12 Read Michel's comments on pre-eclampsia at www.wombecology.com/preeclampsia.html

13 See the following articles:
- Strandberg TE, Andersson S, Järvenpää AL, McKeigue PM. Preterm birth and licorice consumption during pregnancy. *American Journal of Epidemiology*, 2002, Nov1;156(9):803-5
- Hughes J, Sellick S, King R, Robbé IJ. Preterm birth and licorice consumption during pregnancy. *American Journal of Epidemiology*, 2003, Jul15;158(2):190-1; author reply 191
- Strandberg TE, Järvenpää AL, Vanhanen H, McKeigue PM. Birth outcome in relation to licorice consumption during pregnancy. *American Journal of Epidemiology*, 2001, Jun 1;153(11):1085-8

14 Although in some hospitals eating and drinking are not allowed, there really is no scientific basis for this, as research and one systematic review has shown (Goer, et al, 2007). In this review we read: "The likelihood of a fed woman undergoing an unplanned cesarean under general anesthesia dying of pulmonary aspiration calculates to 8 per 10 million or 1 in 1,250,000 ... A study of 13,400 emergency surgeries under general anesthesia reported no deaths from aspiration in patients in reasonably good health (Warner, 1993)."
- Goer H, Sagady Leslie M, Romano A (The Coalition for Improving Maternity Services). Evidence Basis for the Ten Steps of Mother-Friendly Care. Step 5: Does Not Routinely Employ Practices, Procedures Unsupported by Scientific Evidence: The Coalition for Improving Maternity Services. *Journal of Perinatal Education*, 2007, Winter;16(Suppl 1):36S
- Warner MA, Warner ME, Weber JG. Clinical significance of pulmonary aspiration during the perioperative period. *Anesthesiology*, 1993, Jan;78(1):56-62

15 Unfortunately, despite long searching, I cannot as yet locate the reference for this study. (At one point I lost data from a whole computer hard disk and although I'd backed up most of it a few bits and pieces escaped, I'm afraid.) However, the following study into glucose levels in diabetics did find that subjects' pain thresholds decreased significantly on the days (in the study) when they had hyperglycaemia (i.e. an excess of glucose in the blood):

- Thye-Rønn P, Sindrup SH, Arendt-Nielsen L, Brennum J, Hother-Nielsen O, Beck-Nielsen H. Effect of short-term hyperglycemia per se on nociceptive and non-nociceptive thresholds. Department of Endocrinology, Odense University Hospital, Denmark. *Pain*, 1994, Jan;56(1):43-9

In the following study, dextrose limited the duration of analgesia:

- Gage JC, D'Angelo R, Miller R, Eisenach JC. *Does dextrose affect analgesia or the side effects of intrathecal sufentanil?* Department of Anesthesia, Bowman Gray School of Medicine, Wake Forest University, Winston-Salem, North Carolina 27157-1009, USA. jgage@bgsm.edu. Anesth Analg, 1997, Oct;85(4):826-30

16 The following studies noted various positive effects of moving around in labour and using upright positions, including a reduction in the need for pharmacological analgesia, an increased sense of control and increased satisfaction with birth:

- Simkin P, O'Hara M. Non-pharmacological relief of pain during labour: systematic review of five methods. *American Journal of Obstetrics & Gynaecology*, 2002, 186:S131-159
- Spiby H, Slade P, Escott D, Henderson B, Fraser R. Selected coping strategies in labour: an investigation of women's experiences. *Birth*, 2003, 30:189-194
- Albers L, Sedler K, Bedrick E, Teaf D, Peralta P. Midwifery care measures in the second stage of labour and reduction of genital tract trauma at birth: a randomised controlled trial. *Journal of Midwifery & Women's Health*, 2005, 50:365-372

Very specifically, research has shown that upright positions for birth mean a shorter second stage, a much smaller risk of a need for episiotomy, forceps (or ventouse), less pain, easier 'pushing' and fewer fetal heart abnormalities. All in all, being upright seems a very good idea! See:

- De Jonge A, Teunissen T, Lagro Janssen A. Supine position compared to other positions during the second stage of labour: a meta-analytic review. *Journal of Psychosomatic Obstetrics & Gynaecology*, 2004, 25:35-45
- Gupta J, Hofmeyr G. Position for women during second stage of labour (Cochrane Review). In: *The Cochrane Library*, Issue 4. John Wiley & Sons Ltd, 2006
- Johnstone F, Aboelmagd M, Harouny A. Maternal position in the second stage of labour and fetal acid base status. *British Journal of Obstetrics & Gynaecology*, 1987, 94(8):753-757
- Chalk A. Pushing in the second stage of labour: Part 1. *British Journal of Midwifery*, 2004, 12(8):502-508

The only outcome which was found to be better when lying down was blood loss, although it is possible this was because of differences in ease of estimation. (It did not affect outcomes.) See Step 5, Note 9 for my comments on this.

17 Some researchers (Gardberg and Tuppurainen 1994) found that when labour began, 10-15% of women's babies were in the posterior position, but by the end of labour (before the actual birth), this percentage went down to just 6%. Basing their comments on anecdotal evidence only, Sutton and Scott (1996) suggested the number of babies presenting in posterior position is increasing. One systematic review which considered the use of the knee-chest position during pregnancy could not draw any hard and fast conclusions. However, Sutton and Scott's conclusions and recommendations do tie in well with what we already know about the mechanical elements of labour (which are outlined in a 2004 *MIDIRS* article on the subject). The various sources for these documents are as follows:

- Gardberg M, Tuppurainen M. Anterior placental location predisposes for occipito posterior presentation near term. *Acta Obstetrica et Gynecologica Scandinavica*, 1994, 73:151-152
- Sutton J, Scott P. *Understanding and Teaching Optimal Fetal Positioning*. Tauranga, New Zealand: Birth Concepts, 1996 (available from www.amazon.co.uk)
- Hofmeyr G, Kulier R. Hands/knees posture in late pregnancy or labour for fetal malposition (lateral or posterior) (Cochrane Review). In: *The Cochrane Library*, Issue 3. John Wiley & Sons Ltd, 2006
- *MIDIRS* and the NHS Centre for Reviews and Dissemination. *Positions in Labour and Delivery*. Informed Choice for Professionals leaflet, 2004

18 The following researchers found that adopting the knee-chest position for 30 minutes during labour significantly reduced persistent back pain in posterior labours:

- Stremler R, Hodnett E, Petryshen P. Randomised controlled trial of hands-knees positioning for occipitoposterior position in labour. *Birth*, 2005, 32(4):243-251

19 Detailed guidance on massage is provided at www.midwiferytoday.com/articles/ midwifestouch.asp and also in *Beautiful Birth* by Suzanne Yates (Carroll & Brown, 2008). One research study found that women who received massage during labour (abdominal effleurage, sacral pressure and shoulder/back kneading) experienced significantly less pain and anxiety. See:

- Chang M, Wang S, Chen C. Effects of massage on pain and anxiety during labour: a randomised controlled trial in Taiwan. *Journal of Advanced Nursing*, 2002, 38(1): 68-73

Another study found that with massage, women experienced decreased depressed mood, anxiety and pain, less agitated activity, shorter labours, shorter hospital stays and less postnatal depression. I would certainly recommend massage personally... It's one excellent reason to have a doula or other birth assistant, who will be there and willing to perform continuous massage for as little or as much time as you request! See:

- Field T, Hernandez-Reif M. Labour pain is reduced by massage therapy. *Journal of Psychosomatic Obstetrics & Gynaecology*, 1997, 18:286-291

20 One research study has, in fact, confirmed the usefulness of warm packs applied to the perineum (during the second stage) by a caregiver. It's possible that getting into warm water just before the birth has a similarly helpful effect, particularly since waterbirths have also been shown to result in more intact perineums. See:

- Dahlen H. The perineal warm pack trial. Abstract presented at the International Congress of Midwives, Brisbane, 2005
- Geissbuehler V, Stein S, Eberhard J. Waterbirth compared with landbirths: an observational study of nine years. *Journal of Perinatal Medicine*, 2004, 32(4): 308-314

21 Various researchers have demonstrated the benefits of mobility during labour and birth. The following researchers concluded that movement meant that women needed less pain relief and generally ended up feeling more satisfied with their labours:

- Bloom S, McIntyre D, Beimer M. Lack of effect of walking on labour and delivery. *New England Journal of Medicine*, 1998, 339(2):76-79

- MacLennan A, Crowther C, Derham R. Does the option to ambulate during spontaneous labour confer any advantage or disadvantage? *Journal of Maternal and Fetal Medicine*, 1994, 3(1):43-48
- Hemminki E, Saarikoski S. Ambulation and delayed amniotomy in the first stage of labour. *European Journal of Obstetrics, Gynaecology & Reproductive Medicine*, 1983, 15:129-139.

The following studies noted that mobility resulted in more effective contractions, shorter labour, less augmentation, fewer operative deliveries and less fetal distress:

- Flynn A, Hollins K, Lynch P. Ambulation in labour. *British Medical Journal*, 1978, 2(6137):591-593
- Read J, Miller F, Paul R. Randomised trial of ambulation versus oxytocin for labour enhancement: a preliminary report. *American Journal of Obstetrics & Gynaecology*, 1981, 139:669-672
- Albers L, Anderson D, Cragin L. The relationship of ambulation in labour to operative delivery. *Journal of Nurse Midwifery*, 1997, 42(1):4-8

Caldeyro-Barcia R *et al* (1979) showed that movement was beneficial for the baby:

- Caldeyro-Barcia R. Influence of maternal bearing down efforts during second stage on fetal well-being. *Birth & Family Journal*, (1979), 6(i):7-15
- Caldeyro-Barcia R, Giussi G, Storch E. The influence of maternal bearing down efforts and their effects on fetal heart rate, oxygenation and acid base balance. *Journal of Perinatal Medicine*, 1979, 9: 63-67

22 The idea that a labour should begin and then carry on continuously until the baby has been born is not one which has always existed. As well as many anecdotal accounts I have heard about laid-back attitudes towards stop-start labours only 50 years ago. Ina May Gaskin also discovered a Portuguese word *pasmo*, used in a 19th century textbook on midwifery. Basically, *pasmo* meant that labour stopped and everyone went back to their daily lives until it started up again. See:

- Gaskin IM. Going backwards: the concept of 'pasmo'. *The Practising Alidwija*, 2003, 6(8):34-36

23 Actually, research has not yet confirmed this assertion, although the fact that the coccyx can move back when the woman is upright and thereby increase the size of the vaginal opening supports the idea that an upright position is better from the point of view of tearing. Research which has so far been carried out has been inconclusive and has only noted that a) a side-lying position may be slightly better than upright positions, b) that full squats did result in more perineal trauma, and—overall—that c) all-fours, standing, kneeling and semi-recumbent positions were all similar as regards ending up with an intact perineum. However, it must be noted that research carried out will have looked mostly at women who were using some kind of drug-based pain relief—because it is used so frequently. No studies have as yet been conducted exclusively on women who have birthed without any drugs in their system, who are also undisturbed but supported by a sensitive midwife. For the research carried out so far see:

- Shorten A, Donsante J, Shorten B. Birth position, accoucheur and perineal outcomes: informing women about choices for vaginal birth. *Birth*, 2002, 29(1):18-27
- Eason E, Labrecque M, Wells G, Feldman P. Preventing perineal trauma during childbirth: a systematic review. *Obstetrics & Gynecology*, 2000, Mar; 95(3):464-71
- Soong B, Barnes M. Maternal position at midwife-attended birth and perineal trauma: is there an association? *Birth*, 2005, 3:164-169

24 Geissbuehler V, Stein S, Eberhard J. Waterbirth compared with landbirths: an observational study of nine years. *Journal of Perinatal Medicine,* 2004, 32(4):308-314.

25 Both Soong and Barnes' study (2002) and that conducted by Sampselle, *et al* (2005) associated epidurals and commanded pushing with more perineal trauma (i.e. tearing). For research on this issue, see:

- Sampselle C, Hines S. Spontaneous pushing during labour: Relationship to perineal outcomes. *Journal of Nurse Midwifery,* 1999, 44(1):36-39
- Sampselle M, Miller J, Luecha Y, Fischer K, Rosten L. Provider support of spontaneous pushing during the second stage of labour. *Journal of Obstetrics, Gynaecology and Neonatal Nursing,* 2005, 34:695-702
- Soong, B. and Barnes, M. Maternal position at midwife-attended birth and perineal trauma: is there an association? *Birth,* 2005, 3:164-169

26 In the past, midwives and obstetricians sometimes tried to control delivery of the baby's head as he or she was being born. As is explained in one paper (Myrfield *et al* 1977), the physio-logical processes, when left undisturbed, actually create optimal conditions which are, in fact, made suboptimal, when caregivers intervene with their hands at the point of delivery. See:

- Myrfield, K, Brook, C. and Creedy, D. Reducing perineal trauma: implications of flexion and extension of the fetal head during birth. *Midwifery,* 1997, 13(4):197-201

27 The practice of leaving tears unsutured was first recommended by Head in 1993. There are various justifications for leaving first- and even second-degree tears unsutured... Firstly, women complain that suturing is outrageously painful (Salmon 1999, Sanders *et al,* 2002). Secondly, in one study in which women filled out questionnaires 12 months after giving birth, women who had had no suturing for second-degree tears reported *no problems* (Clement and Reed 1999). Thirdly, another study (Lundquist *et al,* 2000) demonstrated that leaving second-degree tears unsutured had a good effect on breastfeeding—presumably because women could sit more comfortably. Another study on suturing for larger second-degree tears (e.g. Fleming *et al,* 2003) had more mixed results, leading to the conclusion that perhaps only tears less than 2cm x 2cm, which are not bleeding—and which definitely don't affect the anus—should be left unsutured. However, a more recent study, which looked at outcomes after a year, (Langley *et al,* 2006) found no significant differences between sutured and unsutured women. See:

- Head, M. Dropping stitches. *Nursing Times,* 1993, 89(33):64-65
- Salmon, D. A feminist analysis of women's experiences of perineal trauma in the immediate post-delivery period. *Midwifery,* 1999, 15(4):247-256
- Sanders, J, Campbell, R. and Peters, T. Effectiveness of pain relief during perineal suturing. *British Journal of Obstetrics & Gynaecology,* 2002, 109:1066-1068
- Clement, S. and Reed, B. To stitch or not to stitch. *The Practising Midwife,* 1999, 2(4):20-28
- Lundquist, M, Olsson, A, Nissen, E. and Norman, M. Is it necessary to suture all lacerations after a vaginal delivery? *Birth,* 2000, 27(2):79-85
- Fleming, V, Hagen, S. and Niven, C. Does perineal suturing make a difference: the SUNS trial. *British Journal of Obstetrics & Gynaecology,* 2003, 110:684-689
- Langley, V, Thoburn, A, Shaw, S. and Barton, A. Second degree tears: to suture or not? A randomised controlled trial. *British Journal of Midwifery,* 2006, 14(9): 550-554

1... Help your mind

1. See page 1 of Desmond Morris' book *Babywatching* (Jonathan Cape 1991).

2. It's not only useful to sort through the 'psychological junk' for your own sake—it's also important for your growing baby. See: www.wombecology.com/maternalemotional.html

3. In fact, systematic reviews of research trials of hypnosis (Leslie, *et al*, 2007; Cyna, *et al*, 2004; Huntley, 2004) found that hypnosis did indeed reduce the need for analgesia, it reduced the level of pain experienced and shortened labour. Both Cyna (2004) and Smith (2003) found that hypnosis reduced the need for augmentation with oxytocin and that the incidence of spontaneous births increased. The CIMS review (the first in the list of references) also noted that no study reported an adverse effect. A couple of articles in *The Practising Midwife* also looked at relevant topics. One recommended hypnosis as a way of reducing the pain of labour and the other one looked at the use of NLP (neuro-linguistic programming) as a means of helping women prepare for labour. Incidentally, the CIMS review also looked at massage and hydrotherapy. See:

   - Leslie MS, Romano A, Woolley D. Step 7: Educates Staff in Nondrug Methods of Pain Relief and Does Not Promote Use of Analgesic, Anesthetic Drugs: The Coalition for Improving Maternity Services. *Journal of Perinatal Education,* 2007, Winter;16(Suppl 1):65S-73S
   - Cyna, A, McAuliffe, G. and Andrew, M. Hypnosis for pain relief in labour and childbirth: a systematic review. *British Journal of Anaesthesia,* 2004, 93(4):505-511
   - Huntley AL, Coon JT, Ernst E. Complementary and alternative medicine for labor pain: a systematic review. *American Journal of Obstetrics & Gynecology,* 2004, Jul; 191(1):36-44
   - Mottershead, N. Hypnosis: removing the labour from birth. *The Practising Midwife,* 2006, 9(3):26-29
   - Spencer, S. Giving birth on the beach: hypnosis and psychology? *The Practising Midwife,* 2005, 8(1):27-29
   - Smith CA, Collins CT, Cyna AM, Crowther CA. Complementary and alternative therapies for pain management in labour. Cochrane Database Systematic Review. 2003, (2):CD003521

4. If you also experienced abuse but your midwife is at a loss as to what to do, there are some pointers at www.midwiferytoday.com/articles/creatingspace.asp If it's your partner experienced sexual abuse you might want to point out another account to him. It's posted at www.midwiferytoday.com/articles/child_is_father.asp

5. Stress in general is something to be taken seriously indeed, not only during pregnancy but even before you're thinking of conceiving. Studies by Khashan, *et al* (2008 and 2009) found that maternal exposure to severe life events, particularly in the 6 months before pregnancy, may increase the risk of preterm and very preterm birth; and that mothers exposed to severe life events before conception or during pregnancy have babies with a significantly lower birthweight. (Note, their conclusions does not say that this *may* happen, but that it does.) Another study by a slightly different team of researchers (Khashan, *et al*, 2008) found that babies of pregnant women exposed to stress during the first trimester were at greater risk of having schizophrenia later on.

   - Khashan AS, McNamee R, Abel KM, Mortensen PB, Kenny LC, Pedersen MG, Webb RT, Baker PN. Rates of preterm birth following antenatal maternal exposure to severe life events: a population-based cohort study. *Human Reproduction*, 2009, Feb;24(2):429-37. Epub 2008 Dec 3

- Khashan AS, McNamee R, Abel KM, Pedersen MG, Webb RT, Kenny LC, Mortensen PB, Baker PN. Reduced infant birthweight consequent upon maternal exposure to severe life events. *Psychosomatic Medicine*, 2008, Jul;70(6):688-94
- Khashan AS, Abel KM, McNamee R, Pedersen MG, Webb RT, Baker PN, Kenny LC, Mortensen PB. Higher risk of offspring schizophrenia following antenatal maternal exposure to severe adverse life events. *Archives of General Psychiatry*. 2008 Feb;65(2):146-52

6 AbouZahr C. Global burden of maternal death and disability. *British Medical Bulletin*, 2003, 67:1-11.

7 Vol 12, No 2.

8 Saito M, Sano T, Satohisa E. Plasma catecholamines and microvibration as labour progresses. *Shinshin-Thaku*, 1991, 31: 381-89. (Also presented at the Ninth International Congress of *Psychosomatic Obstetrics & Gynaecology*. Amsterdam 28; 1 May 1989 (Free communication No 502).

9 Lederman RP, Lederman E, Work B *et al*. The relationship of maternal anxiety, plasma catecholamines and plasma cortisol to progress in progress in labour. *American Journal of Obstetrics & Gynecology*, 1978, 132:495-500.

10 One study did conclude that expectations (which could be the result of visualisation?) did shape birth experience. See:

- Green, J, Coupland, B. and Kitzinger, J. *Great Expectations: A Prospective Study of Women's Expectations and Experiences of Childbirth*. Cambridge: Child Care and Development Group, 1998

11 A useful book to help you visualise might be *Beautiful Birth* by Suzanne Yates (Carroll & Brown, 2008), which talks about visualisation, amongst other things. Doing this is not such a strange idea, when we remember that athletes often prepare for important events (such as the Olympics) in a similar way. There are even psychologists who specialise in helping athletes and other performers, such as musicians... Some people have even argued recently that we should examine our attitudes towards sexuality during labour—er... I mean our attitudes *about* sexuality in labour... which is probably best done beforehand (during pregnancy), not during labour itself! In the following article Ina May Gaskin points out that clitoral stimulation produces endorphin-like effects. (She reports that 20% of labouring women reported orgasm-like experiences.):

- Gaskin, 1. The frequency of reported orgasms in labour and birth in a population of unmedicated women. Abstract No 310, 26th ICM Congress, 2002

The documentary film *Orgasmic Birth*, looks at this in more detail and features interviews with women who've experienced birth positively (only a small minority reporting actual orgasm). In the DVD, the term 'orgasmic' is actually used very broadly, because extreme pain is usually also involved. However, as we've seen all through the book, moving through any pain during labour and birth results in less pain *overall* than women experience when they've had drugs because those involve postnatal consequences. Any pain women experience in labour is usually well-matched by postnatal euphoria and alertness (in both mother and baby, it seems). This gives you and your baby the best possible start to motherhood and your baby the best possible chance for a healthy life, from the moment of birth onwards.

Glossary

In this Glossary I've aimed to provide you with clear and accurate definitions, using personal language sometimes too because I don't think it's helpful to ever become too 'objective' toward the human being who is growing within you. For this reason, instead of the technical term 'fetus', I have often used its literal meaning 'little one' in these definitions. As you will notice, at other points I use the phrase 'your growing baby'.

acceleration a process by which attempts are made to speed up a woman's labour, using one or more different methods

acidaemia high levels of acid in the blood, i.e. a low blood ph

acupuncture a technique which involves inserting tiny needles into key points of a person's body with the aim of restoring health and well-being or eliminating or reducing pain. It is unclear how widely this is used to relieve pain in childbirth (in the UK or in China), but accounts I received suggested it is ineffective and that it prolongs labour. Michel says that the use of acupuncture in labour seems to be a Western idea.

adrenaline (also called 'epinephrine') the hormone which is sometimes called the 'fight-or-flight' hormone because it is produced spontaneously by the body in times of great stress. Strangely enough, although stressful situations generally prevent a good labour and birth, adrenaline is naturally produced as part of a 'fetus ejection reflex'.

adhesions when internal organs or loops of intestine become stuck together. This is possible after any kind of abdominal surgery and it can cause obstructions of the bowel, as well as pain.

AFP test a test which checks the AFP [alpha-fetoprotein] level in a woman's blood

afterpains the contractions which occur as a woman's uterus shrinks back to its pre-pregnancy size

AIMS [Association for Improvements in Midwifery Services] a UK-based organisation at www.aims.org.uk; may be of use to any pregnant woman because its aim is to provide support and information about maternity choices.

alpha-fetoprotein test see 'AFP test'

amnestics drugs administered during labour and birth, which remove the memory of pain, e.g. scopolamine

amnio see 'amniocentesis'

amniocentesis a test which involves inserting a needle into the amniotic sac (through the woman's body, either her abdomen or her vagina) in order to obtain amniotic fluid for testing. The test is clearly highly invasive, it carries a risk of miscarriage and there are false positives and false negatives.

amniotic fluid the clear, odourless, sterile fluid in which your baby floats when he or she is in your womb. As well as nourishing your little one, it also protects him or her from bumps and—oddly enough—is also the place where your little one wees! The fluid is replaced every three hours (by natural processes) which is one reason why it seems important to drink plenty of water.

amniotic sac the sac ('bag') in which your little one develops inside your womb

amniotomy breaking the woman's waters, i.e. the membranes which keep them in, so they flow out. This is sometimes done so as to speed up labour, but it is clearly an intervention.

anaemia a deficiency of red blood cells and/or haemoglobin in the blood; often misdiagnosed in pregnancy.

anaesthesia (general) the use of intravenously-administered drugs to induce loss of consciousness, during which patients are not arousable, even by painful stimulation. Since patients often cannot continue to breathe on their own while anaesthetised, other drugs are used to sustain breathing. A local anaesthetic or a regional anaesthetic (e.g. an epidural) blocks off pain in a specific part of the body and does not result in loss of consciousness

analgesia the use of drugs (familiarly known as 'painkillers') to relieve pain

analgesics drugs which aim to be mild to moderate painkillers e.g. paracetamol and co-dydramol.

antenatal (or 'prenatal') before the birth

antenatal tests a wide range of tests, from taking urine samples to amniocentesis.

anterior the 'front' of a woman's body. Your little one is said to be in an 'anterior' position (or 'anterior presentation', or 'anterior lie') when his or her back is against your front (stomach). This contrasts with a 'posterior' position in which the fetal back lies against the woman's back. An anterior position is more favourable for a smooth labour and birth.

anti-embolism stocking see 'TED anti-embolism stocking'

anti-emetic drugs drugs which prevent a woman from vomiting. Note that thalidomide was an anti-emetic drug. Since these drugs are mainly requested in the first trimester of pregnancy, when all the key parts of the baby's brain and body are forming, their use is highly risky.

Apgar score a score out of 10 given to newborns to indicate health. See page 16.

ARM [artificial rupture of the membranes] a procedure in which the membranes surrounding a woman's waters are broken, with a view to inducing or accelerating labour

arnica a mountain plant used to relieve bruises, stiffness, and muscle soreness. There is no evidence from research to support the idea that the homeopathic arnica remedy is anything more than a placebo.

aspiration (involuntary) breathing in

augmentation of labour stimulation or acceleration of labour, usually by the administration of drugs intravenously (e.g. Pitocin) or by performing an amniotomy, known as ARM

baby carrier an arrangement of material with or without plastic rings and metal pipes, which makes it easy for a mother to carry her newborn baby or young toddler. Useful website: www.thecarryingkind.com

barbiturates sedatives which affect both mother and unborn baby, e.g. Seconal and Nembutol.

Bart's test see 'triple test'

bilirubin lights special lights used to treat newborn jaundice. If it's excessive, jaundice can cause brain damage.

birth canal an unhelpful term which supposedly describes the route your little one travels when he or she is born. Of course, the term is unhelpful because the word 'canal' suggests a hard, straight, man-made passageway, while the reality is a soft, womanly, curvaceous route.

Birthframe a term coined in this book to refer to an account by a woman, man, child or professional which describes any aspect of a pregnancy or birthing experience or experiences

birthing ball another name for a large inflated gym ball, which some women find helpful during labour

birthing centre (also 'birth centre') a small hospital run by midwives which specialises in birth and which aims to create a private and comfortable environment for birthing women

birthing bed one of many items of medical furniture which has been designed over the years and may include reclining features and lithotomy stirrups, amongst other things. In fact, no special furniture is needed when a woman gives birth.

birthing chair see 'birthing bed'
birthing pool a pool (similar to a paddling pool) which may be inflated or assembled (or a permanent fixture) and used at home or in hospital. Birthing pools usually have pumps and heaters which allow water to be put in and heated to an ideal temperature. They are available for hire.
birth plan a word used to describe the paper a woman herself produces, which details her wishes for the birth. In this book the term 'care guide' has been coined because the word 'plan' often triggers negativity in care givers.
blood pressure the force exerted by circulating blood on the walls of blood vessels—one of the main so-called 'vital signs'. It is important to check blood pressure during pregnancy because although it must be high *enough* to ensure that your little one gets enough oxygen (through the placenta), it must also not rise too high, because high blood pressure is one of the symptoms of pre-eclampsia, which *may* (in a few rare cases) be a prelude to the life-threatening condition eclampsia.
bonding a process involving the development of a close, loving relationship, which is said to occur between mother (or father) and newborn babies after the baby's birth
Bradley natural birth classes antenatal classes common in the USA which aim to teach couples how to have a natural birth. The methods recommended are not in harmony with the recommendations in this book since they focus on the use of husband-coaching and alternative forms of pain relief, instead of ways of facilitating birth through non-disturbance.
bradycardia an abnormally slow or unsteady heart rhythm
Braxton Hicks contractions practice tightenings of the womb, which may take place any time from about 6 weeks of pregnancy onwards. These contractions, which were first described by the English doctor John Braxton Hicks in 1872, are not likely to be painful, but may be very noticeable in the later weeks of a woman's pregnancy.
breech when a fetus is in a position where it will be born buttocks first, or feet first. 'Complete breech' means that the baby's hips and knees are flexed so that the baby is sitting cross-legged, with feet beside the bottom. Also see 'frank breech', 'footling breech', and 'kneeling breech', if relevant.
brow presentation when the fetal head is not well 'flexed', i.e. not well tucked into his or her chest. This usually necessitates a caesarean section. Also see 'flexed position'.
Caesar caesarean section
cannula a flexible tube which forms part of a device for an IV
cardiotocograph [CTG] a graph produced by an electronic fetal monitor
carpal tunnel syndrome a condition in which a nerve in the hand becomes compressed at the wrist, causing numbness or pins and needles in the fingers and hands. It is a relatively common, but temporary, problem in pregnancy.
catecholamines hormones such as adrenaline, noradrenaline, and dopamine, produced in the body in response to stresses such as hunger, fear and cold
care guide a term coined in this book to replace the commonly used term 'birth plan'. Like a birth plan, it is a document which details a woman's wishes for her labour and birth.
care provider a midwife, doctor, consultant or obstetrician who is responsible for a pregnant woman's medical care through pregnancy and birth
carotid Doppler machine see 'Doppler machine'
catecholamines hormones and neurotransmitters such as adrenaline, noradrenaline and dopamine, produced by the body in response to stresses such as hunger, fear and cold
catheterise drain off urine using a urinary catheter
catheter a thin, flexible tube which is inserted into the bladder in order to drain off urine

caul the thin, filmy membrane (the amniotic sac) which covers your little one before he or she is born. Being 'born in the caul' simply means that the amniotic sac is still intact when the baby is born. The sac can easily be opened with the fingers at this point and the baby is in no danger.

cephalhemotoma a collection of blood inside one of the bones of the skull. It should not be confused with the common bump, which is under the scalp, outside the skull.

cephalic in a head-down position in the womb (i.e. not breech)

cephalo-pelvic disproportion the situation where a woman's pelvis is supposedly too small (or inappropriately shaped) for the fetal head to pass through. In the past it was frequently given as the reason for an emergency caesarean, but it is now largely discredited in most cases. However, it may still be an issue if a woman has suffered (or is suffering from) scoliosis, kyphosis or rickets. A scan is also often suggested for women with diabetes because this condition often results in an overly large baby.

cerclage the placement of stitches in the cervix to hold it closed

cervix the muscle at the base of the womb. When you go into labour, this muscle will first soften, then shorten and finally open out (like a blossoming flower)—'dilate' in medical jargon—so as to enable your fully-grown baby to leave your womb and enter the world. While you are pregnant, he or she is being kept safe and sound in your womb as a result of this very effective muscle's work.

cholestasis see 'obstetric cholestasis'

chorionic villus sampling a test which aims to identify chromosomal or genetic disorders in a fetus by taking a sample of the chorionic villus (placental tissue). It is carried out earlier than amniocentesis but is equally invasive as a procedure.

choroid plexus cysts [cpc's] these appear in an ultrasound scan as flower-like empty spaces in the developing brain and are a normal stage of fetal brain development

chromosomal analysis a method of checking for genetic disorders which is often recommended for couples who have experienced recurrent miscarriages, or for parents who already have a child with a chromosomal defect. It is also used to evaluate degrees of infertility, mental retardation, oligo/azoospermia or primary amenorrhoea.

CNM [certified nurse midwife] an American term for a qualified midwife

coccyx see 'tailbone'

colostrum a creamy, health-sustaining substance which comes from breasts for the first couple of days after birth, before the thinner milk is produced

commanded pushing when a midwife or doctor instructs a woman to push at certain moments, perhaps according to what they are observing on a monitor, or based on their view of what is happening. It contrasts with 'spontaneous pushing', where a woman pushes spontaneously, based on her intuitive view of timing or her instinctive knowledge of how to give birth.

compression (of the umbilical cord) when the umbilical cord becomes pressed (perhaps during the birth), which may mean the fetus is deprived of oxygen. This is obviously dangerous for the growing baby.

consultant a senior medical expert, typically an obstetrician, working from a hospital in the UK, Australia or Ireland

contractions an unhelpful term to describe the flexing of the uterine muscles when a woman goes into labour and gives birth. The word is unhelpful because it suggests a narrowing and 'drawing in', when in fact an expansion and 'drawing out' is occurring.

contraction stress test [CST] (also called a 'stress test' or 'oxytocin challenge test') a pre-labour procedure which aims to check how well the placenta is functioning and therefore whether a fetus will be able to cope with the reduced levels of oxygen that normally occur during labour contractions. First synotcinon (artificial oxytocin) is injected intravenously, then the pregnant woman is connected up to an electronic fetal monitor. The test is considered risky (and it's expensive) so it is now recommended less often for high risk pregnancies than it was in the past. Also see 'EFM'.

convulsions when a person's body shakes rapidly and uncontrollably, which occurs if muscles contract and relax repeatedly. Convulsions are a symptom of the life-threatening condition eclampsia so are a sign of an emergency treatment.

cord umbilical cord

cord prolapse when the umbilical cord drops down out of the woman's body before the baby is born—a dangerous eventuality because it is likely to lead to cord compression, which can mean the baby is deprived of oxygen and therefore at risk

correlation this means that researchers find a link between two factors, e.g. smoking and birth weight—i.e. a research project may show a clear link (a 'correlation') between the amount a pregnant woman smokes and the subsequent birth weight of her baby

corticosteroids a class of steroid hormones that are synthesised from cholesterol in the adrenal cortex. They are important hormones in that they play a part in the stress response, immune response, the regulation of inflammation, carbohydrate metabolism, protein catabolism, blood electrolyte levels and behaviour.

crown when your little one has travelled down the so-called 'birth canal' and his or her head ('crown') stays visible at the vaginal opening, without slipping back in. This occurs just before the birth.

c-section caesarean section

CTG [cardiotocograph] a graph produced by an electronic fetal monitor

D&C [dilation and curettage] a procedure in which the cervix is artificially dilated (opened) and the lining of the womb (the endometrium) is scraped. This is sometimes done after a miscarriage in the belief that the womb needs to be scraped out so as to avoid heavy bleeding and possible infection.

deep transverse arrest see 'transverse arrest'

deep vein thrombosis [DVT] this occurs when the flow of blood is restricted in a vein and a clot forms. If this clot then becomes dislodged and travels to the lung it may cause death, so DVT is to be taken very seriously.

diabetes see 'gestational diabetes'

diamorphine 100% heroin

dilated open; fully dilated' means a cervix has opened to 10cm

dilation the process by which the cervix opens up (to 10cm) so as to allow a baby to be born. Midwives and doctors usually measure the extent of dilation using their fingers.

dilation and curettage see 'D&C'

discharge secretions produced from small glands in the lining of the vagina and cervix. These change at different times of a woman's menstrual cycle and pregnancy.

domino delivery (short for 'domiciliary, in and out') a home-hospital birthing combination which involves support at home by a midwife in the early stages of labour, a short stay in hospital (where you will be taken by the same midwife), followed by early discharge (again, accompanied by the same midwife)

Doppler machine see 'Sonicaid'

Doptone see 'Sonicaid'

doula a mother figure a woman can rely on before, during or after giving birth

due date see 'EDD'

dystocia a vague term used to refer to an abnormal or difficult labour or birth. It is often the reason given for an emergency caesarean, being expressed as 'failure to progress', although what exactly constitutes a slow labour, or one which is not progressing sufficiently fast, is widely disputed.

eclampsia a serious complication of pregnancy, characterised by convulsions, which may occur before, during or after labour. It usually occurs after the onset of pre-eclampsia, although sometimes no symptoms of pre-eclampsia are found. When it occurs before labour has begun, the fetus needs to be delivered immediately and the mother also requires treatment.
ectopic pregnancy a pregnancy in which the egg fails to travel down to the womb after being fertilised in the fallopian tubes
edema see 'oedema'
ECV [external cephalic version] see 'external cephalic version'
EDD [estimated date of delivery] the day it is predicted your baby may be born
EFM [electronic fetal monitoring] monitoring which involves connecting a woman up to an electronic fetal monitor. It is carried out either intermittently or continuously throughout labour, or during the third trimester, in which case it is called the 'non-stress test'. Two disc-shaped transducers are usually laid on the woman's abdomen in order to measure both the fetal heart rate and uterine contractions (if any). For obvious reasons, this monitoring restricts a woman's movement and gives her a feeling of being observed.
elderly primigravida first-time pregnancy in a woman who is 'older', i.e. over 35
elderly multip an older woman who is having her second or subsequent baby
elective caesarean a caesarean operation which is planned in advance
electrocautery burning the body so as to remove or close part of it. This procedure is frequently used during surgery to stop bleeding of small vessels or for cutting through soft tissue
electronic fetal monitoring (also 'external fetal monitoring') see 'EFM'
embryo your 'baby' from Week 4 of your pregnancy up until the end of Week 8
emergency caesarean a caesarean which is unplanned, which is felt to be necessary during labour; also called an 'in-labour caesarean'
endometriosis (sometimes simply called 'endo') a condition (affecting approx. 2 million women in the UK) in which cells that usually line the womb are found elsewhere in the body, e.g. in the fallopian tubes, the ovaries, the bladder, the bowel, the intestines, the vagina, or the rectum
endometrium the lining of your womb
endorphins the body's natural painkillers, i.e. feel-good hormones which are produced spontaneously during an undisturbed natural labour
enema a procedure in which liquids are introduced into the rectum and colon via the anus with a view to stimulating the expulsion of faeces (poo)
engaged a fetus is considered to be 'engaged' when his or her head drops down into the pelvis, ready for the birth
engorgement a condition which occurs in breastfeeding mothers, where too much milk builds up in the breasts. This may occur when the milk first 'comes in' (about three days after the birth) or later on during breastfeeding. It is rare or is quickly eased when mothers breastfeed consistently on demand (i.e. whenever their baby expresses a wish to feed).
epidemiology the study of factors affecting the health and illness of populations. It is highly regarded in evidence-based medicine for identifying risk factors for disease and determining optimal treatment approaches in clinical practice.
epidural (short for 'epidural anaesthesia') a form of regional anaesthesia which involves injecting drugs through a catheter into the epidural space, in the spine. This form of 'pain relief' may cause loss of sensation and pain because it blocks the transmission of pain signals through nerves in or near the spinal cord. However, it does not always take effect completely, cannot be used throughout labour and may have various other disadvantages.

episiotomy a cut made through the perineum (with a pair of scissors) so as to enlarge the vaginal opening, performed under local anaesthetic and sutured closed after the birth. Rarely performed now in the UK (although this is worth checking), but it is still a routine procedure in many countries of the world. It is a necessary and life-saving procedure if the baby's shoulder gets stuck or in the case of a breech birth which is not going well. Of course, it is also necessary if forceps are used.

ergometrine (also known as 'ergonovine', 'd-lysergic acid' or 'beta-propanolamide') chemically similar to the hallucinogenic drug LSD, this ergoline derivative is commonly used to speed delivery of the placenta after birth and prevent postpartum haemorrhage (i.e. excessive bleeding). In the UK it is usually combined with oxytocin (syntocinon) and called 'syntometrine'.

express to squeeze (milk) out of one's breasts, using a pump or one's hands

external cephalic version [ECV] a manual attempt (by an obstetrician) to turn a fetus who is in the breech position at or after 37 weeks' gestation. It only has a 50% success rate and may result in distress to the fetus if he or she becomes entangled in the umbilical cord. This procedure should only be performed where facilities for an emergency caesarean are immediately available.

external version see 'external cephalic version'

face-to-pubis delivery (also called 'face-to-pubes delivery') a fetus/baby who is still in a posterior position when he or she is being born

faeces poo (excrement)

false positive when a sample is taken and tested and the result is 'positive', when in fact it is 'negative'. Also see 'sample'.

false negative when a sample is taken and tested and the result is 'negative', when in fact it is 'positive'. Also see 'sample'.

female circumcision a procedure in which a girl's clitoris is cut out. Also see 'infibulation'.

fetal adjective referring to an unborn baby (a 'fetus' or 'foetus')

fetal blood sampling a procedure in which a small amount of blood is removed from blood vessels in the umbilical cord or in the fetal liver or heart. As well as being carried out in labour to check fetal oxygen levels, this procedure is sometimes also proposed during pregnancy so as to attempt to diagnose genetic or chromosomal abnormalities, to check for and treat severe fetal anaemia or other blood problems (e.g. Rh disease) or to check for fetal infection. Risks associated with this procedure include bleeding from the sampling site, changes in the fetal heart rate, infection, leaks of amniotic fluid and fetal death.

fetal distress a situation in which the life of an unborn baby appears to be threatened

fetal membranes the thin layers of tissue which surround the embryo or fetus and provide for its nutrition, respiration, excretion and protection. They include the yolk sac, allantois, amnion and chorion.

fetal movement counting the counting of fetal movements a woman may be asked to do when she is overdue; she is usually asked to record these on a 'kick chart'. This is one way of monitoring that her little one is literally still 'alive and kicking'.

fetal scalp blood sampling a widely used in-labour method of taking samples of a fetus' blood (through a mother's cervix) when worrying fetal heart rate patterns occur. The objective of the sampling is to assess the fetal condition. Also see 'fetal blood sampling'.

fetal scalp electrode [FSE] a device which is screwed into the fetal scalp while it is still in the birthing canal; it connects up with a monitor, which monitors the fetal heart rate. A version which uses a sensor rather than a clip is now also available.

fetal scalp monitor a monitoring machine which provides care providers with information about fetal heart activity, using an electrode which is screwed into the fetal scalp. Monitoring of this type can only take place when the woman's cervix is at least 1-2cm dilated and after the membranes have ruptured, either spontaneously or after an amniotomy.

fetal stethoscope (also 'fetoscope' and 'Pinard') a stethoscope shaped like a listening trumpet, which is put on a pregnant woman's abdomen so as to listen to the fetal heartbeat. This type of stethoscope has the advantage that it does not involve the use of ultrasound, unlike the Doppler Sonicaid. See page 195.

fetoscope see 'fetal stethoscope'

fetus (also 'foetus') a word used to describe the baby growing in your womb from the end of Week 8 of your pregnancy, by which time all the major systems and organs will have developed

fetus ejection reflex (also called a 'fetal ejection reflex') a sudden and compelling rush of energy which automatically makes birth simple, active and intuitive

fibroids benign tumours, made up of muscle fibre, that grow in the womb. They can be as small as a pea or as large as a melon and may result in no symptoms, or alternatively may cause heavy bleeding, pain, incontinence or infertility. Fibroids in pregnancy may necessitate a caesarean if they are blocking the baby's passage out of the woman's body.

first stage the stage of labour/birth in which the cervix opens so as to allow the baby to emerge in the second stage

first trimester the first three months of pregnancy

first-degree tear see 'tear'

fizzy-logical birth physiological birth, i.e. a birth which follows physiological processes, which is therefore 'fizzy' (i.e. causes ecstasy) and also 'logical' in that it is safe in rational terms

flexed position when the fetus is curled up and his or her head is tucked into the chest

folic acid known as 'folate' in its natural form, this is one of the B-group of vitamins and is found in small amounts in many foods. Good natural sources include broccoli, brussels sprouts, peas, chickpeas, brown rice and asparagus; it is also often added to processed foods, such as breakfast cereals and bread. Since it is water-soluble, it needs to be consumed daily (because it can't be stored in fat, like some other vitamins). Pregnant women are advised to take a 400 microgram supplement of folic acid until Week 12 of pregnancy so as to help prevent neural tube defects, such as spina bifida.

footling breech birth when one or two feet are born first. This occurs rarely at term, but is relatively common in premature births.

forceps a handheld, hinged instrument made from high-grade carbon steel, used to grasp and apply pressure. In a forceps birth, when a woman's cervix is fully dilated and her bladder has been emptied (perhaps with a catheter) the woman is placed in the lithotomy position, a mild anaesthetic is administered (if an epidural is not already in place) and the two sections of the forceps are individually inserted and locked into position around the baby's head. The fetal head is then rotated to bring the baby to an occiput anterior position (if this is not already the case), an episiotomy is performed, and the baby is pulled out.

forewaters the amniotic fluid which is in front of the fetal head when the baby is engaged. When these waters break the gush is usually dramatic and unmistakable as a leak of amniotic fluid. Also see 'hindwaters'.

frank breech when a baby's bottom is born first, and his or her legs are flexed at the hip and extended at the knees (with feet near the ears). 65-70% of breech babies are born in the frank breech position.

fundal height a measure of the size of a woman's womb (taken from the top of the pubic bone to the top of the 'bump', usually with an ordinary cloth tape measure,

measuring in centimetres) to assess fetal growth and development. Since a 'bump' can also expand to the sides this is obviously rather a crude measurement of fetal growth and it is widely accepted that this measurement becomes increasingly less reliable towards the end of a pregnancy.
gas and air [Entonox] a 50/50 mixture of oxygen and nitrous oxide, only usually available in the UK. See photo on page 131.
general anaesthesia use of drugs to achieve complete unconsciousness in the patient
genetic disorders conditions caused by abnormalities in genes or chromosomes and therefore inherited from parents
gestate grow (fetus)
gestation the period when a baby is growing inside its mother
gestational diabetes diabetes which occurs for the first time during pregnancy
glucose tolerance screening a test to see if a woman has gestational diabetes
glycerine suppositories torpedo-shaped, semi-clear or opaque suppositories containing glycerine, which are used so as to stimulate the expulsion of faeces before birth
GP [general practitioner] a doctor in the UK, Australia or Ireland
Grantley Dick-Reid the author of *Childbirth Without Fear* (originally published in 1942). Grantly Dick-Read apparently devoted his life to investigating why childbirth was painful to most women. In his book he describes how fear is an abnormal reaction to childbirth, and how this fear causes abnormal tension within the muscles of the womb.
haemoglobin [Hb] the iron-containing oxygen-transporting metalloprotein in the red blood cells of the blood
haemoglobin concentration what is tested for in a blood count, in order to check whether or not a woman is suffering from anaemia
haemorrhage excessive bleeding, which is life-threatening
haemorrhoids (also known as 'piles') enlarged and swollen blood vessels in or around the lower rectum or anus. They are very common in pregnancy, especially when the woman experiences constipation, which again underlines the importance of a good diet with plenty of water and roughage.
hCG [human chorionic gonadotrophin] the hormone which pregnancy tests aim to detect
head-down position this means your little one has his or her head pointing downwards in the womb, which is an ideal position for the birth
heparin lock a small tube connected to a catheter which is inserted into a vein in the arm. It allows easy access for IV transfusions.
high blood pressure see 'pre-eclampsia'
hindwater leak see 'hindwaters'
hindwaters the amniotic fluid which is behind the fetal head when the baby is engaged. When these waters break there is usually intermittent trickling which is difficult to distinguish from the odd leak of urine (common at the end of pregnancy), or from thin vaginal discharge. Also see 'forewaters'.
homeopathy a form of complementary medicine developed by Dr Samuel Hahnemann in the 18th century. Homeopathic remedies consist of extremely diluted versions of substances which—when undiluted—would cause symptoms similar to the disease they are aiming to treat. No scientific or clinical studies support the notion that homeopathy is effective.
hormone a chemical messenger which travels in the blood and carries a signal from one cell (or group of cells) to another. Their production and orchestration are crucial to successful birth, but highly susceptible to influence through disturbance.

hydrocephalis a condition caused by the accumulation of an abnormally large amount of cerebrospinal fluid (CSF) in the skull, or cranium

hyperemesis (also known as 'hyperemesis gravidarum' [HG]) severe and continual nausea and vomiting during pregnancy and difficulty eating and drinking (because they cause more nausea). It appears to affect between 0.3% and 1% of pregnant women.

hypertension high blood pressure. This is potentially dangerous in pregnancy if associated with high levels of protein in the urine. Also see 'pre-eclampsia'.

hysterectomy the surgical removal of a woman's womb

iatrogenic problem caused by the diagnosis, manner or treatment of a doctor

ICU [intensive care unit]

ileus temporary paralysis of a portion of the intestines

incision the medical word for 'cut'

incompetent cervix a cervix which tends to open too easily, resulting in repeated premature births or miscarriages

independent midwife a midwife who works independently of the National Health Service (the NHS) in the UK

induced see 'induction'

induction any procedure which triggers the beginning of a woman's labour. Approaches used range from amniotomy to the use of cod liver oil and the use of drugs administered through an IV drip.

industrialised childbirth a term coined by Michel Odent to describe 'managed' childbirth in modern societies

infection the colonisation of a host organism by a foreign species, e.g. bacterium. It may occur through respiration, cuts in the skin, blood infusions (or through the use of contaminated needles), or through gastrointestinal, urinary or sexual routes. Some infections are more dangerous than others during pregnancy. While the common cold and flu are unlikely to cause problems (as long as no commercial remedies are taken), others should be taken very seriously, i.e. chicken pox before 20 weeks' gestation, herpes after 28 weeks' gestation, and toxoplasmosis if it occurs any time during the third trimester. Other infections need to be checked out and possibly treated immediately under the care of a medical expert.

infertility the situation when a couple do not conceive, despite having unprotected sex. It is not usually diagnosed as such until a couple have had sex without contraception for a year.

infibulation [also known as 'Pharaonic circumcision'] the cutting off of the whole clitoris, the whole of the labia minora and the adjacent parts of the labia majora and the stitching of the two sides of the vulva, leaving a small opening for urination and menstruation. Undoubtedly, the most invasive ritual genital mutilation, this is the cause of prolonged labour and means that a birth attendant needs to cut through the sclerous scars for the purpose of enlarging the passage.

inhalation analgesia gas breathed through a mouthpiece or mask, which aims to ease pain, e.g. Entonox—popularly called 'gas and air'. Entonox is a British phenomenon.

in-labour caesarean a caesarean operation which is deemed necessary while the woman is in labour

internal (or internal examination) an internal vaginal examination performed by a care giver to check cervical dilation

intervention any action taken or attempt at communication

interventionist having a preference for intervention

intestinal obstruction partial or complete blockage of the bowel which means that intestinal contents are unable to pass through

intracutaneous within the skin, particularly the dermis

intramuscular injected into a muscle

intrapartum during labour and birth
intra-partum death see 'stillbirth'
intra-uterine death see 'stillbirth'
intravenous drip the fastest way of delivering fluids or medications into veins, achieved through the use of a needle which is inserted into the arm
invasive any action taken which is likely to have a direct effect on a pregnancy or a fetus. Also see 'non-invasive'.
IV [intravenous] abbrev. for a drip inserted into a vein
IVF [in vitro fertilisation] a technique in which egg cells are fertilised by sperm outside the woman's womb
jaundice a yellow colouring of the skin and eyes caused by immature liver function in newborns
kangaroo care a method of caring for premature babies which involves plenty of skin-to-skin contact (between mother and baby), exclusive breastfeeding and medical support (using appropriate technology), when needed
Kegel muscles the muscles which form the 'pelvic floor', which support the pelvic organs, including the vagina, bladder and rectum. For obvious reasons, maintaining use of these muscles is important so as to avoid incontinence.
Kegels term used to describe the exercises you can do so as to strengthen the muscles of your pelvic floor, originally devised by Dr Arnol Kegel
keloid a firm, rubbery lesion of the skin, or shiny, fibrous nodules resulting from overgrowth of tissue at the site of a scar. Although benign and non-contagious, they can cause severe itchiness, sharp pains and in severe cases can affect movement of the skin.
Kettering test see 'triple test'
kick chart see 'fetal movement counting'
kneeling breech position when a fetus is born knees first—an extremely rare eventuality
lactation the process by which a woman produces milk
La Leche League an international organisation originally founded by seven breastfeeding mothers in the USA in 1956 whose aim was and still is to teach or re-teach the art of breastfeeding. See www.llli.org
Lamaze a French obstetrician (Dr Fernand Lamaze) who developed an approach to childbirth in the 1940s, which was an alternative to other managed approaches commonly used at the time. The Lamaze Technique was based on Soviet childbirth practices, which involved performing breathing and relaxation exercises under the direction of a 'monitrice' or midwife. Modern Lamaze antenatal classes in the USA focus on teaching pregnant women techniques to work with labour pain, such as breathing exercises, the use of hot and cold packs, changing positions or using a birthing ball.
lanugo fine, downy hair which can sometimes be seen on a newborn baby's skin. It's nothing to worry about.
laparoscopic surgery (also called 'minimally invasive surgery' (MIS), 'bandaid surgery', 'keyhole surgery' or 'pinhole surgery') a modern surgical technique in which operations in the abdomen are performed through small incisions (usually 0.5-1.5cm) as compared to larger incisions needed in traditional surgical procedures
laparoscopy an operative procedure in which a device (a laparoscope) is inserted through a small incision into the abdomen in order to diagnose or investigate diseases such as endometriosis, pelvic inflammatory disease, ectopic pregnancy, ovarian cysts and appendicitis. It is also used when performing sterilisations.
Leboyer birth an approach developed by Frederick Leboyer (the author of the seminal, poetic book *Birth Without Violence*, first published in French in 1974). A Leboyer birth usually involves the use of dim lighting, soft voices and a warm bath for the newborn straight after the birth.

lithotomy position a common position used for surgical procedures involving the pelvis and lower abdomen. In this position the patient lies on her back with her knees bent and kept spread apart and above her hips through the use of stirrups. Of course, a woman giving birth is not a patient because she is not ill—she is simply a woman—and this position is not suitable for birth. Not only would the baby be forced to travel uphill, but it would also probably be deprived of oxygen because the woman's vena cava would be compressed (reducing blood flow from the placenta) and would be forced to attempt a birth through a narrower opening. Also see 'tailbone'.

lithotomy stirrups U-shaped devices which hold a patient's legs up while she is in the lithotomy position undergoing surgery. See 'lithotomy position'.

LMP [last menstrual period] the first day of your last period, which is used to calculate the day your baby is due to be born

LOA [left occiput anterior] the term used to describe your little one's position when the back of his or her head (the occiput) is pointing down and facing towards the left side of your body, with his or her back round to the front of your body. This is the best position for your baby to be in when you go into labour.

local anaesthetics drugs to block sensation entirely in certain areas of the body, e.g. pudendal and perineal block

lochia the discharge which comes after a baby is born, which contains blood, mucous and placental tissue. Lochia may continue for 4-6 weeks after the birth in three separate stages. In the first stage (which lasts 3-5 days after the birth), the discharge is red because it contains a large amount of blood. In the second stage (which continues until approx. the tenth day after the birth) the lochia is thinner and brownish or pink in colour. (Now the discharge is made up of exuate, erythrocytes, leukocytes and cervical mucous, in case you were wondering!) In the third stage, the lochia is whitish or yellowish-white because it contains far fewer red blood cells and is mainly made up leukocytes, epithelial cells, cholesterol, fat and mucous.

LOP [left occiput posterior] the term used to describe the fetal position when the back of the fetal head (the occiput) is pointing downwards and faces the left side of a mother's body, when the fetal back is round to the back of the woman's body, parallel to her spine. If the baby is still in this position when the woman goes into labour, she is said to have a 'posterior' labour.

lotus birth a birth after which the umbilical cord is not cut. Instead, excess fluids are wiped off the placenta and this is then kept in an open bowl or it is wrapped in a cloth and obviously kept near the newborn baby. Any cloths used to wrap the placenta must allow air to pass through, so that the placenta can air and gradually dry out; sea salt is sometimes applied so as to facilitate this process. (If airtight cloths are used, the placenta would soon start to smell bad.) Sometimes essential oils (such as lavender), or powdered herbs (such as goldenseal or neem) are also applied to the placenta because of their antibacterial properties. This approach to delaying cutting of the umbilical cord is also, rather unromantically, sometimes called 'umbilical nonseverance'. In a partial lotus birth (or in partial umbilical nonseverance) the umbilical cord is left for an hour or so before being cut.

low blood pressure common in early and mid pregnancy and is usually nothing to worry about

lumbar puncture (commonly known as a 'spinal tap') a procedure in which a sample of cerebrospinal fluid is collected in order to check for meningitis, a life-threatening but treatable condition which cannot be diagnosed in any other way. Experts agree that any infant less than 2 months old who has a fever of 38 degrees Celsuis (100.4 degrees Fahrenheit) or greater for no identifiable reason requires a lumbar puncture.

malpresentation the abnormal presentation of a fetus in its mother's womb, i.e. any presentation which is not a head-down position

maternal serum screening a test in which serum is checked, e.g. the alpha-fetoprotein test, the triple screen test or the quad-screen test. Also see 'triple test'.

meconium the sticky, greeny-black substance which results from the storage of waste products in your little one's bowels. It is a mixture of excretions from your baby's alimentary glands, bile pigment, lanugo and cells from his or her bowel wall and is usually passed for the first time shortly after the birth. If it is passed before the birth it is a sign that a fetus is distressed.

membranes see 'fetal membranes'

membrane sweep see 'sweeping'

Mendelson's syndrome inhalation of vomit by anaesthetised patients

Meptid (also called 'meptazinol') a non-addictive analgesic which often makes women feel sick and sometimes also dizzy, used for 'pain relief' in labour

mid-cycle bleeding bleeding which occurs at any time between two periods

milk-ejection reflex the process by which milk in the milk glands of a woman's breasts passes down to her milk ducts when her baby starts feeding. This process, which is stimulated by the hormones prolactin and oxytocin, is also sometimes (unhelpfully) called the 'let-down' reflex. (The baby doesn't feel let down and neither does the woman!)

miscarriage the spontaneous end of a pregnancy before 24 weeks' gestation. Although this is not a subject which is often spoken about amongst women, many must experience it one or more times because some experts believe that it affects as many as 1 in 4 pregnancies, almost always in the first trimester. Useful website: www.miscarriageassociation.org.uk

monitoring any action performed, either formally (using technology) or informally (e.g. listening to sounds) with the aim of checking the progress of a woman's pregnancy, labour or birth and the condition of the little one, inside or coming out!

monochorionic twins who develop in two separate bags ('chorions'), containing two amniotic sacs

morbidity the risk of illness in any particular case

morphines narcotic drugs used for 'pain relief', e.g. pethidine and diamorphine (100% heroin)

mortality the risk of death in any particular case

moxabustion an oriental medicine therapy which uses moxa (the mugwort herb). The mugwort is usually aged and ground to a 'fluff' and then burned at key points on the patient's skin (sometimes in conjunction with acupuncture needles). It probably predates acupuncture, and is used in the hope that it will stimulate blood flow and prevent cold and dampness in the body. No research supports its use in labour or birth.

mucous extractor a device for extracting mucous from a newborn baby's nose, to help him or her breathe in cases where this does not happen spontaneously. Michel has commented that he has very rarely needed to use a mucous extractor after an optimal birth.

mucous plug a mass of capillaries and mucous which fill the 'os', the small hole in the cervix, so as to keep infection out of your womb. It comes away as the cervix begins to open up at the beginning of labour, so noticing some stringy jelly (which may be streaked with blood) is a sign that your labour will begin within the next week or even day.

multipara woman who has been pregnant before

multiple birth the birth of twins, triplets, quadruplets, etc

multiples twins, triplets, quadruplets, etc

myelinated nerves nerves with an electrically insulating layer, which means that messages can travel more effectively

NAD [no abnormalities detected] the phrase a midwife or doctor writes in a new mother's notes if the baby appears to be OK **narcotics** drugs which aim to make pain more bearable, which may cause a woman to lose all alertness and awareness, e.g. Demerol, Nisentil, Dolophine, pethidine, diamorphine (i.e. 100% heroin), pentazocine (Fortral) and meptazinol (Meptid)
neocortex (also sometimes called the 'new brain') the part of our brains in which our rational mind is located
neonatal concerning newborn babies in their first four weeks of life
neotonatologist a specialist who cares for newborn babies at birth and in their first four weeks if they are premature, seriously ill, injured at birth or if they have a birth defect
neurological to do with the nerves
NHS [National Health Service] the health care services which are available free to British citizens, which include provision of maternity care
NICU [Neonatal Intensive Care Unit] a unit within a hospital which cares for babies who are ill or in need of medical support or testing
nitrous oxide a component of 'gas and air'
nocebo effect comments or testing, especially in the antenatal period, which make a woman afraid
non-invasive officially this term refers to any medical procedure which does not penetrate or break the skin or a body cavity, i.e. which does not involve making an incision into the body or the removal of biological tissue. In this book the definition is extended to mean any procedure which does not affect the growing fetus or the successful development of a pregnancy and the outcome of a birth
non-stress test [NST] electronic fetal monitoring which is carried out in the third trimester to check the fetal heartbeat
noradrenaline (also 'norepinephrine') a hormone and neurotransmitter associated with the 'fight-or-flight' response
nuchal fold scan (also 'nuchal fold translucency scan') an ultrasound scan which aims to measure the fold at the back of the fetal neck. This test is sometimes conducted alongside a blood test because fluid in the nuchal fold at 11-14 weeks' gestation may indicate that a fetus has Down's syndrome.
nuchal translucency testing see 'nuchal fold scan'
OB [obstetric] women in North America frequently need to go to an OB Department in a hospital for their antenatal care—which, in the USA, is known as 'prenatal care'
obstetric adjective referring to the field of obstetrics
obstetric cholestasis a rare condition of late pregnancy which occasionally develops when the liver doesn't function as well as it needs to. The main symptom is intense itching, especially on the hands or feet, and the condition is confirmed or ruled out by a blood test. Cholestasis needs to be taken seriously because it can result in stillbirth.
obstetrician a doctor or consultant who specialises in obstetrics
obstetrics the *surgical* medical speciality which relates to anything to do with the care of women (and her babies) during pregnancy and birth, and afterwards. Most obstetricians are also qualified gynaecologists. Note that a midwife is the *non-surgical* speciality which deals with women having babies, which explains why they have to refer women to an obstetrician in cases where, for example, a caesarean is necessary.
occipito-posterior position see 'posterior'
oedema a build-up of excess fluid within body tissues, which causes swelling. This is common in pregnancy and is nothing to worry about unless it is also accompanied by high blood pressure or high amounts of protein in the urine.
oestrogen the primary female sexual hormone

old natural a term used in this book to describe old approaches to natural birth. These focused on complementary therapies for pain relief and coaching in labour by birth attendants. They tended to ignore what facilitates normal, safe birth, which requires no 'support' at all, beyond a sensible medical back-up arrangement, in case help is needed.

Omega 3 fatty acids which are essential for normal growth and which seem to reduce the risk of low birth weight and premature birth. Ideally, Omega-3 should be consumed in food (e.g. in oily fish), but it can also be obtained from supplements.

one-to-one care medical care in which one midwife is assigned to one mother-to-be for pregnancy and/or labour and birth

opiate any drug derived from opium, including pethidine, diamorphine (i.e. heroin), codeine and morphine

opioid a chemical substance that has a morphine-like action in the body

optimal as used in this book, this means a completely physiological birth, without disturbance, which takes place within easy reach of medical support, in case it's needed

optimal fetal positioning an approach recommended by two midwives (Jean Sutton and Pauline Scott), which aims to encourage a fetus into an ideal position for the birth

overdue a woman who is still pregnant (without having given birth yet) beyond her due date, which is generally calculated as being 40 weeks (or 280 days) after the first day of her last menstrual period

ovulation the process by which your body produces eggs (usually one each month), ready for fertilisation by your partner's sperm

oxytocic agent any agent which makes the uterus contract

oxytocin a hormone produced during orgasm, birth and while breastfeeding. During breastfeeding this is the hormone which enables your milk to be released into the milk ducts in your breasts.

oxytocin drip an IV drip which administers an artifical oxytocic, i.e. oxytocin

paediatric registrar a qualified paediatrician working within a hospital

paediatrician a doctor who deals with infants, children and adolescents

palpable possible to touch; 2/5 palpable means that most of the fetal head can be felt by a midwife above the pelvic brim

palpation the process by which a midwife (or other medical expert) uses his or her hands to feel a woman's bump. This is done in an attempt to ascertain the position of the fetus. Surprisingly perhaps, research has found this to be the most reliable way of assessing fetal size.

paralytic ileus a condition in which the bowel stops functioning

pathology the study and diagnosis of disease

pelvic floor the muscle fibres and associated connective tissue which support the pelvic organs. The pelvic floor separates the pelvic cavity from the perineum. Also sometimes called 'Kegels'.

pelvo-cephalic disproportion see 'cephalo-pelvic disproportion'

perinatal period the period around the birth. Technically, this is from 22 completed weeks of gestation (when birth weight is normally 500g) to seven completed days after the birth.

perinatal morbidity this refers to the incidence or prevalence of disease or disability around the time of a baby's birth

perinatal mortality this refers to the number of babies who die in the perinatal period (i.e. before and soon after birth)

perinatal outcome this relates to the baby's health—or otherwise—around the time of a baby's birth and refers to disease, disability and death

perineum the part of the body below the abdomen between the legs, which includes the anus and vagina and is the outlet to the abdomen. If it is 'intact' after birth there has been no tearing.
peritoneum the membrane that lines the abdominal cavity
pessary a pharmaceutical preparation, or a small plastic or silicone medical device which is inserted into the vagina or rectum and held in place by the muscles of the pelvic floor
pethidine an addictive analgesic drug used for 'pain relief' in labour which causes sleepiness in both mother and baby. While some women feel this helps them relax, others find the effect distressing and unhelpful and report that pethidine makes them feel disorientated and distant and that it does not really relieve their pain. As well as causing drowsiness in newborn babies, this drug also weakens a baby's suck, which makes breastfeeding difficult or impossible.
Pharaonic circumcision see 'infibulation'
physiological processes the natural processes the body will normally go through when no interventions of any kind are used and no 'pain relief' is attempted
Pinard stethoscope (sometimes simply called a 'Pinard') a fetal stethoscope shaped like a trumpet, which does not involve the use of ultrasound; named after the French obstetrician Adolphe Pinard (1844-1934)
pitocin synthetic oxytocin, know in the UK as syntocinon. Also see 'synoticinon'.
placenta an organ which develops during the first trimester of pregnancy from the same sperm and egg cells that form your little one. Its function is to transfer nutrients, oxygen, antibodies, and hormones from your own blood to your little one, and to transfer waste back out to your own organs (which will then process it).
placenta abrupto when a woman's placenta prematurely comes away from the uterine wall, suddenly depriving the fetus of oxygen. If symptoms indicate this may have occurred (i.e. bleeding with severe abdominal pain) the mother risks bleeding to death, so must go straight to A&E for emergency care.
placenta accreta the abnormal adherence of part of the placenta into the myometrium (muscle of the uterus). The placenta is said to have grown into the myometrium—a complication of caesareans.
placenta praevia when the placenta lies in the lower part of the uterus and covers part or all of the cervix. If it is only partially covered (Type I or II) a vaginal birth is possible. If the cervix is completely covered (Type III or IV) a caesarean section is necessary because the baby could not otherwise get out of the womb. If you are told you have placenta praevia at or before 20 weeks, the placenta may still work its way higher up as your womb stretches to accommodate your growing baby.
polyhydramnios when there is too much amniotic fluid around the fetus, which occurs in 1 in 250 pregnancies. It may be caused by diabetes or twin-twin transfusion syndrome.
posterior the 'back' of a woman's body. A fetus is said to be in a 'posterior' position (or 'occipito-posterior position') when its back is against the woman's back. This contrasts with an 'anterior' position in which your little one's back lies against your front. An anterior position is more favourable for a smooth labour and birth. Also see 'posterior labour'.
posterior labour a labour which occurs when the fetus is in a posterior position (i.e. its back lies against the mother's back). This generally results in a more painful labour because there are no painfree breaks between contractions. If the woman is conscious and moving about as she wishes it is very possible that the fetus will turn to an anterior position in time for the actual birth. If this does not happen, the baby is said to be born 'face-to-pubis'. This is fine (although much more painful) as long as there is absolutely no commanded pushing, which could cause transverse arrest, necessitating an emergency caesarean.

posterior pituitary the back part of the pituitary gland, which secretes hormones

postmature birth a birth which occurs after 42 weeks of pregnancy (or 43 weeks, according to some definitions). If the placenta is really no longer functioning properly and the baby is truly postmature (i.e. if it is not just a case of the due date having been incorrectly calculated), the newborn baby is likely to be thin and underweight, with slender limbs, dry wrinkled skin and longer hair and nails than usual in a newborn.

postmaturity the condition of a baby born after 42 weeks of gestation or 294 days after the LMP

postnatal after the birth

postpartum after the birth (from the point of view of 'giving birth')

postpartum haemorrhage [PPH] excessive (life-threatening) bleeding which occurs after a woman has given birth. Whether or not this is occurring is usually assessed *visually*, i.e. in rather a subjective, non-scientific manner, by care givers, but it is certainly something to be taken very seriously if bleeding is ongoing and does not stop with treatment (which is usually an injection of syntometrine).

PPH see 'postpartum haemorrhage'

pre-eclampsia (also 'toxaemia' or 'pre-eclamptic toxaemia') a medical condition in which high blood pressure (140/90 or more) occurs at the same time as high levels of protein in the urine (300mg or more per day). It is potentially dangerous for both mother and baby, which explains why it is routinely checked for during antenatal appointments. It's worth knowing that it is much more common in first pregnancies than in subsequent ones. It may also occur immediately postpartum or 6-8 weeks after the birth. Eclampsia—the rare development which occurs in 1 in 2,000 pregnancies—is a much more dangerous progression of this condition.

pre-eclamptic toxaemia see 'pre-eclampsia'

preemie another word for 'premature baby'

pregnancy rhinitis a blocked nose which continues (without other signs of a cold or allergy) for the last six weeks of a pregnancy and until two weeks after the birth. Although it is an inconvenient condition (often resulting in snoring at night!) it is not dangerous and does not require treatment.

premature baby a baby born before 37 weeks of pregnancy are complete

prematurity the condition of being premature

prenatal the American term for 'antenatal'

presenting part the part of your little one which is nearest to your cervix

preterm birth a birth which occurs before 37 weeks of pregnancy, i.e. a premature birth

primal health the basic state of health of a baby at the age of one year. See www.primalhealthresearch.com.

primigravida a woman in her first pregnancy

primipara a woman who has had one baby

progesterone a female hormone which sustains a pregnancy. It has a sedative effect, which explains why you may feel drowsier than when non-pregnant.

prolactin one of the hormones produced when your baby sucks at your breast; this is the hormone which stimulates the production of breastmilk

prolapse see 'uterine prolapse'

prolonged pregnancy a pregnancy which extends beyond 42 weeks. Somewhere between 4-14% of women are thought to experience longer pregnancies.

prostaglandins hormones (often administered in the form of pessaries to induce labour) which may have many actions. They may cause constriction or dilatation of muscles, they may sensitise spinal neurons to pain, affect cell growth and even affect the production of other hormones, amongst other things.

proteinuria the presence of an excess of serum proteins in the urine (which may make the urine look foamy), which is a sign of pre-eclampsia when accompanied by high blood pressure. Also see 'pre-eclampsia'.
protocols routine procedures
pulmonary embolism a blockage in one of the arteries leading to a lung, which may result in difficulty breathing, pain in the chest during breathing. In more severe cases it may result in collapse, circulatory instability and even sudden death.
randomised control trial the type of scientific experiment considered the most reliable within the field of medicine. Randomised control trials involve the random selection of subjects who are allocated different interventions (or not, in the case of the 'control group') in order to test these particular interventions.
raspberry leaf tea a tea made by pouring boiling water over dried raspberry leaves. This infusion is traditionally drunk by pregnant women in the third trimester of pregnancy. Since raspberry leaves contain 'frangine', which strengthens and tones the muscles of the womb, as well as vitamins A, C, E and B, magnesium, calcium and iron, its use is not entirely unscientific and some research studies have apparently confirmed its positive effects in pregnancy and birth. Supplements are available for women who cannot stand the rather strange taste of raspberry leaf tea.
rectum the tube, where faeces (poo) is stored in the body. It is about 20cm long and it culminates in the anus.
regional anaesthetics drugs used to numb a specific area, e.g. epidurals, spinals, saddle blocks and paracervicals
REM sleep [rapid-eye-movement sleep] sleep in which dreaming occurs
resusitaire a neonatal resuscitation unit
rhinitis see 'pregnancy rhinitis'
ring of fire a burning sensation experienced by women as their baby's head presses against the entrance to the vagina, just moments before baby is born
ROA [right occiput anterior] the term used to describe the fetal position when the back of the fetal head (the occiput) is pointing downwards and towards the right side of a mother's body, when the fetal back is round to the front of the woman's body. According to optimal fetal positioning experts Jean Sutton and Pauline Scott, a fetus lying in this position just before labour begins will often drop round to a posterior position for labour... so it is not an ideal position for your little one. (This happened to me, at the end of my first pregnancy, so I believe it! See Index.)
rooming in care of a newborn baby in the mother's bed or in a cot next to it in the same room, rather than in a separate hospital nursery
rooting the head-swaying of a baby searching for a breast
ROP [right occiput posterior] the term used to describe the fetal position when the back of the fetal head (the occiput) is pointing downwards and faces the right side of a mother's body, when the fetal back is round to the back of the woman's body, parallel to her spine. If the baby is still in this position when the woman goes into labour, she is said to have a 'posterior' labour, which is not ideal.
rotation the word used to describe the movement (turning round) of a fetus in the birth canal so as to pass through the pelvis
rushes a term proposed by some American writers—e.g. Ina May Gaskin—to refer to contractions (which is an opening process)
sample a small amount of something (e.g. blood or urine) tested in the assumption that the rest will have the same character-istics. Since this is not always the case, test results are not always totally reliable.
scan see 'ultrasound scan'
SCBU [Special Care Baby Unit]
second stage the stage of birth where the baby is born
second trimester the second three months of pregnancy
second-degree tear see 'tear'
section (also c-section) caesarean section

sedative drugs to encourage women to sleep or rest, e.g. temazepam.
semi-squat a position in which the woman is upright, with her knees slightly bent. Of course, during the second stage of labour women may want to be supported in this position, or hang from something suspended from the ceiling.
sepsis a serious medical condition in which the whole of a person's body becomes inflamed as a result of infection
SGA [small for gestational age] where a fetus appears to be smaller than he or she should be, considering his or her age
shiatsu a traditional Japanese therapy in which pressure is applied by a therapist's hands to a patient's body
shoulder dystocia a term used to describe the situation where a baby's right shoulder cannot be born or where it can only be born with significant expert manipulation
show a discharge of a jelly-like substance, which may be smeared with blood. Also see 'mucous plug'.
small-for-dates (or 'small-for-gestational-age') see 'SGA'
Sonicaid (also 'Doptone', 'Doppler machine' or 'carotid Doppler machine') a device which uses low-frequency ultrasound waves to measure frequencies which are translated into sounds. [See 'ultrasound' too.] It is used to listen to the fetal heartbeat but other sounds will also be heard, e.g. that of blood through the placenta.
sonogram a diagnostic medical image created using ultrasound echo (sonographic) equipment. Women are often given or sold one of these images after having an ultrasound scan.
sphincter part of the body (usually a circular muscle), which closes or opens, as required. There are over 40 sphincters in the human body and they include the anal sphincter (which controls the release of poo) and the epiglottis in the throat, which stops food from going down into the lungs.
spinal (short for 'spinal anaesthesia') a form of regional anaesthesia which involves injecting drugs through a long, fine needle into the cerebrospinal fluid in the spine. This form of 'pain relief' may cause loss of sensation and pain because it blocks the transmission of pain signals through nerves in or near the spinal cord. However, it does not always take effect completely, cannot be used throughout the entire length of labour and may have various other disadvantages. It is widely used in the case of elective caesareans which are carried out before labour begins.
spontaneous abortion the expulsion of an embryo or fetus from a woman's womb, resulting in or caused by its death. Rather upsettingly for many women, a miscarriage is called a 'spontaneous abortion' if it occurs after 20 weeks' gestation. Of course, the word 'abortion' also means the intentional removal of a live embryo or fetus from a woman's womb.
spontaneous pushing see 'commanded pushing'
spotting light bleeding from the vagina between periods or during pregnancy. This may occur in the first month or two after you become pregnant, at the time when you would normally have had your period. In some cases spotting (or any amount of bleeding) indicates a serious problem so it should be checked out with a midwife or doctor. If bleeding is accompanied by severe abdominal pain, the woman needs to go straight to A&E for emergency treatment.
stage one see 'first stage'
stage three see 'third stage'
stage two see 'second stage'
steroid a naturally-produced chemical, such as oestrogen or progesterone
stillbirth a birth in which a baby is born dead, having died after 24 weeks' gestation in the womb ('intra-uterine death'), or during labour ('intra-partum death'). In the UK 1 in 200 babies are stillborn. The risk of stillbirth is higher for multiple pregnancies,

smokers, women over 35, or women who already had medical conditions when they became pregnant. Stillbirth is also more common when there are congenital malformations of the fetus, when there is an antepartum haemorrhage, when babies are born prematurely, when there is a case of rhesus incompatibility or in the case of obstetric cholestasis. Finally, a few cases of stillbirth are caused by birth trauma, untreated infections or immunological disorders (e.g. APS or anti-phospholipid syndrome). Useful website: www.uk-sands.org

stress incontinence accidental leaks of urine (or faeces) after coughing, sneezing or laughing. Urinary stress incontinence is fairly common in late pregnancy, unfortunately!

stress test (ST) see 'contraction stress test'

stretch marks lines which appear as a result of skin stretching. These are initially dark red in colour but eventually fade to a silvery line. Not all women get them and I personally feel that drinking good quantities of water during pregnancy may prevent them.

stripping of the membranes see 'sweeping'

sucking reflex an undrugged baby's innate ability to suck so as to obtain milk from your breasts

suction use of a vacuum extractor, a device which involves putting a kind of 'hat' on a fetus and pulling by suction

supine position when a woman is lying on her back. Also see 'lithotomy position' and 'tailbone'.

suppositories solid medications inserted into a woman's anus, perhaps as an enema, or to induce labour

surfactant a substance which helps to keep lungs from collapsing. Extremely premature babies (e.g. younger than 28 weeks) may lack sufficient surfactant for breathing to be possible.

surrogacy when a woman has a baby on behalf of another woman

suture sew

sweeping when a pregnant woman's amniotic membranes are loosened or broken so as to induce or accelerate labour. In the USA this same procedure is called 'stripping of the membranes'.

syntocinon a synthetic form of oxytocin, sometimes used in a drip to induce or speed up contractions during labour

syntometrine see 'ergometrine'

tailbone (the 'coccyx') the final segment of the human vetebral column, made up of two or three solid bones with rudimentary joints. During birth if the woman is lying down the pressure of the baby passing through the 'birth canal' can make one of these joints break, which can cause considerable pain subsequently. If, on the other hand, the woman is in a forward, leaning-forward position the angles and internal dimensions of the abdomen change dramatically. As the baby passes through the pelvis both the sacrum and coccyx (tailbone) are lifted out of the way, meaning no damage occurs.

tearing see 'tears'

tears damage to a woman's vagina and possibly also other body parts, categorised into four degrees. In a 1st degree tear, there is superficial damage but no tearing of muscles. When 2nd degree tearing occurs, both vaginal walls and muscles may be torn, but the anal sphincter remains intact. In the case of a 3rd degree tear, the tearing extends to the anal sphincter, but the rectum is still intact. A 4th degree tear involves tearing right up to and including the rectum. Tearing is less likely when a woman is completely conscious and if it occurs at all it is less severe and heals more effectively when there is no episiotomy. Tears can be treated fairly easily in the UK, unlike in other parts of the world, where women may become socially ostracised as a result of unrepaired tears.

TED anti-embolism stocking (also called 'Ted hose') a thigh-length stocking which is designed to prevent the formation of blood clots in deep veins in the legs. 'T.E.D.' is a mysterious trademark, but TED stockings are reputedly more effective than other makes

TENS [transcutaneous electrical nerve stimulation] an electronic device that produces electrical signals to stimulate nerves through unbroken skin. These electrical signals are transmitted across two or more electrodes. Although it is widely advertised as a way of relieving pain in labour, there is no evidence to suggest it is effective and it does, of course, inevitably immobilise a woman using it.

third stage the stage of birth where the placenta comes out

third trimester the third three months of pregnancy

third-degree tear see 'tear'

thrombosis when a clot forms inside a blood vessel and blocks the flow of blood

toxaemia see 'pre-eclampsia'

toxoplasmosis a parasitic disease, caught from cats or caused by infected, undercooked meat, which puts a fetus at risk. It sometimes causes flu-like symptoms in its first few weeks.

tranquilisers drugs used to calm someone, e.g. Valium, Vistaril and Penergan

transition the end of the first stage of labour, when the cervix dilates from 7 to 10cm. Symptoms of transition may be extreme and may include longer, stronger contractions, trembling, shaky legs, vomiting, irritability, backache, shiveriness or sweatiness, as well as despair or extreme grumpiness!

transverse arrest when the fetus gets stuck as it is descending the so-called birth canal. This may occur as a result of commanded pushing when the fetus is in a posterior position during the second stage of labour. Also see 'commanded pushing'.

transverse lie when a fetus lies horizontally across its mother's womb. It is common until 27 weeks of pregnancy, by which time the (larger) fetus should have settled into a head-down or breech position, ready for the birth. If the fetus is still lying transverse during labour, a caesarean must be performed.

trimester one of the three periods of pregnancy, lasting approx. three months

triple test (also known as 'triple screen', 'the Kettering test' or 'the Bart's test') a blood test carried out in pregnancy (usually in the second trimester) which aims to detect trisomy 21 (Down's syndrome), trisomy 18 and open neural tube defects by measuring levels of alpha-fetoprotein, hCG and unconjugated estriol in the maternal serum. The test may also detect increased risk for Turner syndrome, triploidy, trisomy 16 mosaicism, fetal death, Smith-Lemli-Opitz syndrome and steroid sulfatase deficiency.

twilight sleep a full-consciousness 'sleep' induced by the injection of morphine and scopolamine, which results in subsequent loss of memory. Used for 'pain relief' a few decades ago, but it fell out of favour because it did not seem effective as a form of pain relief and babies were significantly at risk of asphyxiation.

twin-to-twin transfusion syndrome [TTTS] a serious complication of twin or other multiple pregnancies, where two or more fetuses share a common (monochorionic) placenta. It is also known as Feto-Fetal Transfusion Syndrome (FFTS) and Twin Oligohydramnios-Polyhydramnios Sequence (TOPS).

ultrasound acoustic energy with a frequency above human hearing. Also see 'ultrasound scan' and the photo caption above

ultrasound scan a process in which images are produced using ultrasound (see 'ultrasound' entry above) so as to date and assess a developing pregnancy

umbilical cord the flexible cord which connects your little one to you (inside your womb), which contains umbilical arteries and a vein. It is along this cord that nutrients, oxygen, antibodies and hormones from your own blood pass to your little one, and that waste transfers back to you.

unassisted birth a birth which takes place with no qualified medical staff around
unstable lie this term refers to a fetus who keeps on changing position after 36 weeks. It may be caused by placenta praevia (if the placenta is preventing the fetal head from engaging), or by many other problems including polyhydramnios, prematurity and fibroids.
uterine to do with the womb
uterine prolapse a downward shift in the position of a woman's womb, below its normal abdominal position. Sometimes it results in a womb protruding from outside a woman's vagina.
uterine rupture a life-threatening event in which the womb bursts. This typically occurs during labour or late pregnancy when a scar from a previous caesarean cut bursts open, especially when a labour is induced or augmented artificially.
uterus see 'womb'
vacuum extraction (also 'ventouse delivery') the use of a device, called a vacuum extractor, to pull out a baby. A traction cup is attached to the fetal head, negative pressure is applied and traction is made on a chain passed through a suction tube. Vacuum extraction is an alternative to forceps and does not require an episiotomy.
vacuum extractor (also 'ventouse') see 'vacuum extraction'
vagina the passageway which leads from a woman's womb out of her body. It is commonly thought to include the vulva or female genitals generally, but strictly speaking it only includes the internal tubular passageway.
vaginal discharge see 'discharge'
vaginal exam a check carried out by a midwife to ascertain how dilated a woman's cervix is
varicose veins swollen, irregular-shaped veins which sometimes appear in the legs, particularly on the calves
VBAC [vaginal birth after caesarean] when a woman who has previously had one or more caesareans has a vaginal birth for a subsequent child
vena cava the main vein running down a mother's back, which takes blood from the placenta and therefore also from the fetus. It is easily compressed by the heavy uterus when the mother is lying on her back.
ventouse vacuum extractor. See 'vacuum extraction'.
vernix (also 'vernix caseosa') the creamy substance which can sometimes be found on newborn babies' skin; it protects your little one's skin while he or she is in your womb
version see 'external cephalic version'
vertex position where your little one's presenting part is the occiput of the flexed head, i.e. not the feet (breech)
vitamin K a vitamin which is routinely injected into the newborn baby (or administered orally) to prevent an extremely rare haemorragic disease of the newborn, which occurs only amongst breastfed babies. While formula has added Vitamin K, a few breastfed babies probably do not receive a sufficient quantity of the vitamin because of early problems with breastfeeding after a disturbed birth. After an entirely undisturbed, physiological birth babies will normally receive plenty of colostrum (the early milk), which is rich in this vitamin. Vitamin K is necessary for the synthesis of prothrombin, which helps the blood to clot.
vulva a woman's exterior genitalia (genitals)
water birth a birth in which the woman labours in water (preferably after reaching more than 5cm dilation) and possibly also gives birth under water
waters the amniotic fluid around your baby when he or she is in your womb. Also see 'amniotic fluid'.
Wilkinet a baby carrier which is ideal for a baby's first few weeks because the baby is held firmly against the mother's chest. Useful website: www.wilkinet.co.uk
womb (also 'uterus') the 'bag' of muscle which holds your growing baby and which gradually expands to create a huge bump!

Birthframes index

No.	Name	Features	Page
1	Sylvie Donna	A glimpse into the author's thoughts…	18
2	Sylvie Donna	Experiencing a true fetus ejection reflex	23
3	Sylvie Donna	Difficulties preparing for each birth	27
4	Ashley Marshall	Lotus birth—no cord cutting	36
5	Jo Siebert	Appropriate intervention in pregnancy	39
6	Liliana Lammers	Appropriate intervention during labour	40
7	Anonymous	Infertility through endometriosis	41
8	Anonymous	Adopting a baby	42
9	Anonymous	The experience of surrogacy	45
10	Jenny Sanderson	First-time mother having optimal births	48
11	Nina Klose	'Office drone' having an optimal birth	53
12	Maria Shanahan	Optimal despite fear after a bad first birth	55
13	Michel Odent	Woman with MS giving birth	59
14	Steve and Olga Mellor	Unexpected twin home birth	60
15	Mave Denyer	Vaginal triplet birth in 1961	67
16	Janet Hanton	Vaginal triplet birth in 1999	69
17	Elise Hansen	Vaginal breech birth—'why not?' attitude	73
18	Liz Woolley	Vaginal breech birth after a caesarean	75
19	Laura Shanley	Unassisted footling breech birth	77
20	Nina Klose	A caesarean in retrospect	87
21	Anonymous	Postnatal experience after a caesarean	88
22	Anonymous	Postnatal experience after a caesarean	89
23	Anonymous	A positive experience of a caesarean	89
24	Anonymous	A failed VBAC	91
25	Michel Odent	A successful VBAC	95
26	Sylvie Donna	Difficulty asserting wishes antenatally	104
27	Nuala OSullivan	Posterior labour and face-to-pubis delivery	112
28	Anonymous	Unhelpful interventions	117
29	Michel Odent	Birthing like a mammal	120
30	Bhavna Amlani	Epidural which went wrong	127
31	Deborah Jackson	Importance of no disturbance	135
32	Nina Klose	First perceptions of pregnancy	152
33	Anonymous	Praying for an unborn baby	157
34	Sarah Cave	Avoiding drugs so as to help the baby	173
35	Tanya Kudryashova	Home birth in Russia	175
36	Sylvie Donna	Third baby's postnatal behaviour	186

37	Anonymous	First antenatal appointment	197
38	Bill Anderson	Having a child with Down's syndrome	208
39	Nina Klose	Ultrasound risk assessment	215
40	Karen Low	Antenatal care and classes	222
41	Pauline Farrance	An optimal birth after a managed first birth	225
42	Anonymous	Life-saving intervention	243
43	Tina C from the UK	Hyperemesis (ongoing nausea)	245
44	Jeannette Clark	Managed triplet birth	248
45	Debbie Brindley	Arranging for minimal disturbance	251
46	Christina Mansi	A cascade of intervention	259
47	Christina Mansi	Successful follow-up births	261
48	Sylvie Donna	Intervention refused	262
49	Anonymous	Uncaring treatment of premature labour	276
50	Krisanne Collard	Premature birth and kangaroo care	279
51	Anonymous	An optimal twin birth with the NHS	288
52	Esther Culpin	Breech home birth	288
53	Monica Reid	Stillbirth followed by live births	292
54	Jenny Sanderson	Michel Odent in attendance	301
55	Anonymous	Anger about treatment	303
56	Marion Chatfield	Lack of agreement between caregivers	304
57	Anonymous	Two contrasting experiences	305
58	Jennifer Jacoby	Second birth with a wonderful midwife	306
59	Kathryn Clarke	Harmonious optimal twin birth	313
60	Sarah-Jane Forder	Doula facilitating a smooth hospital birth	315
61	Natalie Meddings	Doula helps woman 'go to another planet'	317
62	Phil Anderton	Man's view on attending births	319
63	David Newbound	Partner as defender	323
64	Alan Low	Partner as fighter and supporter	324
65	Cara Low	Child's account	327
66	Carol Walton	Home birth in the 60s	336
67	Debbie Brindley	A midwife's choices	340
68	Debbie Shaw	Optimal births in hospital in the 1990s	342
69	Georgina Taylor	Horrible hospital birth, lovely home birth	343
70	Justine Renwick	Well-managed twin hospital birth	346
71	Rebecca Wright	Emailed report of a home birth	348
72	Kris Holloway	Home births chosen after working in Mali	348
73	Liliana Lammers	Disturbed hospital birth	352
74	Gemma Shepherd	Painfree home birth	352
75	Clare O'Ryan	Disturbed home birth	355
76	Anonymous	Twin sisters' contrasting experiences	357

77	Michel Odent	Birthing pool tests	360
78	Angela Horn	Experience of using a birthing pool	360
79	Helen Arundell	Late twin pregnancy diary	386
80	Anonymous	Staying fit and healthy in pregnancy	388
81	Ulrike von Moltke	Misguided positioning in labour	393
82	Nina Klose	Discovering how a vaginal birth feels	398
83	Janet Balaskas	Optimal positioning in labour	404
84	Justine Rowan	Thinking through the realities of 'where'	411
85	Nicolette Lawson	Hypnotherapy used for birth	414
86	Beth Dubois	Birth and breastfeeding after sexual abuse	417
87	Anonymous	Shock-start to labour: laughter	428
88	Gaia Pollini	Avoiding other people's negativity	430
89	Anonymous	Woman affected by her partner's doubts	434
90	Michel Odent	Description of typical optimal scenarios	435
91	Liliana Lammers	Three easy births attended by Michel	437
92	Joanne Searle	Problem resolution before labour	439
93	Fiona Lucy Stoppard	'Going to another planet' in labour	444
94	Sue Pakes	Almost painfree births	445
95	Rachel Urbach	Just as Michel said it would be!	447
96	Ruth Clark	Unexpectedly straightforward second birth	447
97	Heba Zaphiriou-Zarifi	Giving birth before the arrival of midwives	451
98	Sylvie Donna	Not to plan, but perfectly fine	453
99	Sarah Buckley	Learning an eco alternative to nappies	480
100	Sarah Hobart	Life after birth	483

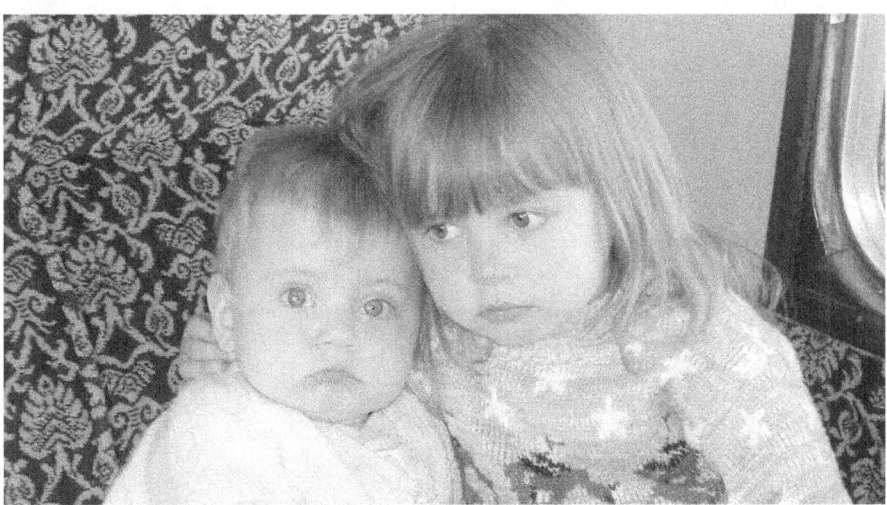

Remember, they're worth it!

Index

This index has been designed to be as useful as it can be.

Quick or relaxed reference...
In cases where a lot of page numbers are listed beside an entry, you will see that some entries are in bold. if you are looking for something in a hurry (e.g. because you quickly want some ideas or information, perhaps after just receiving some news about your situation from a caregiver) only look up the numbers in bold. If you have plenty of time—e.g. when you're in a reflective mood or in the early stages of labour—and really want to review and ponder certain points, you or your partner might like to look up the other entries too.

Birthframes
Where relevant, you are referred to birthframes which are relevant to particular topics. Some contributors have provided information as well as opinions and accounts of their first-hand experience in their birthframes, so it might be worth checking these out too. Numbers refer to the birthframes themselves and page numbers for these can be found in the Birthframes index on pp 582-584.

abdominal pain **378**, 464
abortion 19, 196, 198-199, **205-207**, 213, 221, 236
acceleration of labour—see 'augmentation of labour'
Accordion Method of Preconceptual Care 366
acidaemia 124
active birth **21**, 223, 339, **404**
active management 232-235, 237, 240-242, 405
acupressure 375
acupuncture 6, 98, 104, **132-135**, 241, **306**, 375
addiction 122, 127, 188, 189
adhesions 81
adoption 42-44
adrenal glands 247
adrenaline 252, **429**, 435-436
affirmations 77, 137, 413, **440**
AFP test 215-216, **236**
Africa 13, **18-20**, **199-203**, 348-349, 429, 480
afterbirth—see 'placenta'
afterpains 17, 56
airway obstruction 84
alcohol 144, 166, 175, 368, 476
alertness 7, 12, 14, 15, 37, 85, 121, **190-191**, 253, 256, 456, **466**
allergic reactions 234, 369
all fours—see 'hands-and-knees' position

Index

allicin 381
aloe vera 374
amnestics 121
amniocentesis 103, **206-207**, 216, 236
amniotic fluid 10, 84, 101, **152-153**, 155, 156, 159, 162, 163, 166, 170, 174, **180**, 196, 218, **457**, 458
amniotomy 104, **117-119**, 136, 226, 232, **240**, **241**, 259-262, 270-272, 273, 275, 295, 298, 360, 387, **492-493**
amphetamines 122, 189
anaemia 9, 19, **220**, **383**
anaesthesia 21, 82, 83, 86, 96, 119, **121-127**, **189-194**, 232-235, 237, 240, 241, 244, 249-250, 254, 256, 260, 274, 295, 304, **310-311**, 313, 347, 390, 403, **407**—also see 'epidurals' and 'spinals'
analgesia **21**, 84, 96, **121**, **127-131**, **189-193**, 241, 362—also see specific drugs, e.g. 'pethidine'
animals 52, 101, 102, **120**, 126, 160, 324, 361, **367**, 410, 447, 448, 454
anomaly scan 251
anorexia 188-189
antenatal care **195-258**, 405, 487, 489, 593
anterior position 171, 355, 465—also see 'optimal fetal positioning'
antibiotics 82, 95, 220, **233**, **234**, 247, 375, 381
antibodies 227
Anti-D shot 347
anti-emetic drugs 245, 246, 247
Apgar score **15-16**, 23, 92, **108**, 388
apnoea 281, **284**—also see 'breathing difficulties (baby's)'
appetite 11, 17, **185**, 438, **459-460**
aquanatal classes 223
ARM [artificial rupture of the membranes]—see 'amniotomy'
arnica 132, 319, **379**
AROM [artificial rupture of the membranes]—see 'amniotomy'
aromatherapy **133**, 241, 262
aspirin 368, 385
asthma 188, 358
augmentation of labour **21**, 81, 106, 126, **191**, **234**, 237, **239**, **240**, **259-262**, 270, 272, 275, 336, **359**, 390, 434, **464-465**—also see 'syntocinon', 'pitocin', 'IV' and 'failure to progress'
auscultation 39, 49, 59, 97, 103, **211**, 217, **218-219**, 228, 251, 270, 273, 313, 333, 352, 387, 393, 420, 458—also see 'Pinard' and 'Sonicaid'
autism 188, **189**
backache 10, **20**, 118, 120, 124, 127, 167, 280, 295, 343, 347, **377**, **384**, 386, **394**, 399, 400, 401, 402, 448
Balaskas, Janet 122, 489, 594 and see Birthframe 83

barbiturates 121, 189
baths 49, 133, 137, 138, **139**, **161**, 176, 187, 193, 232, **240**, 262, 266, 269, 272, 275, 278, 286, 293, 297, 325, 329, 345, 353, **359**, 362, 363, **365**, **373**, **381**, 387, **394**, **395**, 401, **407**, 425, 441, 450, 452, 453, **457**, 461, 465
belief suggestions 77-78—also see 'affirmations'
beta-endorphins 100, 102, 151, 153
birth attendants 13, 15, 24-25, 185, **239**, **253**, **301-332**, 340, 348-349, 393, 417-427, 447-450, 451-453, **460**, 489
birth centres 175, 223, **225**, 240, 259, 317, **333**, 357, 358, 398, 418, 487, 489
birthframes 17—and see 'Birthframes Index' on pp 582-584
birthing pool 34, 54, 55, 56, 61, 62, 112-116, 175, 176, 251, 252, **264**, 273, 288, 289, 307, 308, 316, 318, **327**, 328, 333, 340, 343, 348, 353, 354, **359-365**, 398-404, 407, 441, 445, **457**—also see 'water birth'
birthing pool test 359-360
birth partners—see 'birth attendants'
birth plans [called 'care guides' in this book] 6, **18**, 19, 40, **48**, 54, 60, 69, 70, **73**, 75, 86, 90, 91, **117**, 120, 135, **136**, 138, **175**, 176, 177, 178, **196**, 197, **303**, 309, 310, **314**, 316, **321**, **333**, **339**, 341, 342, **345**, 368, **391**, **407**, **408**, **411**, **429**, 432-433, **435**, 445, 448, **453**, **462**, **463**, **472**, **494**, 596—and see Birthframes 45, 51, 52, 56, 67, 69, 75, 84, 86, 88, 96, 97, 98
birth pool—see 'birthing pool' and 'water birth'
birth stories—see 'Birthframes Index' on pp 582-584 or see key words, e.g. 'breech', 'twins', etc.
bleeding 34, 135, **212**, 244, 245, 246, 280, 285, 326, 353, **378**, **382**, **383**, 385, 387, 430, **436**, **466**—also see 'postpartum haemorrhage'
blocked nose **376-377**, 385
blood pressure 16, 21, 25, 41, 82, 83, 84, 85, 87, **123**, 124, 126, 127, **128**, **161**, **196**, 197, **218**, **221**, 226, 228, 230, 246, 252, **336**, 350, **377**, **382**
blood sugar levels 376
bonding 6, 15, 36, 62, **80**, **81**, **102**, **118**, **121**, 177, 184, **187**, **254**, 258, 278, 298, **332**, **472**, 484, **494**, 596
bottom-up position 357
brain damage 381
Braxton Hicks contractions 137, 159, 166, **274**, 275, 307, 347, **384**, 385, 386, 387, 448, **494**
breastfeeding **2**, 6, 7, **13**, **15**, **16**, **17**, **19**, **21**, 23, 25, 30, 37, 47, 49, 56, **66**, 72, 78, 90, 91, 100, 101, **102**, 117, **121**, 122, **123**, 126, 127, 128, 137, **144**, 170, **173**, 176, 177, **179**, **180**, **194**, 197, 226, 229, **253**, **254**, 255, 258, 261, 262, **264**, 269, **271**, **274**, 275, 292, **345**, **369**, 373, **377**, 393, 397, 403, 404, **409**, 416, 418, 419, 434, 453, 454, 455, **457**, **476-478**, 481, **487**, 488, 489, **497**, 502, 504, 506, **507**, **513**, 517, 593, **596**—and see Birthframes 2, 14, 86, 88, 100

breathing difficulties (baby's) **14**, 82, 112, 116, **123**, **127**, 128, 156, 176, 187, 189, **190**, **207**, 238, 242, 244, **254**, 278, 281, **284**, **286**, 342, **350**, 358, **397**
breathing in labour and birth **25**, 82, **84**, 85, 95, 128, **241**, 275, 319, 353, 354, 361, 399, 400, 401, 402, 405, **413**, **414**, 421, 448, 452, **459**, **466**
breathing in pregnancy 249, 276, **368-369**, **375**, 376, **413**, **414**, 430, **466**
breech 12, **40**, 52, 58, **73-79**, 134, **168**, 171, **174**, **212**, 219, **242**, 243, 273, **290-291**, 304, 312, 313, 319, 347, **356**, 431, 448, **494**, 495, 498, **499**, **502**, 512, 513, 515, 516—and see Birthframes 6, 17, 18, 45, 50, 52, 53
brow presentation 360
bruising **7**, 132, 256, **379**
Buckley, Sarah 99-102, 109-111, 123, 128, 212-215, 237, 489, 593 and see Birthframe 99
burning sensation 12, 229—also see 'ring of fire'
caesareans 5, 6, 18, **21**, 24, 39, 40, 56, **58**, 61, **66**, **67**, 69, 70, 71, 73, 75, 77, **80-96**, 102, 118, **119**, 121, **123**, **125**, 175, **188**, **189**, 194, 218, **219**, **234**, **235**, **237**, **239**, 241, 243, 256, 257, 261, **271**, **274**, 276, **290-291**, **303**, 304, 305, **310**, **311**, 312, 313, 319, 320, 322, **335**, **336**, 337, 341, **344**, 345, **359**, **382**, 411, **416**, 430, **433**, 447, **462**, **487**, 492, **494**, **495**, **496**, **497**, 498, 499, **502**, 506, 507, 508, 510, 512, **513**, 515—and see Birthframes 6, 20, 21, 22, 23, 24, 25, 39, 41, 42, 44, 46, 52, 55, 67, 70, 76, 77, 81, 82
calling the midwife 29, 62, 137, 178-179, 228, 307, 325, 342, 347, 398, **400**, 445, 446, **449**, 451, 452, 454, **458**, **460**, 461
camcorders 31, 97, 108, 117, **266**, **320**, 322-323, 328, **462**
cameras 31, 97, **108**, 117, **120**, **266**, 328, **462**
cancer 358
cannula—see 'IV'
cardiotocograph 251—also see 'electronic fetal monitoring'
care guides (pages to take into account while preparing one; main entries are marked in bold) 6, **18**, 40, **48**, 54, 60, 69, 70, **73**, 75, 86, 90, 91, **117**, 120, 135, **136**, 138, **175**, 176, 177, 178, **196**, 197, **252**, **303**, 309, 310, **314**, 316, **321**, **333**, **339**, 341, 342, **345**, 368, **391**, **407**, **408**, **411**, **429**, 432-433, **435**, 445, 448, **453**, **462**, **463**, 472, **494**, **541**, 596—and see Birthframes 45, 51, 52, 56, 67, 69, 75, 84, 86, 88, 96, 97, 98
cascade of hormones 7, 8, **97-102**
cascade of interventions 8, **98**, **99**, 117, 117-118, **188**, **256**, 257, 303, 412, 447—and see Birthframes 46 and 47
catching the baby **14**, 25, 32, 33, 50, 54, 56, 74, 78, **97**, **108**, 116, 136, 176, **269**, **322**, 325, 364, **395**, 454, **463**
catecholamine levels 207
cephalic—see 'head-down position'

cephalo-pelvic disproportion 116, 175, **466**
chemicals 366, 368
chest pain 466
chicken pox **367**, 501
children (toddlers, older children, other children) **4**, **5**, 8, 33, 37, 38, **48**, 67, 70, 81, **85**, 89, 95, 106, 112, 120, 136, 154, **161**, 166, **167**, 179, 227, 228, 231, 247, **266**, 272, 285, 289, 291, 292, **301**, 307, **314**, **321**, **327-330**, **340**, 343, 399, 453, 458, **460**, **461**, 516—also see Birthframe 75
chloroform 122, 232, 233, 234
cholestasis 39, 378
chorionic villi 143
chorionic villus sampling 103, 236
choroid plexus cysts 216
circumcision 194, 236
coaching 234, 275, 319, 345, 407
cocaine 189
coffee 104, 132, 144, 166, 173
colds **385**, 386—also see 'flu'
colostrum 7, 15, 19, 194, 232
commanded pushing 2, **12**, 76, 97, **125**, **241**, 242, **271**, 325, 347, **355-356**, 394, **407-408**, **418**, **423**, 465, **495**, **508**, **512**—also see 'pushing'
complementary therapies 6, 99, 104, **132-135**
compresses 275, 394
conception 9, 10, 41, 42, **48**, 55, 103, **140-144**, **146**, 149, 175, **180**, **181**, **183**, **184**, **188**, 199, **205**, 215, **217**, **242**, 249, 275, 346, 352, **366-368**, 379, 398, 431, 434, **489**, 501, 592, 593
constipation 220, 229, 232, **383**, 389
continuous monitoring—see 'electronic fetal monitoring' and 'monitoring'
contraception 18, 19, 197, **367**
contractions **11**, **12**, 13, **28-29**, 30-34, 59, **78**, 95, **100**, **101**, 102, 105, 117, 119, **123**, 124, 125, 126, 129, 130, 134, 135, 159, 166, **171**, **181**, **190-191**, 227, 228, 229, 232, 234, **240**, 242, **243**, 244, 252, **253**, **259**, 260, **261**, 273, **274-275**, 285, 289, **304**, 306, 307-308, 316, 318, 319, 325, **331**, 336, 342, 343, 344, 347, **352-354**, 355, 356, **359**, 360, 361, **362**, **365**, **379**, **384**, **385**, 389, **390**, **394**, 398, 399, 400, 401, 402, 404, 406, 415, 416, 418, 420, 421, 422, **429**, **434**, **435-436**, **440-441**, **444**, 446, 447, 448, 449, 450, 452, 453, 454, 456, 457, **458-459**, 461, **462-463**, 464, 465, 492, 494, **495-496**, 497, 506, 507, **509**, 511, **512**—and see all birthframes
convulsions **378**, 466
cord—see 'cutting the cord'
cord blood banking 36
cord clamping 83, 436, 450—also see 'cutting the cord'
cord prolapse 40, 291, 304
corticosteroids 375
co-sleeping 40, 424, **476**, **489**

coughing 385
cpc's 216
cravings **144**, 198, 370, **376**
crowning 24, 32, 116, **272**, **275**, 325, 343, 354, 402, **496**
C-sections—see 'caesareans'
CTG 251—also see 'electronic fetal monitoring'
cutting the cord **13**, 34, **35-37**, 56, 63, 83, 123, 176, **179**, **190**, 229, **252**, **269**, **271**, **272**, **290**, 403, 423, **436**, 438, 450, 454, **503-504**, 512, 515—also see 'lotus birth'
Cytotec 420
Daviss, Betty-Anne 612, 615
deep vein thrombosis 82, 85
deformities 211, 245
dehydration 245, 247, **369**, 375, 376
delivery rooms 87, 109, 173, 222, **235**, 252, 288, 304, 314, 316, **340**, 356, 389, **407**, 445
delivery table **275**, 316, **405-406**
Demerol 121, **127-128**, 129, 136
developing countries 13, **18-20**, **199-203**, 348-349, 429, 480
diabetes 196, 358—also see 'gestational diabetes'
diagnosis of labour 28
diamorphine 121, 127-128, **253**
diapers 37, 180, 264, 266, 296, 313, 336, 358, **464**, 472, **479**, **480-482**, 489, **517**
diarrhoea 11, 19, 33, 185, **220**, **350**, 354, 385, 386, **457**
Dick-Reid, Grantly 275
dilation **12**, 25, 28-31, 105, 244, **253**, 313, **354**, 357, **359-360**, 365, 389, **394**, **407**, **412**, **422**, **457**, **461**, **463**, **465**, **495**, **496**, 499, 502, **512**, **513**—and see all birthframes
discharge—see 'vaginal discharge', 'spotting' and 'show'
disturbance 97-138, 251-252, 344, **345**, 352, 355-356, 434, **435-436**, 487, 489
dizziness **144**, **252**, 278, **466**, 504
Doppler machine—see 'Sonicaid'
doubts **53-57**, 58, 121, **456-471**
doulas 36, 95, **268**, **314**, **315-318**, **345**, 350, 360, 436, 437, **475**, **487**, **496**, 516
Down's syndrome 205-210, 213, 216
dreams 9, 78, **144**, 174, 387, **411**, 467
drinking after the birth **17**, 49, 229, 280, **409**, 450, **476**, 481
drinking in labour 94, 106, 228, **239**, **240**, 265, 266, 270, **345**, 390, **457**, **459-460**, **461**
drinking in pregnancy **10**, 103, 132, 139, **143**, 144, 155, 159, 170, 180, 202, 204, **218**, **220**, 245-246, 294, 358, **367**, **368**, **369**, 373, 374, 375, **376**, 378, **379**, **381**, 383, **384**, 492, 501, 511—also see 'coffee' and 'water'

drip **21**, 82, 91, 106, **123**, 126, 226, **234**, **235**, **239**, **240**, 244, 246, 247, 252, **257**, 260, **261**, **270**, **272**, **273**, **275**, 294, 306, 314, **328**, **336**, 344, 347, 360, **375**, **381**, **390**, 399, 494, **500**, **501**, 506, 507

due dates 10, 29, 40, 47, 48, 50, 55, 59, **61**, 62, 70, 75, 112, 120, 137, 138, **140**, **141**, **145**, **148**, 149, 165, 179, **181**, **181-182**, 182, 183, **205**, 215, 227, 248, 262, 263, 279, 282, 289, 294, 302, 313, 315, 317, 342, 353, **367**, **382**, **382**, **384**, 387, 388, 389, 393, 398, 414, 415, 420, **429**, 430, 431, 439, 445, 446, 448, **456**, 484, **496**, **497**, 498, **503**, **506**, **508**—also see 'ultrasound'

dummies 269, 271, 275, 345, **476**

dystocia—see 'failure to progress'

eating after the birth 49, 278, 281, 308, 403, **409**, 431, 438, **464**, **475**—and see Birthframe 100

eating before conception 101, **366-368**

eating during labour 30, 48, **239**, **240**, 340, **345**, **390**, 444, **459-460**, 461

eating in pregnancy 61, **139**. 144, **154**, **155**, **162**, 164, 165, **166**, 168, 171, **177**, 196, 198, **199**, 204, **218**, 248, 293, 315, **369**, **370**, **373**, **374-377**, **382**, **383**, 501

EC [elimination communication] 479, 480-482, 489

eclampsia 196, 199, 218, 382, **378**

ectopic pregnancy 81, 243

ECV 75, 289, **498**

EDD—see 'due dates'

EFM—see 'electronic fetal monitoring'

egg donation 45

elective caesarean 40, 82, 86, 89, 90, **274**—also see 'caesareans'

electrocautery 83

electronic fetal monitoring 6, **18**, **21**, **97**, **103**, 119, 122, 123, 205, **235**, **239**, **240**, 241, 242, 251, **256**, 275, 305, **310**, **335**, **336-337**, 405, **494**, **496**, **497**, 505—also see 'monitoring', 'fetal scalp monitoring' and 'ultrasound'

elimination communication 479, 480-482, 489

elimination timing 479, 480-482, 489

emergency 80, 91, 108, **259**, 266, 272, 289, 301, 306, **311**, **345**, 350, 351, 375, **378**, **382**, **464**

emergency caesareans 86, 87-88, 89, 90, 91, 121, 219, 243, 244, 276, 304, 313, 398, 430—also see 'caesareans'

emotions 368-369, **384-385**, 410-471

endometriosis 41-42

endorphins 77, **100**, **102**, **125**, 128, 131, 151, 153, 252, **257**, 447, **497**

enemas 32, 108, 232, **240**, 270, 274, **497**, 511

engagement **174**, 181, 273, 315, 386

epidurals 1, **20-21**, 39, 76, 82, 84, 92, 119, 121, **122**, **123-127**, 128, 136, 215, **235**, **237**, **244**, 250, 252, **253**, **254**, **257**, 260, **261**, 273, 274, 275, 277, 295, **304-305**, 306, **313-314**, 319, **336**, 350, 352, 356,

398-399, 403, 405, 415, **493**, **497**, 499, 509, 515, 596—also see 'anaesthesia'
epilepsy 358
episiotomy **18**, 95, 118, 119, **125**, 205, **233**, 235, **237**, **239**, 241, **242-243**, 269, 270, 275, 276, 306, 308, **345**, 352, **408**, 412, 415, **497-498**, **499**, **511**. 513
equipment for home birth **265-266**, 339, 350, 395-397, **435**
syntometrine 140, 252, 273
ergot 232, 233
ET [elimination timing] 479, 480-482, 489
ether 232, 233, 234
exercise after pregnancy 220, 221, **223**, 240, 484-486
exercise during pregnancy 63, **65**, 169, **373**, **378-379**, **489**, **502**
expectant management 435—also see 'physiological third stage' and 'third stage'
expressing (breastmilk) 72
external cephalic version 75, 289, 497, 498
eye contact 102, 113, **241**, 408, 462
eye drops **254**, 269
face-to-pubis births 112, 118, **498**, 507, 515
faeces 13, 14, 24, 32, 33, 82, **126**, 153, **180**, 296, **318**, 350, 367, **380**, 398, 497, **498**, **500**, 507, 509, 511
failure to progress **20**, **21**, **94**, **97**, 112, **117**, 226, **357**, 447, **496**
faintness **144**, 246
false labour 28-29—also see 'interrupted labour' and 'failure to progress'
fast labour 23-25, 137, 176, **178-179**, 261, 306-308, 312, 337, 342-343, 344, 346-347, 352-354, 388-389, 445-446, 447, 447-450, **451**, 451-453, **464**
fathers—see 'partners'
fear **1-5**, 9, 12, 37, 40, **52**, 55, 56, 63, 70, 72, 73, 74, **77-79**, 80, 86, 88, 93, **94**, **96**, **97**, **98**, **99**, **101**, **105**, **110**, 114, 117, 137, 138, **157**, **161**, **172**, **187**, **191**, **197-198**, 226, **206**, 209, **219**, 222, 226, **231**, **236**, **240**, **241**, **243**, 246, **256**, 260, **291**, **303**, **310**, 314, 337, **339**, 340, 344, 354, 357, **358**, **375**, 388, **412**, **413**, **415**, **418**, **419**, **428**, **429**, **433**, **438**, **441**, 447, 450, **456**, **465**, **467**, 476, 488, **494**, **500**, **505**, 596—and see Birthframes 19, 88 and 97
female circumcision 19, 194, 236
fertility problems **41-48**, **81**, 102, **141-142**, 243-244, 279, **366-368**
fetal distress 49, 88, **94**, 104, **119**, 123, **153**, 161, 180, 190, **219**, **257**, 320, 333, **337**, 342, **357**, 359, 391, **498**, **504**
fetal monitoring 23-24, 184, 190, 196, **218-219**, **235**, **240**, 251, 260, 269, 270, 273, 272, **275**, 276-277—also see Sonicaid' and 'Pinard'
fetal scalp blood sampling 190
fetal scalp monitoring 190
fetal stethoscope—see 'Pinard'

fetus ejection reflex **12**, **13**, 25, 26, **95**, **101**, 123, 130, **359**, **435-436**, **492**, **499**, 515
fever 124, **126**, 221, 381
fibroids 196
first degree tearing—see 'tearing'
first pregnancy—see 'primiparas'
first stage 11-12, **30-31**, **100-101**, 105-107, 117, 121-135, **186**, 187-193, 237-243, **253**, 256-258, 269, 270, **272**, 273, **290-291**, 295, **356**, **359**, **407**, **457**, **459**, **460**, **499**, 512
first-time mother—see 'primiparas'
first trimester 9, **139-153**, 154, 196, **204-205**, 243-244, **245**, 366-368, **368-371**, **373-385**, 493, **499**, **501**, 504, 507
flashing lights 378
flu 154, 262-263, 293, **385**
fluid retention—see 'oedema'
folic acid 132, 140, **143**, 149, 196, **367**, **371**, 389, **499**
food—see 'eating in pregnancy', 'eating in labour', etc.
footling breech 40, 291, 356, 448
forceps **21**, 54, 83, **95**, **96**, 118, **125**, 126, **188**, **189**, 191, **232-234**, **236**, **237**, **239**, 241, **242**, **243**, 250, 256, **271**, **272**, 306, **311**, **335**, 343, 351, 352, 412, 415, 434, **498**, **499**, 500, **513**
fostering 42-44, 46
fourth degree tearing—see 'tearing'
frank breech 291
freebirth—see 'unassisted birth'
friends **1**, **2**, 45, **48**, 50, 54, 60, 74, 95, **96**, **97**, 112, 113, 136, 137, **138**, **146**, 161, 179, **185**, 223, **240**, 255, 258, 284, 294, 297, 298, 301, 308, 311, **314**, 319, 324, 325, **331**, 349, 352, 353, **368**, **373**, 389, 404, **411**, **423**, **431**, **437**, 438, 450, 453, **458**, 480, 482—also see Birthframe 100
fruit teas 132
fundal pressure 232, 271, 290
futuristic strategy (for obstetrics) 96
gas and air 54, 71, 121, **128**, **129-131**, 173, **189**, 226, 230, 266, 295, 304, 306, 314, 342, 346, 347, 356, 388, 445, 497, **500**, **502**, **505**
Gaskin, Ina May 353, 490
general anaesthesia 81, 82, 121, 124, 232, 234, 260, 274, **304**, **390**—also see 'anaesthesia'
genetic disorders 196
genital mutilation 200, 236
German measles 267
gestational diabetes 196, **220-221**, 358
getting back into shape 17, 409, 484-486
glucose 220, **266**, 314, 390, 460
glucose tolerance test 220

glycerine suppositories 82
going diaperless 479, 480-482, 489
going to another planet 14, **105**, **108**, **123**, 133, 134, **224**, **253**, **395**, **436**, **444**, 516, 517—and see Birthframes 2, 12, 31, 41, 61, 74, 90, 91, 93, 94, 95, 97
going to hospital 29, 31, **40**, 54, 60, **65**, 67, 70, 75, 76, 90, 92, 95, 135, 136, **173**, 194, 204, 215, 217, 221, **222-223**, 224, **226**, **231**, **234-235**, **237**, **240**, 244, 245, 246, 247, 248, 249, 250, **252**, **254**, 258, 259, **260-261**, **262-263**, **265**, 267, 271, 272, **274**, **274-275**, **276-278**, 279-287, 288, **288-291**, 293, 294, 298, 301, **302**, 304, 305, 306, 307, **312**, 313, **316**, 324, 328, 333, **334**, **339**, **342**, 343, 344, **345**, 347, 351, 352, 356, **357**, 360, 387, 389, 393, **394**, 398, **431**, **433**, 445, 446, **461**, **464**, **466**, **492**
haemoglobin 9, **220**
haemorrhage 13, 54, **81**, **102**, **108**, **194**, 312, **326**, **350**, **351**, **382**, **435-436**, **498**, **500**, **508**, 511
haemorrhoids 323, 383
hands-and-knees position 13, 23, 24, 59, 78, 124, 138, **170**, 228, **241**, **265**, **273**, 316, 317, 365, **394**, 395, 422, 435, 438, **465**
headaches **20**, **126**, 191, 206, 232, 250, **252**, **273**, 297, **368**, **384**, 393
head-down position 73, 174, 175, **218**, 251, 273, 289, 296, 304, 312, 341, 448, **495**, **498**, **500**, **503**, 504, 506, **509**, **512**, **513**, 521
heartburn 220, **376**
heart disease 358
heart murmur 197, 260
heparin lock **240**, 314—also see 'IV'
herbs 33, **98**, **104**, **132-133**, 369, **379**, 389
heroin—see 'diamorphine'
hiccups 156
high blood pressure—see 'blood pressure'
high risk pregnancies and labours 5, 27, **58-96**, 102, **103**, **107**, 108, 119, 161, 194, **204**, **205-207**, 211-217, 218-219, 220-221, 233, **235**, **251**, **256**, **264**, **267**, **268**, 273, **288**, **291**, 304, 313, 320, **357**, 358, 381, 390, 406, **412**, 415, **429**, **435**, **465**, **466-467**, **492**, 493, 496, 497, 498—and see Birthframes 1, 2, 3, 5, 13, 15, 16, 17, 18, 19, 24, 25, 26, 34, 35, 36, 41, 43, 44, 45, 46, 47, 48, 49, 50, 51, 52, 56, 59, 67, 70, 74, 75, 79, 82, 88, 95, 98
hindwaters 259-261, 261, 363, 415, **457**—also see 'waters breaking' and 'stress incontinence'
home birth 17, 19, 20, 50, 74, 77, 99, **109**, 128, **129**, 135, **137**, **174**, 175, **178**, 179, 186, **198-203**, 223, 224, **234**, **257**, **264-266**, **267**, **312**, **328**, **333-358**, 360, 364, 381, 418, 419, 420, 423, **433**, **437**, **464**, **488**, 489, 494, 515, 516, 517, 593—and see Birthframes 2, 3, 4, 6, 10, 12, 13, 14, 19, 25, 27, 31, 35, 36, 40, 41, 45, 46, 47, 52, 54, 58, 60, 61, 62, 63, 64, 65, 66, 69, 71, 72, 74, 75, 78, 82, 84, 85, 88, 90, 91, 93, 94, 95, 96, 97, 98

home birth pack 343, 446, 487—also see 'equipment for home birth'
homeopathy 6, 113, 115, **132**, 319, **379**, 386-388, 438, 450
hormones 3, 7, 8, 9, 10, 11, 13, 14, 17, 46, 47, 54, 58, 80, 94, **97-102**, 104, 105, **109-111**, 126, **128**, 143, 144, 157, 180, 181, 188, **191**, 249, **253**, **255**, **256**, **257**, 275, 290, 317, **373**, **375**, 382, **385**, 402, **406**, 419, 424, **429**, **472**, **492**, **494**, **496**, **497**, **498**, **500**, **501**, 504, 505, 506, 507, 508, 512
hospital beds 339, **345**, 389, **405**
hospital birth 1, 5, 12, 15, 19, 29, 30-31, 38, **48**, **52**, 54, 59, 60, 61, 62, 63, **65**, **66**, 67, 82, **86**, 95, **109**, **117**, 130, 131, **175-176**, 179, **189**, 194, 204, 215, **222-223**, **226**, 230, 231, **232-235**, **235-243**, **254-255**, **256-258**, 259, **264-266**, **267-275**, 276, **302**, 305, 306, 307, 308, 310, **312**, **316**, 319, 320, 323, **328**, 331, 333, **334-348**, **349**, **350**, **351**, 352, 354, 355-356, **357-358**, 360, **390**, **405**, 418, 420, 428, **435**, **437**, 446, 447, 452, **461**, **464**, **494**, 495, 487, 489, 501, 505, 509, 516, 517, 593—and see Birthframes 1, 5, 6, 15, 16, 17, 18, 20, 23, 24, 28, 30, 34, 41, 42, 43, 44, 45, 46, 49, 50, 51, 52, 53, 55, 56, 57, 59, 60, 62, 63, 67, 68, 69, 70, 73, 76, 81, 83, 84, 85, 86, 91, 94, 97—and see 'going to the hospital'
hot compresses 275
husbands—see 'partners'
hydration 240—also see 'water', 'amniotic fluid' and 'drinking in pregnancy', 'drinking in labour'
hyperemesis 245-248, 375
hyper-stimulation 243
hypertension—see 'blood pressure'
hypnosis 113, 137, 181, 187, **414**, **414-417**, 447
hypnotherapy—see 'hypnosis'
ice cubes 113, 115, 124, 250, **413**
ICUs [Intensive Care Units] 254, 255, 279-287
incontinence 123, 126, **378-379**, 385
induction 6, **29**, 56, **81**, **98**, 104, 106, 122, **135**, 136, **141**, 145, 182, **184**, **189**, **190**, 215, **217**, 226, **232**, **233**, **234**, **237-238**, **239**, **240**, 248, **256-258**, 261, 262, **270**, **272**, 296, 304, **306-308**, 313, 314, **317**, 320, **384**, 388, 398, 399, **405**, **412**, 415, 418, 420, 430, **493**, **501**, 507, 508, 511, **513**, 596
industrialised childbirth 188, 257
infant mortality **18**, **19**, 40, 80, **198-203**, 214, 244, **283**, 284, 285, **291**, 358, 381, 412, **429**, 504, **507**—also see Birthframe 53
infant potty training 479, 480-482, 489
infection 20, **34**, 47, **81**, 82, 100, 103, 119, 123, **126**, 153, 159, 168, **220**, 231, **254**, **260-261**, **262-263**, 265, 280, 285, 298, 313. **335**, **338**, 339, 357, **380-381**, 390, 415, **457**, 496, 498, **501**, 505, 506, 511, 512
infertility **41-48**, **81**, 102, **141-142**, 243-244, 279, **366-368**

influenza 154, 262-263, 293, **385**
insomnia—see 'sleep'
intact perineum 222, **407-408**, 431, 446, 454—also see 'tearing'
integrated test 216
intensive care 66, 69-72, 276-278, 279-287—also see 'SCBU'
internal examination 31, 40, 59, 103, **119**, 261, **262-263**, 277, **302**, 306, 308, **309**, 352, 357, **408**, 412, **457**, **502**, **513**
interrupted labour 29, 398, **434**, **457**, 464
intervention 1, 2, 4, **5**, 6, 7, 8, **18**, 19, **21**, 27, 34, **39-40**, **52**, 54, 55, 62, 63, 66, 69, 76, 77, 80, 88, **94**, 96, **97**, **98**, **99**, 106, **108**, **110**, 111, **117**, **118-119**, 126, 128, 133, 134, 135, 136, 137, 179, **184**, **188**, **189**, **191**, **194**, 198, 204, **205**, **217**, **218**, 221, **223**, **225**, 226, **232-243**, 245, 249, 251, **253**, **254-258**, 269, 270, 288, **301**, 303, **309-311**, 314, 315, 316, 319, 320, **338**, 340, 342, **344**, 346, 348, 350, 352, 356, 362, **385**, **388**, 398, **408**, 415, 416, 417, 418, 423, **429**, **438**, 447, 455, **458**, 465, **466-467**, 468, 487, 489, 492-493, **502**, 507, 509, 515, 516—also see 'ultrasound' and Birthframes 5, 6, 12, 14, 20, 23, 26, 28, 30, 34, 39, 41, 42, 43, 44, 45, 46, 47, 48, 49, 50, 51, 52, 55, 56, 57, 62, 63, 64, 67, 69, 70, 72, 73, 76, 81, 83, 90, 91, 95, 96
intravenous drip—see 'IV'
intuition 12, 54, 55, **99**, **104**, **110**, **117**, **134**, 173, **177**, 185, **198**, 216, **221**, 225, **257**, **264**, 301, 306, **331**, 374, **391**, 413, 426, **456**, **458**, 460, **466-467**, 495, **499**
invasive tests **205-207**, **211-217**, 249, 258, 336-337—also see 'tests'
in vitro fertilisation—see 'IVF'
IPT [infant potty training] 479, 480-482, 489
iron deficiency **220**, 221, **371**, **383**,
iron supplements **220**, 221, **371**, **383**
itching 128, 39, 373, **378**
IV—see 'drip'
IVF 69, **142**, 243
jabs—see 'vaccinations'
jelly 11, 367
kangaroo care 254, 278, **279-287**
Kegels 378-379
ketones **240**, 246, 247
kickchart 184
kicking 9, 40, 153, **158**, 160, 164, 166, **169**, **184**, **217**, 275, 280, 293, 297, 404, 477, **498**, 502
kidney disease 358
Kitzinger, Sheila 232, 259, 315, 488, 594
kneeling 273, 317, 395, **405**, **407**
!Kung San tribe 53, 437
labour coach 234
Lamaze 224, 275

language **253**, **432-433**, 489
last menstrual period—see 'LMP'
lavender 132, 262
leak—see 'stress incontinence' and 'waters breaking'
leaning forward positions **24**, 30, 32, 33, 49, 71, 76, 116, 117, **119**, **161**, **171**, 228, 231, **240**, **275**, 290, **328**, 353, 354, 362, **365**, 377, **384**, **392**, **394**, **395**, 422, **435**, 450, **459**, **465**, **511**
Leboyer, Frederick 73, **187**
left-handedness 189, **214**
legal issues 14, 59, 63, 160, 163, 179, **257**, **264**, **325**, **334**, **337**, 369, 388, 399, **451**
listeria 367
lithotomy position **239**, 252, **391-392**, 393, 503
lithotomy stirrups 241
LMP **141**, **145**, 185, **367**, 503, 508
LOA 170, **171**, **218**, 448, 503
local anaesthetic 16, **121**, 347, 403, **407**—also see 'anaesthesia'
lochia 34, 85
long labours 29, 98, 106, 228, 230, 269, 322, **339**, **359**, 394, 412, 415, **464-465**—also see 'birth attendants', 'privacy', 'psychological difficulties'—and see Birthframes 46, 52, 93
long-term effects or problems 80, **81**, 462—also see 'primal health'
looking after a new baby **38**, 85, **472-486**
LOP—see 'posterior position'
lotus birth 35, **36-37**, 63, 454
low blood pressure 16, 25, 123, 126, 128, 246, 336—also see 'blood pressure'
low haemoglobin **220**, 221, **371**, 383
low-lying placenta 244, 383—also see 'placenta praevia'
low risk pregnancies 27, 81, 309-311, 340, 381, 412
lumbar puncture 278
lumbar reflexotherapy 133
lung disease 358
malformations 368
malpresentation—see 'position (baby's)'
mammals 12, 100, 101, 105, 111, **120**, 126, 129, 257, 303, **405**, 468
manual removal of placenta 435
massage 30, 113, **135**, 173, 176, 177, 229, **275**, 316, 322, **379**, 389, **394**, 418, **441**, 452, **459**, **465**
mastitis 173
maternal mortality **18**, **19**, 80, **81**, 93, 94, **198-203**, 233, 244, **291**, 358, 412, **429**, 504
meconium 87, **153**, **180**, 215, 269, 333, 398, 399, **504**
media 42, **52**, 60, 70, 161, 167, 178, **236**, 237, 250, **259**, **275**, 297, **338**, 347, **400**, **410**, **411**, **428**, 437, 454, **458**, 480, **487**

membranes 34, 40, 71, 83, 98, 104, 120, 240, 260, 270, 273, 316, 387, 449, **492**, **493**, 494, 498, 499, 504, 507—also see 'amniotomy'
meningitis 381
mess **13**, 14, **265**, **350**, 395, 454, 479
metallic taste **144**, 385, 387
mid-cycle bleeding—see 'spotting' and 'haemorrhage'
midwives' comments and accounts 33, 34, **86**, 127, **190**, **267**, 273, 309, 314, 336, 439, 487, 489—and see Birthframes 17, 45, 52, 67, 72 and see 'Odent, Michel'
migraine 126
miscarriage 47, 133, **145**, **146**, 149, **152**, **204**, 206, 212, **214**, 245, 246, 279, **291**, 343, 346, **353**, **492**, **495**, 496, 501
mobile epidural 124—also see 'epidural'
monitoring 6, **18**, **21**, 39, **49**, **50**, **58**, 66, 85, 87, 92, **94**, 97, 103, **107**, **110**, 113, 115, 118, **119**, 122, **123**, 124, **184**, **190**, 195, 196, **206**, 212, **218-219**, **235**, **240**, 241, 244, 248, **251**, **252**, **256**, 260, **269**, **270**, **272**, **273**, **275**, **276**, 277, 280, 281, 282, 302, 304, 305, 307, 308, **309-311**, 324, **328**, **335**, **336-337**, **345**, 347, 350, 352, 356, 357, **368**, 387, 405, 412, 415, 420, **429**, 437, 494, 495-496, **497**, **498-499**
moods—see 'emotions'
morbidity **18**, 94, 190, **211**, 412—also see 'primal health'
morning sickness **9**, 78, 144, 154, 173, 198, 249, 276, 279, 322, **374-376**, **385**, 389, **501**—also see Birthframe 43
morphine 128, 232, 233, 234
mortality rate **81**, **94**—also see 'maternal mortality', 'infant mortality' and 'stillbirth'
mothering 472-478, **479**, 480-482, 484-486
movement in labour and birth 97, 115, 124, **125**, 126, 127, 134, **239**, **240-241**, 270, 274, 307, 309, 317, 340, **345**, 353, 354, 355, 360, 381, **391-392**, **395**, 396, 399, 400, **405-406**, 410, 412, 422, **435**, 447, **458**, **459**, **464**, **465**
moxabustion 75
MS—see Birthframes 13 and 74
mucous extractor 50
mucous plug 49—also see 'show'
multiple birth—see 'twins' and 'triplets'
multiple sclerosis—see Birthframes 13 and 74
multivitamins 371—also see 'supplements'
music in labour 55, 228, 231, **264**, **265**, **272**, **274**, 305, 340, **345**, 360-361, 362, **441**, **444**, **459**, **461**, **464**
music in pregnancy 297, **368**, **411**, 442, **444**
NAD 15
narcotics 121, **127-131**
natural infant hygiene 479, 480-482, 489

nausea **9**, 78, 113, **127**, **128**, **144**, 154, **198**, 249, 276, 279—also see Birthframe 43
neglect 106
nesting 185, **467-468**
Newton, Niles 80
NICU [Neonatal Intensive Care Unit] 141—also see 'SCBU'
NIH [natural infant hygiene] 479, 480-482, 489
nocebo effect **110**, 236, 241
noise in labour and birth 23, 56, 115, **190**, 194, **228**, **241**, **269**, **275**, **309**, 328, **345**, 356, 361, **391**, **394**, 400, 401, 402, **410**, **459**, **465**—and see Birthframes 27 and 31
noise in pregnancy 160, 161, **162**, 328,
non-stress test 307, 347, 387—also see 'monitoring', 'due dates', 'overdue' and 'postmaturity'
nosebleeds 385
nuchal fold scan 249, 430
nuchal translucency testing 236
number of people at the birth—see 'birth attendants' and 'privacy'
obstetric cholestasis **39**, 378
Odent, Michel **4**, **5**, 12, 13, 14, 27, 28, **29**, 33, **49**, **58**, 78, **80**, 83, **94**, **95-96**, **98**, **99**, 101, **105**, **107**, 123, **131**, **133**, 134, 179, **188**, **191**, 192, **199**, 202, **205**, **206-207**, **211**, **217**, **219**, **220**, 223, **224**, **243**, **256**, **257**, **286**, **301**, **309**, 313, **318**, **321**, **323**, 353, **356-357**, **359**, **364**, **366**, **375**, **474**, **488**, 492, 501, 505, 515, 516, 517, 592, 593—and see Birthframes 2, 6, 10, 12, 13, 25, 27, 29, 41, 46, 47, 48, 52, 54, 61, 64, 65, 77, 90, 91, 93, 95, 98
oedema [excessive swelling] 123, 243
older mothers 18, 27, 204, 206, 224—and see Birthframes 1, 2, 3, 13, 16, 34, 35, 39, 44, 51, 80, 89, 95
olive oil 379
Omega-3 fish oil supplements **132**, 139, **371**
onset of labour 10, **11**, 23, **28-29**, 49, **94**, 95, **100-101**, 102, 173, **185**, 227, 232, 244, 259, 261, 276, **317**, 324, 343, 347, **382**, **382**, **384-385**, 389, 428, 439, 444, 445, 448, 453, **456-471**—also see 'waters breaking', 'show' and 'contractions'
opiates 19, 84, 121, **127-129**, **189**, 234
optimal birth 1, 2, 3, 5, **6-7**, **8**, 52, 58, **95-96**, —also see the whole of the chapter: 10... Understand 'optimal'
optimal fetal positioning **160-161**, **167**, **170**, **171**, 377, **391-392**, 389, 393, 446
orgasm 36, 78, 80, **141**, 159, **379-380**, **385**, 446
overdue 29, 55, 112, 114, 138, **140**, 149, **179-186**, 215, 248, 262, 294, 306, 355, **384**, **456**, **498**, 506—also see 'due dates'
ovulation **140**, **141**, **142**, 144, **145**, 183, 205, 214, **366**, **367**
oxytocin (or 'oxytocics') 13, 29, **80**, 100, **101**, **102**, 104, 123, 128, 181, **191**, **201**, 235, 237, 240, 252, 273, **429**, **436**, **463**, 496, 498

pain 1, 2, **3**, **4**, 7, **11**, **12**, **13**, 17, 27, 30, 33, 34, 41, **84**, **86**, 97, **98**, 100, 101, 105, 108, 110, **111**, **117**, 119, **121**, **122**, 123, 124, 125, 126, 127, 130, 132, 133-134, **138**, 144, **157**, 159, 164, **167**, **171**, **190**, **191**, **224**, 227, 228, **241**, 243, 246, 247, 250, **253**, **254**, **256**, **259**, 260, 261, **266**, 268, **269**, **275**, 277, **291**, 292, 295, **304**, **307**, 314, 315, 318, 319, 325, 331, 338, **339**, 340, 347, 348, 351, **352-354**, 356, **359**, 361, **362**, 365, **379**, 380, **382**, **384**, 385, 386, 389, **390**, 393, **394**, 398, 400, 402, **404**, **408**, **413**, **415**, 418, 420, 421, 422, **429**, **431-432**, **438**, 440, **441**, **444**, 445, 446, **447**, 448, 449, 453, **454**, **455**, **457**, **459**, **460**, **462-463**, **465**, **466**, **476**, **492**, **493**, 494, **497**, **499**, 500, **502-503**, 509, **511**, 596—and see Birthframes 2, 10, 13, 19, 20, 21, 22, 30, 34, 41, 71, 73, 74, 78, 81, 82, 85, 88, 93, 94, 95
pain relief 1, 2, 3, 6, **7**, **20**, **21**, 39, **65**, 85, **86**, 94, 97, **98**, **99**, 108, **121-135**, **191**, **223**, **232-235**, **237-238**, **241**, **253**, **256**, **266**, 268, **270**, **273**, 282, 284, **289**, 304, 306, 315, 319, **336**, **340**, 342, 344, **345**, **346**, 361, **362**, 388, **391**, **408**, 412, **414-416**, 445, 446, **455**, **456-457**, **458**, **459**, **462-463**, 487, 488, 489, **493**, 494, **497**, **500**, 502, **504**, 505, 506, **507**, **510**, **512**
palpation 23-24, 49, **196**, 212, **218**, 219, 251, 273, **384**, 431, 458
paracervicals 121
paralysis 20, 126, **127**
partners 18, 54, 56, 74, 75, 76, 82, **96**, 109, 117, 118, **120**, 127, **135**, 140, 141, 142, **146**, 157, 158, 159, **164**, 173, 175, 176, 177, **178**, 179, 183, 205, 206, 214, 216, 222, **234**, 245, 246, 247, 260, 261, 262, **264**, 269, **270**, **271**, **272**, **275**, 279, 280, 281, 282, 286, 288, 289, 290, **291**, 294, 306, 313, **314**, 316, **318-326**, **331**, 333, 335, 352, 357, 362, **366**, **367**, 368, 380, 401, 402, 403, **410**, **413**, **417**, **418**, 419, 420, 422, 423, 424, 425, 428, **429**, 430, **432**, **433**, 434, **435-436**, **438**, 439, 445, 448, 449, 450, **451**, 452, 453, 454, **457**, **458**, **474**, **475**, 480, 484, **485**, **494**, 516—and see Birthframes 1, 13, 14, 19, 35, 41, 43, 50, 53, 62, 63, 64, 88, 89, 92, 93, 96, 97, 98
Pelosi technique 83
pelvic floor 80, 86, 89, **353**, 421
penicillin 233
people at the birth **14**, 54, 97, 99, 105, 107, **108**, 129, 133, **233**, 273, 270, **301-332**, 350, **407**, 429, **458**, **460**, **462**—and see Birthframes 1, 31, 34, 41, 56, 57, 58, 60, 61, 62, 63, 64, 65, 69, 72, 73, 75, 86, 89, 90, 91, 97, 96
peppermint tea 132, **133**
perineal block 121
perineal massage **379**, 389
perineal trauma—see 'perineum' and 'tearing'
perineum 12, 13, 16, **18**, 34, **86**, 89, 222, 362, **365**, **379**, 389, 402, 403, **407-408**, 454, **497**, 507

periods 9, 41, 55, 140, **141**, 142, 143, **144-145**, 148, 183, **185**, 205, 227, 261, 277, **295**, 353, **367**, **382**, 440, 445, 506
pessaries 226, 230
pethidine 121, **127-128**, 129, 136, **253**, **507**
photographs 72—also see 'cameras' and 'camcorders'
physiological third stage 13, **34**, 235, 252, 267, 271, 272, 273, 290—also see 'third stage' and 'placenta'
piles—see 'haemorrhoids'
Pinard 24, 49, **103**, 156, 169, **195**, **211**, **217**, **218**, **219**, 251, **269**, **270**, **273**, 313, **499**, **507**
Pithiviers 4, 28, 206, 217, 221, 223, 243, 259, 286, 359, 364
pitocin—see 'syntocinon'
placenta **9**, **13**, 16, 31, 33, **34**, **36-37**, 54, 81, **84**, 100, 101, **102**, **108**, 116, 117, 135, 136, 137, 151, 152, 154, 156, 157, 158, 159, **161**, 162, 166, 168, **170**, 177, **180**, **194**, 196, **212**, 220, 226, 229, **233**, **235**, **237**, 244, 252, 257, **265**, **266**, **267**, 269, **271**, **272**, **273**, **274**, 290, 341, 346-347, 354, **369-370**, **374**, **375-376**, **382**, **383**, **397**, 399, **403**, 406, 423, 430, **435-436**, **447**, 450, **454**, **463**, 464, **492**, **494**, 495, **498**, **503-504**, **507**, 508, 512, 513—also see 'third stage' and all birthframes
placenta abrupta 244, 378, 382
placenta praevia 81, 196, 212, 244, **382**, **383**
poo 13, 14, 24, 32, 33, 82, **126**, 153, **180**, 296, 318, **350**, **367**, **380**, 398, 401, **480-482**, **497**, 498, 507
position (baby's) 24, **119**, **167**, 196, 251, 273, 341, 355, 356, 357, 360, 393, **394**, 446, **465**, 458—also see 'LOA', 'posterior position' and 'breech'
positions (for labour or birth) **239**, **241**, **391**, **392**, **394**, **395**, **396**, 489—also see 'squatting' and all birthframes
posterior position 30, 112, **125**, 131, **135**, **167**, **170**, **171**, 355, **394**, **465**, **493**, **498**, **506**, **507**, **509**, 512, 515—and see Birthframes 1 and 27
postmaturity 183-185, 262, 303, 317, 320, 355, **384**, 388
postnatal depression 81, 260, 278, 283, 414, 472, **475**
postnatal care 50, 424-427, **436**, **472-482**
postnatal pain 7, 13, 20, 34, 86, 121, 125-127, **178-179**, **188-194**, 256, 345, 389, 394, **408**, 432, 441, 456, **472-479**, **484-486**—and see Birthframes 3, 20, 21, 22, 23, 24, 25, 30, 34, 42, 46, 49, 50, 55, 86, 98
postpartum haemorrhage 13, 54, **81**, **102**, **108**, **194**, **201**, **233**, **234**, **244**, **259**, **267**, **273**, 312, 326, **350**, 351, **382**, **435-436**, **498**, **500**
posture 10, **167**, **377**, 384
PPH [postpartum haemorrhage]—see 'postpartum haemorrhage'
practical issues 267-275, **264-266**, 365, 366-368, 371, 373-374
preconceptual detox 366
pre-eclampsia 189, 196, **218**, **220**, **382**, 415
preemies—see 'premature babies'

pregnancy pillow 377
pregnancy rhinitis 376-377, 385
pregnancy rocker 377
pregnancy scares **27**, **380-384**
pregnancy test **144-145**, 319
premature babies 47, **170**, 223, **254-255**—also see 'premature labour', 'kangaroo care', and Birthframes 16, 35, 42, 44, 49, 50, 89
premature labour 104, 135, **163**, **170**, 174, 214, **220**, **214**, 223, **429**, **508**—also see 'premature babies', 'kangaroo care', and Birthframes 16, 35, 42, 44, 49, 50, 87, 88, 89
prematurity—see 'premature labour', 'premature babies' and 'kangaroo care'
prepping 124, **240**
presentation—see 'position (baby's)'
primal health **188-189**, **508**, 593
Primal Health Research Data Bank **188-189**, **487**
primal period 188
primiparas [first-time mothers] 12, 172, 204, **221**, **224**, **237**, **297**, 312, **497**, **508**—and see Birthframes 1, 6, 10, 14, 17, 31, 34, 35, 40, 41, 43, 44, 46, 50, 53, 59, 60, 69, 72, 80, 84, 86, 88, 93, 94, 95
privacy **12**, 50, 66, **94**, **96**, **97**, **98**, **105**, **107**, **108**, **109-111**, **131**, 146-147, **224**, 256, **257**, **259**, **266**, **273**, 291, 296, **309**, 322, **323**, **331**, **332**, **340**, **350**, 356, **359**, **441**, 446, **458-459**, **461**, **466**, 489, 494—and see Birthframes 10, 13, 25, 29, 45, 52, 56, 61, 67, 75, 83, 90
progesterone **100**, **101**, 151, 154, **508**, 510
prolactin **100**, **102**, 191, **504**, **508**
prophylactic obstetrics 233
prostaglandin pessaries **98**, 226, **240**,
prostaglandins 101—and see Birthframe 13, 86
protein in the urine **196**, **218**, **382**, 497, 501, **508**, **509**
protocols **18**, **19**, 82, 97, 199, **222**, **235**, **242**, **243**, **259**, **310**, **333**, **339**, **340**, 342, **345**, 381, **461**
psychological difficulties 7, **81**, **99**, 104, 110, 111, 146, **185**, **187**, **198**, **236**, **310**, 340, 365, **375**, 376, 380, **384**, **410-471**, **472**, 488—and see Birthframes 82, 85, 86, 88, 89, 92, 97, 98
pudendal block 121, 503
puerperal sepsis 233, **510**
pulse 84, 85, **184**, **275**—and see Birthframe 46
pushing 11, **24**, **25**, 29, 32, **33**, 50, 53, 54, 56, 62, 71, 76, 77, 78, 92, **101**, 116, 117, 118, 124, **125**, **130**, 138, 176, 229, **237**, **241**, 242, 262, **271**, 275, 296, 304, 305, 318, 325, 328, 342, 343, 344, 347, 354, 355-356, 362, **391**, 393, **394**, **398-399**, 401-402, 404, **407-408**, 418, 422, 423, 431, **437**, 444, 445, 449, **465**, **495**, **510**—also see 'commanded pushing'
quad-screen test 236, 504
quinine 232

Rank, Otto 187
raspberry leaf tea **132**, 319, **379**, 389, **509**
rebirthing—see Birthframe 88
rectal analgesia 84
reflexology 317
regional anaesthesia 121—also see 'anaesthesia' and 'epidurals'
regurgitation 84
rest-and-be-thankful phase 12, 362
resting in pregnancy 160-161
retained placenta 347
rhesus negative 347
rhinitis 376-377, 385
ringing in the ears 466
ring of fire 12, 33
risk assessment **3**, **6**, 7, 13, 39, 40, 46, **58-96**, 102, 103, **107**, 108, 119, **121**, 123, 132, **134**, 152, **188**, 189, 194, 198, **204**, **205**, **206-207**, **211**, **213**, **215**, 218, **220**, **221**, 226, 235, **251**, **256**, 260-261, 262-263, **264**, **267**, **268**, 273, **288**, **291**, 304, 305, 310-311, 313, **320**, 323, 328, 339, 340, 341, 348, 357, 358, 359, **367**, **373**, 374, 377, **380**, 381, 390, **394**, 399, 406, **412**, 415, **429**, **435**, **465**, **466-467**, **492**, **493**, **495-496**, **497**, **498**, 504, **506**, 510, 512, 516, 596
ROA 170
rooming in 269, **271**, 272, 274, **345**, 393
rooting 155, 316—also see 'breastfeeding'
ROP 170
rubella 196, 367
rupture of the membranes—see 'waters breaking'
saddle blocks 121
safety 4, **6**, 12, **13**, 14, **39**, 50, **58**, 66, 77, 80, **81**, **94**, **95**, 97, **98**, 102, **108**, **109**, **110-111**, 112, **117**, **123**, 130, 131, **138**, 139, 153, 175, **178**, **179**, 198, **198-203**, **211**, 212, 214, 223, **225**, **234**, **236**, **238**, **242**, **251**, **256**, **258**, **269**, 270, 273, 286, **288**, **289**, 303, 312, 317, **321**, **331**, **333**, **334**, **336-337**, **338**, 340, **350**, 351, 353, 357, **365**, 388, **392**, 405-406, **407**, **411-413**, **417**, 418, 420, 421, 422, 424, **433**, **439**, **447**, **451**, **456**, **458**, 459, **463**, 468, 476, 495, **499**, **506**
salt-replacement therapy 375—also see Birthframe 43
sanitation **19**, 95, 199-203, 335-336
scalp monitor—see 'fetal scalp blood sampling'
scans—see 'ultrasound'
SCBU 254, 255—and see Birthframes 16, 42, 44, 49, 50
schizophrenia 154, 189
scopolamine 121, 233
screening tests 19, 196, 236—also see 'tests'
second degree tearing—see 'tearing'

second stage 11, **31-33**, 107, 108-111, 117-120, 121-135, **171**, 178-179, 187-193, 237-243, **253**, 256-258, 262, **269**, 270, 271, **272**, 273, 291, 322, 325, **345**, **362**, **379**, **407**, **422**, **435-436**, 437, **457**, **459**, **464**, **466**, 509, 51, 512—and see all birthframes
second trimester 9, **154-164**, 207, **368-380**, **501**, 510
sedation 84, **121**, **127-128**, 189, 233, **493**, 508, **510**
semi-squatting—see 'squatting'
sepsis 233, **510**
septic workup 254
septicaemia 381
serum screening 236
sex 3, **7**, **14**, **50**, 54, 80, 86, **95**, **98**, 105, **109**, **126**, **140**, **141**, **142**, **159**, 164, **178**, 183, **185**, **318**, 368, **379-380**, **385**, 387, **407-408**, **410**, **457**, **480**, **489**, 498, **501**—also see Birthframe 86
sexual abuse 410—and see Birthframe 86
SGA—see 'small for gestational age'
shaving (pubic hair) 240, **270**, **274**, 277
shiatsu 104, **132**, 135, 241, **510**
show **11**, 28, 135, 324, 342, 347, **382**, 387, 448, **457**, **466**, 510
showers 74, **161**, **269**, **278**, **338**, **345**, **381**, **394**, 401, **441**, 445, 453, **465**
side-effects 1, 4, 5, **7**, 17, **20**, **21**, 80, **81**, **96**, **98**, 101, 102, **103**, 110, **121**, **122**, 124, **125-126**, **127-128**, 129, 130, 131, 134, 157, 159, **187**, 188, **194**, **214**, **220**, 221, **245**, 246, **252**, 254, **273**, 311, 322, 324, 325, **361**, 367, 374, 389, **391**, **413**, **417**, 437, **457**, **458**, **460**, **462**, **505**, 507
skincare during pregnancy 373-374, 378
skin-to-skin contact —see 'kangaroo care' and 'bonding'
sleep **9**, 15, 23, 30, 38, 40, 55, 71, 72, 90, 93, 100—also see 'dreams' and 'tiredness'
slow labours—see 'long labours', 'failure to progress', 'disturbance', 'birth attendants' and 'privacy'
small for dates—see 'small for gestational age'
small for gestational age **166**, 177, 212, **221**, **384**, **510**
smoking 45, **139**, 144, **159**, **166**, 168, 204, **218**, 294, 358, **368**, 369, **374**, 496
snoring 376-377
Sonicaid 31, **103**, 104, 107, **211**, 212, **218**, **219**, 236, **251**, **273**, 293, 496, **499**, **510**, **514**
Special Care Baby Unit 254, 255—and see Birthframes 16, 42, 44, 49, 50
speech development 214
spina bifida 132, **143**, 149, 215, **217**, 367
spinals 6, 118, 119, **121**, 250, 319, 393, 509, **510**
spinal taps 254, **504**
spontaneous labour—see 'onset of labour'
spontaneous pushing—see 'pushing'

spots before the eyes 378, 466
spotting 144, **382**—and see Birthframe 42
squatting 12, **13**, 24, 32, 33, 50, 76, **78**, 229, 231, **241**, 261, 262, 316, 354, **361**, **389**, **391**, **405**, **407**, **408**, **465**, 510
SROM—see 'waters breaking'
stage—see 'first stage', 'second stage', 'third stage'
staples 274
STDs [sexually transmitted diseases] 196
steroids 247, **248**, 249, 260, 375, **496**, **510**, 512
stillbirth 39, 291, **378**, 502, 505-506, **510-511**—and see Birthframe 53
stirrups 124, **239**, **241**, 493, **503**
stitches **16**, 23, 34, 54, 77, **84**, 89, 91, 92, 116, **130**, 222, **274**, 308, 342, 343, 347, 388, 389, **408**, 445, 450, **495**, **497-498**
Strep B [Streptococcal (GBS) infection] 19, 196, 381
stress 66, **100**, **126**, **165**, **169**, **191**, 204, 207, 232, **243**, 271, 283, 310, 320, **492**, **494**, **496**—also see 'fetal distress' and Birthframe 33
stress incontinence 263, **511**
stretch marks 10, **374**, **511**
students 251-252, 272, 296, 325—and see Birthframes 73, 75, 81, 91
suck (baby's) **7**, **12**, 14, 15, 25, 33, 56, 57, 91, **102**, **121**, **126**, **127**, **131**, 154, 155, 156, 158, 160, **164**, **170**, 176, **190**, **191**, **193**, 253, 274, 354, **476**, **511**—also see Birthframe 86
suction—see 'ventouse'
suctioning **83**, **269**, 358, 402
suggestibility 97, 205, **221**, 241, **269**, **272**, 388, **436**, **458**
suicide **188**, **189**
supine position **18**, **119**, 124, **141**, **161**, 167, **168**, **171**, 176, 177, **239**, **393**, 412, 503, **511**
supplements **132**, 139, **140**, 196, **220-221**, 269, **271**, 367, **371**, **499**, 506, 509
supported squat—see 'squatting'
suppositories 82, 124, **500**, **511**
surrogacy 446, **511**—and see Birthframe 9
suturing—see 'stitches'
swaddling 37, 226, **269**, 474
sweating 16, 76, 160, **385**, 386, 484, **512**
sweeping the membranes **240**, 261, 317, 504, **511**
swelling **123**, 198, 243, **338**, 402, **407**, **497**, 500, 513—also see 'oedema' and Birthframe 75
syntocinon 59, 106, 126, **239**, **240**, 270, 272, 275, 306, 360, 390, 507—also see 'augmentation'
syntometrine 34, 54, 71, **237**, **252**, **271**, **272**, **273**, 302, **498**, **511**
T-18 216, 512
tailbone 12, 32, 495, 503

talking in labour and birth 29, 40, 49, **97**, 105, **106**, **108**, 113, **138**, **269**, **280**, **301**, 304, 307, **317**, 324, **355**, **394**, **395**, 400, **408**, 420, **454**, **462**, **465**
talking through problems 147, 162, **171**, **172**, 179, 183, 184, **247**, **260**, **276**, 283, **285**, 291, 292, **298**, 299, 304, 307, **314**, **321**, **376**, **410**, **411**, 413, 429, **432**, **433**, **439**, **440**, 454, 462
tandem feeding 478
tearing 7, **16**, **18**, 23, 25, 34, 57, 67, 83, **95**, **126**, 130, 262, 302, 308, 347, 348, 362, **365**, **379**, 402, 403, **407-408**, 423, 431, 450, 499, **511**
teenagers 99, 116, **131**, **188**, **224**
television 42, **52**, 60, 66, 120, **161**, **236**, 259, **275**, **338**, 347, 400, **410**, **428**, **458**
temperature changes (in women) 30, 84, 85, 101, 126, 159, 160, 171, 182, **190**, **214**, **254**, **261**, **263**, 357, **359**, **365**, **378**, **385**, **457**, **466**, 494
TENS 6, 39, 54, **132**, **133-134**, **241**, 306, 319, 333, **388**, 447, 449, **512**
teratogens 245
term 69, **174**, 177, 216, **254**, 262, **284**, 285, 290, 298, 381, **383**, 499, **508**
termination—see 'abortion'
tests 2, 39, 41, 75, 90, **100**, **103**, **104**, 142, **143**, 144,-145, 146, **195-258**, 269, 279, 313, **359-360**, **381**, 430, **472**, 489, **492**, **495-496**, **497**, **498**, **500**, **504**, **505-506**, **508**, **509**, **511**, **512**, 596
thalidomide 245, 299, **374**, 493
third degree tearing 126, 511—also see 'tearing'
third stage **34**, 102, 107, **108**, 136, 178, **201**, 232, 235, 237, **252**, **267**, **269**, 270, **272**, **273**, 290, 326, **345**, 351, **359**, **435-436**, 447, 512—and see all birthframes
third trimester **10**, **132**, 139, 163, **165-186**, **368-390**, **379**, 497, **501**, 505, 509, 512
thirst 17, 124, 250—also see 'water', 'drinking in pregnancy', 'drinking in labour' and 'drinking after the birth'
thrombosis 82, 85, 496, 512
tiredness **9**, **10**, 69, 85, 113, 115, 116, **144**, 154, **191**, 229, 291, 247, 250, **272**, 278, **284**, 295, 298, **375**, **376**, 386, 387, 389, 404, 415, 431, 432, **450**, 455, **465**, **468**, 482—also see 'sleep' and 'nausea'
toxaemia 358, **508**, 512
toxoplasmosis 367, 501, 512
tranquilizers 121, 512
transcutaneous electrical nerve stimulation—see 'TENS'
transferring to another hospital 70, 72, **84**, 333
transition 115, 117, 137, 354, **355**, 401, 422, **512**
transverse arrest 496, 507-508, 512
transverse lie 512
trial of labour 95, 290-291
trimester—see 'first trimester', 'second trimester', 'third trimester'
triple test **215**, **236**, 493, 502, **504**, **512**

triplets 2, 11, 58, **66-72**, 143, 171, 212, 301, 488, 515, 516—and see Birthframes 15, 16, 44, 49
Trisomy 205-210, 213, 216, 512
TV—see 'television'
twilight sleep 233, 234, **512**
twin monitor 66, 273
twins 2, 11, 29, 30, 42, 58, **60-65**, 143, 171, 182, 212, **217**, 253, **257**, 301, 312, 357, 376, 447, 477, 488, 507, **512**, 515, 516, 517—and see Birthframes 5, 14, 30, 35, 42, 44, 45, 51, 56, 59, 67, 70, 79, 81, 87, 88
Tylenol 121, 385
ultrasound 39, 42, 61, 63, 69, 71, 103, 104, 149, 156, 159, 196, 198, **206**, **211-217**, 218, **219**, **221**, 234, **236**, 243, 244, 245, 246, 248, 249, **251**, **256**, **273**, 276, 279, 293, 294, 298, **310-311**, 313, 325, **335**, 346, 353, **384**, 393, 398, 430, 489, 495, **499**, **505**, **507**, 509, **510**, **512**, 514, 516—and see Birthframes 26, 35, 37, 39, 45
unassisted birth [birth with no medical person in attendance, either intentionally or by accident] 19—also see Birthframes 19, 35, 96, 97
upright positions **12**, **13**, 32, 78, **111**, 167, **239**, 270, **273**, **391**, **392**, **407**, 410, **463**, **465**, **466**, **510**—and see Birthframes 40, 52, 67, 75, 83, 90
urinary tract infections 380-381
urine **13**, 28, 74, 82, 85, 103, 123, 144, 153, 196, **218**, 226, 246, 247, **263**, 279, 378, **380-381**, 494, **497**, **500-501**, **508**, **509**, 511
ursodeoxycholic acid 39
uterine prolapse 379, **513**
uterine rupture **81**, 92, **513**
vaccinations 269, 323, 347, **472**, 593
vacuum extraction—see 'ventouse'
vaginal birth after caesarean—see 'VBAC'
vaginal breech birth—see 'breech'
vaginal discharge **11**, 34, **142**, **144**, 367, 496, 501, **503**, **510**
vaginal examination—see 'internal examination'
Valium 121, 512
varicose veins 383, **512**
VBAC 37, 96, **433**, 473, 488, 489, 513—and see Birthframes 18, 20, 22, 24, 25, 47, 82
vena cava 24, **161**, 377, **513**
ventouse **21**, 95, **234**, **237**, **239**, 242, 243, 256, 272, 311, 412. 415, **513**
vernix **16**, 36, **158**, 174, 181
vertex—see 'head-down position'
visitors 85, **475**—also see 'birth attendants'
visualisation **17**, 137, 138, 157, 163, **268**, 269, 346, 353, 398, **408**, 413, **414**, 424, 431, **440-441**, **422**, 444, **446**, 447, **465**
Vitamin B6 375
Vitamin E oil 379, 389

Vitamin K 87, 269, **273**, **472**, **513**

vitamins—see 'supplements'

vomiting 24, 30, 75, 76, 84, 127, 128, 130, **144**, 154, 173, 252, **265**, 273, 276, 279, 294, 295, 342, **374-376**, 387, 389, **390**, **395**, 402, 445, 453, 454, **457**, 460, **464**, **493**, **501**, 504, 512—also see Birthframe 43

water 10, 17, 19, 20, **91**, 92, 124, 133, **139**, **143**, 159, 170, 177, 180, 187, 200, **202**, **218**, 245, **265**, 269, 271, 280, 293, 297, 325, 344, 368, **369**, **373**, **374**, **375**, 376, **378**, **384**, **390**, **409**, **441**, 453, **457**, **459**, 460, 464, 465, 476, **492**, **499**, 500-501, 511—also see 'amniotic fluid', 'amniotomy', 'membranes' and 'waters breaking'

water birth 6, **31**, 33, 34, 54, 55, 56, 62, 115, 116, 176, **251**, 262, **275**, **289**, **291**, 308, 318, 327, 333, **340**, 353, 354, **359-365**, **394-395**, 400, **407**, **441**, 445, **457**, **459**, 465, 487, **494**, 513, 593—and see Birthframes 82, 86, 95, 97, 98

waters breaking **11**, 23, 30, 36, 62, 63, 67, 69, 70, 71, 74, 75, 78, 115, 135, 173, 176, 215, 229, 260, **262-263**, 305, 313, 324, 342, 343, 344, 353, 356, 357, 381, 386, 389, 398, 399, 415, 428, 444, 445, 449, **457**, **466**, **499**, **500-501**, 513—also see 'amniotomy', 'hindwaters' and 'stress incontinence'

weakness 466

weighing the baby 87, 92, **177**, **190**, **192**, 269, 271, 274, 381, 450

weight gain and loss 63, 246, 263, **291**, 358, **366**, 372, **373**, **376**, 390, **409**, 454—and see Birthframe 100

working during pregnancy 18, **147**, **165**, 199, 247, 277, 389, 445

World Heath Organization 1, 93, 239, 435

worry 9, 23, 25, **27**, **29**, **52**, **54**, **58**, 63, **71**, 73, 77, **97**, 113, 123, 131, 169, **178-179**, **181-186**, **195-207**, **204**, **206**, 207, **213**, 216, **219**, **221**, 224, 225-243, 244, 249, 260, **269**, **279**, **293**, 306, 312, **320**, **321**, 328, **338**, 342, **350**, 355, 361, 362, **370**, 372, 373, 376, **378**, **382**, **383**, **384**, **385**, 386, 390, 394, **414**, 418, 419, 422, 423, 427, **430**, **433**, **439**, 445, 448, 450, 451, **457**, **459**, 460, **461**, **464**, **472**, 497, 498, 504, 596—also see 'fear' and 'nocebo effect' and Birthframes 85, 86, 92, 94, 95, 97

yoga 340, 413

zinc 220, **371**, **383**

If you need more information, do your own research using any of the websites recommended in the Useful contacts section (see page 490) or Google (www.google.co.uk). Of course, you also need to discuss any medical issue with your caregiver(s) so that you can reach agreement on appropriate approaches and also ensure that you receive full support while you're in labour and giving birth. In this respect, remember the importance of writing a care guide—look up 'care guides' in this index!—and perhaps get your prospective caregiver to sign it, as confirmation that all points have been agreed. If you can't reach agreement, you can always seek support from another health care professional.

You need to feel relaxed with your midwife. If you find someone you're in tune with, you'll have a real advocate and companion.

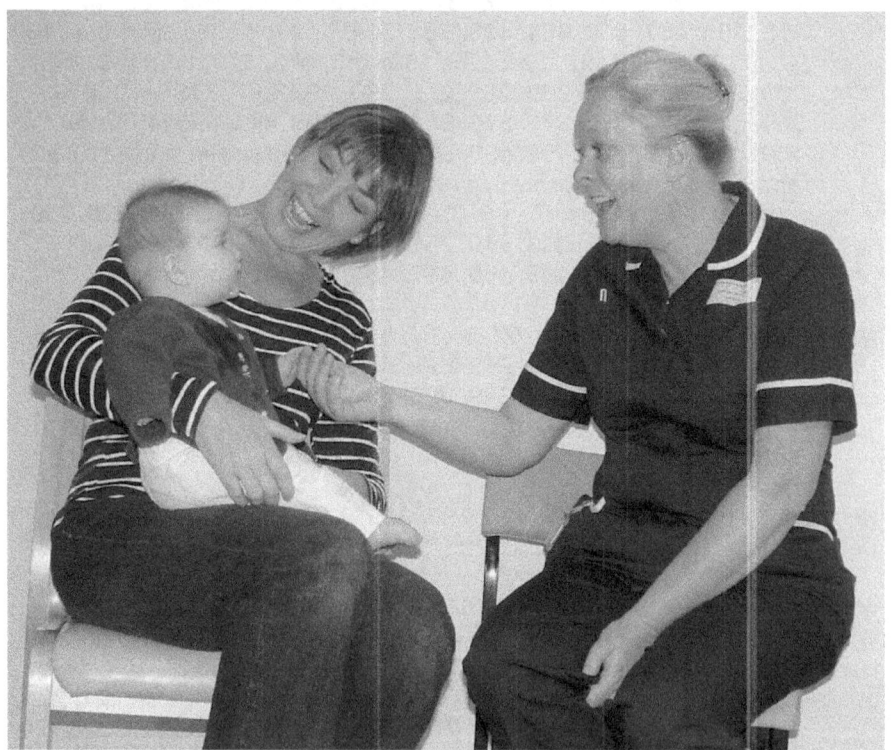

After searching the Index and any other relevant places, if there's anything you want to discuss, remember your midwife is the best person. That's what she's there for.

About the author

Before she started having children, Sylvie Donna worked in companies or taught English, mostly to working adults. She also trained teachers, or managed courses, departments—or a whole language centre in one case. She taught or organised courses for middle and top-level managers (as well as clerical or research staff) in Europe, North Africa, South Asia, South East Asia, the Middle East and the Far East. Her first book—*Teach Business English* (Cambridge University Press 2000)—is a synthesis of her experience in this field. After her third baby was born, Sylvie worked from home for a while, writing and editing, or marking Master's assignments. She now works full-time at Durham University (teaching potential or actual postgraduates) and she also marks MA assignments and supervises dissertations for Birmingham University.

Sylvie started researching issues surrounding pregnancy and childbirth when she conceived her first child at the age of 37. (The reason she started checking things is explained in Birthframe 1.) Perhaps it was because of her long experience of working with managers and directors, that Sylvie found the confidence to challenge her caregivers when she disagreed with them!

Anyway, Sylvie eventually found the support she needed and all went smoothly, thanks to her thorough preparation and a little bit of luck! Then, a few days after the birth she read *Birth Reborn* by Michel Odent (Souvenir Press 1994) and it struck a note of recognition in her—for the first time she was reading about the kind of birth she'd experienced. She then felt fortunate to have the author agree to attend the birth of her second child. The experience of birthing with Michel Odent in attendance prompted her to think through more issues, which she was then able to put to the test on a very modest scale when she gave birth to her third child, with NHS midwives in attendance.

Having had the idea to write a book to help other women and families, Sylvie was inspired to complete this enormous project when she advertised for contributions and support. Numerous women, men and children (including many professionals) responded to her requests or advertisements and helped with research. The research itself has convinced Sylvie that natural birth is what pregnant women need to 'relearn', if we are to build harmonious and happy families and societies, and a constructive future for humankind.

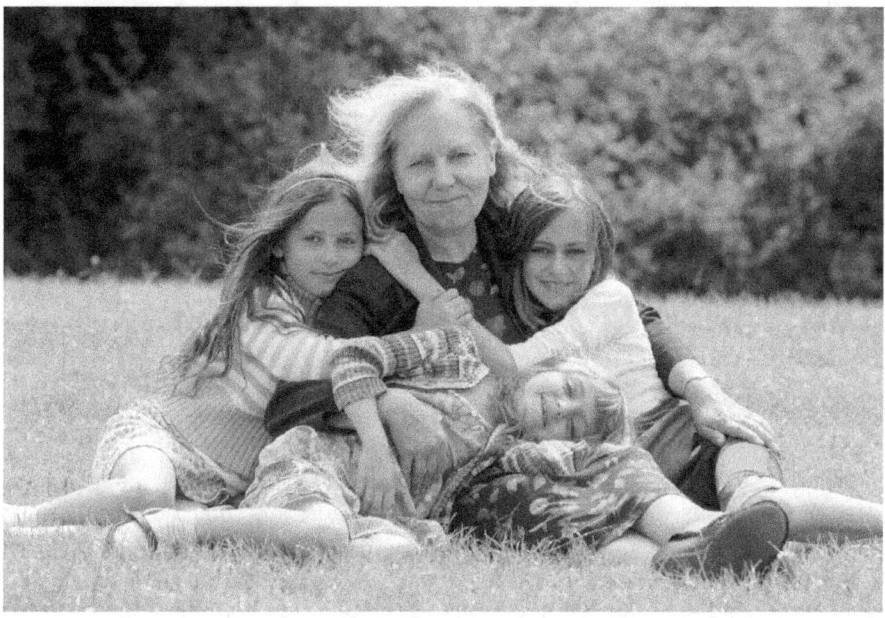

Sylvie with her three daughters, when they were 7, 9 and 11

What inspired this book?

While she was pregnant with her own three children, the author and editor of this book, Sylvie Donna, kept on meeting women who'd had difficult experiences. She started trying to work out what could have gone wrong for these women. It seemed to her that too many women were being traumatised temporarily, if not for the rest of their lives, by childbirth. Sadly, the memory of giving birth was leaving these women feeling disappointed, alienated or betrayed. Their babies, partners and families were affected too.

For many people Sylvie met, pregnancy was more of an obstacle course of tests and worries, than a time of wonder and waiting. Somehow, amongst all the antenatal appointments, risk assessment and birthing pool hire, the baby-to-be got thrown out with the as yet non-existent bath water. And many women told her how the birth they'd planned went wrong in the end. From some of the women, who were the 'statistics' of care gone wrong, she heard horrendous stories of pain and trauma. Many women simply described their feelings of disempowerment as they were 'managed' through the maternity system. For others it was the breastfeeding or the bonding which didn't work out...

What was it, she wondered, that made things go wrong? Listening carefully to countless women, she started making connections between behaviour in pregnancy and birth, and outcomes. She realised that things often start going wrong in pregnancy for no good reason, other than fear. She also discovered—through women's personal accounts—that drug-based pain relief often ended up causing more pain than it ever relieved, if postnatal pain was counted too.

While she was realising these things, she also became increasingly aware that very few women see the chain of events which they set up for themselves by accepting or even requesting certain treatment while they're pregnant, in labour, giving birth and even afterwards. For example, how many women are aware that having an induction of labour increases their risk of having all kinds of other interventions? How many women would choose to have an epidural if they knew what it really involved and if they knew what consequences there might be for either herself or her newborn baby? How many women have found out about and thought through the potentially harmful effects of other forms of drug-based pain relief? How many women have been able to carefully compare postnatal scenarios after a vaginal birth and a caesarean, considering emotional, physical and practical aspects of the experience? Most importantly, Sylvie wondered, how many women know that research shows that a great deal of care offered antenatally and during labour flies in the face of research recommendations—although NICE guidelines suggest this should be recitified?

A book was definitely needed so as to raise awareness of these issues amongst pregnant women. Sylvie decided she would describe the principles she'd deduced—i.e. the ways of making things work out so that birth is optimally healthy and happy for both mother and baby—as well as the father. When collecting material for this book she discovered that other women have discovered these principles too. And they've discovered how much better things can be. You can too.

What this book can do for you...

There are many books written about childbirth, each one valuable because each author adds a unique dimension to resonate with changing times. In academic circles, many hours are spent detailing important issues, but in so doing, the basics can get left behind. Sylvie has done a great job of bringing a resonant dimension, the literature, and common sense together in one book for parents who are as new at this process as are their newborns. She has created a prescription for healthy birth in a 10-step approach to keep parents focused on what is important in a potentially disastrous birth environment. The liberal use of anecdotes from other parents is reminiscent of the group prenatal care approach that has swept North America in its warm appeal because learning from other parents is often better than from professionals who don't understand well what the average parent needs.

Sylvie's book should ring a bell not only with the parents for whom it was intended, but also as a 10-step refresher course for professionals to remember what it is like to be in parents' shoes. She has gracefully unravelled the problems that health professionals and hospital policies have imposed on normal, healthy birth and provided us with a book that encapsulates anything you wanted to know about keeping your birth normal and healthy, with some extras you may never have thought about.

Betty-Anne Daviss

Midwife, Perinatal Epidemiology Consultant &
Adjunct Professor at the Pauline Jewett Institute of
Women's and Gender Studies, Carleton University, Ottawa, Canada
Former Project Manager, Safe Motherhood/Newborn Initiative,
International Federation of Gynecology and Obstetrics

Also available from Fresh Heart:

- *Surprising, Inspiring Birth* by Sylvie Donna (a little book of birth stories to give your partner, relatives and friends to read—to inspire them!
- *Birth Your Way: Choosing birth at home or in a birth centre* by Sheila Kitzinger
- *Birthing Normally After a Caesarean or Two* by Hélène Vadeboncoeur
- *Birth Pain: Power to Transform* by Verena Schmid
- Various books for caregivers...

See the website for more info. All books are available from www.amazon.co.uk.

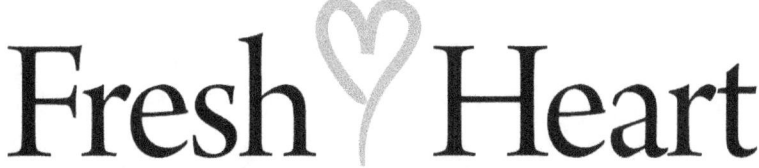

www.freshheartpublishing.co.uk

www.ingramcontent.com/pod-product-compliance
Lightning Source LLC
Chambersburg PA
CBHW080718300426
44114CB00019B/2413